Precision Medicine and Human Health

Edited by

Farzana Mahdi
Era University
Lucknow
India

&

Abbas Ali Mahdi
Era University
Lucknow
India

Precision Medicine and Human Health

Editors: Farzana Mahdi and Abbas Ali Mahdi

ISBN (Online): 978-981-5223-58-3

ISBN (Print): 978-981-5223-59-0

ISBN (Paperback): 978-981-5223-60-6

First published in 2024.

need for a court order if at any point you breach any terms of this License Agreement. In no event will any delay or failure by Bentham Science Publishers in enforcing your compliance with this License Agreement constitute a waiver of any of its rights.

3. You acknowledge that you have read this License Agreement, and agree to be bound by its terms and conditions. To the extent that any other terms and conditions presented on any website of Bentham Science Publishers conflict with, or are inconsistent with, the terms and conditions set out in this License Agreement, you acknowledge that the terms and conditions set out in this License Agreement shall prevail.

Bentham Science Publishers Pte. Ltd.
80 Robinson Road #02-00
Singapore 068898
Singapore
Email: subscriptions@benthamscience.net

BENTHAM
SCIENCE

CONTENTS

FOREWORD

Precision Medicine seems to be a new adage in the world of Medical Science. However, a careful analysis of human civilization from across the globe suggests that almost every civilization has been health-conscious and requires medical attention. Historically, the most reliable and single source of all the medicines were plants, which were carefully selected, propagated and used in different forms. American Indians in the USA used plant-based medicines for relieving pain. Approximately, 40% of all modern drugs are plant-based. Among the 252 essential chemicals designated by the World Health Organization, 11.1% are sourced from plants, while 8.7% originate from animals. Currently, the United States employs approximately 19,000 FDA-approved prescription drugs, with several of them having their origins rooted in the animal kingdom. This suggests that almost 50% of all the drugs are either from plants or animals and perhaps many more may be discovered in due course of time.

The concept of precision medicine has already gained momentum over the world. Simultaneously, medical science has made remarkable progress using the data from the field of Omics, cell and tissue engineering, and gene therapy. The progress and success with molecular taxonomy and tissue expressions in genetic variants have brought confidence in precision diagnosis, efficient prognosis, prevention and effective treatment. We do not have a cure for all the diseases, but are on the right track of passing on the benefits of new knowledge and technology to the patients and their families.

The book **Precision Medicine** contains well organized 20 chapters covering a wide range sub-disciplines. An overview of several important topics in addition to a critical appraisal on precision medicine has been provided. This initial attempt in the country shall pave the way for more such books on specialized sub-disciplines in future. Advances in today's medical sciences has provided a scope for new drug molecules, next generation vaccines, stem cell and gene therapy, robotic surgery and other high-end medical intervention. A careful analysis of drug molecules and finding the drug target in the body without any side effects are the areas that still warrant relentless research and innovation.

The present book on precision medicine is the brain child of Farzana Mahdi and Abbas Ali Mahdi, who have shown exemplary courage, determination and concern to provide the best possible care to the patients. Era University has a well-known and highly respected medical college. During the upsurge of Covid-19, more than 3200 patients were cured and the success rate was 98.5%. This is an achievement that has been duly acknowledged by the honourable Governor of Uttar Pradesh.

Farzana Mahdi and Abbas Ali Mahdi are hard core academicians, distinguished biochemists, capable administrators and great mentors. Both believe in quality research and transparent dealing with excellent academic records to their credit; publishing papers in high impact factor journals. They are well connected with the global body of scientists and keep an eye on the emerging advancements in the area of biomedical research. Farzana Mahdi has successfully helmed the Era University as a Vice Chancellor during the pandemic of Covid-19, and Abbas Ali Mahdi is the current Vice Chancellor of the university.

It is gratifying to mention that all the chapters in the book, one way or the other are related to Precision Medicine. I am very hopeful that this book would fuel the thoughts of academicians, clinicians and researchers alike transgressing all the sub-disciplines of biomedical research eventually culminating into a better human health care system.

Rameshwar N. K. Bamezai
Former Vice Chancellor, SMVD University, J & K
Former Hon. Director, Delhi School of Public Health
Institution of Eminence
University of Delhi
Delhi-110007
India

PREFACE

Writing a book on an upcoming topic like precision or personalized medicine (PM) in the context of human health is both rewarding as well as challenging. The origin of such a book is related to an International Symposium that was held on June 24, 2022, at the Department of Molecular and Personalized Medicine, Era University, Lucknow.

During the course of extensive deliberation, it became clear that we need in-depth additional information, not only regarding the diseases and their causative factors, but also about the overall background of the patients encompassing lifestyle, nutrition, age, comorbidity, previous history of the disease, demography, epidemiology, living condition, environmental, social and economic status, gender, marital status, physical and physiological attributes, mutational landscapes of the diseased gene, genetic background, upbringing, region, religion, faith, culture, tradition, familial dis/harmony, marital incompatibilities and overall awareness towards a disciplined and healthy life. Longevity has always been an enticing proposition for mankind since the dawn of civilization. The quest to live forever is still cherished in almost all the societies of the world. The dollar wellness industry thrives on this psyche and that would continue to grow because the demand for such products never seems to be ending.

As the situation stands now, much of the medical issues may be circumvented employing the approach of molecular and personalized medicine. This will require additional biomedical research, keeping in view the patient's background information and careful titration of the prescribed medicaments. Perhaps, many medicines may not be needed and only a few ones would be enough since the diagnosis will be based on the hard core molecular and "ics" data facilitating the physicians and clinicians to make the correct decision at the right time. With concerted efforts on this line, precision medicine will not only see the light of day but will provide health to all even in the fall flung areas of the country harvesting the power of digitalization, telecommunication and Artificial Intelligence. It is envisaged that the proposed health card (*made at the time of birth as proposed in the first chapter*) of the patient will carry all the relevant background data in the form of a QR code only to be accessed by authorized clinicians and physicians across the globe. This simple but reliable trick would provide past medical records instantly and do away with many social evils, false claims and impersonation augmenting much-needed transparency in the human health care system.

The present narrative embodied in this book is a biological and biomedical symphony based on research, innovation, experience, and detailed deliberation emerging from the conference, symposium and scientific meetings all culminating in the PM. This encompasses different aspects of life that we come across rather routinely not realizing that many of these events affect our health. Of course, the vicissitudes of life also prove to be blessings in disguise, making a person, careful, strong and optimistic. In conclusion, the growing consensus is that one should be aware of the wide conundrum of health issues and follow the path of a disciplined life. This may not guarantee health, happiness, overall wellness and much-desired longevity. Nonetheless, it would drastically reduce the disease burden and occurrence of negative events in life that in turn would percolate down the ladder leading to robust health. Finally, if we seek peace in life, then we must start believing that peace begins from the self which in turn can be spread in the family, society, state, country, continents, and finally across the world. Needless to mention, a peaceful and relaxed person is a lot less prone to diseases and infection than the one who has an agitated mind. Thus, those of us who preach peace but do not practice will not be able to see the desired results.

This book, **Precision Medicine and Human Health**, has a total of twenty chapters spread across the spectrum of disciplines. The book includes some of the areas that were less represented earlier in the medical literature. The first chapter dealing with precision medicine provides a critical appraisal encompassing all the key areas that relate to human healthcare systems. For example, emotions, social interactions and life experiences culminating into overall happiness play an important role in the life of a person. Thus, an emotionally strong and happy person is usually healthy. Since everybody, whether diseased or healthy, has a unique genome, this uniqueness must be utilized in selecting the drug molecule, dose, and its long-term effects. Healing and cure strategies should address the root cause of the problem and not the symptoms only to provide short-term relief. Similarly, repurposing of the drug should be explored to cover a much wider number of diseases, cutting down the cost of the development of medicine. Finally, clinicians and doctors should be sensitized to the concept of precision medicine and its sub-disciplines. The medical field, besides being a deep, very deep science is also an art starting from how to deal with diverse types of patients of different backgrounds and educate them by instilling a sense of confidence and then to cure the disease. Clinical psychologists and genetic counsellors particularly in a hospital set up can play their roles too to achieve this goal. Healing requires a combination of medical treatment and a positive environment to achieve faster recovery and long-term benefits for patients.

The second chapter deals with the significance of epigenetics, gene function and putative change or modification in the DNA's sequence. Genes are prone to changes that are brought about by a number of mechanisms encompassing gene conversion, exon/intron reshuffling, alteration in the mutational landscape, and copy number variation. In addition, repeat DNA sequences tend to expand or shrink changing the topology of adjacent genes resulting in their altered functions. Alterations in gene activity, especially those that are brought on by epigenetic errors, frequently cause genetic diseases. Researchers are particularly interested in how epigenetic modifications and mistakes affect gene function, protein synthesis, and human health. It is envisaged that a deeper understanding of the epigenetic modification of the genome or its aberration would augment our understanding of the function of the normal and diseased human genomes.

The third chapter is on Hepatocellular carcinoma (HCC) which is the most common malignancy and is the third leading cause of cancer-related death worldwide. Most HCC patients are diagnosed at the middle or advanced stage, thereby losing surgical resection opportunities. Due to disease heterogeneity, standard treatments such as chemotherapy or radiation are effective only in some patients. Tumors can have underlying genetic differences and may express different proteins across the spectrum of patients. At this juncture, how the PM can provide a better alternative is indeed thought-provoking. Precision medicine relies on matching a patient's molecular profile to an effective and targeted therapy. In clinical practice, the shift from stage oriented to a therapeutic-oriented approach is necessary to direct the selection of HCC treatment towards the potentially most effective option on an individual basis. The clinical application of discoveries in tumor biology holds the promise to improve the treatment outcomes for cancer patients on a large scale. This chapter discusses precision medicine for HCC management and highlights the completed or ongoing clinical trials of novel therapies for treating patients with advanced HCC.

The fifth and sixth chapters are devoted to protein biochemistry encompassing its various forms under varying physical and physiological conditions including folding and misfolding resulting in a wide range of debilitating disorders. These diseases are characterized by the deposition of insoluble plaques consisting of amyloid fibrils rich in β-sheet structures. Many natural proteins form amyloid fibrils or aggregated disease-specific proteins causing human diseases. The role of amyloids and their mechanism of formation, as well as the methods for detecting various types of aggregates, has been examined and discussed. Despite visible progress in the field of biochemistry, we still have questions regarding the aggregation and co-aggregation of protein molecules. Proteins are functional in their three-dimensional forms. The free amino group of the protein in the body when interacting with the carbonyl group of the reducing sugar follows the Maillard reaction to produce hazardous by-products, referred to as advanced glycation end products (AGEs). Studies have shown different aggregation pathways leading to fibril formation. Thus, the development of large number of therapeutic proteins is envisaged to complement the requirement of precision medicine.

Chapter seven relates to Helicobacter pylori in the human gut biomes playing an important role in our health and wellbeing. *Helicobacter pylori* (*H. pylori*) is a Gram-negative, microaerophilic, and slow-growing bacteria, colonized in more than half of the world's population. This bacterium has co-evolved and migrated with humans from East Africa, the first birthplace of *Homo sapience*, about 58,000 thousand years ago. Special properties of *H. pylori*, like urease, helical shape, and motile flagella, make it a successful resident in the human stomach under extreme stress conditions. The presence or absence of *H. pylori* in the stomach has a good and/or bad relationship with humans depending on host genetic susceptibility, immune responses, and environmental conditions. Usually, *H. pylori*-infected people are asymptomatic; however, about 20% of infected people develop gastric diseases like peptic ulcer (10-15%), gastric adenocarcinoma (1-3%) and mucosa-associated lymphoid tissue (MALT) lymphoma (1%) that are common to elder people. On the other hand, people who have no *H. pylori* infection are more susceptible to other diseases like gastric esophageal disease (GERD), oesophagus carcinoma, diabetes mellitus, and asthma. Clinical manifestations in the infected individuals greatly vary geographically due to the high level of genetic diversity in the bacterial genome and several virulence factors. Eradication of *H. pylori via* antibiotics and proton pump inhibitors is the complete cure for the disease. However, an increase in resistance against antibiotics and lack of effective vaccines are still some challenges to combat the infection. In this context, the effective precision medicine would be the vaccine. This chapter provides an insight into host-pathogen interactions, persistence, prevalence, and pathogenesis of this bacterium in the context of human health and precision medicine.

Chapter eight is devoted to breast cancer which is most common among females. Current data shows more than 1 million women worldwide are affected about ~400 000 patients die every year. Partial success has been achieved by mammography and adjuvant treatment. However, incidences and mortality both are increasing. Of the several sub-categories, one is triple-negative breast cancer (TNBC). This is defined by a lack of expression of oestrogen and progesterone receptors and human epidermal growth factor receptor 2 (HER-2). Several approaches have been undertaken both for speedy and accurate diagnosis and precise treatment. In this context, the precision medicine approach may be of great relevance in ameliorating the suffering of the patients from the menace of breast cancer. However, it may be noted that several drug molecules and strategies need to be developed to cover different stages of breast cancer before a respite may be achieved.

Chapter nine focuses on depression, a pervasive, arduous psychological condition with profound neurological ramifications. Many individuals suffering from depression undertake a recurring or persistent therapy that correlates to a decline in cognitive processing. The underpinning of the exact aetiology and pathogenesis of melancholy is probably the outcome of a variety of mechanisms. These include physiological, behavioural, and socioeconomic variables, all playing their roles. Multiple therapies, medications and medical interventions are employed but depression has yet to find its match in the context of precision medicine. One option is to search for a more effective drug molecule befitting to all the symptoms of depression. The other approach is to find a cure from herbal formulation. In any event, both approaches need additional research, innovation, and development for ultimate effective interventions.

One of the aspects of precision medicine is to make use of artificial intelligence (AI) which is discussed in chapter ten. The digital ecosystem of AI will have global outreach evoking expert opinion from clinicians in serious conditions of the patients. The AI is envisaged to be the game changer, particularly in case of cancer, which is described as a heterogeneous cellular conglomeration comprising many dissimilar subtypes. The AI involves the use of deep learning which is a part of artificial intelligence (AI) that permits an algorithm to learn itself via the knowledge acquired from a large set of instances that determine the predicted outcomes. The use of AI is continuously growing for the prognosis of various diseases enabling pathologists to accurately diagnose various diseases, and classify them into grades and subtypes keeping in view the process of invasion, mutations, and metastases. AI also contributes to the area of precision medicine to overcome drug resistance and relapse of diseases. This chapter outlines various illustrations for the uses of AI in oncology research, together with circumstances in which deep learning has adequately addressed the difficulties that were earlier assumed to be unsolvable. AI also focuses on resources and datasets that can assist in developing interconnections with AI's intricacies in disease investigation. The expansion of advanced computational methodologies and AI are envisaged to facilitate interactomes studies and help significantly gain insights into the field of oncology fulfilling the concept of personalized medicine.

Chapter eleven relates to Fibromyalgia Syndrome (FMS) which has attracted much attention, especially with the gene discovery pushing towards a newer understanding of disease biology. Potential candidate genes found to be associated with fibromyalgia are SLC64A4, TRPV2, MYT1L, and NRXN3. Fibromyalgia is a widespread musculoskeletal pain disorder accompanied by fatigue, sleep, memory and mood issues. FMS amplifies painful sensations by affecting the way the brain and spinal cord process painful and non-painful signals. Some targeted treatments are now available improving the FMS patients on a short-term basis. This chapter highlights the key breakthroughs focusing on technologies that touch upon personalized or precision medicine in FMS. If FMS is related to brain and spinal cord functioning, work on this line using animal models would prove to be a rewarding proposition as the use of human patients would pose a logistic problem.

The time code is expressed in the form of circadian clocks composed of many transcription, co-activator, and co-repressor factors. These aspects have been covered in Chapter twelve. The transcription-translation feedback loops generated collectively by these factors regulate daily ~24-hour rhythms in physiology, metabolism, and behaviour across divergent phyla. Genome-wide studies reflect that chronic disruption of circadian rhythms provides a plinth for the occurrence and progression of multiple diseases across our lifespan. Increasing epidemiological and experimental evidences are confirming that circadian clocks are compromised in cancer and several other diseases. Altered expressions of circadian clock components are likely to be associated with the onset and progression of cancer and cardiovascular diseases. The concept of targeting circadian clocks at the molecular level is rapidly evolving and opening a new therapeutic window in cancer. Here, we discuss the approaches and recent advancements that have been made for the identification and development of clock-modulating small molecules bearing drug-like properties for the therapeutic management of cancer. Thus, this chapter is envisaged to augment the concepts of precision medicine in general and circadian-related system anomalies in particular.

Of the several diseases that have become the cause of concern, Multiple Sclerosis (Mus) is one that is an autoimmune inflammatory disease affecting roughly 2.8 million people worldwide which is covered in Chapter thirteen. Mus is a highly heterogeneous disease in term of course, clinical symptoms and drug response. The exact pathogenesis and aetiology of this disease remain unknown. The lack of successful treatment can be explained by the heterogeneous nature of MuS with patients exhibiting widely disparate clinical features and progression pattern resulting in phenotypic heterogeneity. With the introduction of *Omics* approaches, personalized medicine has gained momentum revealing hitherto unseen elements of illness causation, initiation and progression. This chapter highlights the potential role of genomics, transcriptomics, proteomics and metabolomics in MuS for possible identification of biomarkers facilitating and augmenting the concept of precision medicine.

The chapter fourteen deals with the clinical challenge related to metastasis of cancer cells to distant organs forming a secondary tumor. Many cancers are prone to metastasis due to epithelial-mesenchymal transition (EMT), which confers motility and invasive properties to the tumor. EMT is also responsible to chemotherapy resistance and facilitates metastasis by generating cancer stem cells (CSCs). Therefore, the EMT may be an important candidate for therapeutic potential for personalized cancer treatment. This chapter discusses approaches for the design of EMT-based personalized therapies in cancer, summarize the evidence for some of the proposed EMT targets, and review the potential advantages and limitations of each approach.

Yet another rather common cancer is the oral cancer covered in Chapter fifteen. Oral cancer is a type of head and neck cancer mainly caused by poor oral hygiene, alcohol and tobacco abuse, and promotes HPV infection. The conventional approaches for the treatment of oral cancer often rely on surgery, chemotherapy and/or radiotherapy. Now, the precision medicine, with the advent of newer diagnostic techniques, enables healthcare professionals to diagnose the disease early and treat the patient with appropriate medicines with the optimized dose. Targeting specific proteins, such as EGFR and HER2 to suppress tumor growth or make cancer cells more susceptible to the immune system's combat mechanism is also discussed. In addition, this chapter has an overview of various drugs that are being used to treat patients who are positive for HER2 and EGFR. Various challenges and limitations of precision medicine and future prospects for research in this area are highlighted.

The chapter sixteen and seventeen are devoted to herbal medicine. The treatment using plant based medicaments has been prevalent in almost every civilization such as Sumerian, Maya, Red Indian of USA, Greek, Roman and Egyptian for the past seven thousand years. India is blessed with rich medicinal plant biodiversity. Food harnessing and garnishing have become standard practice to enhance the taste and look. Some of the herbs are used directly as food whereas others are used as food additives. Simultaneously, a large number of Phytoconstituents have been characterized for their medicinal properties. In these chapters, Phytoconstituents used for herbal formulation have been discussed with their detailed properties. It is envisaged that such information would be of great use to ameliorate the diseases ensuring better health complementing the concept of personalized medicine.

The Chapter eighteen deals with the human habitat where there is paucity of oxygen (hypoxia). Hypoxia is a condition wherein an organism or a cell of an organ does not receive adequate levels of oxygen to carry out normal life processes. The ability to sense oxygen level and respond appropriately is termed "oxygen sensing" that is used to describe the biological effects of hypoxia. Hypoxia is involved with multiple diseases from high altitude pulmonary oedema to cancer. The oxygen sensing molecular networks is crucial for survival and has a notable impact on human health systems. A very important niche of hypoxia is the study of environmental stressor also called high-altitude hypoxia. High-altitude hypoxia holds multiple molecular similarities with diabetes, cancer, obesity and other diseases like COPD. In addition, unregulated exposure to hypobaric hypoxia is known to directly cause high altitude illnesses like HAPE/HACE. Acclimatization with the high altitude is known to prevent the occurrence of high-altitude illnesses. This chapter highlights the occurrence of hypobaric hypoxia, its socio-economic impact, molecular underpinnings and correlation with inflammation, cancer, diabetes, obesity and possible therapeutic approaches to these diseases.

Chapter nineteen discusses the advances in nanotechnology and its therapeutic potential. This chapter highlights the promising role of Nanomaterial in Precision oncology where the conventional therapy dwindles. Moreover, the emerging role of Precision Medicine in dentistry genetic diseases and Cystic fibrosis is highlighted which was once a nightmare but now is completely curable with the boon of Precision Nanomedicine. Chapter twenty provides an overview of the current state of the art in nanotechnology-based drug delivery systems and their potential applications. It discusses the various types of nanoparticles that are currently being used or developed for drug delivery, including liposomes, dendrimers, and polymeric nanoparticles, and highlights their advantages and disadvantages. It also covers some of the key challenges and risks associated with the use of nanotechnology in drug delivery, such as toxicity and regulatory issues. Finally, the article explores the future prospects of nanotechnology in drug delivery and highlights some of the areas where further research and development are needed. It is envisaged that this technology will facilitate augmentation of precision medicine for better human health care across the spectrum of diseases.

In this book, chapters have been linked with PM. The book also highlights hitherto less trailed aspects of Ayurveda, a treasure trove of our country. Logic dictates that if already available tried and tested herbal formulations are given as an additive or supplementary medicaments to the patients, that may speed up the process of healing with no or minimal side effect. Simultaneously, research may be conducted to uncover active factors from the still uncharacterized medicinal plants and herbs, synergizing their strength to make them more potent to be used as drug supplement. It is envisaged that the book will provide a conceptual framework for clinician, doctors and researchers in the field of biomedical research augmenting the human health care system and providing additional impetus for future research and innovation complementing the Precision Medicine.

Farzana Mahdi
Era University, Lucknow, India

&

Abbas Ali Mahdi
Era University, Lucknow, India

DEDICATION

Dedicated
To
Late Professor Dr. Mahdi Hasan
PhD, DSc, FNA, FASc, FNASc, FAMS, AvH, DAAD-Germany
Padma Shri, Government of India

List of Contributors

Armiya Sultan	Department of Biotechnology, Jamia Millia Islamia, New Delhi, India
Anamika Gangwar	Defence Institute of Physiology & Allied Sciences (DIPAS), Defence R & D Organization (DRDO), Timarpur, New Delhi, India
Allal Ouhtit	Biological and Environmental Sciences, College of Arts and Sciences, Qatar University, Qatar
Anam Farooqui	Centre for Interdisciplinary Research in Basic Sciences, Jamia Millia Islamia, New Delhi, India
Baby Tabassum	Toxicology, Lab, Department of Zoology, Govt Raza P.G. College, Rampur-(U.P.) 244901, India
Chirag N. Patel	Chemical Biology Laboratory, Center for Cancer Research, National Cancer Institute, National Institute of Health, Frederick, USA
Deepti Kaushik	School of Biotechnology, Gautam Buddha University, Greater Noida, India
Deepti Singh	Molecular Cancer Genetics & Translational Research Lab, Section of Genetics, Department of Zoology, Aligarh, India
Farhan Jalees Ahmad	Department of Pharmaceutics, School of Pharmaceutical Education and Research, Jamia Hamdard, New Delhi, India
Fayaz Malik	Indian Institute of Integrative Medicine, Sanat Nagar, India
Farhan Ali	Internal Medicine, Yakima Valley Memorial Hospital, WA, USA
Ghizal Fatima	Department of Biotechnology, Era University, Lucknow, India
Hifzur R. Siddique	Molecular Cancer Genetics & Translational Research Lab, Section of Genetics, Department of Zoology, Aligarh, India
Ifrah Fareed	Interdisciplinary Biotechnology Unit, Aligarh Muslim University, Aligarh, India
Khalid Umar Fakhri	Genome Biology Lab, Department of Biosciences, Jamia Millia Islamia, New Delhi, India
Kanu Priya	Department of Life Sciences, School of Basic Sciences and Research, Sharda University, Greater Noida, India
Kajim Ali	Department of Biotechnology, Era's Lucknow Medical College & Hospital, Era University,, Uttar Pradesh, India
Loveleena Kour Anand	Indian Institute of Integrative Medicine, Sanat Nagar, India
Mohd. Tashfeen Ashraf	School of Biotechnology, Gautam Buddha University, Greater Noida, India
Mohammad Hashim	Department of Biochemistry, Mohammad Ali Jauhar University, Rampur-(U.P.) 244901, India
Mohd Adil	Centre for Interdisciplinary Research in Basic Sciences, Jamia Millia Islamia, New Delhi, India
Mohammad Faheem Khan	Department of Chemistry, Era University, Lucknow-226003, India

Mir Shahid Maqbool	Indian Institute of Integrative Medicine, Sanat Nagar, India
Monalisa Mukherjee	Amity Institute of Click Chemistry Research and Studies, Amity University, Uttar Pradesh, India
Md Zubbair Malik	Department of Genetics and Bioinformatics, Dasman Diabetes Institute, Dasman, Kuwait City, Kuwait
M. Moshahid Alam Rizvi	Genome Biology Lab, Department of Biosciences, Jamia Millia Islamia, New Delhi, India
Mohammad Afsar Khan	Molecular Cancer Genetics & Translational Research Lab, Section of Genetics, Department of Zoology, Aligarh, India
Mohd Yasir Khan	Department of Biotechnology, Jamia Millia Islamia, New Delhi, India
Nimisha Gupta	Department of Biotechnology, School of Chemical and Life Sciences, Jamia Hamdard, Jamia Nagar, New Delhi, India
Nida Idrees	Toxicology, Lab, Department of Zoology, Govt Raza P.G. College, M.J.P. Rohilkhand University, Bareilly, Rampur- (U.P.) 244901, India
Nida Jamil Khan	Department of Biosciences, Jamia Millia Islamia, New Delhi, India
Navin Kumar	School of Biotechnology, Gautam Buddha University, Greater Noida, Uttar Pradesh, India
Najma	Centre for Interdisciplinary Research in Basic Sciences, Jamia Millia Islamia, New Delhi, India
Piyush Bhati	School of Biotechnology, Gautam Buddha University, Greater Noida, India
Rupali Ghosh	Department of Biotechnology, School of Chemical and Life Sciences, Jamia Hamdard, Hamdard Nagar, New Delhi, India
Radhika Chaurasia	Amity Institute of Click Chemistry Research and Studies, Amity University, Uttar Pradesh, India
Rafat Ali	Centre for Interdisciplinary Research in Basic Sciences, Jamia Millia Islamia, New Delhi, India
Romana Ishrat	Centre for Interdisciplinary Research in Basic Sciences, Jamia Millia Islamia, New Delhi, India
Rizwan Hasan Khan	Interdisciplinary Biotechnology Unit, Aligarh Muslim University, Aligarh, India
Robeena Sarah	Toxicology, Lab, Department of Zoology, Govt Raza P.G. College, M.J.P. Rohilkhand University, Bareilly, Rampur- (U.P.) 244901, India
Saima Wajid	Department of Biotechnology, School of Chemical and Life Sciences, Jamia Hamdard, Hamdard Nagar, New Delhi, India
Sugandh Kumar	School of Medicine, University of California San Francisco (UCSF), San Francisco, USA
Subhojit Paul	Defence Institute of Physiology & Allied Sciences (DIPAS), Defence R & D Organization (DRDO), Timarpur, New Delhi, India

Swaraj Mohanthy	Defence Institute of Physiology & Allied Sciences (DIPAS), Defence R & D Organization (DRDO), Timarpur, New Delhi, India
Syed Tasleem Raza	Department of Biochemistry , Era's Lucknow Medical College and Hospital, Lucknow, India
Saliha Rizvi	Department of Biochemistry, Era University, Lucknow, India
Sher Ali	Department of Personalized and Molecular Medicine, Era University, Lucknow, India
Sadia Malik	Interdisciplinary Biotechnology Unit, Aligarh Muslim University, Aligarh, India
Sumbul Yasmeen	Interdisciplinary Biotechnology Unit, Aligarh Muslim University, Aligarh, India
Tassaduq Hussain Wani	Department of Biological Sciences, The University of North Carolina at Charlotte, Charlotte, USA
Tahira Sultan	Department of Clinical Biochemistry, University of Kashmir, Srinagar, India
Tajalli Ilm Chandel	Interdisciplinary Biotechnology Unit, Aligarh Muslim University, Aligarh, India
Waseem Ahmad Ansari	Department of Biotechnology, Era's Lucknow Medical College & Hospital, Era University,, Uttar Pradesh, India
Yogesh Kumar	Department of General, University Medical Centre Hamburg-Eppendorf, Visceral and thoracic surgery, Hamburg, Germany
Yasmin Ahmad	Defence Institute of Physiology & Allied Sciences (DIPAS), Defence R & D Organization (DRDO), Timarpur, New Delhi, India

CHAPTER 1

Personalized Medicine (PM) A Critical Appraisal

Syed Tasleem Raza[1,*], Saliha Rizvi[2], Allal Ouhtit[3], Farhan Ali[4] and Sher Ali[5]

[1] *Department of Biochemistry, Era's Lucknow Medical College and Hospital, Lucknow-226003, India*

[2] *Department of Biotechnology, Era University, Lucknow-226003, India*

[3] *Biological and Environmental Sciences, College of Arts and Sciences, Qatar University, Qatar*

[4] *Internal Medicine, Yakima Valley Memorial Hospital, WA-98902, USA*

[5] *Department of Personalized and Molecular Medicine, Era University, Hardoi Road, Lucknow-226003, India*

Abstract: Personalized medicine, also referred to as precision medicine, deals with a clinical model that delineates patients into different groups based on their ethnicity, lifestyle, food habits, medical history, drug reaction, comorbidity, the robustness of the immune system, age, gender, and proneness to infection, overall psyche and attitude towards life. Further, emotions, social interactions and life experiences culminating into overall happiness play an important role in the life of a person. Thus, an emotionally strong and happy person is usually healthy. Taking all these above factors into consideration and with accurate diagnosis, a drug may be prescribed more in tune with the uniqueness of the patient's genome. Since everybody, whether diseased or healthy, has a unique genome, this uniqueness must be utilized in deciding the drug, dose and its long-term effects. Healing and cure should address the root cause of the problem instead of working only on the symptoms to provide short-term relief. In addition, repurposing of the drug which is not an old concept should also be carefully explored because with this approach, a large number of already available drugs may be used for a much wider number of diseases than the medicine originally developed for. This will also help reduce the cost of the development of medicine. Finally, clinicians and doctors should be sensitized to the concept of precision medicine and its less obvious sub-disciplines. This is envisaged to provide better, more accurate diagnosis and may result in better treatment. The medical field, besides being a deep science is also an art starting from how to deal with diverse types of patients of different backgrounds and educate them all the way to instill a sense of confidence and then to prescribe the medicine to cure the disease. Seemingly, within the realm of precision medicine, it is a huge task. However, it is possible to collect and analyze diagnostic data to reach a consensus. This would require the involvement of clinical psychologists and genetic counselors in a hospital setting ensuring that patient care is holistic, taking

* **Corresponding author Syed Tasleem Raza:** Department of Biochemistry, Era's Lucknow Medical College and Hospital, Lucknow-226003, India; Tel: 9839179527; E-mail: tasleem24@gmail.com

Farzana Mahdi & Abbas Ali Mahdi (Eds.)

into account both the physical and psychological aspects of health. This integrated approach can lead to improved patient care and long-term well-being.

Keywords: Demography, Epidemiology, Genome heterogeneity, Human psyche, Pain management, Precise medicine, System biology.

INTRODUCTION

Every human genome is unique as mentioned earlier with respect to its organization, gene expression, regulation, signal transduction, immune system, and response towards different drugs. The genome is a dynamic ensemble of several attributes and constantly adopts and adjusts to maintain cellular homeostasis. During the course of duplication of about 7 billion diploid sequences in a single cell, the genome must ensure that it remains error-free. However, the genome is constantly getting affected by the environment and therefore the possibility of newer mutations may not be ruled out. It is therefore relevant to uncover genetics and environmental bases of diseases. How the concept of PM is viewed across the globe, is another important issue because the world has become small though the healthcare system has become big. Since quality management of patients is possible only when we have a deeper understanding of the disease heterogeneity together with the genome heterogeneity of the patients, we have included demography, epidemiology, ethnicity and genome heterogeneity in our discussion. Finally, we have taken into consideration the prevalent healthcare system and its management, not only in India but in other countries as well. It is envisaged that our attempt at PM will enhance awareness of this theme evoking sufficient interest amongst clinicians and doctors to become more multidisciplinary in their approaches, bringing several healthcare systems on a single platform. This will be a win-win situation for both doctors and researchers. Since medicine is manufactured by pharmaceutical companies, it would be befitting to keep them in the loop so that more fruitful results are obtained. In the context of PM, drug repurposing and titration are two main aspects that must be seriously considered as a topic of research. When adequate data is available on this line, innovation will continue to trickle into the realm of the human healthcare system. Finally, we all agree that prevention is better than cure; we should therefore try to sensitize the masses to make a change in their lifestyle from an unhealthy one to a healthy one. If this calls for some sacrifice at a personal level, so be it. It has been largely believed that our life revolves around genetics and environment with a ratio of 50:50. However, a recent closer scrutiny suggests that the role of genetics is only 10% and the rest all is the environmental impact. Thus, the scope of the environment in the human health care system is expanded with new found knowledge. Clearly, the environment includes a lot more things than we have envisaged so far. Cancer now is considered a preventable disease but 1 million Americans and more than 10 million people worldwide are at risk of cancer. Significantly, 5-10% of cancers have a genetic basis; the remaining ones are based on lifestyle and environmental factors. The lifestyle includes cigarette smoking, diet (fried food meat), alcohol, sun exposure, environmental pollutants, infections, stress, obesity, and lack of physical inactivity. About 25-30% of cancer-related deaths are due to tobacco alone, 30-35% are linked with diet, about 15-20% are due to infections and the rest are because of radiation, noise pollution, lack of sleep, and substance abuse. Prevention is possible in most of the cases, like quitting the use of tobacco, regular uptake of fruits and nuts, moderate or better still, no use of alcohol, restricted intake of calories, use of whole grains, use of timely vaccination, avoidance of too much sun exposure, regular exercise and routine medical checkup. Such changes amongst masses may reduce the genome heterogeneity facilitating the development of PM. There has been a history behind the origin of precision medicine but the concept is now gaining momentum with the availability of better research tools, more awareness, and faster communication.

ORIGIN AND CONCEPT OF PERSONALIZED MEDICINE (PM)

A teenage boy and his grandmother would not buy the same clothes because their bodies will have different size requirements. However, during sickness, they may receive the same medical treatment and so will everyone else. At this juncture, the differences and now fully established genome heterogeneity are not taken into consideration.

That's because even the world's best scientists and doctors do not fully understand how different people develop diseases and respond differently to treatments. The "one-size-fits-all" approach in medicine has been going on but this has never been rationalized let alone challenged. Why population study, demography, epidemiology, population structure, genetic makeup, genotypes, mutational load, food habits, region, religion, susceptibility and resistance, liking and disliking, thought processes, customs and tradition, choice of mating partners, day-to-day activities, the timing of food intake and retiring to bed, disciplined/ undisciplined lifestyle and change in the weather are not taken into consideration before prescribing the medicine. This is because what is practiced by the doctors is what they have been taught. Perhaps doctors do not have time to think beyond their defined hours of duty. During their studies, they were not asked not to think and use their own imagination. The so-called common sense is highly uncommon, because, in the majority of the cases in every field, this is simply lacking. Thus, based on broad population averages, and decade-old drug trials, medicine is prescribed. There is no information on how the same medicine in two different persons will be metabolized. However, after the intake of the drug, this can be ascertained by analyzing urine samples from the patients. Nonetheless, this approach has never been part of the drug trial. This traditional practice often misses its mark because each person's genome makeup and genetic background are very different from the other persons. These points are important because they all affect our health. The concept based on precision medicine is moving us closer to a more precise, predictable and powerful healthcare system that is customized for an individual patient. Our growing understanding of genetics and genomics would allow us to gain an insight into health drive, disease and drug responses in each person. This would enable doctors to ensure better disease prevention, more accurate diagnoses, safer drug prescriptions and more effective treatments for many diseases. Thus, personalized medicine is going to stay because its time has come.

ISSUES RELATED TO PM

There are several issues that are related to precision medicine. These are highlighted here under with the assumption that they evoke the imagination of clinicians and doctors.

Shift the Emphasis in Medicine from Reaction to Prevention Because Prevention is Better than Cure

If the disease symptom is detected early, perhaps the disease may easily be managed. Besides, textbook knowledge, overall experience plays a great role in correct diagnosis. This is particularly important for some very serious or accidental cases. Based on the blood or urine analysis, medicine is prescribed but hardly ever, attempts are made to uncover the causative factors taking cellular homeostasis into consideration. This includes genetic background, lifestyle, ethnicity, resistance or susceptibility to the diseases, past medical history, and physical and emotional quotients that may be collectively or individually responsible for altered blood or body chemistry. Even the living and work conditions tend to affect the health of a person. When there are too many variables, finding a consensus becomes a challenge. However, concerted attempts on this line would start showing the results. Thus, challenges may be taken more like an opportunity to nurture and nourish this upcoming branch of biomedical science.

Susceptibility Prediction of an Individual to Diseases

Susceptibility of an individual to a disease may be due to several reasons including genetics, environment, allergy, compromised immune system, age, gender, emotional quotient, wrong diagnosis and incorrect medicine or its wrong dose. Thus, improved disease detection (genetic analysis), family background information, and disease history including genomepatri may all be helpful. Some people are severely affected by a mere change in weather since the environment itself continues to change with respect to the presence of virus, bacteria, allergens, pollutants and a variety of immunogens. Similarly, food allergy is equally common resulting in food phobia amongst the affected people. Not withstanding these challenges, this area deserves exploration for a broader understanding of the genome interaction with the environment and vice versa. For example, if a strong association of food or pollen allergy with a particular ethnicity is established, that would accordingly facilitate the prognosis and diagnosis. The development of data on this line would then allow focusing on other variables in search of consensus. Eventually, this work is envisaged to uncover the much-desired population structure in the context of the occurrence of diseases and disease susceptibility.

Pre-empt Disease Progression

Disease pre-emption involves prior appropriation of the diseases. Thus, if a disease is diminished even up to 50%, that too will be helpful. The aim is not to allow the disease to spread and cripple the person. For example, if a person develops oral cancer and shows leukoplakia, should he be immediately rushed to the Operation Theater? Perhaps not, if the oral cancer may be controlled by drugs, the surgical operation may be avoided. Better still, if the awareness program is conducted on a war footing, particularly in the village set up to apprise the ignorant ones about the danger of tobacco consumption, this menace may largely be reduced. Disease pre-emption may not be feasible for all diseases. However, wherever possible, that should be done. Similarly, prenatal diagnosis will help in the context of suspected genetic anomalies. A severe case may be considered for medical termination of pregnancy after due deliberation and consultation of the doctors with parents. While pursuing this area, a patient's medical history may faithfully be recorded which will be part of the medical database for futuristic medicine.

Customization of Strategies for Disease-prevention

A large number of infectious diseases and the ones that are waterborne may be managed by awareness programs and community health services. The doctors may aim to reach the far-flung areas in a mobile van to spread the message and educate the masses on how not to get infected by taking certain precautions. In extreme conditions, water can be boiled and filtered before its use or supplemented with chlorine tablets. The water source or the wells in the village may be sanitized with a recommended dose of potassium permanganate. The diseases that are caused due to unhygienic conditions may be curtailed by practicing overall sanitation. This requires a large-scale awareness program focusing on far-flung areas of the country. In principle, this aspect may further be facilitated by print and electronic media focusing particularly on the uneducated people of the society. Simultaneously, local, state, and central governments may gear their machinery to ensure that basic living facilities are available in the far-flung areas of the country.

Prescribe more Effective but Economical Drugs

When multiple drugs are available for the treatment of a particular disease, it is prudent to prescribe those that are both highly efficient and cost-effective. At this juncture, doctors have to exercise their ethical prerogative together with medical ones using their high level of civility and wisdom. It may be noted that not all cheap medicines are ineffective and not all expensive ones are highly effective. Behind the prescription of drugs, several other factors remain operative. However, to maintain the sanctity of the medical practice, those factors are not highlighted here with the assumption that overall ethics should be followed. Further, a large number of herbal formulations are available in the market and many of these may turn out to be more effective compared to allopathic drugs. For example, skin eruption and acne are largely treated with expensive ointment and allopathic drugs. The patients perhaps have more faith in such expensive items. However, this can be taken care of with Neem extract capsules readily available in the market. It not only cures acne but rejuvenates and enhances the overall health of the skin. There are many wellness products based on herbal formulations that have been discussed in other chapters of this book.

Development of Smart Drug Strategies for Patients

The development of smart drug strategies involves deliberation and debate about all the available medicines including drug molecules that are sitting ideally in the database. The best possible and most effective ones should be chosen carefully and prescribed judiciously. If combination therapy is needed in allopathy, Unani, or Ayush, then it may be favorably considered later. It all depends on the psyche of the caregiver, the disease condition of the patient, and the overall awareness of the patient's family. For a patient suffering from any disease, the immediate step on the part of the family member is to find a secure clinic or a hospital setup. Often such a decision is taken in a hurry and thus, it may not always be the correct one. However, an efficient medical setup manned by experienced and qualified doctors would prove to be a real boon for the patient. Thus, together with the smart drug strategy on the part of the doctors, the smart choice of the clinic/hospital on the part of the patient (or family members) is equally important.

Strict Exclusion of Drugs with Possible Side Effects

Drug prescriptions must be made exclusively for the benefit of the patients and not for drug companies. "Which drug, how much, and for whom" should always be taken into consideration even though the doctor's decision may not match with the medical representative's feedback. Needless to mention, a medical representative works for the drug company but not for the doctors or patients. Thus, doctors are supposed to safeguard the interests of the patients and not that of the drug companies. It is well known that only some patients react to the drug and show side effects. Thus, if the population (ethnicity) is delineated into a genetical group and linked with the side effects of a drug, which would be of great help. This calls for research and innovation because this is a gap amongst different sub-disciplines of PM. Food allergy, pollens, fumes, chemicals, dust, building material, paints and varnish, all react to drug molecules. However, they all have different effects on different individuals. This aspect also needs to be strengthened keeping in view the allergy part of the patients and drug sensitivities and tolerance.

Broad Based Intelligent Clinical Trials with Reduced Time, Cost, and Failure Rate of the Pharmaceuticals

It is not clear if, during drug trials, population structure, occurrence of the diseases, robustness of the immune system and remedy for side effects are taken into consideration. However, simultaneous drug trials across the spectrum of ethnicity will provide a wealth of health information. Thus, the drug trial scope needs to be broadened and augmented in light of the newfound knowledge focusing on personalized medicine. If the patient's diagnostic parameters are fed into the robotic system (Artificial Intelligence, AI), along with the drug specification, AI may use the best possible algorithm to decipher the rate of drug metabolism across the patients and recommend the most effective dose of the medicine and its likely alternative. This will surely cut down the time and failure rate of pharmaceutical clinical trials. This approach may eliminate the trial-and error inefficiencies that inflate healthcare costs and undermine patient care. For meaningful clinical trials, the use of artificial intelligence (AI), machine learning (ML), and deep learning (DL) may be exploited for data analysis collected from the field to hasten the process. However, an AI-based robust platform needs to be developed coupled with advanced algorithms. Thus, ambiguity must be eliminated wherever this is possible to ensure intelligent clinical trials.

Drug Titration

Whenever possible, drug titration must be conducted to decide precise doses for different patients keeping in view the patients' overall background (POB) that has already been highlighted earlier. The drug titration approach has been found to be very effective in type 2 diabetes. While titration of the drug is advocated, one must equally be concerned with the toxicological part and the side effects. Safe prescription and secure limits, both are important. Drug titration should also be done with combination therapy wherever possible to arrive at the most effective dose for the patients. Along with the allopathic drug, herbal and homeopathic ones may also be considered either as the main option or an alternative one. This may prove to be cost-effective and a lot less unsafe for fragile and weak patients. In principle, all these are possible but in an actual case scenario, an allopathic doctor would avoid entering into the domains of Homeopathy, Ayush, or Unani Systems. This is partly because the allopath doctor has no idea about the efficacy of such drugs away from his field and or because s/he does not have faith in other systems. However, if this concept is propagated, slowly and gradually, this would take off and ameliorate the suffering of the patients because these alternative forms of medicine are more economical.

Psychosomatic and Spiritual Health

Finally, playing on the psychology of the patients by providing them reassurance and timely medical counseling irrespective of the severity of the disease and treatment outcome would prove to be highly effective. Emotional reassurance to the patients would complement the efforts of the doctors and caregivers. Thus, positivity on the part of the caregiver must be reflected all the time in their thoughts, actions and communication. The positive vibes will provide additional reassurance to the patients speeding up the healing process. Incidentally, this simple and single aspect is always neglected because not many people are aware of this concept or believe in the positivity of mode, mind and miracles. This less-explored domain makes it more attractive and worth pursuing. It has been proved beyond doubt that sincere and systematic prayers bless the patients and the healing process is speeded up. Perhaps, this aspect may be included in the medical curriculum so that doctors in actual case scenarios may remain aware of this aspect and use their knowledge for critical patients.

Civility of the Patients and their Family Members

While doctors and nursing staff are there to take care of the patients, it is implied that patients and their family members would show respect to them because it is the benevolent hands of God through which these caregivers operate on a 24x7 basis. Mutual respect, trust, and faith must be the hallmark of the human health care system. This is particularly important in the Indian scenario as cases of assault on doctors have been reported on time and again even in some big hospitals and famous Institutes. Society should strongly condemn flaunting wealth, strength, and power to ensure a calm and secure environment in clinics and hospitals. It's crucial to recognize that healthcare professionals and support staff are essential members of our community. This is the least that a civic society can do to the healthcare personnel.

Skill Up-gradation

Doctors must be encouraged to acquire new knowledge about the latest scientific/medical developments so that they are able to make correct decisions for the patients. Acquiring new skills and experiences gained in the process of clinical practice must be judiciously used all the time to augment the caregiving system. It is generally found that the doctor's prescription is based on a variety of medical tests but often, such tests are not required. Unfortunately, this unhealthy practice is done in the name of healthy treatment. Some of the tests are outrageously expensive or made expensive in the name of advanced and better health care. Thus, the doctors may be sensitized to these issues. In addition, patients should also be educated with basic facts about their diseases and treatment. This will help patients follow the advice of their doctors and remain aware of their responsibility. More than that, it would instill a sense of confidence amongst the patients and provide much-needed hope for a speedy recovery.

Health and Hygiene

Different doctors with the same degree and training adopt different approaches for the cure and management of the patients. In certain conditions, a consensus amongst the medical fraternity would go a long way to address this issue of patient care and follow-up. This is true for serious ailments where more than one opinion is required. Finally, adhering to ethics and moving away from any undue temptation would perhaps bring much-needed hygiene to the health care system because health and hygiene complement each other. Thus, system hygiene is equally important if not more since that would instill confidence amongst the patients. It is known that people working in the hospital setup are often infected. This is because standard hospital SOP is not followed faithfully. The standard SOP needs to be followed every day, every time, and all the time. Compromise in the SOP of a hospital setup would culminate in the health compromise defeating the very purpose of an efficient health care system.

Advanced Scientific Approach

The more we know the basis of the disease using advanced scientific analyses, the better we are in terms of diagnosis, prognosis and prescription of the medicine. Similarly, with respect to surgical operation, only the best possible approach may be employed ensuring minimal tissue trauma and maximum healing without compromising on the quality. The frequent use of robotic surgery backed/coupled with artificial intelligence (AI), involving local and global surgeons may prove to be lost less traumatic and perhaps more economical. Robotic surgery requires a full-fledged setup and equipment besides well-trained doctors. However, this one-time expenditure would reduce the undue burden on surgeons allowing them to exercise their own surgical prerogative. Overall automation will have its own reward in handling a large number of patients, particularly in the event of an endemic or epidemic. Hospital management must focus on the overall work of its caregivers which include doctors, nurses and other supporting staff. Undue workload must be avoided to ensure the overall well-being and happiness of the caregivers in any hospital set-up.

HISTORICAL PERSPECTIVE OF PM

In ancient times 1550 BC, as per Greek mythology, the first evidence of medicine used for an individual's health is found in the Odyssey written by Homer [1]. Menelaus was the king of Sparta, the brother of Agamemnon, and the husband of Helen, who helped lead the Greeks in the Trojan War. The king of Sparta offered Odysseus'son, Telemachus, assistance and provided information on the whereabouts of his father. Telemachus was very sad when he visited Menelaus and Helen in search of his father after the Trojan War [1]. Helen puts a drug into the wine, which eases the grief or anger and makes him forget his woes. This drug came from Egypt [1]. The adaptation of that ancient "Egyptian medicine" to an individual's health status was further elucidated in the Classical period from Herodotus when the practice of medicine was divided into different categories. With this, every doctor became a specialist for one disease and one body part [1]. This is the first evidence of personalized medicine, as doctors realized that separating the diseases according to the human body parts can help them to achieve a deeper understanding of illness. Greeks were fascinated by this approach to medicine, and with the result; they elucidated Egyptian medicine in their treatises with admiration [1]. Only after the appearance of Hippocratic medicine in the fifth century did Egyptian medicine start to be omitted from the Greek books [1]. Although "Hippocratic medicine" shares similarities with the Egyptians, the former did not undermine the latter. In contrast, Hippocrates used the knowledge of Egyptian medicine and advanced it by removing the magico-religious part and making it more rational [1]. During ancient times, physicians took into consideration the patient's needs and beliefs in order to have a successful treatment [2]. Hippocrates believed that "diseases might be treated from their origin" and "the treatment should address the cause of the disease." Therefore, they focused more on the personalized approach to the disease and eliminated all the surrounding superstitions prevalent at that time [3]. Thus, Hippocrates was ahead of his time and gave direction on the PM (now genomic) medicine. He suggested that every human is distinct, and this affects both the disease prediction and the treatment [3]. Accordingly, Hippocrates is considered to be the father of Western Medicine and thus, personalized medicine has come a long way attracting a lot of our attention.

However, despite the availability of ancient wisdom, modern medicine employed a broad approach based on clinical data from heterogeneous populations instead of focusing on each patient. Physicians used standardized approaches based on the knowledge of the earlier patients/diseases to decide on a therapeutic regimen. Clinical trials were only aiming for standardized treatment rooting out 20% of the population that was not going to respond to a treatment or even show adverse effects possibly due to differences in their genetic makeup [2]. This meant that medicine had no room for idiosyncrasy (from ancient Greek idosugkrasia/ idiosynkrasia, "a peculiar temperament, habit of the body, *e.g.*, blend of humors." Idiosyncrasy defined the way that physicians conceived diseases in the nineteen century). This approach began to change in the 1870s, when discoveries made by researchers in Europe allowed the advent of "scientific medicine," a precursor to the evidence-based medicine practiced now.

GENETICS AND ENVIRONMENTAL BASIS OF DISEASE

As mentioned earlier, we are the product of genes and environment. The question is how much is the contribution of genetics and how does the environment affect us? The old concept that both factors (genes and environment) play 50:50 roles is no longer valid because of enormous genome variability emerging from across the sub-disciplines. We inherit genes from our parents together with the mutations if they are there and have no control over them. Also, newer sporadic mutations are added with the passage of time. However, if parents are screened for deleterious or serious mutations prior to the birth of the child, remedial measures may be undertaken. That would also uncover newer sporadic mutations. Thus, knowing the mutational landscape of a person, particularly one with a history of genetic, infectious, and metabolic diseases, would help to decide the right course of action. Genome analysis in the context of its organization, gene expression, mutation, regulation, conversion, and duplication may all prove to be useful for taking measures to ameliorate the disease. Several genetic diseases may not be cured. In such a situation, alternative measures may be adopted. Besides the involvement of genetics, environments tend to play huge roles in causing diseases. This is true for infectious and waterborne diseases including cancer.

Precision Medicine and Cancer

We discuss cancer as an example to highlight the fact that genetics remain, mute spectators, when the environment takes over. A perusal of the literature shows that there are more than 200 different types of cancer. Some of them are mean whereas others are standard deviations with respect to their etiology. The mean ones pose more challenges for their treatment but the ones falling in the category of standard deviation genetic heterogeneity and variation are less difficult to manage. This aspect is further complicated when metastasis sets in. Breast cancer, glioblastoma, meningioma, prostate, and cervical cancers show variation in their etiology, and thus a consensus is not there when prescribing a precision medicine. This is because when cancer progression takes place, it is difficult to predict the extent to which the body will be affected. There is no technique available that can allow us to know the exact number of cells that have been affected across the tissues in the body. Early detection is therefore a lot less demanding, providing an opportunity for better and more manageable treatment.

Similarly, in case of oral cancer (another example), a patient having leukoplakia approaches a doctor much later during the disease progression. Clearly, oral cancer is largely caused because of the use of chewing tobacco and ignoring health advisories. A large number of such patients are made aware of the danger of using tobacco and its ill effects. However, they still choose to stick to their conventional lifestyle. All such patients are a drain on the (fragile) healthcare system. The only remedy is that the tobacco-related products must be banned. Society will continue to pay a price if we do not ban the production of such items. This does not require rocket technology, instead only will power and determination on the part of the government to take this step.

INHERITANCE OF BIOLOGICAL TRAITS

The biological traits are inherited from the parents and thus genotype /phenotype are largely decided by the genetic makeup of an individual. However, genetic makeup continues to interact with the environment making a change as and when required adopting the latter. If a person is subjected to extreme conditions such as the Chernobyl accident in the former USSR or Bhopal gas exposure, the genome is altered in a big way increasing the load of mutation affecting even eukaryotic transcriptional machinery. Thus, a study on the mutational load in the context of diseases would provide a wealth of information narrowing down the search for causative gene(s) for the disease. In addition, the genome also acquires sporadic mutations and some of them may prove to be devastating. Based on the interactions among hundreds of genes and their networks (interactomes), along with external factors such as diet, exercise, clean or unclean environment, and a healthy disciplined lifestyle, a genome tends to change all the time adjusting and re-adjusting with new environmental conditions. The unseen, unrecognized, and un-assessed conditions alter the blood chemistry and cause high cholesterol levels, an aberrant carbohydrate metabolism, deficiency in vitamins and minerals, and abnormal signal transduction. All these are linked with the unhealthy lifestyle when the health advisories are ignored. The biological complexity of the human body in the context of disease can be better understood by employing systems genetics, molecular biology, genomics, proteomics, and metabolomics. This is altogether a different discipline requiring comprehensive research at the single cell and specialized tissue levels including the organelles. It may seem to be a far-fetched idea but if we are able to develop for example a well-defined synthetic cell, exactly the way as nature does, it would enhance our understanding several folds. However, system biology is still evolving like personalized medicine. Yet another approach that is currently being used is the molecular mining of the databases employing powerful statistical and bioinformatics tools. Geneticists, mathematicians, physicists, and computer scientists are generating newer insights as to how genetic complexity drives health and diseases. Thus, personalized medicine has now metamorphosed from an interdisciplinary discipline into a multidisciplinary one involving several sub-disciplines. The fact that we have no control over the sporadic mutation in a gene will continue to complicate the health issue. However, mutational landscapes can be mapped and the most susceptible regions in the genome may be identified. Once this is achieved, at least some causative factors may be eliminated by correlating a genotype with a phenotype. Genetic disease may erupt due to a variety of reasons. For example, a stretch of DNA that is used to bind with the protein is no longer available because of mutation. The DNA protein binding is highly specific and a change in the DNA will hamper the binding. This in turn will impede the subsequent reactions and other biochemical steps in the cascade. Thus, from the available database, if we are able to uncover the regions of the genomes that are implicated in biochemical reactions, we can decipher the outcome of such mutations and then correlate that genotypic abnormality with the phenotypic one. Molecular mining of the available data and genotype-phenotype correlation have not been pursued extensively. Unlike a wet research lab, molecular data mining does not require large-scale research paraphernalia. The molecular mining of databases will go a long way to set things right generating consensus on genotype-phenotype correlation of a disease not withstanding sporadic mutations. This aspect of science is acknowledged globally, but not many attempts have been made on this line. Perhaps data mining, gene hunting, genome dissection, and genotype-phenotype correlation call for much deeper involvement of the researchers. Accordingly, it is envisaged that the result would augment the area of PM. The other example related to the involvement of the environment is the prevalent genotoxicity in animals, plants, and humans. For example, arsenic is present in Ganga in UP and fishes in the water are affected. Arsenic is also present in water in Bihar and Bengal. Those who are not aware of this fact will tend to use contaminated water affecting their health largely due to ignorance. Studies conducted on the fishes treated with Arsenic and then provided Neem extract have shown remarkable results. The Neem extract seems to ameliorate the ill effects of Arsenic in the fish. A systematic large-scale study on this line would provide a remedy for the genotoxicity of Arsenic present in the environment. The Neem extract may not be used on a large number of fish in water bodies owing to logistic constraints. However, this can be used for humans. Not withstanding available data from the fish, detailed human studies need to be conducted to prove this point beyond doubt.

STATUS OF PM ACROSS THE GLOBE

The emergence of personalized medicine (PM) has raised some concerns in the context of human healthcare systems. Usually, PM is expensive and health budgets are limited thus, quality healthcare delivery is not feasible. Not withstanding the cost, many countries, including those in Southeast Asia (SEA) where resources are not unlimited have started to pursue this promising concept. Here, we examine the PM adoption in SEA, highlight the challenges and assess the possibilities for its future development.

A perusal of literature from four countries encompassing Indonesia, Malaysia, Singapore, and Thailand offers much for us to learn and infuse in the list of our priority. The PM program needs to address the healthcare system, governance, access, awareness, implementation, collection and annotation of the large scale data. In an actual case scenario, if a hospital keeps the record of the newly born babies in a health booklet (HB) exclusively designed for this purpose; much vital health related background information may be obtained through this single source embedded in the simple QR code. Any subsequent health related issues may be entered into the HB only to have a complete reliable history of the individual. While the financing and implementation mechanism may be worked out with the government machinery, it must also involve the masses in the country. This would require the sensitization and creation of awareness about the PM at the country and the countryside levels; for example, a country like India that has brought awareness of the usefulness of the Aadhar Card can easily achieve this goal. The PM program and policies may vary across the states. As most of the PM programs are resource-intensive and the available funding is limited, its potential needs to be widened to minimize existing health disparities. Low PM awareness in the society and the absence of the financial and political support are the fundamental barriers. There is a clear need to broaden the awareness of the PM especially amongst policymakers. Multi-stakeholder, multi-country strategies need to be prioritized in order to leverage resources and expertise. As the situation stands now, adopting PM remains in its infancy in several countries including SEA ones.

To achieve an effective PM adoption, it is imperative to balance equity issues across diverse populations while improving efficiency in healthcare.

Philosophically speaking, if a fraction of funds used for war is diverted to PM related research, the world would become a much better and safer place. Games of the war have been played since time immemorial but human civilization now can change the course of history by agreeing not to agree on war in any form for any place on earth. **No war on earth** policy would ensure survival of the planet and in turn survival of mankind. However, this requires re-sizing the egos of the world leaders and innate urge to make this world a safer, better and happier place. There are several sub-disciplines that affect our life, health and happiness.

SUB-DISCIPLINES OF PM

- Environment
- Nutrition and Food Habits
- Life Style
- Physical Activities, Religious Faith and Marital Status
- Connectivity with Nature

Body and brain in a person operate based on the genetic constitution and available environment. However, both may be trained and reconditioned. Thus, if a person is aware of how to live a disease-free life, he can do that to a large extent. For sure, life and death cannot ever be controlled but all the bad habits may easily be avoided. If one is living in a toxic or polluted environment, that too can be changed and one can move out to a better environment.

Environment

As mentioned earlier, the above several sub disciplines are related to personalized medicine. For example, a person living in the foothills or mountainous regions is physically more active by default owing to difficult and demanding terrains. He gets much better air, water and food for his/her sustenance. With the results, s/he remains almost free from diseases. Nature ensures a more robust immune system for all such persons as they remain connected with nature and follow the traditional healthy way of life. Compared to such people, their urban counterparts are exposed to a variety of challenges even for their survival on a daily basis. This is because resources for life support systems are limited but demands are unlimited. For a common urban man, a less clean and unhealthy environment to live in and often inadequate sleep coupled with equally unhealthy and often unhygienic food result in a saggy immune system. While this may not be true for all those who are less fortunate face the brunt. There are many other such constraints that a common man faces by default. As the situation stands now, everything cannot be changed. However, awareness of the people would play many positive roles and despite living in an urban setup, a person can avoid all such unhealthy (seemingly unavoidable) activities. Partaking clean and healthy food on time, going to sleep on time, and being aware of the surroundings should be manageable. Thus, all of us should be acutely aware of the environment where we live, and how we live. Perhaps these issues may be made part of the academic curriculum at the school level to enhance awareness amongst the students.

Nutrition and Food Habits

Food is a basic necessity for all living beings. With the passage of time, the nutritional quotient has witnessed a drastic change. However, food and its actual nutritional value often do not match. Then again, food processing and cooking take away some or major parts of the nutrition. Too deep-fried food, too much oil and spices, and too much salt may appeal to the taste bud of a person. However, such food items are not healthy, more so when these are consumed on a regular basis. Many of us would not find much merit in boiled vegetables or soup on a routine basis and would surely reject it. However, such items are healthy, easy to digest, and provide enough nutrition. This does not mean that one should give up oil, spice or salt altogether. That only means one should practice moderation for all such items. Today, the world has become a village, and information technology has progressed so much that any news can reach the world in no time. Despite the availability of a huge influx of useful information on any subject, people remain or perhaps try to remain ignorant. Pampering the taste buds and resorting to some enticing liquid diet (alcoholic drink) may appear to be a tempting proposition. However, all such temptations are bad for the brain, body and soul. Similarly, taking food on time, every time and maintaining a gap between evening supper and bedtime is very crucial. A gap of 4 hours between the food and bedtime is ideal. If that is not possible, at least 2-3 hours gap must be religiously followed. This will ensure good health, good night sleep and the next day, a fresh and very good morning. A great deal of literature is available illustrating which food should be avoided in the night and which one should not be combined with other one. Thus, acquiring an understanding of food and nutrition and following a healthy regimen will go a long way to ensure good health and an equally strong immune system protecting a person from sporadic diseases.

Lifestyle

"Early to bed, early to rise makes a person healthy, wealthy, and wise" is an old adage. However, when it comes to practice, very few people stick to this dictum. This requires discipline, a habit that requires conditioning of the mind, body, and soul. A very strong will perhaps would allow a person to recondition his body and brain but this would not happen to many people. Developing a strong willpower particularly, at a later stage of life is difficult if not impossible. A change in lifestyle requires sacrificing a large number of pleasure-seeking activities instead of accepting the simple and healthy ones. This would include partaking food on time, retiring to bed early, leaving the bed before sunrise; and re-adjusting and recalibrating life's routine activities on a regular basis which may be difficult for everyone. Quitting smoking, avoiding late night work, excluding rude food, shunning the use of alcohol, resorting to simple food, starting the day early morning, moderate exercise, avoiding toxic and negative people's company, keeping the word, becoming a man of honor, working hard, being punctual and polite in dealing, not harming any living soul, not being judgmental, believing in human, humanity and supreme power, resisting violence and backbiting are all part of the lifestyle. Such a large-scale change will require a re-orientation of the body, brain, and belief. In addition, this would also require re-sizing of the ego. Most of the time, the human ego impedes the process of acquiring healthy attributes. However, if one believes in humility, it is possible to achieve it. If one is able to alter the lifestyle by altering a few things, he would be bountifully blessed throughout life and would become an icon of inspiration.

Physical Activities and Religious Faith

A man ceases to play because he grows old and a man ceases to grow old because he plays. This shows that the process of aging is affected by physical activities. Physical activities tend to affect physiological activities. This in turn affects all our body organs ensuring that our metabolism and all the systems operate optimally and are able to maintain cellular homeostasis. Thus, irrespective of age, gender, ethnicity, food habits, lifestyle, region, religion, faith, choice of mating partner, and overall status of health, physical activities will always be useful. This simple logic is accepted by many and thus they enjoy bounties of health. However, a large number of people, although aware of it, do not practice. Once again, creating awareness on this line will help secure the future of many people. Because physical activities will help keep a person healthy, this will reduce the burden on the health care system allowing a person to perform more optimally. Similarly, marital status and education tend to affect life and usually provide awareness, stability and in turn good health. While having faith or no faith in religion is a personal choice, it is usually found that a religious person is more disciplined. Achieving awareness through religion in any direction including health is almost free and highly beneficial. It is said and largely believed that prayer moves the mountain. Whether it does so or not is immaterial but what it does, however, is that the person who regularly prays is more at peace and disciplined. However, this cannot be generalized because our personality and perception are the results of so many variables and each variable tends to fluctuate with time and space. It is equally connected with social setup, upbringing, culture, and tradition.

Connectivity with Nature

When we look around, we find an order and this order is provided by nature. However, owing to our activities, this order is disturbed and suddenly we realize that nature is no longer interested in maintaining equilibrium. We are aware that many areas in the world are submerged in water. Many are covered with snow and equally large parts of the earth are flooded with untimely and unexpected rain. Nature does what it wants to do without making noise. However, nature does provide enough warning to us. Philosophically speaking, nature revolves around the innate energy that is neither created nor destroyed. Only it changes to appear in different forms. The best way to live on the planet Earth is to respect nature and not indulge in committing atrocities on it. Clearing 30% of the Amazon forest is surely not a good idea and does not stand for any justification. The world's 25% oxygen is used to be produced by that part of the forest. One can have many such examples but that should not be part of this book. What needs to be emphasized here is that we should respect nature, remain connected with it, and do not commit atrocities in any form on it or on any living being. Polluting the environment, rivers, a large number of water bodies and contaminating wells are all open atrocities on Nature. When our environment or surroundings are polluted, we cannot remain healthy and that would not guarantee us health and happiness. A large number of countries in the world have strict rules to protect the environment. Such rules are laid down in our countries also. However, they are not enforced as strictly as required. Thus, still, there is a room for environmental improvement and this can be achieved through more awareness, some sacrifice and some precautionary measures. Recycling and reuse of our abfall (trash) is a tried and tested approach to minimize the environmental pollution.

PATIENTS DIVERSITY AND DISEASE HETEROGENEITY

The concept of PM is not a new one as it dates back to ancient times as mentioned earlier. The first evidence of individual targeting medicine appeared in ancient times thousands of years ago. Various therapeutic approaches have been established since then. In the context of PM, ethnicity-specific data across the spectrum of society is needed. The lack of information from the heterogeneous genomes was felt more during COVID-19 pandemic. Such limitations that came to light baffled the researchers, caregivers and doctors world over who witnessed enormous heterogeneity and differential response from amongst the COVID-19 patients. Even after the vaccination of one or two doses, persons not only redeveloped the symptoms but many died. Similarly, the patients who were treated showed different responses to the same medicine. Yet again, some people took much longer to recover whereas others made it rather quickly. Owing to the heterogeneous and uniquely different genomes, similar treatment was not effective for all the Covid-19-affected individuals. Here comes the need to delineate and stratify the population based on ethnicity, and genomic makeup so that treatment may be given while keeping in view the dissimilarity of the genomes. It is clear that the "journey" of personalized medicine that was started long ago is not yet completed though important milestones have been achieved. What needs to be done in view of the long-term perspective is to develop a comprehensive PM platform for research and innovation involving both the doctors and researchers. The highly focused approach along the line would generate vital information encompassing key factors related to the healthcare system. This would also provide a chance to repurpose the already available drug molecules to enhance their wider but personalized use. Simultaneously, large-scale data already available in the database may be analyzed systematically and possible side effects of the drugs may be recorded. If a drug has a side effect in a patient from a given ethnic group, does that mean all the individuals of that ethnicity would show the same side effect? What would be the effect of that drug on other individuals belonging to other ethnicities? Clearly, an answer to this question is possible when the effect of drug molecules across the ethnicity is monitored and faithfully recorded. This way, the drug molecules useful for repurposing may also be segregated in tune with their past prescriptions

DEMOGRAPHY, EPIDEMIOLOGY, ETHNICITY AND GENOME HETEROGENEITY

Demography is the statistical study of human populations that deals with the analysis, examination and measurement of the dimensions and dynamics of populations. It covers whole societies or groups defined by criteria such as education, nationality, religion, and ethnicity. In the present scenario, we do not expect all the individuals to be the same in any respect. Thus, during an outbreak of a disease, different individuals will react in different ways. The Covid-19 pandemic is a recent example. In any demographic setup, there could be several ethnic groups. Each group may still have heterogeneous genomes. Depending upon the size of the population, the choice of the mating partner, faith and religious beliefs, lifestyle, and food habits, the demography remains a dynamic component. This would be reflected showing differences in the resistance or susceptibility to the diseases. For example, black women in the USA tend to show 40% more instances of breast cancer than white ones. The genetic variability operative in almost every population warrants the development of health parameters that can cater to the requirement of precision medicine. Thus, data from all the above-mentioned disciplines would be relevant to develop contours of precision medicine. Similarly, genome heterogeneity is an equally dynamic component. Genomes tend to change in response to a large number of factors including that of the environment as mentioned earlier. Epidemiology deals with the study of the distribution and determinants of health-related states or events in a given population. Epidemiology is useful for uncovering and controlling health-related problems. Thus, the demography, epidemiology, ethnicity, and genome heterogeneity all put together present an ensemble of health-related homeostasis. Clearly, lopsidedness on the part of any component becomes the cause of the imbalance of homeostasis. A deeper understanding of all these aspects would facilitate strengthening the concept of personalized medicine facilitating the human healthcare system.

GLOBAL ADAPTATION OF PM

Driven by a spectrum of genomic breakthroughs, personalized medicine (PM) has now become a central theme across healthcare systems, but this is truer for the United Kingdom (UK), the United States (US), and the European Union (EU). Thus, it has yet to gain global momentum. It is known as an emerging field in which the application of specific biological markers, often genetic, enables diagnosis, and disease is more accurately targeted at the individual patient. By providing "the right treatment to a patient at the right time", a paradigm shift in healthcare from the current "one-size-fits-all" to a more personalized approach can be realized. Despite its high cost, many countries have started to adopt this novel PM concept including Southeast Asia (SEA) as mentioned earlier. At the same time, these healthcare systems are striving towards universal health coverage (UHC) to ensure everyone has access to needed health services without undue financial hardship. The financial constraint remains as one of the main challenges in attaining and maintaining UHC. Adopting an expensive PM would place increasing strain on the already constrained health budget. Incidentally, the PM program does not provide an immediate return nor does it provide a quick cure to the patients. However, this should not be an impediment to undertaking the PM-related research. The initial efforts and expense on PM would yield a rich dividend in due course of time because a very new type of data is envisaged to emerge that in turn would percolate down through the ladder to the patient care level.

CURRENT HEALTH CARE SYSTEM AND ITS MANAGEMENT

In a majority of clinical setups, doctors themselves do not always indulge in research and innovation and they use the available information in their area of specialization. Although this cannot be generalized at the global level, this is largely true for Indian sub-continents. The prevalent human health care system is often erratic and not perfect. This requires extensive critical auditing across the country. The mushrooming of a large number of medical colleges in the country makes auditing even more challenging. However, in principle, the healthcare system requires research and innovation to move on to newer areas of medicine and better treatment. Better treatment is possible only when we have a better diagnostic platform.

On the research and innovation fronts, several sub-disciplines of PM need to be pursued. For example, in a heterogeneous demography, how the level of resistance or susceptibility to a disease is different compared to a homogenous demography? Similarly, how two different populations living in two very different environments will respond to a pandemic or infectious disease? The overall lifestyle, food habits, hygienic conditions, social structure, and many more such attributes are all envisaged to show variation amongst the set of populations for a disease. The challenge then is to delineate levels of such variation whether it has a genetic basis, caused due to lifestyle, food habits, or overall living conditions (OLC). This calls for research on a well-defined ethnic population that experiences frequently occurring diseases. Since several variables are to be addressed and linked with an occurrence of the disease, this requires a team of doctors and researchers. More than that, government blessings would be equally or more important for financial support. Not withstanding these challenges, a large number of young students can use this platform to acquire skills related to PM. Similarly, doctors will get an opportunity to learn more about the root cause and genetic basis of disease and the role played by one or more such factors of OLC. Thus, the creation of the PM platform would be a win-win situation both for doctors and researchers. During Covid-19, the epidemiological need was felt for the development of strategy for cure and tracking of infection. Large-scale data emerging from the sub disciplines of PM would enable us to assess the outcome of the prescribed drugs on a defined population. The ultimate aim is to develop a clear picture of a population structure encompassing OLC so that doctors may offer better diagnosis, prognosis, with less or no side effects and less expensive treatment to the patients. On the line of Janam patri and now genome patri, right from the time of birth, a health booklet may be made available to each citizen. This would continue to record all the health related variables including the serious ones. As mentioned earlier, with a QR code embedded on the health booklet, a doctor can access all the information. It would then be possible for the doctor to exercise his clinical prerogative in accordance with the best possible treatment. This proposal seems to be a huge one and also the most demanding. However, this is not impossible because at the time of birth, only once this arrangement is required to be made. Thus, a health booklet for a healthy life should be the slogan immediately after the confirmation of the pregnancy.

EVIDENCE BASED MEDICINE

In the early 1950s, scientists realized the need for "evidence-based medicine." The prediction of drug response to ensure the safety of the patient and a better outcome gave birth to the field of today's "personalized medicine." Discoveries in the field of molecular biology contributed to a better understanding of drug response [4]. Further, human genome mapping proved to be a breakthrough providing a better understanding of people's genetic make-up. Although individuals are 99.1% identical, the remaining 0.9% of inter individual genetic variability is responsible for the observed variation within the humans.

The purpose of PM is to combine modern medicine with molecular advances in order to target patients individually and improve the effectiveness of the therapeutic approaches [5]. The conventional approach of using candidate genes alone is not sufficient to explain the differences in disease risks between different ethnic groups and also within individuals. This realization led to the whole genome approach. The evolution of different genotyping technologies over the years has allowed focusing on specific regions of the genome enabling deeper coverage and understanding of the variants. Therefore, it enabled medical practitioners to identify and treat patients based on their unique genetic characteristics.

Today, the four humors of Hippocrates, blood, phlegm, yellow bile, and black bile, which determined the treatment of each individual, have been complemented with the four building blocks (A, T, G, and C) of the DNA enabling improved medical predictions. Cutting-edge biochemical advances including single nucleotide polymorphisms (SNPs), genotyping, and biochips have made personalized medicine a reality. Variations such as SNPs, insertions and deletions, and copy number variations of genes in the human genome play a distinctive role in the manifestation and progression of diseases such as cancer, diabetes, neurodegenerative and cardiovascular diseases [6]. Hence, much emphasis is given on the development of biomarkers as a way of predicting certain diseases and also identifying patient subgroups that respond only to specific drugs.

However, environmental factors can also act as triggers and/or cofactors as mentioned earlier. Therefore, predicting response to drugs and treatment based only on genetic information without taking into account the environmental determinants can lead to poor or false results [6]. Combining the human genome, environmental factors, disease assessments, and medication in order to achieve a better therapeutic outcome is the exact vision that personalized medicine is aiming to achieve. It is obvious that the journey of personalized medicine is still continuing. Several problems are still around the patient's needs, which require to be circumvented. We may focus on the major discoveries from the past to the present, point out milestones that helped personalized medicine, underline the current problems that physicians still face, and give insights into the future, augmenting the healthcare systems globally.

UNDERPINNINGS OF TARGETED THERAPY

The concept of personalized medicine will remain insipid unless we focus on the history of pharmacotherapy. This will help us achieve targeted medicine for individuals' needs. For example, the incident of malaria was first recorded in 2700 BC listed in an ancient Chinese medical record. Despite concerted efforts made by researchers to control this menace, malaria is still a serious and fatal disease. As the situation stands now, malaria will continue to appear one way or the other because we cannot rid of the mosquitoes. Malaria affected 228 million people resulting in 405,000 deaths globally in 2018. This is more common in Africa and some Asian countries. We know the diagnosis, prevention, and treatment of this disease. However, the medical assistant may not reach people who live in far-flung areas or the government may not have a sufficient budget to deal with this requirement. Thus, in the context of personalized medicine, some tried and tested precautions would prove to be a lot more beneficial. These include not allowing stagnant water around, If a pond nearby is infested with mosquito larvae, Gambusia fish may be used. While this fish may not be an attractive food for human consumption, in the same pond, the culture of Gambusia along with edible fish may be maintained if the water bodies are available. This strategy will allow dual benefits; fish production and control of mosquito proliferation. Prevalence of malaria is higher in the tropical climate because the global mortality rate ranges from 0.3 to 2.2% whereas for tropical environments, the same is 11–30%.

Besides this biological control, herbs have been used to treat malaria. This includes Qinghai in the second century BC in China and the Cinchona tree in the 16th century in Peru [7]. In 1926, one of the most effective drugs, pamaquine, an 8-aminoquinoline was used to treat acute malaria. Despite the effectiveness of this antimalarial drug, its administration raised concerns about its safety [8]. During 1930 and 1940, about 250 cases of acute hemolytic anemia were reported after providing this drug to patients [9]. In view of the side effects, this was not found to be suitable for the control of malaria. In 1943, scientists started investigating alternative therapeutic regimens to encounter the adverse effects of pamaquine. The search led to the identification of primaquine, which also belongs to 8-aminoquinolines [8]. The Primaquine, an 8-(4-amino-1-methyl-butylamino) 6-methoxyquinoline was first used during the Korean War as an antimalarial drug to eliminate the long latency of *P. vivax* infection [10]. Not withstanding its effectiveness, primaquine was still found to cause hemolytic anemia [8]. In 1956, Carson *et al.* discovered that the cause of hemolytic anemia was due to a deficiency in the G6PD enzyme [8]. The G6PD enzyme gene is an X chromosome linked. In human females, where of the two X chromosomes, one is inactivated. Thus, only one copy of the gene of G6PD remains active. Since the human male has only one X chromosome and the other one is Y. G6PD is adequately dosage compensated in both genders. However, if the gene for G6PD is mutated in males, the level of this enzyme will be affected. Interestingly it may seem, that the phenomenon of gene dosage compensation was reported by Murray Barr and Ewert Bertram in 1949 [11]. However, the G6PD deficiency was established during 510 BC [12] when Pythagoras, even though he was not a physician [13], had observed Malaria. The advances in molecular diagnostics revealed that there are a lot of mutations in the gene but people remained asymptomatic and only in a few cases, such as after the administration of primaquine triggered severe side effects [13]. Taken together, it would be useful to uncover all the mutations in G6PD genes among individuals who show reduced levels of G6PD enzyme. This is an example of how basic research can enrich the repertoire of the PM. According to WHO, primaquine is now used to cure liver infection caused by malaria (*P. vivax* and *P. ovale*) and prevent relapse. To eliminate hemolytic anemia and to achieve a better therapeutic outcome, the World Health Organization WHO has provided guidelines for primaquine administration to reduce the risk in people with G6PD deficiency. For example, for the prevention of malaria in normal adults, the therapeutic approach is to administer 0.25–0.50mg/kg body weight daily for a duration of 14 days. However, for people with G6PD deficiency, the dosage to be used is 0.75 mg/kg body weight once a week for 8 weeks with close monitoring of the patients [14].

Thus, the association between antimalarial drugs and G6PD deficiency opened a new perspective toward personalized medicine. The incidence of reported cases of malaria is still large (228 million globally in 2018) while diseases such as Ebola and Cholera, which are of a similar magnitude, are being managed properly resulting in a decrease in the infected population. This could be because 90% of the population infected by malaria originated in Africa. For example, the Ebola virus appeared in 1976 in central Africa but the outbreak in 2014–2016 was the one that alerted the scientific community as the virus managed to spread quickly from West Africa to urban areas and across borders transforming it into an epidemic. Another aspect could be the inadequacy of resources in developing countries. Lack of food and medical supplies hinders the treatment, proving that the environment is also a co-factor in disease progression and subsequent management or cure. So physicians should consider every continent and every patient individually according to their origin and take into account their environment to achieve improved therapy.

THE PHARMACOGENETIC EVOLUTION

The biochemical health sciences started evolving during the 1940s and 1950s together with the development of instrumentation and new research methods. The scientific field is responsible for the research of different patients' responses to the drugs and the minimization of the adverse effects caused also by variability on the metabolizing enzymes is known as 3 Years of Ebola Virus Disease Outbreaks. Thus, here again, personalized medicine comes into the picture reminding us that doctors have to play much larger roles in the treatment of patients.

The research process was fueled by the availability of some key equipment useful for pharmacogenetics. With the mass spectrometers, cytochrome P450 (CYP450) was identified in 1958 and later in 1965, this P450 (CYP450) turned out to be a novel drug metabolizing enzyme [15]. This is yet another example showing the gap between physicians and the knowledge regarding pharmacogenetics that can be put to use to achieve personalized medicine [16]. The enzyme that belongs to the CYP450 family is responsible for the metabolism of 20% of the drugs encompassing antiarrhythmic, antidepressants, antipsychotics, beta-blockers, and analgesics [17]. The discovery of CYP2D6 in 1969 itself was dramatic because different concentrations of nortriptyline were observed in the plasma of the patients, indicating differences in their metabolism [18].

In 1977, an adrenergic-blocking drug debrisoquine was used to treat hypertension [19]. This drug showed variations in response to treatment [20]. Today, debrisoquine is mostly used as a marker to determine the activity of the CYP2D6 enzyme in patients. More specifically, debrisoquine and its 4-OH-metabolite are measured in urine with gas chromatography and high-performance liquid chromatography (HPLC) methods in order to find the individual's CYP2D6 genotype [21]. Thus, CYP2D6 genotype analysis can be exploited for predicting the phenotype of each patient. This, in turn, will uncover the response to specific drugs metabolized by the CYP2D6 enzyme [22]. It is now known that multiple variants of CYP2D6 exist. The administration of several drugs to patients depending on the association with specific SNPs and DNA is possible. However, it may be noted that depending solely on SNP may not serve the purpose unless a clear-cut association between SNP and drug metabolism is established beyond doubt across the wide spectrum of patients. If this challenge is met, it will bring us a step forward to personalized medicine.

Another important advancement regarding the application of personalized medicine in cancer therapy is the discovery of the HER-2 gene. Breast cancer can be divided into different subtypes depending on the tumor and the patient's predisposition and genetic background [23]. More specifically, the HER-2 gene

(Human Epidermal Growth Factor Receptor 2) encodes a tyrosine kinase receptor that takes part in signaling pathways both in normal and in malignant breast cells and is strongly associated with a lower response to cancer treatment and survival rate [24]. The HER-2 gene became clinically relevant in 1987 when Salmon *et al.* [24] reported a lower survival rate in women with breast cancer carrying the mutated gene. It was discovered that in the majority of patients carrying the mutation, the overexpression of this gene was associated with chemotherapy resistance, poor patient prognosis [25], high risk of cancer progression, and a low survival rate [26]. Patients that are carrying the HER-2 gene amplified have a distinctive molecular signature that can distinguish these types of cancers from other breast cancers [23]. A lot of studies were conducted in order to reverse these adverse effects of the HER-2 gene overexpression and eventually achieved with the use of monoclonal antibodies targeting the tyrosine kinase receptor [24]. A great example is the antibody trastuzumab which inhibits tumor growth when used as monotherapy. However, in combination with cisplatin, carboplatin, docetaxel, and ionizing radiation, this shows synergistic effects. Similarly, it shows additive effects when used with doxorubicin, cyclophosphamide, methotrexate, and paclitaxel [24]. Several clinical trials have proved the efficacy of trastuzumab resulting in establishing routine HER-2 testing in breast cancer patients and changing dramatically the therapeutic approach to those carrying the mutation [23]. This gene is a great milestone of applied personalized medicine, clearly showing that the right choice of a drug, based on the genetic background of a patient, can have positive effects on life. It is therefore important to identify the most innovative diagnostic methods that can be used to predict if individuals are at a high risk for a given disease, thus enabling early prognosis and application of preventive therapies. After the Genome Wide Association Studies (GWAS), thousands of genetic variants were linked to several complex diseases overcoming the statistical limitations. GWAS enabled disease prediction combining multiple genetic factors with the use of polygenic risk scores. Although polygenic risk score is a promising new tool, its application has not reached clinical accuracy yet. However, several discoveries have indicated its potential utility in disease prediction, such as cancer, Alzheimer's disease, Parkinson's disease (PD), and cardiovascular disease (CVD). This observation suggests the impact of personalized medicine on the healthcare system. Thus, if we understand the cause of the problem, we can solve it. Finding the cause will require innovative research and development on an adequate number of samples from the patients fulfilling medical and ethical requirements.

FUTURE PROSPECTS OF PM

Let us have a quick look at the future prospects of the PM in light of the ever-growing scientific advancement. Since the dawn of civilization, the practice of medicine has largely been reactive. Even today, we usually wait until the onset of the disease and then try to treat and cure it. Often, we do not fully understand the genetic and environmental factors that cause major diseases such as cancer, Alzheimer's and diabetes, autism, Parkinson's, split personality and depression, infertility and high blood pressure. These are a few examples but cancer alone has more than 200 different types and each one has its own unique etiology, genesis, and genetics as mentioned earlier. Cancer is caused by a variety of reasons involving a number of mechanisms despite the fact the body tries to cope up with the onslaughts of circumstances. Clearly, our efforts to treat these diseases are often imprecise, unpredictable, ineffective, and not always economical. Further, the patient would suffer even more if the medicine has side effects. We all have unique genomes that are amply supported by the fact that some drugs have side effects on one person but not on all persons. Similarly, a drug may be useful for one person but not for the other ones. In the case of a dreaded disease, we can well imagine the emotional trauma that patients and family members both experience.

The drugs and treatments we devise are tested on broad-based populations and prescribed using statistical averages. Consequently, they work for some patients but not for many others owing to genetic and several non-genetic differences in the population. Startling may it seem, the prescription drug available now in the market works only for half of those who take it, which means, factors responsible for the disease are hampering the drug activity. Knowing these factors and refining our diagnostic approaches would go a long way to ensuring health for all. Health for all is not the responsibility of the government only; this is also an individual and social responsibility. Awareness about the health and health care systems, specialized doctors, accurate diagnostics backed by genome, proteome, and metabolome analyses, and help in the form of a second opinion are some of the options that would make the patient's care less painful. In addition, the medicine should be as economical as possible. Many drug companies may not subscribe to this view because they make a huge investment in developing a drug molecule. While this may be true, what is equally true is that in a large number of instances, less expensive, homeopathic or herbal medicaments are very powerful and may be prescribed thus regulating/avoiding the exorbitant price without health compromise. This calls for gearing up the healthcare personnel to be aware of such alternative medicines. In this context, Ayush, Unani, Homeopathy, and Siddha systems need in-depth exploration, repurposing, and exploitation focusing on research and innovation. When diagnosis is largely based on the blood, tissue, or metabolic profiles and other factors are overlooked, that may be less accurate. The majority of the doctors who deal with a large number of patients may not uncover the root cause of the problems. Often they are overworked and undervalued which is true for most of the cosmopolitan cities. Thus, they treat the symptoms and not the disease. Today, drugs are available for every known symptom. However, what remains obscure behind the symptoms (root cause) must be uncovered which is where additional research and innovation is required. It is this aspect that will bridge the gap between conventional medicine and personalized/precision medicine.

CONCLUDING REMARKS

In principle, personalized medicine is based on each patient's unique genetic makeup including factors that have been mentioned earlier. The genetic makeup itself is affected and modulated by these factors. If we are able to broaden the conventional approaches, that would fulfill the aspiration of personalized medicine. As the situation stands now, healthcare providers may start focusing on several aspects mentioned earlier though not necessarily in the same order if the concept of PM is to be materialized.

ACKNOWLEDGMENT

The authors are grateful to the Era University administration for providing infrastructural support and facilities.

We also acknowledge our colleagues for their critical comments and inputs on the draft. Very special thanks to Abbas Ali Mahdi and Farzana Mahdi for their encouragement, academic indulgence, and valuable support.

REFERENCES

[1] Jouanna J. Greek medicine from hippocrates to galen. Jacques: Bril 2012. [http://dx.doi.org/10.1163/9789004232549]

[2] Fierz W. Challenge of personalized health care: To what extent is medicine already individualized and what are the future trends? Med Sci Monit 2004; 10(5): RA111-23. [PMID: 15114285]

[3] Sykiotis GP, Kalliolias GD, Papavassiliou AG. Pharmacogenetic principles in the hippocratic writings. J Clin Pharmacol 2005; 45(11): 1218-20. [http://dx.doi.org/10.1177/0091270005281091] [PMID: 16239353]

[4] Vogenberg FR, Isaacson Barash C, Pursel M. Personalized medicine: Part 1: Evolution and development into theranostics. P&T 2010; 35(10): 560-76. [https://doi.org/10.3389/fgene.2020.569175] [PMID: 33424917]

[5] Mini E, Nobili S. Pharmacogenetics: Implementing personalized medicine. Clin Cases Miner Bone Metab 2009; 6(1): 17-24. [PMID: 22461093]

[6] Agyeman A, Ofori-Asenso R. Perspective: Does personalized medicine hold the future for medicine? J Pharm Bioallied Sci 2015; 7(3): 239-44. [http://dx.doi.org/10.4103/0975-7406.160040] [PMID: 26229361]

[7] Talapko J, Škrlec I, Alebić T, Jukić M, Včev A. Malaria: The past and the present. Microorganisms

2019; 7(6): 179.
[http://dx.doi.org/10.3390/microorganisms7060179] [PMID: 31234443]

[8] Howes OD, Williams M, Ibrahim K, *et al.* Midbrain dopamine function in schizophrenia and depression: A post-mortem and positron emission tomographic imaging study. Brain 2013; 136(11): 3242-51.
[http://dx.doi.org/10.1093/brain/awt264] [PMID: 24097339]

[9] Beutler E. The hemolytic effect of primaquine and related compounds: A review. Blood 1959; 14(2): 103-39.
[http://dx.doi.org/10.1182/blood.V14.2.103.103] [PMID: 13618370]

[10] Ashley EA, Dhorda M, Fairhurst RM, *et al.* Spread of artemisinin resistance in Plasmodium falciparum malaria. N Engl J Med 2014; 371(5): 411-23.
[http://dx.doi.org/10.1056/NEJMoa1314981] [PMID: 25075834]

[11] Barr ML, Bertram EG. A morphological distinction between neurones of the male and female, and the behaviour of the nucleolar satellite during accelerated nucleoprotein synthesis. Nature 1949; 163(4148): 676-7.
[http://dx.doi.org/10.1038/163676a0] [PMID: 18120749]

[12] Relling MV, Evans WE. Pharmacogenomics in the clinic. Nature 2015; 526(7573): 343-50.
[http://dx.doi.org/10.1038/nature15817] [PMID: 26469045]

[13] Luzzatto L, Arese P. Favismand glucose-6-phosphate dehydrogenase deficiency. N Engl J Med 2018; 378(1): 60-71.
[http://dx.doi.org/10.1056/NEJMra1708111] [PMID: 29298156]

[14] Policy brief. Testing for G6PD deficiency for safe use of primaquine in radical cure of *P. Vivax* and *P. ovale*.2016. https://www.who. int/malaria/publications/atoz/g6pd-testing-pq-radical-cure-vivax/en/

[15] Estabrook RW. A passion for P450s (remembrances of the early history of research on cytochrome P450). Drug Metab Dispos 2003; 31(12): 1461-73.
[http://dx.doi.org/10.1124/dmd.31.12.1461] [PMID: 14625342]

[16] Rogers JF, Nafziger AN, Bertino JS Jr. Pharmacogenetics affects dosing, efficacy, and toxicity of cytochrome P450–metabolized drugs. Am J Med 2002; 113(9): 746-50.
[http://dx.doi.org/10.1016/S0002-9343(02)01363-3] [PMID: 12517365]

[17] Yang S, Paik K, McGrath GS, *et al.* Functional topology of evolving urban drainage networks. Water Resour Res 2017; 53(11): 8966-79.
[http://dx.doi.org/10.1002/2017WR021555]

[18] Mahgoub A, Dring LG, Idle JR, Lancaster R, Smith RL. Polymorphic hydroxylation of Debrisoquine in man. Lancet 1977; 310(8038): 584-6.
[http://dx.doi.org/10.1016/S0140-6736(77)91430-1] [PMID: 71400]

[19] Silas JH, Lennard MS, Tucker GT, Smith AJ, Malcolm SL, Marten TR. Why hypertensive patients vary in their response to oral debrisoquine. BMJ 1977; 1(6058): 422-5.
[http://dx.doi.org/10.1136/bmj.1.6058.422] [PMID: 837136]

[20] LLerena A, Dorado P, Peñas-Lledó EM. Pharmacogenetics of debrisoquine and its use as a marker for CYP2D6 hydroxylation capacity. Pharmacogenomics 2009; 10(1): 17-28.
[http://dx.doi.org/10.2217/14622416.10.1.17] [PMID: 19102711]

[21] Siest G, Jeannesson E, Visvikis-Siest S. Enzymes and pharmacogenetics of cardiovascular drugs. Clin Chim Acta 2007; 381(1): 26-31.
[http://dx.doi.org/10.1016/j.cca.2007.02.014] [PMID: 17362901]

[22] Burstein HJ. The distinctive nature of HER2-positive breast cancers. N Engl J Med 2005; 353(16): 1652-4.
[http://dx.doi.org/10.1056/NEJMp058197] [PMID: 16236735]

[23] Slamon D, Eiermann W, Robert N, *et al.* Adjuvant trastuzumab in HER2-positive breast cancer. N Engl J Med 2011; 365(14): 1273-83.
[http://dx.doi.org/10.1056/NEJMoa0910383] [PMID: 21991949]

[24] Harari D, Yarden Y. Molecular mechanisms underlying ErbB2/HER2 action in breast cancer. Oncogene 2000; 19(53): 6102-14.
[http://dx.doi.org/10.1038/sj.onc.1203973] [PMID: 11156523]

[25] Gajria D, Chandarlapaty S. HER2-amplified breast cancer: Mechanisms of trastuzumab resistance and novel targeted therapies. Expert Rev Anticancer Ther 2011; 11(2): 263-75.
[http://dx.doi.org/10.1586/era.10.226] [PMID: 21342044]

[26] Chasioti D, Yan J, Nho K, Saykin AJ. Progress in polygenic composite scores in alzheimer's and other complex diseases. Trends Genet 2019; 35(5): 371-82.
[http://dx.doi.org/10.1016/j.tig.2019.02.005] [PMID: 30922659]

CHAPTER 2

An Integrative Approach to Bioinformatics and Epigenetics Toward Personalized Medicine

Anam Farooqui[1], **Najma**[1] and **Sher Ali**[2,*]

[1] *Centre for Interdisciplinary Research in Basic Sciences, Jamia Millia Islamia, New Delhi-110025, India*

[2] *VC Office, Era University, Lucknow-226003, India*

Abstract: Studies on epigenetics have shown cell control, gene function, and putative change or modification in the DNA's sequence. Genes are prone to changes that are brought about by a number of mechanisms encompassing gene conversion, exon/intron reshuffling, alteration in the mutational landscape, and copy number variation of the genes. In addition, repeat DNA sequences tend to expand or shrink changing the topology of adjacent genes resulting in a change in their functions. Alterations in gene activity, especially those that are brought on by epigenetic errors, frequently cause genetic diseases. Researchers are particularly interested in how epigenetic modifications and mistakes affect gene function, protein synthesis, and human health. Precise mapping and evaluation of epigenetic biomarkers will enhance treatment approaches by enabling more accurate and early diagnosis prior to a change in the genetical landscape. This chapter covers the topics of genomics, bioinformatics and epigenetic clocks that pave the way to personalized medicine. It is envisaged that a deeper understanding of the epigenetic modification of the genome or its aberration would augment our understanding of the function of the normal and diseased human genomes.

Keywords: Disease diagnosis, Epigenetic modification, Epigenetic clocks and protein misfolding, Gene expression, Precision medicine.

INTRODUCTION

The fields of medicine and healthcare are rapidly expanding, ushering in a continuous stream of advanced treatments aimed at enhancing patients' well-being. Nevertheless, alongside these advancements, we are confronted with the challenges of side effects and limited treatment effectiveness. This has prompted a critical re-evaluation of the traditional "one-size-fits-all" approach to healthcare.

* **Corresponding author Sher Ali:** VC Office, Era University, Lucknow-226003, India;
E-mail: profsali55@gmail.com

In response, healthcare management is undergoing a transformation towards a more personalized approach. This shift is driven by the realization that previous methods, such as genomics, proteomics, and transcriptomics, while impressive, have not provided a complete understanding of why some individuals exhibit altered characteristics. To truly revolutionize healthcare management and personalized medicine, there is an urgent need for a comprehensive, systematic approach that integrates various disciplines. This integration cannot be achieved without proactive collaboration between bioinformatics, epigenetics, and genomics.

Recent developments in epigenomics and the emerging field of omics offer promising paths for enhancing clinical care. These fields enable us to directly connect biomarkers to observable traits or characteristics, potentially leading to more effective and personalized treatments. Several variables are now driving epigenomic medicine research. The first is the field's overall high level of interest. Second, reference epigenomes are continuously being characterized to advance and amplify research efforts. The third is the accessibility of effective tools for characterizing epigenomes, such as next-generation sequencing (NGS).

Bioinformatics and computational biology have provided effective methods for understanding epigenetic mechanisms and analysing epigenomic data. These are becoming increasingly crucial in unraveling the mysteries of gene regulation both in normal and diseased conditions. Bioinformatics tools and techniques aid in the field of epigenetics in a variety of ways. The most important one is to understand the biology of diseases caused by the epigenome enabling optimization of therapies. The large-scale analysis of epigenetic datasets has affected almost all the fields of the human health care system including cancer and various heritable alterations.

In this chapter, we aim to shed light on the significance of epigenetic data and its possible use in personalized medicine. Specifically, we delve into topics such as epigenetic alterations of the human genome, epigenetic biomarkers, personalized medicine, and the pivotal role of bioinformatics in advancing the field of personalized medicine. This chapter is envisaged to enhance our better understanding of bioinformatics and epigenetics towards personalized medicine leading to improved diagnosis, prognosis, and therapeutics of a diseased phenotype.

EPIGENETIC ALTERATIONS OF THE HUMAN GENOME

Our genes play a significant role in our health, but the gene expression itself is modulated by our behaviour, like what we eat and the level of exercise that we do, and the environment to which we are exposed [1]. The field of epigenetics deals with how cells regulate gene activity without altering the DNA sequence. In Greek, "epi-"means "on or above," and "epigenetic" refers to factors other than the genetic code [2]. It is, thus, the study of how environmental factors and behaviour can alter the functions of the gene (Fig. **1**). While epigenetic changes are reversible and do not alter our DNA sequence as genetic changes do, they can alter how our body interprets a DNA sequence [3]. Because epigenetic modifications regulate whether genes are switched on or off, they have an impact on protein production in cells. This regulation ensures that each cell generates only the proteins required for its activity. Proteins that promote bone formation, for example, are not generated in muscle cells. Patterns of epigenetic change vary amongst persons, the tissues within an individual, and even between the cells within a tissue [4]. Environmental factors such as a person's nutrition and exposure to contaminants can affect the epigenome.

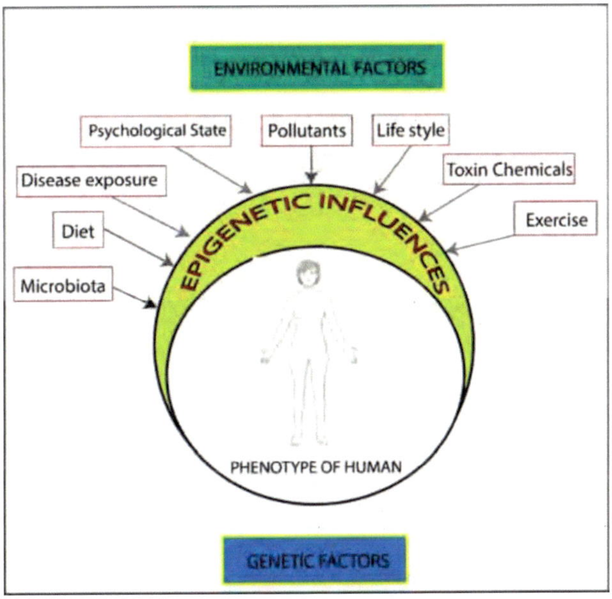

Fig. (1). The phenotype of humans is influenced by environmental factors and genetic factors.

Epigenetic alterations can be passed down *via* families or acquired in response to the environment. Decisions about one's way of life enhance exposure to factors (such as pollution and cigarette smoke) that alter our epigenome [5]. Monozygotic or 'identical' twin studies have revealed insightful information into the genetics and environmental factors that control epigenetic pathways, indicating that our genes cannot be solely responsible for regulating the development of complex phenotypic traits. Similar to this, biochemical signals from the womb during fetal development or hormones released after puberty cause epigenetic alterations that alter the control of certain genes, affecting many important developmental processes [6].

DNA methylation is a common form of epigenetic alteration. DNA methylation is the process by which small chemical groups termed methyl groups (containing one carbon atom and three hydrogen atoms- CH_3) are attached to DNA-building units (Fig. **2**). When methyl groups are found on a gene, it is switched off or silenced, and no protein is produced [7]. Despite inheriting the same genetic material and growing up in the same environment, identical twins frequently show differences in the occurrence of diseases including diabetes, autism, and some types of cancer [6]. Monozygotic twins' DNA methylation patterns change from one another more frequently as they age and in adult twins with different medical backgrounds, suggesting that lifestyle decisions and environmental factors have a significant impact on the epigenome [8].

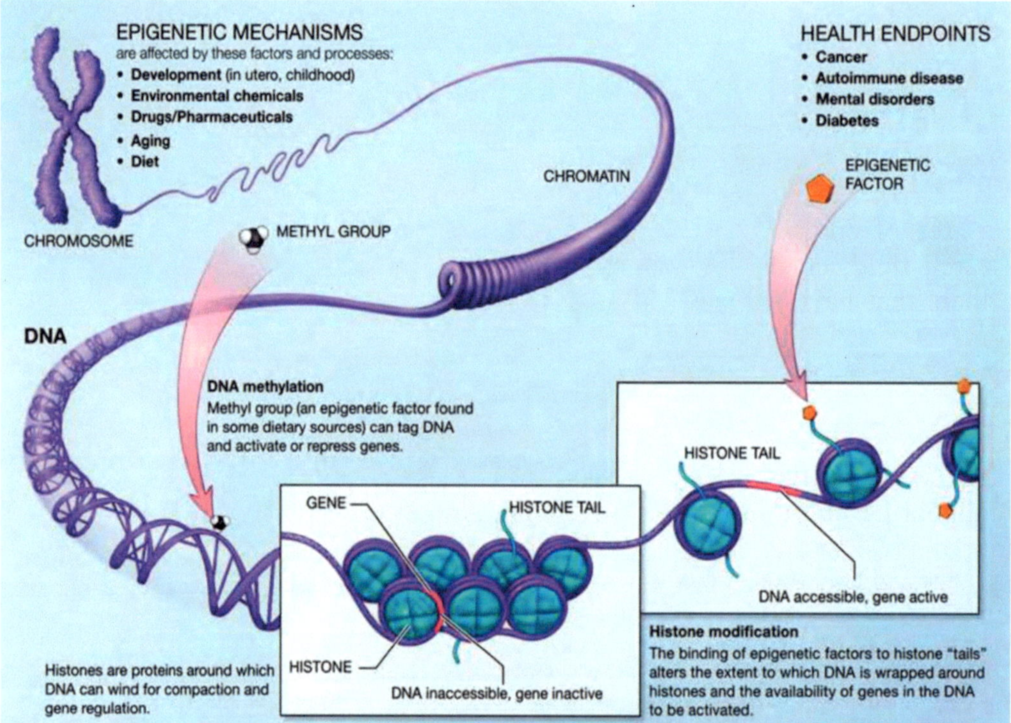

Fig. (2). Epigenetic mechanisms. Adapted from the national institutes of health.

Histone modification is another prevalent epigenetic alteration (Fig. **2**). Histones are the structural proteins found in the nucleus of cells. The shape of chromosomes is determined by DNA wrapping around the histones. Histones can be altered by adding or removing chemical groups such as methyl or acetyl groups (each consisting of two carbon, three hydrogen, and one oxygen atom). The chemical groups determine how firmly the DNA is coiled on histones which influences the extent to which a gene can be switched on or off [9].

Another type of epigenetic alteration is Non-coding RNAs (ncRNAs), that have lately been recognized as participants in chromatin remodelling, especially implicated in the heterochromatin formation and transcriptional or post-transcriptional gene silencing [10].

Abnormal gene expression or inactivation may result from errors in the epigenetic process, such as the alteration of the incorrect gene or the failure to add a chemical group to a specific gene or histone. Genetic disorders are frequently brought on by altered gene activity, including that brought on by epigenetic mistakes. Epigenetic defects have been linked to diseases like cancer, metabolic issues, and degenerative conditions. The association between the genome and chemical molecules that alter it is still being researched by scientists. They are particularly interested in how gene activity, protein synthesis, and human health are affected by epigenetic alterations and errors [11].

PROSPECT OF EPIGENETIC BIOMARKERS

The area of epigenetics has evolved into a thriving and interesting scientific research field, encouraging collaborations between commercial and academic partners that have resulted in the identification of numerous major epigenetic biomarkers for a wide spectrum of serious and life-threatening diseases [12]. Precise mapping and assessment of epigenetic biomarkers will improve therapeutic interventions by allowing diagnosis during the early phases of disorder progression, far before genetic changes have occurred. In glioblastoma, epigenetic modifications linked with tumorigenesis can be discovered in neighbouring non-tumor cells, despite the fact that they appear to be genetically 'normal' [13]. In an *in vitro* lung cancer model, researchers also discovered that epigenetic changes occur before typical genetic abnormalities [14]. Epigenetic-based diagnostics that may identify early disease signs offer an opportunity for clinical intervention before symptom progression affects the quality of life, and patients are still reasonably healthy and may be treated successfully. These highly targeted biomarkers can aid in the individualization of disease management by enabling more accurate monitoring of treatment response and medication alterations to improve treatment outcomes, lessen the potentially harmful side effects of some medications, and promote the efficient use of healthcare resources [5].

EPIGENETICS AND PERSONALIZED MEDICINE

Many issues pertaining to a person's health and disease can be addressed by studying the genome and the data it contains. Because the Human Genome Project (HGP) is now complete, whole-genome DNA sequence information is now available. This marked the beginning of an exciting new era in genetic medicine. It is already obvious that genes alone cannot fully explain key elements of human development and aging or forecast our susceptibility to the majority of complicated diseases [15]. Specific pharmaceuticals must be utilized for individuals who are not responding to regular treatments as expected and have a very low rate of disease management success [16]. Epigenetic alterations are frequently linked to a wide variety of diseases, including bone and skin diseases associated with autoimmune disorders, neurodegenerative diseases such as schizophrenia and cancer. As was already mentioned, one of the most significant alterations causing disease is DNA methylation. DNA methylation regulates a wide range of biological activities, including gene expression, X-chromosome inactivation, imprinting, chromatin architecture, and others [17]. A methyl group (-CH3) is typically added to cytosine in gene promoter regions with CpG islands, which are sequences of large repeating CpG dinucleotides that occupy 60% of the promoter region. Cancer and other diseases have been linked to CpG dinucleotide methylation [18]. Several conditions have been linked to ubiquitination too, including Parkinson's disease, Angelman syndrome, and mental retardation. Therefore, it is believed that epigenetic changes have a significant impact on both healthy and diseased organisms [17].

Epigenetics and epigenetic factors are rapidly gaining prominence as leading components in the key pathways that initiate and advance a wide range of life-threatening and severe hereditary ailments [5]. Technologies that take advantage of our growing understanding of epigenetic mechanisms have the potential to transform approaches to healthcare and medicine around the world. It will be necessary to conduct both genetic and epigenetic diagnostic tests to fully realize the promise of personalized medicine [19]. Patients with diseases that have epigenetic origins may not respond well to conventional therapy. For these patients, researchers are more likely to uncover patient-specific treatments known as personalized or genomic medicines [17]. Adding more detail to this, healthcare professionals use the results of prognostic and diagnostic tests that use genomic data or DNA to diagnose disorders or diseases to assess a patient's risk of disease, determine the right dosage for a patient based on variations in metabolism, and decide whether the patient will benefit from a particular drug intervention for the management of a disease [20]. Contrarily, personalized medicine uses a patient's unique genetic profile to forecast disease, prevent disease through medicinal interventions, and make lifestyle and disease management decisions based on the requirements of each particular patient [21]. Furthermore, genetic screening is critical for personalizing treatment for a patient. Patients are given genomic or personalized medicines after collecting genomic information and associated data such as levels of RNA, proteins, and other metabolites, which are critical factors in medical decision-making for personalized medicine [20, 21]. For accurate disease management and prediction, genomic methods like the discovery of DNA sequence variants, transcriptomics, proteomics, and metabolomics are helpful. These strategies provide practical methods for bridging epigenetics with personalized medicine. Genomic applications can be employed at several key checkpoints to personalize a patient's medical care as they progress from a healthy to a diseased state [17, 15].

Pharmacogenomics examines a range of biological aspects of drug metabolism, such as drug transporters, the role of receptors, and drug-metabolizing enzymes with polymorphisms that influence the drug response in several diseases. All of these aspects are regulated by epigenetic mechanisms [16]. The idea of a precise medicine for a specific patient at a precise concentration and time is made clearer by pharmacogenomics. It also refutes the idea that "one medicine fits everyone." When it comes to many drug reactions, a number of variables, including diet, age, body weight, sex, genetic behaviour, infections, concurrent drugs, and organ function, must be taken into account because they cannot be avoided during the course of disease treatment. Additionally, the care of a problem is highly focused on the integration of relevant evidence connected to medical informatics and personalized medicines [17].

Pharmacokinetics (PK) and pharmacodynamics (PD) are very helpful for comprehending varied drug responses (conventional and/or personalized therapies). The quantitative assessments of drug exposure and effect are combined in these two fields. The analysis of phenotypic markers (epigenetic markers) valuable for customized treatment is made possible by pharmacokinetics data, which are linked to drug exposure and drug level monitoring. The polymorphic genes of the CYP450 family that encode the drug-metabolizing enzymes cytochrome P450 and glucuronyl transferase [22], as well as the hundreds of genes that encode the drug transporters, are frequently implicated in drug response variability [23].

There are not many personalized medications on the market right now. Conventional cancer medicines are ineffective for some patients with late-stage non-small cell lung cancer (NSCLC) who have rearrangements in the anaplastic lymphoma kinase (ALK) gene. Therefore, the 5% of patients who will respond to crizotinib (Xalkori®), an anti-cancer drug that inhibits ROS1 (c-ros oncogene 1) and ALK, are used because they have a chromosomal rearrangement that results in a gene fusion (ALK and EML4, echinoderm microtubule-associated protein-like 4) that causes carcinogenesis [17]. There are over 1,600 molecular diagnostic tests available that target numerous ailments. Genetic testing is advised for a number of diseases that could be addressed with personalized therapy [24]. Studies have revealed that the reasons why many patients do not respond to first-line medicines include variations in the genes that encode drug targets, transporters, and metabolizing enzymes such as cytochrome P450 and glucuronyl transferase [25]. There are molecular diagnoses for a large number of malignancies that help doctors better manage their patients' conditions and increase their chances of survival. For instance, the results of the BRAF genetic test are used to categorize melanoma cases. Additionally, ALK and BRAF gene changes can be targeted during molecular therapy since non-small cell lung tumors often test positive for these mutations [26].

The number of genetic changes that fuel carcinogenesis varies among malignancies; melanoma has the greatest rate (73%), while thyroid cancer has the second-highest incidence (56%). In terms of driver mutation incidence, lung cancer comes in second at 41%, followed by gynaecological cancers at 31%, gastrointestinal cancers at 25%, and both ovarian and head and neck cancers at 21% [26]. In contrast to the 13% risk experienced by the general female population, people with mutations in the BRCA1 or BRCA2 genes have a 36 to 85% likelihood of developing breast cancer [27]. The cell surface protein known as human epidermal growth factor receptor 2 (HER2) is overexpressed in about 30% of breast cancer cases, and the usual therapy is ineffective in these patients who have HER2-overexpressing tumors [28]. But when paired with chemotherapy, the antibody medication trastuzumab can reduce the recurrence of HER2-positive cancers by 52%, a response that is better than chemotherapy by itself [29]. Cetuximab (Erbitux®) and panitumumab (Vectibix®) can be used to treat metastatic colon cancer in individuals with a KRAS mutation, although it is advised that only those with a normal KRAS gene use these medications in combination with chemotherapy [30].

Therefore, based on a person's unique genomic profile, medications employed in personalized medicine can be used to manage these conditions. The FDA has approved a large number of medications that are utilized in customized medicine. Given that every patient is different, there are a number of challenges for the scientists and researchers who are examining genetic abnormalities and their phenotypic expression [17].

BIOINFORMATICS AND GENOMICS IN PERSONALIZED MEDICINE

As mentioned earlier, the translation of each patient's genome into digital data, which is subsequently processed, saved, and retrieved as required, is a prerequisite for the real practice of personalized medicine. To achieve this, a combination of genetics, bioinformatics, and personalized medicine is required (Fig. **3**). This might sound simple, yet it is very complex to comprehend. Yet, all of this is extremely fascinating since personalized medicine opens up a nearly unlimited number of previously unimaginable possibilities. It means that diseases long thought to be incurable, such as cancer, can now be cured. This new approach to medicine also provides many possibilities for treating rare diseases that were previously too expensive to explore. We can now research, treat, and possibly cure various diseases as a result of these technologies [31].

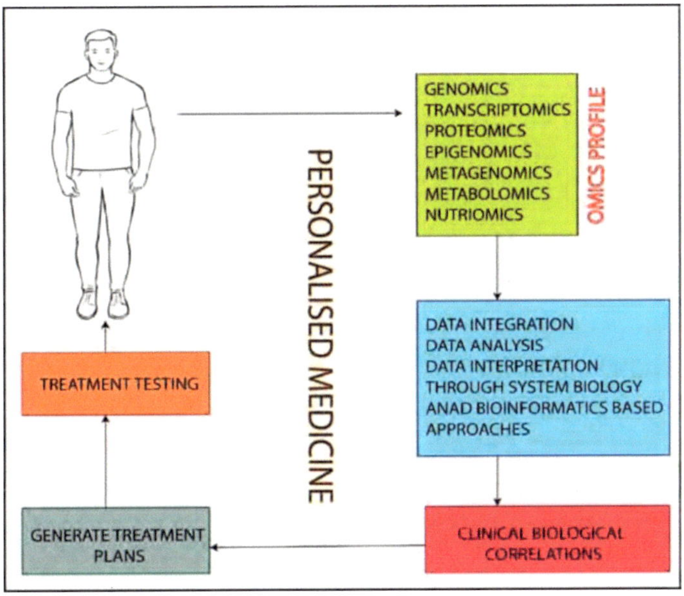

Fig. (3). A basic framework of personalized medicine.

For a better understanding of biological mechanisms, systems biology has emerged as a result of the availability of huge omics (genomics, transcriptomics, proteomics, epigenomics, metagenomics, metabolomics, nutrigenomics, *etc.*) data sets [32]. Systems biology seeks to understand complicated biological interactions by comprehensively integrating data from diverse disciplines (holism instead of the more traditional reductionism). Systems biology, in contrast to addressing a collection of elements as a single entity leading to an outcome, depends on experimental and computational methodologies to provide insight into biological phenomena [33]. It is generally acknowledged that to understand biological systems, several dimensions must be taken into account at once [34]. Modern biology and medicine are being advanced through systems techniques. Predictive, preventive, customized, and participatory medicine are all expected to be made possible by the use of deterministic networks for both normal and disordered phenotypes (personalized medicine) [35].

Human health appears to have a promising future. A longer lifespan with a higher quality of life in later years is another projected benefit of personalized medicine. Personalized medicine is expected to become more prevalent in the near future, but not as swiftly as some in the scientific community and the media may anticipate [33]. Parallel to a rising two-tiered global health system, a similar two-tiered phenomenon is observed regarding our capacity to generate and analyze omics data, which may further prolong the transition to personalized care. Despite technological progress, the collection and management of omics data (storage and computational resources) remain costly [36]. This suggests that access to personalized medication might only be available in wealthy nations. This is reflected by a widening disparity in our capacity to produce and understand omics data. In omics techniques, data management, integration, analysis, and interpretation are becoming the bottlenecks rather than data collection [37]. It is vital to close the gap between high-throughput technology advancements and our capacity for data management, integration, analysis, and interpretation.

Therefore, everyone must contribute to the effort if these potentials are to be fully realized. The movement toward better patient outcomes, cheaper costs, and greater quality healthcare cannot be slowed down at the moment. This very well means that one's life may rely on the success of genomics, bioinformatics, and personalized medicine [33].

BIOINFORMATICS CHALLENGES FOR PERSONALIZED MEDICINE

Though, personalized medicine promises to tailor treatments to the patients' specific genotype towards better patient outcomes, cheaper costs, and greater quality healthcare, many challenges need to be addressed to make this concept a reality [38]. The era of genomic medicine is rapidly approaching, and patients and physicians will have access to genetic information to personalized medical care. Soon the evaluation of 500,000–100,0000 variant markers with associated trait data [39], and complete genome sequencing will be available for less than $1000 [40]. A thorough clinical evaluation of a patient using a personal genome has been carried out by one group [41], and the 1000 Genomes Project is now sequencing the genome of 1000 people [42]. Individual genomic data will flood the bioinformatics industry in the upcoming years. The bioinformatics community must deal with serious problems brought on by this enormous data flow. If we take 1000 human genomes for sequencing each having 7 billion diploid sequences, the total sequences will be $7x10^{12}$ nucleotides. The challenge for bioinformatics expert would be to fish out the so-called culprit sequence from these enormous data and then ensure that the one picked up is the real one and not a candidate of sequences polymorphism. Thus, delineating mutation with polymorphism and correlating the same with diseased loci will continue to be resource intensive and demanding proposition. However, these issues are circumvented amicably; the reward will be enormous because one can then find the drug molecule corresponding to this sequence alteration. While challenges have no limit, the human ingeniousness is also enormous. Thus, the quest for precision medicine is challenging but not impossible. This only needs efforts, optimism and large scale indulgence on the past of researchers in the collaborative mode.

Processing Large-scale Genomic Data

This is one of the major challenges that must be addressed. Microarray-based genotyping techniques, which could only examine regions of known variation, are being replaced by sequencing technologies as they become more widely available and more cost-effective [43]. With an error rate of less than one per 100 kb, a full genome or a few dozen exomes may now be sequenced in about two weeks [40]. Even with such low error rates, there might still be a lot of mistakes; for example, a 3 GB human genome would contain about 30,000 incorrect variant calls. These technologies' high error rates present substantial difficulties for applications, such as finding new variations. One thousand somatic mutations every generation and between 100,000 and 300,000 previously unknown SNPs are predicted in each freshly sequenced genome [44]. As new genomes are sequenced, the projected number of mutations may decline; yet, the sheer volume of errors makes variant finding an unlikely challenge.

Because of the false positive rate, whenever a novel variant is detected, it must be confirmed. Furthermore, other types of variation, such as small insertion-deletion variants (indels), copy number variations (CNVs), and structural variants (SVs), are more challenging to discover with high-throughput sequencing. In order to detect these types of alterations in clinical applications, new algorithms for calling indels, CNVs, and SVs from read data will be critical. Even high-quality sequence reads must be placed in their genomic context to discover variations, which is an active area of research because different mapping and aligning algorithms, for example, sometimes produce inconsistent findings [42]. Sequences are typically mapped to a genomic reference sequence rather than *de novo* assembly because this process is slower and more difficult due to repeated regions [45]. The size of the genome affects how quickly some algorithms, such BLAST [46] or Smith-Waterman [47], can be executed. While a single query might only take a few seconds on a single CPU, aligning 100 million of them would take more than three years on a single CPU [46, 47].

Analysis of the Functional Impact and the Effects of Genetic Variation

This is another challenge that is faced in the field of bioinformatics. Following the processing of genomic data, it is necessary to examine how genetic differences affect both function and overall health. The statistical correlations of SNPs with a variety of significant common diseases have been evaluated using genome-wide association studies (GWAS). These techniques are yielding novel insights, but few variants have been defined, and it has been challenging to comprehend the functional connection between linked polymorphisms and phenotypic features [48]. A SNP is, by definition, a single nucleotide variant with an allele frequency greater than 1% in the human population. Data management, retrieval, and quality control are crucial concerns for estimating the effects of SNPs. The number of known SNPs has exponentially expanded during the past few years. The most complete source of SNP data from various organisms is the dbSNP database [49]. A complete collection of germline mutations in genes linked to human hereditary disorders is available in the Human Gene Mutation Database (HGMD). More than 76000 mutations from about 2900 genes are available in the free version for educational and non-profit users. The SwissVar is a database of 56 000 mSNPs from more than 11 000 genes that have been manually annotated (mSNPs) [50]. The Online Mendelian Inheritance in Man (OMIM) database of human SNPs and their relationships with Mendelian disorders is another notable source of SNP data [51]. The PharmGKB database provides manually curated relationships between genes and medications, as well as a catalog of genetic variations known to influence drug response, including >40 VIPs and over 3400 annotated drug-response variants [52]. The Sanger Institute's Catalogue of Somatic Mutations in Cancer (COSMIC) has 25000 distinct somatic mutation data relating to human cancer gathered from the literature. Several computer approaches for predicting harmful missense SNPs have been developed in recent years [53]. These methods have used a variety of approaches, including empirical rules [54], Hidden Markov Models (HMMs) [55], Neural Networks [56], Decision Trees [57], Random Forests [58].

Amino acid sequence, protein structure, and evolutionary data are frequently used as input features by prediction algorithms. The hydrophobicity, charge, polarity, and bulkiness of the altered residues are among the physicochemical characteristics that the amino acid sequence features depend on [59]. Protein structural data describes the mutation's structural surroundings and has been used to successfully foresee the change in protein stability after a mutation [60]. Because essential amino acids are frequently conserved in protein families, alterations at conserved positions tend to be harmful. This is one of the most significant characteristics for the prediction of the impact of missense SNPs [61]. Experimental testing is necessary to confirm genetic predictions because prediction approaches do not provide any information about the pathophysiology of the disorders. There is a need for quick and precise approaches to gene prioritizing because laboratory validation is costly and time-consuming. The concept of similarity to genes associated with the biological process of interest (guilt-by-association) is currently the most successful approach. Protein-protein interaction (PPI) data, functional annotation, biological pathway data, and literature are the sources of the input data for the various gene prioritization techniques. Additionally, new techniques are required to assess the effects of synonymous, insertional, and deletional SNPs. Additionally, it is necessary to identify functional genomic areas, such as splicing sites and promoter regions, in order to examine the impact of intronic SNPs [38].

Bringing Systems and Data Together to Capture Biological Complexity

The common "one-SNP, one-phenotype" method used in most studies is insufficient since personalized medicine involves complex phenotypes. It is believed that gene-gene and gene-environment interactions are the main causes of the majority of medically significant phenotypes [62]. For instance, the response to a medicine is frequently influenced by a number of pharmacokinetic and pharmacodynamic interactions, which together comprise a strong and tolerant system with many highly polymorphic enzymes [63]. This intricacy makes it likely that a drug-response phenotype of interest will be influenced by a variety of environmental factors and genes [38]. In order to keep complexity algorithms manageable given the magnitude of the genomic datasets, dimensionality reduction techniques including principal components analysis, information gain, and multifactor dimensionality reduction will be crucial [64]. Finding multilocus connections with disorders like hypertension and familial amyloid polyneuropathy type I using some of these techniques has been fruitful [65]. A recent review categorizes and discusses numerous additional feature selection methods for bioinformatics [66]. These techniques can be quite useful when working with enormous datasets, but they don't take into account any outside information sources or the biology underlying the relationships [38].

By integrating molecular data from several levels of biology, such as genomes, transcriptomes, metabolomes, proteomes, and functional and regulatory networks, systems biology and network approaches deal with the problem of complexity [67]. A disease or drug response phenotype can be viewed as a widespread disruption of networks from their steady state [68]. This method combines research findings from networks to draw conclusions about which genes, or groups of genes, and other genetic markers are more likely to be linked. These methods are encouraging, but bioinformaticians must be cautious of a few traps as they move forward. In particular, when one inaccurate assumption can spread *via* several data sources and exacerbate the error, methods must be based on high-quality data to avoid the "garbage-in, garbage-out" phenomena. For instance, moving annotations based on resemblance can occasionally succeed, but it can also accidentally link a paralog to the wrong function. The risk is the same for molecules that are identical chemically; two comparable molecules may biochemically act significantly differently. Finally, assumptions must be carefully considered. For instance, a method that links gene expression with medication targets must take into account the fact that the majority of medicines bind proteins, not DNA or RNA [38].

Interpreting the Data with Proper Clinical Relevance

This is another challenge that needs to be addressed. Applying the research findings to better patient care is its biggest obstacle. A lot of this research has not yet been applied in clinical settings. In fact, a lot of doctors are not ready to use patient genetic testing in their practices, and it is not apparent how to best use study findings to advance patient care [69]. Pharmacogenomics is one of the fields where bioinformatics can have the most clinical influence. An early example of prospective pharmacogenomics application is a trial for Alzheimer's disease utilizing rosiglitazone, an approved Type II diabetes medicine. The hypothesis was that ApoE4 non-carriers would outperform ApoE4 carriers. The preliminary Phase II pharmacogenetic-based data appeared to suggest that non-ApoE4 carriers outperformed placebo [70]. Subsequent research of ApoE4-stratified patients found no substantial advantages. However, the concept of prospective gene-based stratification for therapeutic trials remains promising for the future [71]. Prospective gene-stratification hypotheses must be developed for future trials, which will necessitate the development of new bioinformatics approaches [70]. Because novel medications will lack established gene interactions, techniques for predicting drug-target or drug-gene interactions will be critical [72].

Personalized medicine education and training for clinicians, routine pharmacogenetic testing, and additional clinical studies to demonstrate the effectiveness of pharmacogenetic-based prescriptions are all necessary updates to the existing state of medical practice. Eventually, bioinformatics needs to create strategies that explore the genome in a clinical setting and enable doctors to practice personalized medicine [19]. There are two possible approaches that can be adopted. Both require the development of databases. One database must have a single disease and all the available information on that disease from across the world encompassing all *omics,* clinical parameters, updates on the disease (like OMIM), and all possible variants and mutational load. For a clinician, a search of such a single database on a single disease, all the relevant information will be available. The clinician can take the available information from the database to decide the future course of action and prescribe the most appropriate drug. The other possible database may include all the diseases, their corresponding omics-related information, and mutational load. Clearly, such a composite database would be much more elaborate but would prove to be rewarding. As of now, we do not have a database exclusive to precision medicine. This is because PM involves so many attributes and information from different disciplines, collecting all such details at one place from across the world will take time. Further, clinicians need to be sensitized with the concept of precision medicine and its future prospects. Acceptance of PM concept by the clinicians would speed up the process of progress and perhaps then the much desired dream would be fulfilled.

EPIGENETICS AND DNA METHYLATION AGING CLOCKS

Age is one of the biggest risk factors for a number of human diseases, including cancer, metabolic, neurological, and cardiovascular disorders, which are all on the rise as the population ages. This added weight poses a significant socio-economic, economic, and public health concern. The rate of aging varies among people, though. In addition to individual variability in diseases susceptibility and mortality, there is a significant interindividual diversity in the rate of aging [73]. Important possibilities for prioritizing prevention and intervention would arise from identifying those people who are most at risk for age-related illnesses and death. In order to effectively predict the risk of age-related diseases and death, molecular targets are of great interest as clinical biomarkers. Cellular senescence, genomic instability, telomere attrition, and mitochondrial dysfunction are some of the biomarkers that have been linked to a variety of age-related illnesses and death. They appear to reflect key features of biological age [74].

It is generally recognized that as people age, a variety of molecular changes take place within the cells and tissues. Age-related changes in DNA methylation patterns have been demonstrated; as a result, they might constitute a fundamental mechanism underlying human aging. DNA methylation measures have been used to create epigenetic indicators of aging also referred to as the epigenetic clock.

The fundamental question of why we age, as well as other long-standing issues in many fields, may be answered with the use of epigenetic biomarkers [75].

Bocklandt *et al.* of UCLA's team made the first reliable demonstration that salivary DNA methylation levels could produce age predictions with an average accuracy of 5.2 years in 2011 [76]. The Hannum epigenetic clock, which consists of 71 indicators that precisely predict age based on blood methylation levels, was reported by Trey Ideker and Kang Zhang at the University of California, San Diego [77]. Steve Horvath, a UCLA professor of human genetics and biostatistics, created the first multi-tissue epigenetic clock, known as Horvath's epigenetic clock. Horvath spent more than 4 years gathering publicly accessible Illumina DNA methylation data and choosing appropriate statistical techniques. Horvath's epigenetic clock represents a major advance in the field of epigenetics because it is broadly applicable and uses the same set of 353 CpGs and prediction algorithm regardless of the organism's DNA source, that it does not need to be adjusted or calibrated. With the use of the same aging clock, this trait enables comparison of the ages of various bodily parts. Soon after, the Intrinsic Epigenetic Age Acceleration (IEAA), an estimator based on the cellular makeup of the blood, was created as a derivative of Horvath's clock [78].

Few years later, a second generation of epigenetic clocks appeared, which had better age estimation than the first. This was accomplished by including both environmental and epigenetic variations, such as smoking or chronological age, as well as DNA methylation and other epigenetic variations. GrimAge and PhenoAge clocks stand out among these others. GrimAge employs the mortality risks associated with aging along with the smoking variant among other risk factors, whereas PhenoAge uses the chronological age as a factor in its epigenetic clock. GrimAge is superior to other epigenetic clocks at "predicting death" because it takes environmental variations into consideration. In addition to facilitating the diagnosis of some diseases, new age estimation technologies are constantly being developed [79].

The Horvath's epigenetic clock has been applied in various fields of biology. It has been used to assess epigenetic age acceleration in genetic investigations. The difference between DNA methylation age and chronological age can be used to calculate age acceleration. Blood from older patients has a broad sense of heritability (measured by Falconer's formula) of age acceleration of about 40%, although it seems to be much higher in infants [78]. The prefrontal region of the brain showed a similar 41% age acceleration in older participants [80].

The association between a high body mass index (BMI) and the DNA methylation ages of human blood, liver, muscle, and adipose tissue was examined using the epigenetic clock [81]. For the liver, there was a discernible relationship (r = 0.42) between BMI and the acceleration of epigenetic age. A significantly larger sample size (n = 4200 blood samples) showed a weak but statistically significant connection (r = 0.09) between BMI and intrinsic age acceleration of blood [82]. The same extensive investigation discovered an association between blood epigenetic age acceleration and several metabolic syndrome biomarkers, including glucose, insulin, triglyceride, C-reactive protein, and waist-to-hip ratio. On the other hand, a decreased rate of blood's epigenetic aging was linked to high levels of HDL cholesterol. Additionally, there is evidence that physical exercise may mitigate the effects of greater body mass index, waist-to-hip ratio, and waist size on accelerated epigenetic clocks [83].

In female breast tissue next to breast cancer tissue, DNAm age is older than chronological age. Because normal tissue adjacent to other cancer types does not show the same age acceleration effect [78]. This study implies that normal female breast tissue ages quicker than other regions of the body [84].

Both positive and negative effects of age acceleration are seen in cancer tissues. For the majority of tumor types, there is no discernible correlation between age acceleration and tumor morphology (grade/stage). On average, the age acceleration of cancer tissues with mutant TP53 is less than that of cancer tissues without it. Furthermore, compared to cancer tissues with low age acceleration, those with high age acceleration typically exhibit fewer somatic mutations [78]. Age acceleration and numerous genetic abnormalities in cancer tissues are strongly correlated [85].

The risk of numerous chronic diseases, which are normally linked to aging, is raised in people with Down syndrome. Trisomy 21 may cause tissues to age more quickly biologically, according to clinical signs of accelerated aging; however there isn't much molecular data to support this theory. Trisomy 21 dramatically increases the age of blood and brain tissues, according to the epigenetic clock (on average by 6.6 years) [86].

Numerous neuropathological parameters that are related to Alzheimer's disease were shown to be correlated with the epigenetic age acceleration of the human prefrontal cortex. Additionally, it was discovered to be connected to a loss in both global and memory performance in people with Alzheimer's disease [80]. Blood's epigenetic age is related to how well elders' brain functions. Overall, these findings clearly imply that it is possible to determine the biological age of the brain using the epigenetic clock [87].

It has been discovered that Huntington's condition accelerates the epigenetic aging of certain human brain areas [88].

As indicated by the increasing incidence and variety of age-related disorders at very early age, Human Immunodeficiency Virus-1 (HIV) infection is linked to clinical symptoms of accelerated aging. However, it has proven challenging to find evidence of an accelerated aging effect at the molecular level. HIV-1 infection significantly accelerated the aging process in blood (5.2 years) and brain (7.4 years) tissue, according to an epigenetic clock analysis of human DNA from HIV+ individuals and controls [89]. According to a large-scale study, the granulocyte ratio of people with Parkinson's disease shows (very mild) signs of accelerated aging [90].

Epigenetic aging is accelerated by menopause. The menopause-related loss of female hormones speeds up the aging of blood and perhaps other tissues on the basis of epigenetic factors. The higher epigenetic age acceleration of blood has been demonstrated to be related to early menopause [91].

It is clear that the aging-related epigenetic alterations detected by DNA methylation clocks are widespread and suggestive of genomic, cell biology, and tissue changes taking place over the course of a life. These molecular changes may lead to a high-resolution and precise understanding of age-related disease and physiology [92, 93].

CONCLUSION

With personalized medicine, it is possible to transform a "one-size-fits-all" approach to prevention, pharmacological therapy, and diagnostics into an individualized one. Of course, there are similarities amongst all of us but not without differences. Both personalised and precision medicine relies on circadian or aging clocks. By conquering the hurdles and working together, personalised medicine will thrive in the future, providing promise for a better quality of life and enhanced longevity.

ACKNOWLEDGEMENTS

A.F. is financially supported by the Indian Council of Medical Research under SRF (Senior Research Fellowship) (Project No. ISRM/11(50)/2017).

REFERENCES

[1] Toraño EG, García MG, Fernández-Morera JL, Niño-García P, Fernández AF. The Impact of External Factors on the Epigenome: *In Utero* and over Lifetime. BioMed Res Int 2016; 2016: 1-17. [http://dx.doi.org/10.1155/2016/2568635] [PMID: 27294112]

[2] R R. Published, Epigenetics: Definition & Examples, livescience.com. Available from: https://www.livescience.com/37703-epigenetics.html (Accessed Jan. 24, 2023).

[3] Berger SL, Kouzarides T, Shiekhattar R, Shilatifard A. An operational definition of epigenetics: Figure 1. Genes Dev 2009; 23(7): 781-3.

[http://dx.doi.org/10.1101/gad.1787609] [PMID: 19339683]

[4] CDC. What is Epigenetics? | CDC Centers for Disease Control and Prevention, 2022. Available from: https://www.cdc.gov/genomics/disease/epigenetics.htm (Accessed Jan. 24, 2023).

[5] Team DDW. Epigenetics - Unlocking The Potential for Personalised Medicine Available from: https://www.ddw-online.com/epigenetics-unlocking-the-potential-for-personalised-medi-ine-586-201710/ (Accessed Jan. 28, 2023).

[6] Castillo-Fernandez JE, Spector TD, Bell JT. Epigenetics of discordant monozygotic twins: Implications for disease. Genome Med 2014; 6(7): 60. [http://dx.doi.org/10.1186/s13073-014-0060-z] [PMID: 25484923]

[7] Moore LD, Le T, Fan G. DNA methylation and its basic function. Neuropsychopharmacology 2013; 38(1): 23-38. [http://dx.doi.org/10.1038/npp.2012.112] [PMID: 22781841]

[8] Martino D, Loke Y, Gordon L, *et al.* Longitudinal, genome-scale analysis of DNA methylation in twins from birth to 18 months of age reveals rapid epigenetic change in early life and pair-specific effects of discordance. Genome Biol 2013; 14(5): R42. [http://dx.doi.org/10.1186/gb-2013-14-5-r42] [PMID: 23697701]

[9] Handy DE, Castro R, Loscalzo J. Epigenetic modifications. Circulation 2011; 123(19): 2145-56. [http://dx.doi.org/10.1161/CIRCULATIONAHA.110.956839] [PMID: 21576679]

[10] Al Aboud NM, Tupper C, Jialal I. Genetics, Epigenetic Mechanism. StatPearls. Treasure Island, FL: StatPearls Publishing 2022. http://www.ncbi.nlm.nih.gov/books/NBK532999/ [Online].

[11] López V, Fernández AF, Fraga MF. The role of 5-hydroxymethylcytosine in development, aging and age-related diseases. Ageing Res Rev 2017; 37: 28-38. [http://dx.doi.org/10.1016/j.arr.2017.05.002] [PMID: 28499883]

[12] Yuan J, Hegde PS, Clynes R, *et al.* Novel technologies and emerging biomarkers for personalized cancer immunotherapy. J Immunother Cancer 2016; 4(1): 3. [http://dx.doi.org/10.1186/s40425-016-0107-3] [PMID: 26788324]

[13] Raiber EA, Beraldi D, Martínez Cuesta S, *et al.* Base resolution maps reveal the importance of 5-hydroxymethylcytosine in a human glioblastoma. NPJ Genom Med 2017; 2(1): 6. [http://dx.doi.org/10.1038/s41525-017-0007-6] [PMID: 29263824]

[14] Vaz M, Hwang SY, Kagiampakis I, *et al.* Chronic cigarette smoke-induced epigenomic changes precede sensitization of bronchial epithelial cells to single-step transformation by KRAS Mutations. Cancer Cell 2017; 32(3): 360-376.e6. [http://dx.doi.org/10.1016/j.ccell.2017.08.006] [PMID: 28898697]

[15] Ginsburg GS, Willard HF. Genomic and personalized medicine: Foundations and applications. Transl Res 2009; 154(6): 277-87. [http://dx.doi.org/10.1016/j.trsl.2009.09.005] [PMID: 19931193]

[16] Pirmohamed M. Pharmacogenetics: Past, present and future. Drug Discov Today 2011; 16(19-20): 852-61. [http://dx.doi.org/10.1016/j.drudis.2011.08.006] [PMID: 21884816]

[17] Rasool M, Malik A, Naseer MI, *et al.* The role of epigenetics in personalized medicine: challenges and opportunities. BMC Med Genomics 2015; 8(S1) (Suppl. 1): S5. [http://dx.doi.org/10.1186/1755-8794-8-S1-S5] [PMID: 25951941]

[18] Available from: https://core.ac.uk/reader/37882817?utm_source=linkout (Accessed: Jan. 28, 2023).

[19] Strianese O, Rizzo F, Ciccarelli M, *et al.* Precision and personalized medicine: How genomic approach improves the management of cardiovascular and neurodegenerative disease. Genes 2020; 11(7): 747. [http://dx.doi.org/10.3390/genes11070747] [PMID: 32640513]

[20] Bilkey GA, Burns BL, Coles EP, *et al.* Genomic testing for human health and disease across the life

cycle: Applications and ethical, legal, and social challenges. Front Public Health 2019; 7: 40. [http://dx.doi.org/10.3389/fpubh.2019.00040] [PMID: 30915323]

[21] Goetz LH, Schork NJ. Personalized medicine: Motivation, challenges, and progress. Fertil Steril 2018; 109(6): 952-63. [http://dx.doi.org/10.1016/j.fertnstert.2018.05.006] [PMID: 29935653]

[22] Phillips KA, Veenstra DL, Oren E, Lee JK, Sadee W. Potential role of pharmacogenomics in reducing adverse drug reactions: A systematic review. JAMA 2001; 286(18): 2270-9. [http://dx.doi.org/10.1001/jama.286.18.2270] [PMID: 11710893]

[23] Huang Y, Anderle P, Bussey KJ, *et al.* Membrane transporters and channels: Role of the transportome in cancer chemosensitivity and chemoresistance. Cancer Res 2004; 64(12): 4294-301. [http://dx.doi.org/10.1158/0008-5472.CAN-03-3884] [PMID: 15205344]

[24] NIH wants to hear about genetic tests. Available from: https://www.science.org/content/article/nih-wants-hear-about-genetic-tests (Accessed Jan. 28, 2023).

[25] Mangravite LM, Thorn CF, Krauss RM. Clinical implications of pharmacogenomics of statin treatment. Pharmacogenomics J 2006; 6(6): 360-74. [http://dx.doi.org/10.1038/sj.tpj.6500384] [PMID: 16550210]

[26] WSJ - Major shift in war on cancer," friends of cancer research. Available from: https://friendsofcancerresearch.org/news/wsj-major-shift-in-war-on-cancer/ (Accessed Jan. 28, 2023).

[27] BRCA gene mutations: Cancer risk and genetic testing fact sheet - NCI. Available from: https://www.cancer.gov/about-cancer/causes-prevention/genetics/brca-fact-sheet (Accessed Jan. 28, 2023).

[28] Piccart-Gebhart MJ, Procter M, Leyland-Jones B, *et al.* Trastuzumab after adjuvant chemotherapy in HER2-positive breast cancer. N Engl J Med 2005; 353(16): 1659-72. [http://dx.doi.org/10.1056/NEJMoa052306] [PMID: 16236737]

[29] Romond EH, Perez EA, Bryant J, *et al.* Trastuzumab plus adjuvant chemotherapy for operable HER2-positive breast cancer. N Engl J Med 2005; 353(16): 1673-84. [http://dx.doi.org/10.1056/NEJMoa052122] [PMID: 16236738]

[30] Lièvre A, Bachet JB, Le Corre D, *et al.* KRAS mutation status is predictive of response to cetuximab therapy in colorectal cancer. Cancer Res 2006; 66(8): 3992-5. [http://dx.doi.org/10.1158/0008-5472.CAN-06-0191] [PMID: 16618717]

[31] How bioinformatics and genomics shape personalized medicine. Available from: https://genomealberta.ca/genomics/how-bioinformatics-and-genomics-s-ape-personalized-medicine.aspx (Accessed Jan. 28, 2023).

[32] Hood L, Flores M. A personal view on systems medicine and the emergence of proactive P4 medicine: Predictive, preventive, personalized and participatory. N Biotechnol 2012; 29(6): 613-24. [http://dx.doi.org/10.1016/j.nbt.2012.03.004] [PMID: 22450380]

[33] Alyass A, Turcotte M, Meyre D. From big data analysis to personalized medicine for all: Challenges and opportunities. BMC Med Genomics 2015; 8(1): 33. [http://dx.doi.org/10.1186/s12920-015-0108-y] [PMID: 26112054]

[34] Loos R, Schadt E. This I Believe: Gaining New Insights Through Integrating 'Old' Data 2012. Available from: https://www.frontiersin.org/articles/10.3389/fgene.2012.00137 (Accessed: Jan. 28, 2023). [http://dx.doi.org/10.3389/fgene.2012.00137]

[35] Hood L, Flores M. A personal view on systems medicine and the emergence of proactive P4 medicine: predictive, preventive, personalized and participatory. N Biotechnol 2012; 29(6): 613-24. [http://dx.doi.org/10.1016/j.nbt.2012.03.004] [PMID: 22450380]

[36] Hardy BJ, Séguin B, Goodsaid F, Jimenez-Sanchez G, Singer PA, Daar AS. The next steps for

genomic medicine: Challenges and opportunities for the developing world. Nat Rev Genet 2008; 9(S1) (Suppl. 1): S23-7.
[http://dx.doi.org/10.1038/nrg2444] [PMID: 18802418]

[37] Mardis ER. The $1,000 genome, the $100,000 analysis? Genome Med 2010; 2(11): 84.
[http://dx.doi.org/10.1186/gm205] [PMID: 21114804]

[38] Fernald GH, Capriotti E, Daneshjou R, Karczewski KJ, Altman RB. Bioinformatics challenges for personalized medicine. Bioinformatics 2011; 27(13): 1741-8.
[http://dx.doi.org/10.1093/bioinformatics/btr295] [PMID: 21596790]

[39] Available from: https://www.pnas.org/doi/10.1073/pnas.0903103106(Accessed Jan. 27, 2023).

[40] Drmanac R, Sparks AB, Callow MJ, *et al.* Human genome sequencing using unchained base reads on self-assembling DNA nanoarrays. Science 2010; 327(5961): 78-81.
[http://dx.doi.org/10.1126/science.1181498] [PMID: 19892942]

[41] Ashley EA, Butte AJ, Wheeler MT, *et al.* Clinical assessment incorporating a personal genome. Lancet 2010; 375(9725): 1525-35.
[http://dx.doi.org/10.1016/S0140-6736(10)60452-7] [PMID: 20435227]

[42] Abecasis GR, Altshuler D, Auton A, *et al.* A map of human genome variation from population-scale sequencing. Nature 2010; 467(7319): 1061-73.
[http://dx.doi.org/10.1038/nature09534] [PMID: 20981092]

[43] Ng SB, Buckingham KJ, Lee C, *et al.* Exome sequencing identifies the cause of a mendelian disorder. Nat Genet 2010; 42(1): 30-5.
[http://dx.doi.org/10.1038/ng.499] [PMID: 19915526]

[44] A map of human genome variation from population scale sequencing. Nature 2010; 467: 1061-73.
[http://dx.doi.org/10.1038/nature09534]

[45] Shendure J, Ji H. Next-generation DNA sequencing. Nat Biotechnol 2008; 26(10): 1135-45.
[http://dx.doi.org/10.1038/nbt1486] [PMID: 18846087]

[46] Altschul SF, Gish W, Miller W, Myers EW, Lipman DJ. Basic local alignment search tool. J Mol Biol 1990; 215(3): 403-10.
[http://dx.doi.org/10.1016/S0022-2836(05)80360-2] [PMID: 2231712]

[47] Smith TF, Waterman MS. Identification of common molecular subsequences. J Mol Biol 1981; 147(1): 195-7.
[http://dx.doi.org/10.1016/0022-2836(81)90087-5] [PMID: 7265238]

[48] Frazer KA, Murray SS, Schork NJ, Topol EJ. Human genetic variation and its contribution to complex traits. Nat Rev Genet 2009; 10(4): 241-51.
[http://dx.doi.org/10.1038/nrg2554] [PMID: 19293820]

[49] Sherry ST, Ward MH, Kholodov M, *et al.* dbSNP: The NCBI database of genetic variation. Nucleic Acids Res 2001; 29(1): 308-11.
[http://dx.doi.org/10.1093/nar/29.1.308] [PMID: 11125122]

[50] Mottaz A, David FPA, Veuthey AL, Yip YL. Easy retrieval of single amino-acid polymorphisms and phenotype information using SwissVar. Bioinformatics 2010; 26(6): 851-2.
[http://dx.doi.org/10.1093/bioinformatics/btq028] [PMID: 20106818]

[51] Hamosh A, Scott A F, Amberger J S, Bocchini C A, McKusick V A. Online Mendelian Inheritance in Man (OMIM), a knowledgebase of human genes and genetic disorders. Nucleic Acids Res 2005; 33(1): 514-7.
[http://dx.doi.org/10.1093/nar/gki033]

[52] Thorn CF, Klein TE, Altman RB. PharmGKB: The pharmacogenomics knowledge base. Methods Mol Biol 2013; 1015: 311-20.
[http://dx.doi.org/10.1007/978-1-62703-435-7_20] [PMID: 23824865]

[53] Karchin R. Next generation tools for the annotation of human SNPs. Brief Bioinform 2009; 10(1): 35-52.
[http://dx.doi.org/10.1093/bib/bbn047] [PMID: 19181721]

[54] Ramensky V, Bork P, Sunyaev S. Human non-synonymous SNPs: server and survey. Nucleic Acids Res 2002; 30(17): 3894-900.
[http://dx.doi.org/10.1093/nar/gkf493] [PMID: 12202775]

[55] Thomas PD, Kejariwal A. Coding single-nucleotide polymorphisms associated with complex vs. Mendelian disease: Evolutionary evidence for differences in molecular effects. Proc Natl Acad Sci USA 2004; 101(43): 15398-403.
[http://dx.doi.org/10.1073/pnas.0404380101] [PMID: 15492219]

[56] Bromberg Y, Yachdav G, Rost B. SNAP predicts effect of mutations on protein function. Bioinformatics 2008; 24(20): 2397-8.
[http://dx.doi.org/10.1093/bioinformatics/btn435] [PMID: 18757876]

[57] Krishnan VG, Westhead DR. A comparative study of machine-learning methods to predict the effects of single nucleotide polymorphisms on protein function. Bioinformatics 2003; 19(17): 2199-209.
[http://dx.doi.org/10.1093/bioinformatics/btg297] [PMID: 14630648]

[58] Calabrese R, Capriotti E, Fariselli P, Martelli PL, Casadio R. Functional annotations improve the predictive score of human disease-related mutations in proteins. Hum Mutat 2009; 30(8): 1237-44.
[http://dx.doi.org/10.1002/humu.21047] [PMID: 19514061]

[59] Capriotti E, Fariselli P, Casadio R. A neural-network-based method for predicting protein stability changes upon single point mutations. Bioinformatics 2004; 20(1): 63-8.
[http://dx.doi.org/10.1093/bioinformatics/bth928]

[60] Zhou H, Zhou Y. Distance-scaled, finite ideal-gas reference state improves structure-derived potentials of mean force for structure selection and stability prediction. Protein Sci 2002; 11(11): 2714-26.
[http://dx.doi.org/10.1110/ps.0217002] [PMID: 12381853]

[61] Agrahari AK, Pieroni E, Gatto G, Kumar A. The impact of missense mutation in PIGA associated to paroxysmal nocturnal hemoglobinuria and multiple congenital anomalies-hypotonia-seizures syndrome 2: A computational study. Heliyon 2019; 5(10): e02709.
[http://dx.doi.org/10.1016/j.heliyon.2019.e02709] [PMID: 31687525]

[62] Manolio TA, Collins FS, Cox NJ, *et al.* Finding the missing heritability of complex diseases. Nature 2009; 461(7265): 747-53.
[http://dx.doi.org/10.1038/nature08494] [PMID: 19812666]

[63] Wilke RA, Reif DM, Moore JH. Combinatorial pharmacogenetics. Nat Rev Drug Discov 2005; 4(11): 911-8.
[http://dx.doi.org/10.1038/nrd1874] [PMID: 16264434]

[64] Hahn LW, Ritchie MD, Moore JH. Multifactor dimensionality reduction software for detecting gene–gene and gene–environment interactions. Bioinformatics 2003; 19(3): 376-82.
[http://dx.doi.org/10.1093/bioinformatics/btf869] [PMID: 12584123]

[65] Soares ML, Coelho T, Sousa A, *et al.* Susceptibility and modifier genes in Portuguese transthyretin V30M amyloid polyneuropathy: complexity in a single-gene disease. Hum Mol Genet 2005; 14(4): 543-53.
[http://dx.doi.org/10.1093/hmg/ddi051] [PMID: 15649951]

[66] Saeys Y, Inza I, Larrañaga P. A review of feature selection techniques in bioinformatics. Bioinformatics 2007; 23(19): 2507-17.
[http://dx.doi.org/10.1093/bioinformatics/btm344] [PMID: 17720704]

[67] Kohl P, Crampin EJ, Quinn TA, Noble D. Systems biology: An approach. Clin Pharmacol Ther 2010; 88(1): 25-33.
[http://dx.doi.org/10.1038/clpt.2010.92] [PMID: 20531468]

[68] Auffray C, Chen Z, Hood L. Systems medicine: The future of medical genomics and healthcare. Genome Med 2009; 1(1): 2.
[http://dx.doi.org/10.1186/gm2] [PMID: 19348689]

[69] McGuire AL, Burke W. An unwelcome side effect of direct-to-consumer personal genome testing. JAMA 2008; 300(22): 2669-71.
[http://dx.doi.org/10.1001/jama.2008.803] [PMID: 19066388]

[70] Roses AD. The medical and economic roles of pipeline pharmacogenetics: Alzheimer's disease as a model of efficacy and HLA-B(*)5701 as a model of safety. Neuropsychopharmacology 2009; 34(1): 6-17.
[http://dx.doi.org/10.1038/npp.2008.153] [PMID: 18923406]

[71] Gold M, Alderton C, Zvartau-Hind M, *et al.* Rosiglitazone monotherapy in mild-to-moderate Alzheimer's disease: Results from a randomized, double-blind, placebo-controlled phase III study. Dement Geriatr Cogn Disord 2010; 30(2): 131-46.
[http://dx.doi.org/10.1159/000318845] [PMID: 20733306]

[72] Hansen NT, Brunak S, Altman RB. Generating genome-scale candidate gene lists for pharmacogenomics. Clin Pharmacol Ther 2009; 86(2): 183-9.
[http://dx.doi.org/10.1038/clpt.2009.42] [PMID: 19369935]

[73] Niccoli T, Partridge L. Ageing as a risk factor for disease. Curr Biol 2012; 22(17): R741-52.
[http://dx.doi.org/10.1016/j.cub.2012.07.024] [PMID: 22975005]

[74] Crimmins E, Vasunilashorn S, Kim JK, Alley D. Biomarkers related to aging in human populations. Adv Clin Chem 2008; 46: 161-216.
[http://dx.doi.org/10.1016/S0065-2423(08)00405-8] [PMID: 19004190]

[75] Gensous N, Bacalini MG, Franceschi C, Meskers CGM, Maier AB, Garagnani P. Age-Related DNA methylation changes: Potential impact on skeletal muscle aging in humans. Front Physiol 2019; 10: 996.
[http://dx.doi.org/10.3389/fphys.2019.00996] [PMID: 31427991]

[76] Bocklandt S, Lin W, Sehl ME, *et al.* Epigenetic predictor of age. PLoS One 2011; 6(6): e14821.
[http://dx.doi.org/10.1371/journal.pone.0014821] [PMID: 21731603]

[77] Hannum G, Guinney J, Zhao L, *et al.* Genome-wide methylation profiles reveal quantitative views of human aging rates. Mol Cell 2013; 49(2): 359-67.
[http://dx.doi.org/10.1016/j.molcel.2012.10.016] [PMID: 23177740]

[78] Horvath S. DNA methylation age of human tissues and cell types. Genome Biol 2013; 14(10): R115.
[http://dx.doi.org/10.1186/gb-2013-14-10-r115] [PMID: 24138928]

[79] Levine ME. Assessment of epigenetic clocks as biomarkers of aging in basic and population research. J Gerontol A Biol Sci Med Sci 2020; 75(3): 463-5.
[http://dx.doi.org/10.1093/gerona/glaa021] [PMID: 31995162]

[80] Levine ME, Lu AT, Bennett DA, Horvath S. Epigenetic age of the pre-frontal cortex is associated with neuritic plaques, amyloid load, and Alzheimer's disease related cognitive functioning. Aging 2015; 7(12): 1198-211.
[http://dx.doi.org/10.18632/aging.100864] [PMID: 26684672]

[81] Horvath S, Erhart W, Brosch M, *et al.* Obesity accelerates epigenetic aging of human liver. Proc Natl Acad Sci USA 2014; 111(43): 15538-43.
[http://dx.doi.org/10.1073/pnas.1412759111] [PMID: 25313081]

[82] Quach A, Levine ME, Tanaka T, *et al.* Epigenetic clock analysis of diet, exercise, education, and lifestyle factors. Aging 2017; 9(2): 419-46.
[http://dx.doi.org/10.18632/aging.101168] [PMID: 28198702]

[83] Kresovich JK, *et al.* Associations of body composition and physical activity level with multiple

measures of epigenetic age acceleration. Am J Epidemiol 2020; Nov; 190(6): 984-93. [http://dx.doi.org/10.1093/aje/kwaa251] [PMID: 33693587]

[84] Sehl ME, Henry JE, Storniolo AM, Ganz PA, Horvath S. DNA methylation age is elevated in breast tissue of healthy women. Breast Cancer Res Treat 2017; 164(1): 209-19. [http://dx.doi.org/10.1007/s10549-017-4218-4] [PMID: 28364215]

[85] Levine ME, Hosgood HD, Chen B, Absher D, Assimes T, Horvath S. DNA methylation age of blood predicts future onset of lung cancer in the women's health initiative. Aging 2015; 7(9): 690-700. [http://dx.doi.org/10.18632/aging.100809] [PMID: 26411804]

[86] Horvath S, Garagnani P, Bacalini MG, *et al.* Accelerated epigenetic aging in Down syndrome. Aging Cell 2015; 14(3): 491-5. [http://dx.doi.org/10.1111/acel.12325] [PMID: 25678027]

[87] Horvath S, Zhang Y, Langfelder P, *et al.* Aging effects on DNA methylation modules in human brain and blood tissue. Genome Biol 2012; 13(10): R97. [http://dx.doi.org/10.1186/gb-2012-13-10-r97] [PMID: 23034122]

[88] Horvath S, Langfelder P, Kwak S, *et al.* Huntington's disease accelerates epigenetic aging of human brain and disrupts DNA methylation levels. Aging (Albany NY) 2016; 8(7): 1485-512. [http://dx.doi.org/10.18632/aging.101005] [PMID: 27479945]

[89] Horvath S, Levine AJ. HIV-1 Infection Accelerates Age According to the Epigenetic Clock. J Infect Dis 2015; 212(10): 1563-73. [http://dx.doi.org/10.1093/infdis/jiv277] [PMID: 25969563]

[90] Horvath S, Ritz BR. Increased epigenetic age and granulocyte counts in the blood of Parkinson's disease patients. Aging (Albany NY) 2015; 7(12): 1130-42. [http://dx.doi.org/10.18632/aging.100859] [PMID: 26655927]

[91] Levine ME, Lu AT, Chen BH, *et al.* Menopause accelerates biological aging. Proc Natl Acad Sci 2016; 113(33): 9327-32. [http://dx.doi.org/10.1073/pnas.1604558113] [PMID: 27457926]

[92] Bell CG, Lowe R, Adams PD, *et al.* DNA methylation aging clocks: challenges and recommendations. Genome Biol 2019; 20(1): 249. [http://dx.doi.org/10.1186/s13059-019-1824-y] [PMID: 31767039]

[93] Bergsma T, Rogaeva E. DNA methylation clocks and their predictive capacity for aging phenotypes and healthspan. Neuroscience Insights 2020; 15: 11. [http://dx.doi.org/10.1177/2633105520942221] [PMID: 32743556]

CHAPTER 3

Precision Medicine in Improving Treatment Outcomes in Hepatocellular Carcinoma: Clinical Outcomes and Advancements

Deepti Singh[1], **Mohammad Afsar Khan**[1] and **Hifzur R. Siddique**[1,*]

[1] *Molecular Cancer Genetics & Translational Research Lab, Section of Genetics, Department of Zoology, Aligarh Muslim University, Aligarh-202002, India*

Abstract: Liver cancer ranks sixth among the most commonly diagnosed malignancies and 90% of liver cancer cases are of Hepatocellular carcinoma (HCC). Treatment options for HCC include resection, radiotherapy, and systemic therapies with chemotherapeutic drugs. The late diagnosis of HCC prevents successful treatment by surgical resection. Further, conventional treatment modalities such as chemotherapy and radiotherapy are ineffective in all patients as tumors are heterogeneous. The heterogeneous nature of tumors enables them to have genetic variations and express specific proteins in different patients. This inherent variability of cancer creates the need to move to a growing field of medicine, *i.e.*, precision/personalized medicine. Precision medicine is based on complementing the molecular profile of a patient to a targeted therapy. In clinical practice, the transition from a stage-based approach to a targeted therapy-based approach is necessary for determining the most appropriate treatment plan for a patient. The clinical outcomes for patients could be improved on a large scale if the discoveries in tumour biology are applied efficiently in clinics. This chapter discusses the research on precision medicine for improving treatment outcomes in HCC patients, especially advanced cancers. It also includes the clinical studies of novel therapeutics used for the targeted therapy of advanced liver cancer patients. Concisely, we summarize the recent studies on the applications of precision and personalized medicine.

Keywords: Cancer management, Clinical trials, Hepatocellular carcinoma, Precision/personalised medicine, Targeted therapy.

* **Corresponding author Hifzur R. Siddique:** Molecular Cancer Genetics & Translational Research Laboratory, Section of Genetics, Department of Zoology, Aligarh Muslim University, Aligarh-202002 India; Phone No. +91-57--2700920 (Ext-3456); Fax: +91-571-2702607; E-mail: hifzur.zo@amu.ac.in

Farzana Mahdi & Abbas Ali Mahdi (Eds.)

INTRODUCTION

Among the various cancer types, liver cancer ranks sixth among the most frequently diagnosed malignancies and the third leading cause of death globally [1]. Among other primary liver cancers, 90% of cases are of HCC and result from exposure to a carcinogen, alcohol abuse, obesity, and hepatitis B and C viral infections [2 - 4]. HCC is characterized by uncontrolled growth, low resection capability, recurrence, inadequate response to treatment, and poor prognosis. Currently, >850,000 cases of HCC are diagnosed annually, and it is anticipated that this incidence will rise to 1 million cases in the future [3, 5]. Further, the mortality rate due to HCC is the highest among other cancers [2]. Due to the high incidence and mortality rate, HCC is not easily manageable despite improvements in diagnosis and therapies.

Surveillance programs in developed nations have facilitated the timely detection of HCC in ~40-50% of affected patients, thereby allowing potentially remedial treatments [3, 6]. However, intermediate- and advanced-stage HCC patients are manageable only with loco-regional, ablation, and systemic treatments. Generally, ~50% of patients are treated with systemic therapies (chemotherapeutic drugs) during disease progression [3, 6]. Sorafenib/Nexavar is a Tyrosine Kinase Inhibitor (TKI) used to treat advanced HCC patients. It has been reported that the administration of sorafenib increased the overall survival from 8 to 11 months. Moreover, Sorafenib is associated with a tolerable safety profile and manageable side effects [7, 8]. From 2007 to 2016, Sorafenib remained the only chemotherapeutic treatment option for late-stage HCC patients. However, recent randomized Phase III clinical studies have demonstrated improvement in treatment outcomes in patients given Lenvatinib as a frontline treatment [7] followed by the second-line treatment of Regorafenib [8], Cabozantinib [10], and Ramucirumab [11] after the patients have experienced HCC progression on Sorafenib. Currently, the second-line treatment for HCC management is Regorafenib. Recently, Immunotherapy is another emerging personalized therapeutic option for HCC patients, for instance, a monoclonal antibody (Nivolumab) targeting the immune checkpoint protein 1 (PD-1). The use of Nivolumab in Phase I/II study resulted in favorable responses and survival rates in patients who have undergone treatment with Sorafenib [12], granting increased FDA approval. Despite extensive efforts, several kinase inhibitors, including Brivanib and Erlotinib, and treatments such as Doxorubicin and radio-embolization using Yttrium 90 (90Y)-microspheres, have failed to demonstrate a significant improvement in the survival rate for patients with unresectable HCC [13]. Also, therapeutic outcomes in patients receiving systemic therapies have been reported to be low.

In the past decade, research evidence has highlighted that every individual's cancer is unique, indicating that their response to conventional therapies (like chemotherapy and radiation) may vary significantly [14]. The conventional treatment methods are often too simplistic and may result in treatments that are expensive, not effective, and associated with significant side effects, causing patients to experience adverse outcomes. Therefore, precision medicine is a more effective approach that aims to shift away from the "one-size-fits-all" approach to cancer therapy. Precision medicine involves developing specialized treatments for each specific cancer subtype by critical analysis of various types of data, including genetic, metabolomic, transcriptomic, proteomic, and other relevant patient data. The majority of healthcare facilities worldwide rely on the BCLC staging system to determine the most effective therapeutic approach for HCC patients [15, 16]. A detailed analysis/investigation of tumor burden, liver function, and overall health status guides in selecting the most specific and personalized treatment option for HCC patients [15]. However, due to the late diagnosis of patients, only a few patients (one-third) are eligible for curative-intent treatments. The majority of HCC patients are diagnosed in the advanced stage, leaving only limited treatment options, resulting in poor treatment outcomes.

The implementation of precision medicine against HCC challenges the traditional "one-size-fits-all" approach to treatment. It focuses on the molecular targets specific to a patient's tumor biology to develop individualized treatment plans. Precision medicine recognizes that each patient's cancer is unique, and treatment should be tailored to their specific needs to achieve better outcomes (Fig. **1**) [17, 18]. In this regard, molecular insight into the disease biology can enable HCC management and help advance the therapies through a complete understanding of the disease etiology; an approach termed a biomarker-driven approach. This approach is crucial at this hour when HCC incidence is increasing alarmingly. This chapter discusses precision medicine for advanced-stage HCC management from the perspective of its clinical implications.

THERAPEUTIC APPROACHES EFFECTIVELY MANAGING HEPATOCELLULAR CARCINOMA (HCC)

In the past decade, various staging systems have been proposed for HCC [19 - 21]. Among them, the BCLC staging system is the most widely used for patient staging and treatment administration [22 - 24]. In developed countries, treatment options including liver resection, transplantation, or localised ablation are possible only in ~50% of the patients, which could be diagnosed at early stages (BCLC stage 0-A) [24]. The available therapeutic options for early-stage HCC have shown a median overall survival of over 60 months [24]. However, it has been reported that ~70% of such patients experience cancer relapse within five years of treatment, and this limitation has not been overcome to date [25]. Further, patients in the intermediate (BCLC stage B) stage who have preserved liver functions, *i.e.*, the Child-Pugh class A stage, have been reported to respond well to transarterial chemoembolization (TACE). This has been confirmed in two clinical studies that compare the approach with the best palliative care [26, 27]. In addition, one meta-analysis [28] confirmed this approach's outcomes, which showed an estimated median overall survival of 108-130 weeks in patients. Further, these results have not been reported to improve with any combination of therapies. For instance, the treatments employing a combination of TACE with tyrosine kinase inhibitors such as Sorafenib or Brivanib did not improve patient outcomes. Nevertheless, the majority of HCC patients, ~50%, receive systemic treatments in due course. It has been documented that HCC patients with progression on TACE and those with BCLC stage C HCC (*i.e.*, advanced stage) most likely benefit from Sorafenib [29]. Among the various drugs, Lenvatinib is the first-line systemic treatment [9], and Regorafenib, Cabozantinib, and Ramucirumab are the second-line drugs [8, 10, 11] that have been reported to deliver survival advantage to advanced-stage HCC patients.

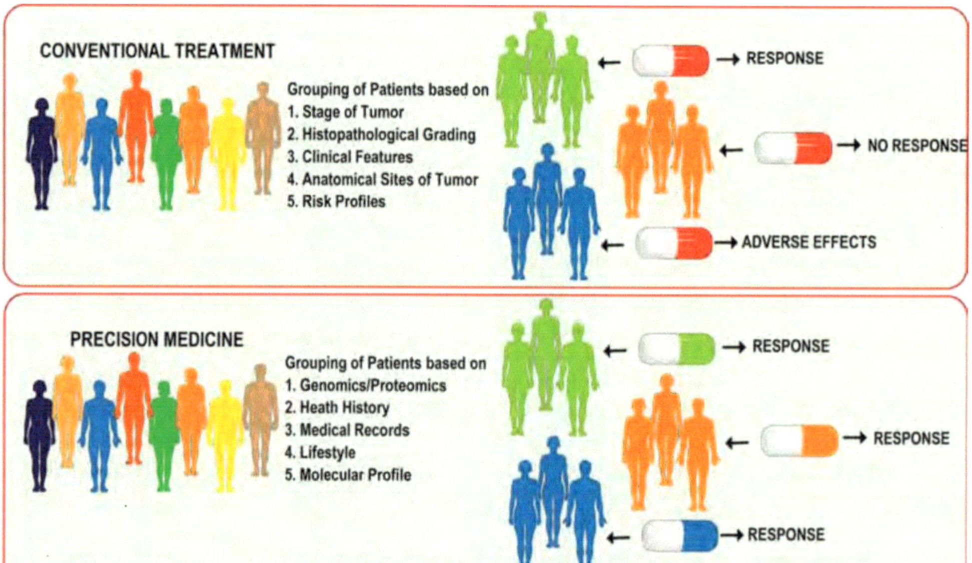

Fig. (1). A schematic illustration of precision medicine generating better treatment outcomes/response. Precision medicine enables the proper therapeutic intervention to reach the patient at the right time.

This therapeutic approach has been tested in clinical trials and yielded a median survival of ~one year. Another second-line drug with treatment benefits proven in

Phase I/II trials is Nivolumab. Nivolumab has a better overall response and survival rate in Phase I/II trials of this agent [12]. In the end, patients diagnosed with BCLC-stage D or end-stage HCC are mainly recommended appropriate help in pain management along with nutritional and moral support. The international and national guidelines for better managing HCC have been updated based on research evidence encompassing most of the therapies tested for HCC.

FIRST-LINE SYSTEMIC TREATMENTS FOR ADVANCED HCC MANAGEMENT

The treatment of HCC is difficult as most patients have an end-stage diagnosis. The end-stage diagnosis limits the survival benefits of conventional systemic chemotherapy. For instance, a Phase III trial comparing Doxorubicin to a PIAF regimen (Cisplatin, IFNα2b, Doxorubicin, Fluorouracil) in unresectable HCC patients. The treatment groups were compared for adverse events and median survival. The median survival in the Doxorubicin-treated and PIAF-treated groups was 6.83 and 8.67 months, respectively. Further, the overall response was 10.5% and 20.9% in the Doxorubicin and PIAF group, respectively. The adverse events, including Neutropenia, thrombocytopenia, and hypokalemia, were observed prominently in the PIAF arm compared to Doxorubicin [30]. The results of another randomized Phase III trial that compared the effectiveness and safety of Doxorubicin alone and in combination with Sorafenib in advanced HCC and Child-Pugh A disease demonstrated that Sorafenib administration with Doxorubicin had a greater median time to disease progression and progression-free survival [31]. In addition, the comparison of Doxorubicin with FOLFOX4 (Fluorouracil, Leucovorin (Folinic acid), and Oxaliplatin) also showed negative results and adverse effects/toxicity [32].

Sorafenib, a Multikinase Inhibitor

Sorafenib/Nexavar is an orally administered multikinase inhibitor and is presently the recommended first-line treatment option for advanced HCC patients. Clinical trials, including Phase III SHARP trial in 2007, have shown that Sorafenib significantly improves overall survival. In the SHARP trial, Sorafenib improved the median overall survival from 7.9 months in the placebo to 10.7 months. Further, patients receiving Sorafenib had a median time to disease progression of 5.5 months compared to 2.8 months (control group). This was an excellent discovery for better and more effective advanced-stage HCC management. Similarly, another Phase III randomized study in advanced-stage HCC patients from the Asia-Pacific region demonstrated survival benefits and less progression in the Sorafenib-treated group [33]. However, these trials showed grade 3 adverse effects such as diarrhea, fatigue, vomiting, hand-foot skin reactions, and hypertension, which were manageable and resulted in treatment discontinuation in only 10-15% of patients [29, 33].

Surprisingly, the Sorafenib-associated dermatologic adverse effects that appeared within 60 days of treatment initiation were correlated with better survival outcomes [34]. An exploratory pooled analysis of the two Phase III clinical studies, SHARP and the Asia-Pacific testing Sorafenib, revealed a survival benefit in all the subgroups of HCC patients [35]. However, the benefit was significant in the HCC patients having the disease confined to the liver or those having a lesser neutrophil-to-lymphocyte ratio, and those with Hepatitis C virus [35]. A multicentre study investigated Sorafenib's overall safety and efficacy and demonstrated that it is beneficial for HCC patients having Child-Pugh class A, BCLC stage B, and C disease progressing after loco-regional therapy as they have a more prolonged overall survival rate and time to disease progression. Further, these groups had acceptable safety profiles with mild to moderate adverse effects [36, 37].

Sorafenib is clinically effective as it targets both cancer cells and the heterogeneous cell population of the tumor microenvironment. Sorafenib targets ~40 kinases, such as Vascular Endothelial Growth Factor Receptors (VEGFRs), Epidermal Growth Factor Receptors (EGFRs), and Platelet-Derived Growth Factor Receptor-β (PDGFRβ). Further, it also targets cell proliferation modulators including RAF1, BRAF, and c-KIT [38]. Due to the efficacy of this drug against advanced-stage HCC, its clinical efficacy is explored in other trials. A Phase II SPACE trial tested the efficacy and safety of Doxorubicin-eluting beads (DEB)-TACE plus Sorafenib in intermediate-stage HCC patients. The results demonstrated that the combination was technically feasible but did not improve the time to unTACEable progression (TTUP) [39]. Similarly, in a randomised placebo-controlled Phase III trial, the combination of DEB-TACE and Sorafenib was not effective in improving progression-free survival in HCC patients [39, 40]. Clinical trials have demonstrated that other agents have not been clinically superior to Sorafenib. These include Brivanib, Sunitinib, Linifanib [41 - 44]. Their disappointing results were mainly due to overinterpreting the results of Phase II studies concerning their therapeutic efficacy, mainly due to the flaws in study design, toxicity profile, and lack of biomarker-driven approach [13].

Another Phase III clinical trial, called SARAH, was conducted to evaluate the safety and effectiveness of Sorafenib in comparison to selective internal radiotherapy (SIRT) with yttrium-90 in patients with HCC. This was an open-labelled, randomized, controlled trial that aimed to investigate which treatment approach would be more effective and safe for advanced HCC patients. The results showed that the overall survival did not differ significantly between the two treatment groups, Sorafenib and SIRT with yttrium-90 [45]. The SIRveNIB73 trial comparing the therapeutic effectiveness of radioembolization and Sorafenib in locally advanced HCC patients revealed that the overall survival is similar in both treatment groups. However, the radioembolization group had improved toxicity profile and quality of the patient's life [45, 46].

Lenvatinib

Lenvatinib is another tyrosine kinase receptor inhibitor that targets VEGFR, FGFR, PDGFRs, KIT, and RET [47]. In 2018, Lenvatinib was approved by the US FDA as a first-line systemic treatment option for advanced HCC. The effectiveness of lenvatinib against advanced-stage HCC was evaluated through Phase II and III clinical trials, aimed at exploring its safety and effectiveness as a treatment option for HCC patients [9, 48]. A Phase III clinical trial was conducted to compare the overall survival rates in advanced HCC patients who received either Sorafenib or Lenvatinib as their first-line treatment. The results demonstrated that patients receiving Lenvatinib had a median overall survival of 13.6 months, which was similar to those receiving Sorafenib (12.3 months) [7]. Despite its therapeutic efficacy in the clinical setting, Lenvatinib is associated with multiple adverse effects, such as hypertension, reduced appetite, and reduced body weight [9, 48]. Due to the associated adverse effects, ~10% of the patients administered Lenvatinib and Sorafenib had to undergo treatment discontinuation, thereby affecting the patient's life.

The Lenvatinib-associated adverse effects include liver failure, hemorrhage, and respiratory failure. However, only 2% of patients suffered from these adverse effects compared to Sorafenib (1%). This evidence establishes the potential of lenvatinib as an alternative chemotherapeutic option to Sorafenib for treating HCC patients having cancer progression following TACE.

SECOND-LINE TREATMENTS FOR ADVANCED-STAGE HCC MANAGEMENT

After the approval of Sorafenib as a first-line treatment for HCC, there has been a growing necessity to explore and develop second-line treatment options for patients experiencing disease progression despite treatment with Sorafenib. Second-line therapy is typically used for patients who are unable to tolerate first-line treatments or those experiencing disease progression despite initial treatment.

Regorafenib

Regorafenib is a second-line drug that has structural similarities to Sorafenib. However, they have slightly different inhibitory targets. Regorafenib targets

VEGFR kinases, Angiopoietin 1 receptor (TIE2), RET, and KIT [49]. A multicentre, open-labeled Phase II safety study has reported that Regorafenib has acceptable tolerability and therapeutic efficacy in intermediate or advanced-stage HCC patients with progression following Sorafenib [50]. The positive outcomes observed with Regorafenib in patients who had disease progression on Sorafenib led to the development of the first randomized, double-blind, placebo-controlled Phase III trial demonstrating the survival benefits of Regorafenib, which ultimately led to its FDA approval as a second-line treatment option for HCC. The RESORCE trial observed that Regorafenib improved the overall survival in patients, increasing it from 7.8 months to 10.6 months [51]. This trial was performed explicitly on HCC patients who tolerated Sorafenib ($\geq$ 400mg daily) for more than 20 days in the 28 days treatment cycle [51].

An exploratory analysis was conducted to evaluate the efficacy of sequential treatment with Sorafenib followed by Regorafenib after the RESORCE trial had shown that Regorafenib improved overall survival in HCC patients. The results revealed that the median survival from the initiation of Sorafenib treatment to death was 26 months in patients receiving Regorafenib, whereas it was 19.2 months for patients receiving a placebo [52]. Further, the adverse events rates were found to be manageable and similar in both treatment arms. Although Regorafenib and Sorafenib have markable similarities, the mechanism responsible for this survival benefit has not been established clearly. Regorafenib also targets other pathways involved in various carcinogenesis aspects, such as growth, progression, invasion, and metastasis [49].

Cabozantinib

Cabozantinib is a small molecule multitarget TKI that EMA and the FDA have approved for treating advanced HCC. It has a specific activity for hepatocyte growth factor receptor MET. MET is involved in HCC progression and the development of Sorafenib resistance in patients [53]. A randomized Phase III trial showed that treatment with Cabozantinib has an overall survival of 10.2 months which was two months more compared to placebo. Further, Cabozantinib also prolonged the progression-free survival from 1.9 to 5.2 months. Despite overall and progression-free survival, Cabozantinib was associated with adverse effects in 68% of patients compared to placebo (36%). Palmar-plantar erythrodysesthesia, hypertension, increased levels of AST, fatigue, and diarrhea were among the reported adverse events. These events were manageable by implementing dose modification strategies and providing supportive care [53]. Further, the cost-effectiveness studies revealed that Cabozantinib is an effective treatment option but not cost-effective [54].

Ramucirumab

Ramucirumab, a monoclonal antibody that blocks the binding of VEGF to its receptor, is effective against advanced HCC [55]. A phase II and biomarker study has demonstrated that Ramucirumab has anticancer effects against late-stage HCC with a manageable toxicity profile. The anti-tumor effects of Ramucirumab against advanced-stage HCC were reported first in a Phase II pilot study [56]. Based on phase II results, a randomized, double-blind phase III trial was performed to check the Ramucirumab's safety and efficacy in advanced HCC patients receiving Sorafenib as a first-line treatment [57]. In the REACH trial, 565 patients were included and were randomly assigned to receive either Ramucirumab (283 patients) or placebo (282 patients). The primary endpoint was median overall survival, which was 9.2 months in the Ramucirumab arm and 7.6 months in the placebo arm. The trial concluded that Ramucirumab did not have a significant promising effect in improving survival over a placebo. A separate Phase III trial, REACH-2, was conducted to evaluate the effectiveness of Ramucirumab in patients with advanced HCC and with AFP levels of 400 ng/mL or higher. The trial revealed that patients in the Ramucirumab group had a median overall survival of 8.5 months, compared to 7.3 months in the placebo group. The primary endpoint of overall survival was met, and Ramucirumab demonstrated a better tolerability profile and manageable safety profile [58]. Similarly, Ramucirumab in another REACH-2 trial also improved the overall survival of the Japanese patient population [59]. This trial revealed the effectiveness of Ramucirumab in the Japanese HCC patient population.

Immune Checkpoint Inhibitors

HCC is characterized by inflammation in a microenvironment, thereby infiltrating the tumor microenvironment with immune cells such as killer T-cells, Myeloid cells, and Killer cells. Tumor behavior and immune response are determined by the crosstalk between the immune system and the tumor microenvironment [60, 61]. Conditions associated with improved overall survival in HCC include enhanced infiltration of immune-related cells such as T-cells and low levels of macrophages. In contrast, the prognosis of HCC may worsen when the tumor microenvironment becomes immunosuppressive, which is characterized by the presence of immunosuppressive T-cells, tumor-associated macrophages (TAMs), and myeloid-derived suppressor cells (MDSCs). The escape of cancer cells from the immune surveillance machinery is mediated by several immune checkpoint molecules such as T lymphocyte antigen-4 (CTLA-4) and programmed cell death (PD-1), programmed cell death-Ligand 1 (PD-L1) expressed on T cells [62, 63]. Immunotherapeutics involve the use of immune checkpoint inhibitors, which function by blocking the immunosuppressive pathways. Several immunotherapeutic drugs are used to prevent cancer cells from escaping the immune surveillance machinery, such as Ipilimab (monoclonal antibody to CTLA-4), Nivolumab (monoclonal antibody to PD-1), and Atezolizumab (monoclonal antibody to PD-L1).

Combination of Molecular Targeted Therapies

Recently, combination therapies are gaining global attention where a combination of molecular targeted therapies and immunotherapies are used. Studies have shown the promising effectiveness of Lenvatinib and Pembrolizumab in Renal cell carcinoma (RCC) patients, thereby being regarded as a promising therapeutic intervention by the FDA [64, 65]. This combination is now being evaluated in an open-label Phase 1b study to assess the tolerability and safety of this combination in HCC patients (NCT03006926). Similarly, the combination of Regorafenib and Pembrolizumab is under evaluation in advanced liver cancer patients (NCT03347292). Molecularly targeted therapies using multi-targeting TKIs and other kinases would be beneficial in generating the therapeutic response. For instance, Lenvatinib and Regorafenib showed promising therapeutic efficacy in targeting the tumor microenvironment, promoting immune response and tumor regression [64, 65].

A PROOF OF CONCEPT FOR PRECISION MEDICINE

The results of precision medicine-based clinical trials have been promising, resulting in opting for these therapeutic strategies for advanced-stage HCC (Fig. **2**). However, these results were based on studies done without selecting the patient population using a biomarker-mediated approach. The field of oncology is undergoing rapid changes where molecularly targeted therapies are designed based on the biomarker-selected patient population. However, the biomarker-selected approach is not in everyday use in HCC. However, some attempts have been made to investigate the biomarker-selected approach for HCC patients.

MET-RTK

The MET-RTK has been linked to the pathogenesis of HCC. Increased expression of MET and its ligand, hepatocyte growth factor (HGF), has been associated with the development of Sorafenib resistance and poor prognosis [53]. A subgroup analysis was performed on HCC patients in a Phase II study that evaluated the safety and effectiveness of Tivantinib (ARQ 197), a small-molecule MET inhibitor, in 71 patients with advanced HCC who had already received Sorafenib treatment. A correlation was found between high expression of MET and the median time to progression with Tivantinib. Also, 66% of Tivantinib patients had progressive disease compared to 72% in the placebo group [66]. This concept needed confirmation in a Phase III trial. Therefore, a phase III study was conducted to confirm the results of Phase II in MET-high HCC patients administered with Sorafenib previously. However, the trial results did not reveal any significant improvement in the overall survival of patients who received Tivantinib compared to the placebo. The median overall survival was 8.4 months in the Tivantinib group and 9.1 months in the placebo group [67]. The correlation between high expression of MET and median survival in advanced HCC patients created an idea of whether high MET could be a negative marker of prognosis.

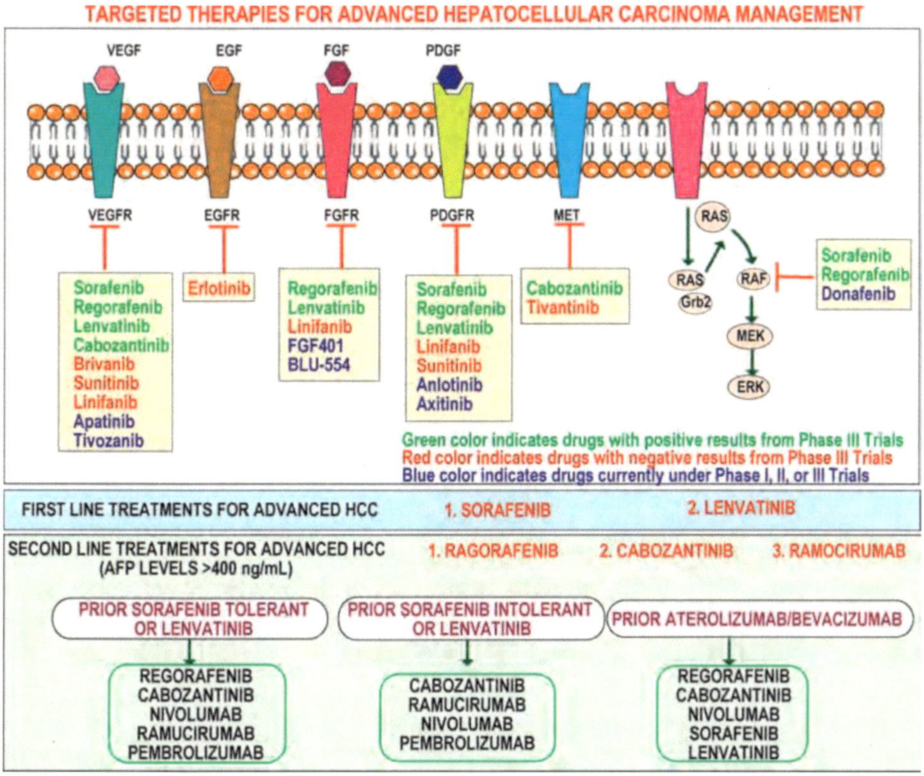

Fig. (2). A schematic illustration of several molecular targeted therapies approved/under trial for managing advanced Hepatocellular carcinoma. Sorafenib, lenvatinib, regorafenib, cabozantinib, and ramucirumab yielded positive results from phase III trials. Sunitinib, linifanib, erlotinib, rivanib, and tivantinib yielded negative results from phase III trials. Apatinib, tivozanib, BLU-554, FGF-401, Anlotinib, axitinib, and donafenib are still under development in phase I, II, or III trials.

Another Phase 2 study with Tivantinib has reported its MET-independent action mechanism [68]. In this context, there are several ongoing clinical studies analysing the effectiveness of MET inhibitors as monotherapy or in combination with other treatments, including immunotherapy, in advanced HCC patients.

The FGF19-FGFR4 Axis

The Fibroblast Growth Factor (FGF) family has at least five different RTKs and at least 22 ligands. These ligands and receptors are potential targets for cancer inhibition [69]. Aberrant FGFR2 is a therapeutic target in several cancer types [70, 71]. Among the FGFRs, the potential target for anticancer treatment is FGFR4—the binding of FGF19 to its receptor, FGFR4 stimulates the proliferation of hepatocytes [72]. The amplification of FGF19 is observed in 5-10% of HCC. Further, the oncogenic role of FGF19 has also been implicated in driving resistance to Sorafenib [73], thereby becoming a therapeutic target for FGFR kinase inhibitors [74 - 76]. Several clinical studies have been designed and conducted to establish the therapeutic potential of FGFR4 Kinase inhibitors in managing HCC, including Fisogatinib (NCT02508467), H3B-6527 (NCT02834780), and FGF401 (NCT02325739) [77, 78].

Intracellular Kinases: mTOR

Previous studies have primarily focused on developing drugs targeting RTKs for HCC treatment. However, recent preclinical and clinical research has also explored intracellular kinases as potential targets for therapy. For instance, mTOR, a serine/threonine protein kinase, regulates several pathways involved in cell division, growth, proliferation, and apoptosis. It is a downstream molecule activated during RTK signaling, involved in HCC progression [79, 80]. Everolimus is an mTOR complex (mTORC1) inhibitor. It has been investigated in a randomized clinical trial EVOLVE-1 in patients having cancer progression after Sorafenib. However, the results were not promising, as the overall survival did not differ significantly [43]. Other mTOR inhibitors with broad inhibitory activity are being tested in clinical trials, including dual mTORC1 and mTORC2 inhibitors and inhibitors targeting the mTOR-PI3K (NCT03059147) [80, 81]. Refametinib is an oral, allosteric MEK inhibitor tested for its safety and efficacy in a phase II study (NCT01204177) conducted on Asian HCC patients. The trial was performed in a biomarker-selected population. The results revealed that patients having RAS mutations benefited more from Refametinib/Sorafenib combination treatment [82].

Further, two phase II clinical studies have also evaluated the clinical benefit of Refametinib in patients having RAS mutations (NCT01915589 and NCT01915602). A Phase II study examining the safety and efficacy of Refametinib alone and in combination with Sorafenib in patients with RAS-mutant HCC revealed that the median overall survival was 12.7 months in the combination group of patients with RAS mutations [83].

Immunotherapeutic Approaches: Future of Precision Medicine

An increased understanding of the tumor-host interaction has resulted in developing novel cancer immunotherapeutics. Several inhibitors targeting immune checkpoint molecules have been approved to treat cancers [84]. Despite their therapeutic effectiveness, only 20-50% of the patients respond to treatment due to differences in their tumor types. Further, immunotherapy may result in severe and permanent autoimmune adverse effects [85]. Therefore, using a biomarker-driven approach to target patients with immunotherapy would be beneficial. Presently, the immunotherapeutic marker that has been approved as a diagnostic and complementary test is PD-L1. Immunohistochemical examination of PD-L1 expression is commonly used in various cancer types, including but not limited to lung and bladder cancer [86]. Pembrolizumab (an immune checkpoint inhibitor and FDA-approved drug) is used for treating solid tumors with microsatellite instability. However, the percentage of patients responding to the treatment was only 40% [87].

In contrast, the phase I/II study in HCC patients revealed that the responses to Nivolumab did not correlate with the expression of PD-L1 on tumor cells, thereby creating the need to identify alternative HCC biomarkers [12]. Sia *et al.* [88] examined the molecular characteristics of immune cells infiltrating HCC to determine the use of agents inducing immune responses against liver cancers [88]. The study reported that 25% of HCCs have markers of inflammatory response. In the study, similar results were observed as previously reported, with immune cell infiltration, PD-1, PD-L1 expression, and active IFNγ signaling [88]. However, the study also reported an immune exclusion phenotype in 25% of HCCs, characterized by mutations in CTNNB1, lower immune infiltration, and overexpression of PTK2, an oncogenic pathway that may contribute to poor infiltration of immune cells into the tumor [89]. A phase III trial (CheckMate 459) is being conducted to evaluate the efficacy of Nivolumab in comparison to the first-line drug Sorafenib for HCC patients. If this trial demonstrates promising results, Nivolumab might become a first-line therapeutic option for advanced HCC patients (NCT02576509).

A summary of the various ongoing trials of molecular targeted therapy for HCC has been presented in Table. (**1**). Identifying biomarkers and biomarker-mediated patient selection is essential for better managing HCC or any other cancer type. It would help improve the therapeutic response in advanced HCC patients.

CONCLUDING REMARKS

Hepatocellular carcinoma (HCC) is a global health concern accounting for ~90% of liver cancers. HCC incidence might soon surpass 1 million cases annually. The late diagnosis of HCC is responsible for the poor prognosis in patients and makes systemic therapies ineffective; however, these patients survive ~1 year using effective multikinase inhibitors. Immune checkpoint inhibitors have recently gained widespread attention for HCC management due to their promising results in clinical trials. Further, a combination of molecular targeted therapies and immunotherapies are emerging as new therapeutic approaches against HCC. The combination therapies make the therapeutic approach more beneficial. With recent research advancements, there is hope that these therapeutic interventions will increase the potential of systemic HCC treatments and enhance patient survival beyond two years. This could be possible if a biomarker and patient-driven approach is followed. In this regard, precision medicine is based on using an individual/patient-driven approach that enables the correct therapeutic decision-making and disease management. A better understanding of the liver microenvironment and heterogeneity of the tumor will therefore be helpful for improved treatment efficacy.

ABBREVIATIONS

GLOBOCAN	Global Cancer Observatory
HCC	Hepatocellular Carcinoma
FDA	Food and Drug Administration
BCLC	Barcelona Clinic Liver Cancer
SHARP	Study of Heart and Renal Protection
RTKs	Receptor Tyrosine Kinases
TACE	Transarterial chemoembolization
PD-1	Programmed Death protein-1
TKI	Tyrosine kinase Inhibitor
EGFR	Epidermal Growth Factor Receptor
AFP	Alpha-Fetoprotein
CTLA-4	Cytotoxic T-lymphocyte–associated Antigen-4
HGF	Hepatocyte Growth Factor
MET	Mesenchymal Epithelial Transition
mTOR	Mammalian Target of Rapamycin
PI3K	Phosphoinositide 3-Kinase
IFNγ	Interferon gamma

ACKNOWLEDGMENTS

The authors thank the Department of Zoology, A.M.U, India, for providing the necessary facilities. DS and MAK express gratitude to UGC-India [524/ (CSIR-UGC NET JUNE 2019)] and CSIR-India [09/112(0599[/2018-EMR-I] for providing Fellowships, respectively. HRS is thankful to the UGC-India [Grant no. F.30-377/2017(BSR)] and DST-SERB, India (Grant no. EMR/2017/001758), New Delhi, for financial help.

FUNDING

The University Grants Commission (UGC) supported this work under Grant [F.30-377/2017(BSR)] and the Department of Science and Technology-Science and Engineering Research Board (DST-SERB), New Delhi, India, under Grant [EMR/2017/001758].

REFERENCES

[1] Available from: https://gco.iarc.fr/today/data/factsheets/cancers/11-Liver-fact-sheet.pdf (Accessed on 02 Jan 2023).

[2] Zucman-Rossi J, Villanueva A, Nault JC, Llovet JM. Genetic landscape and biomarkers of hepatocellular carcinoma. Gastroenterology 2015; 149(5): 1226-39. [http://dx.doi.org/10.1053/j.gastro.2015.05.061] [PMID: 26099527]

[3] Llovet JM, Kelley RK, Villanueva A, *et al.* Hepatocellular carcinoma. Nat Rev Dis Primers 2021; 7(1): 6. [http://dx.doi.org/10.1038/s41572-020-00240-3] [PMID: 33479224]

[4] Choi HY, Siddique HR, Zheng M, *et al.* p53 destabilizing protein skews asymmetric division and enhances NOTCH activation to direct self-renewal of TICs. Nat Commun 2020; 11(1): 3084. [http://dx.doi.org/10.1038/s41467-020-16616-8] [PMID: 32555153]

[5] Torre LA, Bray F, Siegel RL, Ferlay J, Lortet-Tieulent J, Jemal A. Global cancer statistics, 2012. CA Cancer J Clin 2015; 65(2): 87-108. [http://dx.doi.org/10.3322/caac.21262] [PMID: 25651787]

[6] Bruix J, Sherman M. American Association for the Study of Liver Diseases. Management of hepatocellular carcinoma: An update. Hepatology 2011; 53(3): 1020-2. [http://dx.doi.org/10.1002/hep.24199] [PMID: 21374666]

[7] Kudo M, Finn RS, Qin S, *et al.* Lenvatinib *versus* sorafenib in first-line treatment of patients with unresectable hepatocellular carcinoma: A randomised phase 3 non-inferiority trial. Lancet 2018; 391(10126): 1163-73. [http://dx.doi.org/10.1016/S0140-6736(18)30207-1] [PMID: 29433850]

[8] Singh D, Khan MA, Akhtar K, Arjmand F, Siddique HR. Apigenin alleviates cancer drug Sorafenib induced multiple toxic effects in Swiss albino mice *via* anti-oxidative stress. Toxicol Appl Pharmacol 2022; 447: 116072. [http://dx.doi.org/10.1016/j.taap.2022.116072] [PMID: 35613639]

[9] Bruix J, Qin S, Merle P, *et al.* Regorafenib for patients with hepatocellular carcinoma who progressed on sorafenib treatment (RESORCE): A randomised, double-blind, placebo-controlled, phase 3 trial. Lancet 2017; 389(10064): 56-66.

[http://dx.doi.org/10.1016/S0140-6736(16)32453-9] [PMID: 27932229]

[10] Abou-Alfa GK, Meyer T, Cheng AL, *et al.* Cabozantinib in patients with advanced and progressing hepatocellular carcinoma. N Engl J Med 2018; 379(1): 54-63. [http://dx.doi.org/10.1056/NEJMoa1717002] [PMID: 29972759]

[11] Zhu AX, Park JO, Ryoo BY, *et al.* Ramucirumab *versus* placebo as second-line treatment in patients with advanced hepatocellular carcinoma following first-line therapy with sorafenib (REACH): a randomised, double-blind, multicentre, phase 3 trial. Lancet Oncol 2015; 16(7): 859-70. [http://dx.doi.org/10.1016/S1470-2045(15)00050-9] [PMID: 26095784]

[12] El-Khoueiry AB, Sangro B, Yau T, *et al.* Nivolumab in patients with advanced hepatocellular carcinoma (CheckMate 040): An open-label, non-comparative, phase 1/2 dose escalation and expansion trial. Lancet 2017; 389(10088): 2492-502. [http://dx.doi.org/10.1016/S0140-6736(17)31046-2] [PMID: 28434648]

[13] Llovet JM, Hernandez-Gea V. Hepatocellular carcinoma: Reasons for phase III failure and novel perspectives on trial design. Clin Cancer Res 2014; 20(8): 2072-9. [http://dx.doi.org/10.1158/1078-0432.CCR-13-0547] [PMID: 24589894]

[14] Burney I, Lakhtakia R. Precision Medicine: Where have we reached and where are we headed? Sultan Qaboos Univ Med J 2017; 17(3): 255-e258. [http://dx.doi.org/10.18295/squmj.2017.17.03.001] [PMID: 29062546]

[15] Forner A, Reig M, Bruix J. Hepatocellular carcinoma. Lancet 2018; 391(10127): 1301-14. [http://dx.doi.org/10.1016/S0140-6736(18)30010-2] [PMID: 29307467]

[16] Galle PR, Forner A, Llovet JM, Mazzaferro V, Piscaglia F, Raoul JL, *et al.* European association for the study of the liver easl clinical practice guidelines: Management of hepatocellular carcinoma. J Hepatol 2019; 70: 817.

[17] Zehir A, Benayed R, Shah RH, *et al.* Mutational landscape of metastatic cancer revealed from prospective clinical sequencing of 10,000 patients. Nat Med 2017; 23(6): 703-13. [http://dx.doi.org/10.1038/nm.4333] [PMID: 28481359]

[18] Zheng H, Pomyen Y, Hernandez MO, *et al.* Single-cell analysis reveals cancer stem cell heterogeneity in hepatocellular carcinoma. Hepatology 2018; 68(1): 127-40. [http://dx.doi.org/10.1002/hep.29778] [PMID: 29315726]

[19] Kudo M, Chung H, Osaki Y. Prognostic staging system for hepatocellular carcinoma (CLIP score): Its value and limitations, and a proposal for a new staging system, the Japan Integrated Staging Score (JIS score). J Gastroenterol 2003; 38(3): 207-15. [http://dx.doi.org/10.1007/s005350300038] [PMID: 12673442]

[20] Sobin LH, Compton CC. TNM seventh edition: What's new, what's changed. Cancer 2010; 116(22): 5336-9. [http://dx.doi.org/10.1002/cncr.25537] [PMID: 20665503]

[21] Yau T, Tang VYF, Yao TJ, Fan ST, Lo CM, Poon RTP. Development of hong kong liver cancer staging system with treatment stratification for patients with hepatocellular carcinoma. Gastroenterology 2014; 146(7): 1691-1700.e3. [http://dx.doi.org/10.1053/j.gastro.2014.02.032] [PMID: 24583061]

[22] Llovet J, Brú C, Bruix J. Prognosis of hepatocellular carcinoma: The BCLC staging classification. Semin Liver Dis 1999; 19(3): 329-38. [http://dx.doi.org/10.1055/s-2007-1007122] [PMID: 10518312]

[23] Bruix J, Sherman M. Management of hepatocellular carcinoma: An update. Hepatology 2011; 53(3): 1020-2. [http://dx.doi.org/10.1002/hep.24199] [PMID: 21374666]

[24] Galle PR, Forner A, Llovet JM, *et al.* Electronic address: Easloffice@easloffice.eu; European Association for the Study of the Liver. EASL Clinical Practice Guidelines: Management of

hepatocellular carcinoma. J Hepatol 2018; 69(1): 182-236. [http://dx.doi.org/10.1016/j.jhep.2018.03.019] [PMID: 29628281]

[25] Bruix J, Takayama T, Mazzaferro V, *et al.* Adjuvant sorafenib for hepatocellular carcinoma after resection or ablation (STORM): A phase 3, randomised, double-blind, placebo-controlled trial. Lancet Oncol 2015; 16(13): 1344-54. [http://dx.doi.org/10.1016/S1470-2045(15)00198-9] [PMID: 26361969]

[26] Llovet JM, Real MI, Montaña X, *et al.* Arterial embolisation or chemoembolisation *versus* symptomatic treatment in patients with unresectable hepatocellular carcinoma: a randomised controlled trial. Lancet 2002; 359(9319): 1734-9. [http://dx.doi.org/10.1016/S0140-6736(02)08649-X] [PMID: 12049862]

[27] Lo CM, Ngan H, Tso WK, *et al.* Randomized controlled trial of transarterial lipiodol chemoembolization for unresectable hepatocellular carcinoma. Hepatology 2002; 35(5): 1164-71. [http://dx.doi.org/10.1053/jhep.2002.33156] [PMID: 11981766]

[28] Llovet J, Bruix J. Systematic review of randomized trials for unresectable hepatocellular carcinoma: Chemoembolization improves survival. Hepatology 2003; 37(2): 429-42. [http://dx.doi.org/10.1053/jhep.2003.50047] [PMID: 12540794]

[29] Llovet JM, Ricci S, Mazzaferro V, *et al.* Sorafenib in advanced hepatocellular carcinoma. N Engl J Med 2008; 359(4): 378-90. [http://dx.doi.org/10.1056/NEJMoa0708857] [PMID: 18650514]

[30] Yeo W, Mok TS, Zee B, *et al.* A randomized phase III study of doxorubicin *versus* cisplatin/interferon alpha-2b/doxorubicin/fluorouracil (PIAF) combination chemotherapy for unresectable hepatocellular carcinoma. J Natl Cancer Inst 2005; 97(20): 1532-8. [http://dx.doi.org/10.1093/jnci/dji315] [PMID: 16234567]

[31] Abou-Alfa GK, Johnson P, Knox JJ, *et al.* Doxorubicin plus sorafenib *vs* doxorubicin alone in patients with advanced hepatocellular carcinoma: A randomized trial. JAMA 2010; 304(19): 2154-60. [http://dx.doi.org/10.1001/jama.2010.1672] [PMID: 21081728]

[32] Qin S, Bai Y, Lim HY, *et al.* Randomized, multicenter, open-label study of oxaliplatin plus fluorouracil/leucovorin *versus* doxorubicin as palliative chemotherapy in patients with advanced hepatocellular carcinoma from Asia. J Clin Oncol 2013; 31(28): 3501-8. [http://dx.doi.org/10.1200/JCO.2012.44.5643] [PMID: 23980077]

[33] Cheng AL, Kang YK, Chen Z, *et al.* Efficacy and safety of sorafenib in patients in the Asia-Pacific region with advanced hepatocellular carcinoma: A phase III randomised, double-blind, placebo-controlled trial. Lancet Oncol 2009; 10(1): 25-34. [http://dx.doi.org/10.1016/S1470-2045(08)70285-7] [PMID: 19095497]

[34] Reig M, Torres F, Rodriguez-Lope C, *et al.* Early dermatologic adverse events predict better outcome in HCC patients treated with sorafenib. J Hepatol 2014; 61(2): 318-24. [http://dx.doi.org/10.1016/j.jhep.2014.03.030] [PMID: 24703956]

[35] Bruix J, Cheng AL, Meinhardt G, Nakajima K, De Sanctis Y, Llovet J. Prognostic factors and predictors of sorafenib benefit in patients with hepatocellular carcinoma: Analysis of two phase III studies. J Hepatol 2017; 67(5): 999-1008. [http://dx.doi.org/10.1016/j.jhep.2017.06.026] [PMID: 28687477]

[36] Iavarone M, Cabibbo G, Piscaglia F, *et al.* Field-practice study of sorafenib therapy for hepatocellular carcinoma: A prospective multicenter study in Italy. Hepatology 2011; 54(6): 2055-63. [http://dx.doi.org/10.1002/hep.24644] [PMID: 21898496]

[37] Ganten TM, Stauber RE, Schott E, *et al.* Sorafenib in patients with hepatocellular carcinoma—results of the observational INSIGHT Study. Clin Cancer Res 2017; 23(19): 5720-8. [http://dx.doi.org/10.1158/1078-0432.CCR-16-0919] [PMID: 28698202]

[38] Wilhelm SM, Adnane L, Newell P, Villanueva A, Llovet JM, Lynch M. Preclinical overview of

sorafenib, a multikinase inhibitor that targets both Raf and VEGF and PDGF receptor tyrosine kinase signaling. Mol Cancer Ther 2008; 7(10): 3129-40. [http://dx.doi.org/10.1158/1535-7163.MCT-08-0013] [PMID: 18852116]

[39] Lencioni R, Llovet JM, Han G, *et al.* Sorafenib or placebo plus TACE with doxorubicin-eluting beads for intermediate stage HCC: The SPACE trial. J Hepatol 2016; 64(5): 1090-8. [http://dx.doi.org/10.1016/j.jhep.2016.01.012] [PMID: 26809111]

[40] Meyer T, Fox R, Ma YT, *et al.* Sorafenib in combination with transarterial chemoembolisation in patients with unresectable hepatocellular carcinoma (TACE 2): a randomised placebo-controlled, double-blind, phase 3 trial. Lancet Gastroenterol Hepatol 2017; 2(8): 565-75. [http://dx.doi.org/10.1016/S2468-1253(17)30156-5] [PMID: 28648803]

[41] Cheng AL, Kang YK, Lin DY, *et al.* Sunitinib *versus* sorafenib in advanced hepatocellular cancer: Results of a randomized phase III trial. J Clin Oncol 2013; 31(32): 4067-75. [http://dx.doi.org/10.1200/JCO.2012.45.8372] [PMID: 24081937]

[42] Johnson PJ, Qin S, Park JW, *et al.* Brivanib *versus* sorafenib as first-line therapy in patients with unresectable, advanced hepatocellular carcinoma: results from the randomized phase III BRISK-FL study. J Clin Oncol 2013; 31(28): 3517-24. [http://dx.doi.org/10.1200/JCO.2012.48.4410] [PMID: 23980084]

[43] Zhu AX, Kudo M, Assenat E, *et al.* Effect of everolimus on survival in advanced hepatocellular carcinoma after failure of sorafenib: the EVOLVE-1 randomized clinical trial. JAMA 2014; 312(1): 57-67. [http://dx.doi.org/10.1001/jama.2014.7189] [PMID: 25058218]

[44] Cainap C, Qin S, Huang WT, *et al.* Linifanib *versus* Sorafenib in patients with advanced hepatocellular carcinoma: Results of a randomized phase III trial. J Clin Oncol 2015; 33(2): 172-9. [http://dx.doi.org/10.1200/JCO.2013.54.3298] [PMID: 25488963]

[45] Vilgrain V, Pereira H, Assenat E, *et al.* Efficacy and safety of selective internal radiotherapy with yttrium-90 resin microspheres compared with sorafenib in locally advanced and inoperable hepatocellular carcinoma (SARAH): An open-label randomised controlled phase 3 trial. Lancet Oncol 2017; 18(12): 1624-36. [http://dx.doi.org/10.1016/S1470-2045(17)30683-6] [PMID: 29107679]

[46] Chow PKH, Gandhi M, Tan SB, *et al.* SIRveNIB: Selective Internal Radiation Therapy *Versus* Sorafenib in Asia-Pacific Patients With Hepatocellular Carcinoma. J Clin Oncol 2018; 36(19): 1913-21. [http://dx.doi.org/10.1200/JCO.2017.76.0892] [PMID: 29498924]

[47] Llovet JM, Montal R, Sia D, Finn RS. Molecular therapies and precision medicine for hepatocellular carcinoma. Nat Rev Clin Oncol 2018; 15(10): 599-616. [http://dx.doi.org/10.1038/s41571-018-0073-4] [PMID: 30061739]

[48] Ikeda K, Kudo M, Kawazoe S, *et al.* Phase 2 study of lenvatinib in patients with advanced hepatocellular carcinoma. J Gastroenterol 2017; 52(4): 512-9. [http://dx.doi.org/10.1007/s00535-016-1263-4] [PMID: 27704266]

[49] Wilhelm SM, Dumas J, Adnane L, *et al.* Regorafenib (BAY 73-4506): A new oral multikinase inhibitor of angiogenic, stromal and oncogenic receptor tyrosine kinases with potent preclinical antitumor activity. Int J Cancer 2011; 129(1): 245-55. [http://dx.doi.org/10.1002/ijc.25864] [PMID: 21170960]

[50] Bruix J, Tak WY, Gasbarrini A, *et al.* Regorafenib as second-line therapy for intermediate or advanced hepatocellular carcinoma: Multicentre, open-label, phase II safety study. Eur J Cancer 2013; 49(16): 3412-9. [http://dx.doi.org/10.1016/j.ejca.2013.05.028] [PMID: 23809766]

[51] Bruix J, Qin S, Merle P, *et al.* Regorafenib for patients with hepatocellular carcinoma who progressed on sorafenib treatment (RESORCE): a randomised, double-blind, placebo-controlled, phase 3 trial.

Lancet 2017; 389(10064): 56-66.
[http://dx.doi.org/10.1016/S0140-6736(16)32453-9] [PMID: 27932229]

[52] Finn RS, Merle P, Granito A, *et al.* Outcomes of sequential treatment with sorafenib followed by regorafenib for HCC: Additional analyses from the phase III RESORCE trial. J Hepatol 2018; 69(2): 353-8.
[http://dx.doi.org/10.1016/j.jhep.2018.04.010] [PMID: 29704513]

[53] Goyal L, Muzumdar MD, Zhu AX. Targeting the HGF/c-MET pathway in hepatocellular carcinoma. Clin Cancer Res 2013; 19(9): 2310-8.
[http://dx.doi.org/10.1158/1078-0432.CCR-12-2791] [PMID: 23388504]

[54] Sieg M, Hartmann M, Settmacher U, Arefian H. Comparative cost-effectiveness of cabozantinib as second-line therapy for patients with advanced hepatocellular carcinoma in Germany and the United States. BMC Gastroenterol 2020; 20(1): 120.
[http://dx.doi.org/10.1186/s12876-020-01241-y] [PMID: 32316925]

[55] Ding XX, Zhu QG, Zhang SM, *et al.* Precision medicine for hepatocellular carcinoma: Driver mutations and targeted therapy. Oncotarget 2017; 8(33): 55715-30.
[http://dx.doi.org/10.18632/oncotarget.18382] [PMID: 28903454]

[56] Zhu AX, Finn RS, Mulcahy M, *et al.* A phase II and biomarker study of ramucirumab, a human monoclonal antibody targeting the VEGF receptor-2, as first-line monotherapy in patients with advanced hepatocellular cancer. Clin Cancer Res 2013; 19(23): 6614-23.
[http://dx.doi.org/10.1158/1078-0432.CCR-13-1442] [PMID: 24088738]

[57] Zhu AX, Park JO, Ryoo BY, *et al.* Ramucirumab *versus* placebo as second-line treatment in patients with advanced hepatocellular carcinoma following first-line therapy with sorafenib (REACH): a randomised, double-blind, multicentre, phase 3 trial. Lancet Oncol 2015; 16(7): 859-70.
[http://dx.doi.org/10.1016/S1470-2045(15)00050-9] [PMID: 26095784]

[58] Zhu AX, Kang YK, Yen CJ, *et al.* Ramucirumab after sorafenib in patients with advanced hepatocellular carcinoma and increased α-fetoprotein concentrations (REACH-2): a randomised, double-blind, placebo-controlled, phase 3 trial. Lancet Oncol 2019; 20(2): 282-96.
[http://dx.doi.org/10.1016/S1470-2045(18)30937-9] [PMID: 30665869]

[59] Kudo M, Okusaka T, Motomura K, *et al.* Ramucirumab after prior sorafenib in patients with advanced hepatocellular carcinoma and elevated alpha-fetoprotein: Japanese subgroup analysis of the REACH-2 trial. J Gastroenterol 2020; 55(6): 627-39.
[http://dx.doi.org/10.1007/s00535-020-01668-w] [PMID: 32107609]

[60] Singh D, Khan MA, Siddique HR. Role of p53-miRNAs circuitry in immune surveillance and cancer development: A potential avenue for therapeutic intervention. Semin Cell Dev Biol 2022; 124: 15-25.
[http://dx.doi.org/10.1016/j.semcdb.2021.04.003] [PMID: 33875349]

[61] Abd El Aziz MA, Facciorusso A, Nayfeh T, *et al.* Immune checkpoint inhibitors for unresectable hepatocellular carcinoma. Vaccines 2020; 8(4): 616.
[http://dx.doi.org/10.3390/vaccines8040616] [PMID: 33086471]

[62] Singh D, Khan MA, Siddique HR. Specific targeting of cancer stem cells by immunotherapy: A possible stratagem to restrain cancer recurrence and metastasis. Biochem Pharmacol 2022; 198: 114955.
[http://dx.doi.org/10.1016/j.bcp.2022.114955] [PMID: 35181312]

[63] Pinato DJ, Guerra N, Fessas P, *et al.* Immune-based therapies for hepatocellular carcinoma. Oncogene 2020; 39(18): 3620-37.
[http://dx.doi.org/10.1038/s41388-020-1249-9] [PMID: 32157213]

[64] Fukumura D, Kloepper J, Amoozgar Z, Duda DG, Jain RK. Enhancing cancer immunotherapy using antiangiogenics: opportunities and challenges. Nat Rev Clin Oncol 2018; 15(5): 325-40.
[http://dx.doi.org/10.1038/nrclinonc.2018.29] [PMID: 29508855]

[65] Khan KA, Kerbel RS. Improving immunotherapy outcomes with anti-angiogenic treatments and *vice versa.* Nat Rev Clin Oncol 2018; 15(5): 310-24.
[http://dx.doi.org/10.1038/nrclinonc.2018.9] [PMID: 29434333]

[66] Santoro A, Rimassa L, Borbath I, *et al.* Tivantinib for second-line treatment of advanced hepatocellular carcinoma: A randomised, placebo-controlled phase 2 study. Lancet Oncol 2013; 14(1): 55-63.
[http://dx.doi.org/10.1016/S1470-2045(12)70490-4] [PMID: 23182627]

[67] Rimassa L, Assenat E, Peck-Radosavljevic M, *et al.* Second-line tivantinib (ARQ 197) vs placebo in patients (Pts) with MET-high hepatocellular carcinoma (HCC): Results of the METIV-HCC phase III trial. J Clin Oncol 2017; 35(15_suppl) (Suppl. 15): 4000.
[http://dx.doi.org/10.1200/JCO.2017.35.15_suppl.4000]

[68] Basilico C, Pennacchietti S, Vigna E, *et al.* Tivantinib (ARQ197) displays cytotoxic activity that is independent of its ability to bind MET. Clin Cancer Res 2013; 19(9): 2381-92.
[http://dx.doi.org/10.1158/1078-0432.CCR-12-3459] [PMID: 23532890]

[69] Babina IS, Turner NC. Advances and challenges in targeting FGFR signalling in cancer. Nat Rev Cancer 2017; 17(5): 318-32.
[http://dx.doi.org/10.1038/nrc.2017.8] [PMID: 28303906]

[70] Javle M, Lowery M, Shroff RT, *et al.* Phase II Study of BGJ398 in patients with fgfr-altered advanced cholangiocarcinoma. J Clin Oncol 2018; 36(3): 276-82.
[http://dx.doi.org/10.1200/JCO.2017.75.5009] [PMID: 29182496]

[71] Konecny GE, Finkler N, Garcia AA, *et al.* Second-line dovitinib (TKI258) in patients with FGFR2-mutated or FGFR2-non-mutated advanced or metastatic endometrial cancer: A non-randomised, open-label, two-group, two-stage, phase 2 study. Lancet Oncol 2015; 16(6): 686-94.
[http://dx.doi.org/10.1016/S1470-2045(15)70159-2] [PMID: 25981814]

[72] Wu X, Ge H, Lemon B, *et al.* FGF19-induced hepatocyte proliferation is mediated through FGFR4 activation. J Biol Chem 2010; 285(8): 5165-70.
[http://dx.doi.org/10.1074/jbc.M109.068783] [PMID: 20018895]

[73] Gao L, Wang X, Tang Y, Huang S, Hu CAA, Teng Y. FGF19/FGFR4 signaling contributes to the resistance of hepatocellular carcinoma to sorafenib. J Exp Clin Cancer Res 2017; 36(1): 8.
[http://dx.doi.org/10.1186/s13046-016-0478-9] [PMID: 28069043]

[74] Sawey ET, Chanrion M, Cai C, *et al.* Identification of a therapeutic strategy targeting amplified FGF19 in liver cancer by Oncogenomic screening. Cancer Cell 2011; 19(3): 347-58.
[http://dx.doi.org/10.1016/j.ccr.2011.01.040] [PMID: 21397858]

[75] Finn RS, Aleshin A, Zhao D, *et al.* Abstract 3858: Gains in FGF19 are predictive of response to the fibroblast growth factor receptor (FGFR) small molecule tyrosine kinase inhibitor BGJ 398 *in vitro*. Cancer Res 2012; 72(8_Supplement) (Suppl. 8): 3858. [abstract 3858].
[http://dx.doi.org/10.1158/1538-7445.AM2012-3858]

[76] Guagnano V, Kauffmann A, Wöhrle S, *et al.* FGFR genetic alterations predict for sensitivity to NVP-BGJ398, a selective pan-FGFR inhibitor. Cancer Discov 2012; 2(12): 1118-33.
[http://dx.doi.org/10.1158/2159-8290.CD-12-0210] [PMID: 23002168]

[77] Hagel M, Miduturu C, Sheets M, *et al.* First selective small molecule inhibitor of FGFR4 for the treatment of hepatocellular carcinomas with an activated FGFR4 Signaling Pathway. Cancer Discov 2015; 5(4): 424-37.
[http://dx.doi.org/10.1158/2159-8290.CD-14-1029] [PMID: 25776529]

[78] Joshi JJ, Coffey H, Corcoran E, *et al.* H3B-6527 Is a Potent and Selective Inhibitor of FGFR4 in FGF19-Driven Hepatocellular Carcinoma. Cancer Res 2017; 77(24): 6999-7013.
[http://dx.doi.org/10.1158/0008-5472.CAN-17-1865] [PMID: 29247039]

[79] Villanueva A, Chiang DY, Newell P, Peix J, Thung S, Alsinet C, *et al.* Pivotal role of mTOR signaling

in hepatocellular carcinoma. Gastroenterology 2008; 135(6): 1972-83. [http://dx.doi.org/10.1053/j.gastro.2008.08.008]

[80] Matter MS, Decaens T, Andersen JB, Thorgeirsson SS. Targeting the mTOR pathway in hepatocellular carcinoma: Current state and future trends. J Hepatol 2014; 60(4): 855-65. [http://dx.doi.org/10.1016/j.jhep.2013.11.031] [PMID: 24308993]

[81] Janku F, Yap TA, Meric-Bernstam F. Targeting the PI3K pathway in cancer: Are we making headway? Nat Rev Clin Oncol 2018; 15(5): 273-91. [http://dx.doi.org/10.1038/nrclinonc.2018.28] [PMID: 29508857]

[82] Lim HY, Heo J, Choi HJ, *et al.* A phase II study of the efficacy and safety of the combination therapy of the MEK inhibitor refametinib (BAY 86-9766) plus sorafenib for Asian patients with unresectable hepatocellular carcinoma. Clin Cancer Res 2014; 20(23): 5976-85. [http://dx.doi.org/10.1158/1078-0432.CCR-13-3445] [PMID: 25294897]

[83] Lim HY, Merle P, Weiss KH, *et al.* Phase II Studies with Refametinib or Refametinib plus Sorafenib in Patients with *RAS* -Mutated Hepatocellular Carcinoma. Clin Cancer Res 2018; 24(19): 4650-61. [http://dx.doi.org/10.1158/1078-0432.CCR-17-3588] [PMID: 29950351]

[84] Smyth MJ, Ngiow SF, Ribas A, Teng MWL. Combination cancer immunotherapies tailored to the tumour microenvironment. Nat Rev Clin Oncol 2016; 13(3): 143-58. [http://dx.doi.org/10.1038/nrclinonc.2015.209] [PMID: 26598942]

[85] Weber JS, Yang JC, Atkins MB, Disis ML. Toxicities of immunotherapy for the practitioner. J Clin Oncol 2015; 33(18): 2092-9. [http://dx.doi.org/10.1200/JCO.2014.60.0379] [PMID: 25918278]

[86] Masucci GV, Cesano A, Hawtin R, *et al.* Validation of biomarkers to predict response to immunotherapy in cancer: Volume I — pre-analytical and analytical validation. J Immunother Cancer 2016; 4(1): 76. [http://dx.doi.org/10.1186/s40425-016-0178-1] [PMID: 27895917]

[87] Marcus L, Lemery SJ, Keegan P, Pazdur R. FDA Approval Summary: Pembrolizumab for the treatment of microsatellite instability-high solid tumors. Clin Cancer Res 2019; 25(13): 3753-8. [http://dx.doi.org/10.1158/1078-0432.CCR-18-4070] [PMID: 30787022]

[88] Sia D, Jiao Y, Martinez-Quetglas I, *et al.* Identification of an immune-specific class of hepatocellular carcinoma, based on molecular features. Gastroenterology 2017; 153(3): 812-26. [http://dx.doi.org/10.1053/j.gastro.2017.06.007] [PMID: 28624577]

[89] Spranger S, Bao R, Gajewski TF. Melanoma-intrinsic β-catenin signalling prevents anti-tumour immunity. Nature 2015; 523(7559): 231-5. [http://dx.doi.org/10.1038/nature14404] [PMID: 25970248]

CHAPTER 4

Protein Structures, Aggregation, Misfolding, Induction Factors and Precision Medicine

Sadia Malik[1], **Sumbul Yasmeen**[1] and **Rizwan Hasan Khan**[1,*]

[1] *Interdisciplinary Biotechnology Unit, Aligarh Muslim University, Aligarh, 202002, India*

Abstract: The aggregation of protein is a complex process influenced by various factors resulting in a wide range of debilitating disorders. These are characterized by the deposition of insoluble plaques consisting of amyloid fibrils rich in β-sheet structures. Many natural proteins form amyloid fibrils and build-up misfolded or aggregated disease-specific proteins in the tissues causing human diseases. The present chapter deals with protein structures, aggregation, misfolding, induction factors, and their involvement in human disease and implications in precision medicine. We have discussed the role of functional amyloids in portraying the mechanism of its formation, highlighting the method of detection of diverse types of aggregates. Moreover, we also contextualized therapeutic strategies to combat the process of aggregation keeping in view that this is a broad field of research that ranges from biophysics to clinical trials. Despite visible progress in the field of biochemistry, we still have questions regarding the aggregation and co-aggregation of protein molecules. However, with the present level of knowledge, it is envisaged that accurate treatments against diseases related to aggregation would be feasible in near future.

Keywords: Human diseases, Induction factor, Protein aggregation, Protein misfolding, Precision medicine, Proteins structures.

INTRODUCTION

Protein misfolding is a detrimental process that is interconnected with aggregation and is known to be involved in a large variety of localized, systemic, non-neuropathic, and neurodegenerative diseases [1, 2]. Owing to its implications in several human diseases, these processes have attracted much attention and have become a dynamic field of research. In some cases, the disease arises when a specific protein adopts a misfolded conformation or encounters trafficking impairment and is no longer functional, resulting in loss-of-function diseases [3]. In contrast, if misfolding and aggregation occur concomitantly resulting in a pathological state then this is regarded as a gain-of-function diseases [4]. Alth-

* **Corresponding author Rizwan Hasan Khan:** Interdisciplinary Biotechnology Unit, Aligarh Muslim University, Aligarh, 202002, India; Tel: +91-571-2720388; Fax: + 91-571-2721776; E-mail: rizwanhkhan1@gmail.com

Farzana Mahdi & Abbas Ali Mahdi (Eds.)

ough protein polymerization can be a physiological process in case of the formation of muscles F-actin filament. However, in several instances, native protein oligomerization has been reported to be connected to specific pathological conditions underlying several human disorders [5, 6]. The diseases in which the misfolded protein aggregates formed are termed "Protein misfolding diseases". The accumulation of diverse proteins in various organs of a human body is the hallmark of protein misfolding disorders (PMDs). Table **1** comprises the list of human diseases linked with the misfolded proteins. The most known protein misfolding disease (PMD) is Amyloidosis, which is known to be caused by the building up of insoluble amyloid fibrils in the extracellular space [7]. Amyloidosis are difficult to diagnose and complicated to study because one or more organs like heart, liver, kidney, pancreas, and the central nervous system may be involved [8]. In localized amyloidosis, intracellular or extracellular deposition of amyloid takes place only in the organ/tissue where the precursor protein synthesis occurs [9]. For example, the accumulation of Aβ and α-synuclein occurs outside of the cells, whereas insoluble toxic protein aggregates of misfolded SOD1 form inside the cells [10]. In contrast to localized amyloidosis, all the systemic amyloidoses remain extracellular. Their onset occurs when the expression and secretion of the precursor protein take place at one site but it gets deposited at distinct sites. The diverse systemic disorders include light chain amyloidosis (AL), heavy chain amyloidosis (AH), secondary amyloidosis (AA), lysozyme amyloidosis (ALys), familial amyloid polyneuropathy (FAP or ATTR), dialysis-related amyloidosis (Aβ2M), *etc* [11].

Table 1. List of human diseases linked with protein misfolding and aggregate formation.

Serial Number	Neurodegenerative Diseases	Aggregating Proteins	Nonneuropathic Systemic Amyloidosis	Aggregating Proteins	Nonneuropathic Localized Diseases	Aggregating Proteins
1	Alzheimer's disease	β-Amyloid (plaques),Tau (neurofibrillary tangles)	Light chain amyloidosis	Immunoglobulin light chain	Type II diabetes	Amyloin (IAPP)
2	Parkinson's disease	α-Synuclein	Heavy chain amyloidosis	Immunoglobulin heavy chain	Medullary carcinoma of thyroid	Calcitonin
3	Dementia with Lewy bodies	α-Synuclein	Lysozyme amyloidosis	Mutants of lysozyme	Injection-localized amyloidosis	Insulin
4	Huntington's diseased	Huntington with polyQ Expansion	Senile systemic amyloidosis	Wild-type transthyretin	Cataract	γ-Crystalline
5	Spongiform encephalopathies	Prion protein or fragments thereof	Familial amyloidotic polyneuropathy	Mutants of transthyretin	Lattice corneal dystrophy	Mainly C-terminal fragments of kerato epithelin
6	Amyotrophic lateral sclerosis	Superoxide dismutase	Cardiac arrhythmias	Fragments of serum amyloid A protein	Corneal amyloidosis associated with trichiasis	Lactoferrins

(Table 1) cont.....

7	Spinocerebellar ataxia	Ataxins with polyQ Expansion	Hemodialysis-related amyloidosis	β2-microglobulin	Atrial amyloidosis	Atrial natriuretic factor
8	Frontotemporal dementia	Hyperphosphorylated TDP-43	Fibrinogen amyloidosis	Variants of fibrinogen α-chain	Aortic medial amyloidosis	Medin
9	Familial British dementia	ABri	Finnish hereditary amyloidosis	Fragments of gesolin mutants	Pulmonary alveolar proteinosis	Lung surfactant protein C
10	Familial Danish dementia	ADan	Cystatin amyloidosis	Cystatin C	Cutaneous lichen amyloidosis	Keratins

When the proteinaceous deposits occur on the neuronal cells resulting in progressive damage to the neurons, then this leads to the onset of neurodegenerative diseases. One of the most studied neurodegenerative disorders is Alzheimer's disease (AD) that affect sizable older populations. AD is a fatal diseases caused by 40-42 amino acids long amyloid beta aggregates [12]. Others include widespread illnesses like Parkinson's disease, Huntington's disease, transmissible spongiform encephalopathies (TSE), and amyotrophic lateral sclerosis (ALS) [13 - 15]. Fig. (**1**), illustrates the diagrammatic representation of the several organs of the human body that are affected by neuropathic as well as non-neuropathic diseases.

Despite diversity at a molecular level, all the proteins have a common property of rapid and spontaneous self-assembly into functional three dimensional structures. However, native conformation is not the only fold available to a polypeptide chain but an alternative state termed as Amyloid may represent primordial of protein folding. Studies have shown that folding of protein and fibril formation are competitive processes that operate parallelly. Basically, the intermediate states determine the diversion of molecules between the folding and aggregation landscapes. We still have a lot to learn to better understand the balance that lies between protein folding and aggregation. The complete understanding regarding the structural properties of different stages of all the proteins folding and aggregation is a major task.

Thus, studying protein aggregation is important to understand the structural and mechanistic basis of the conformational changes and factors that promote the precursor states' conversion into aggregates. In the current review, we tried to delineate the mechanism of amyloid aggregation and the underlying factors that assist in *in vivo* and *in vitro* aggregation of proteins. The strategies to combat protein aggregation have also been discussed. There are several organs that are affected due to protein aggregation as illustrated in the following diagram.

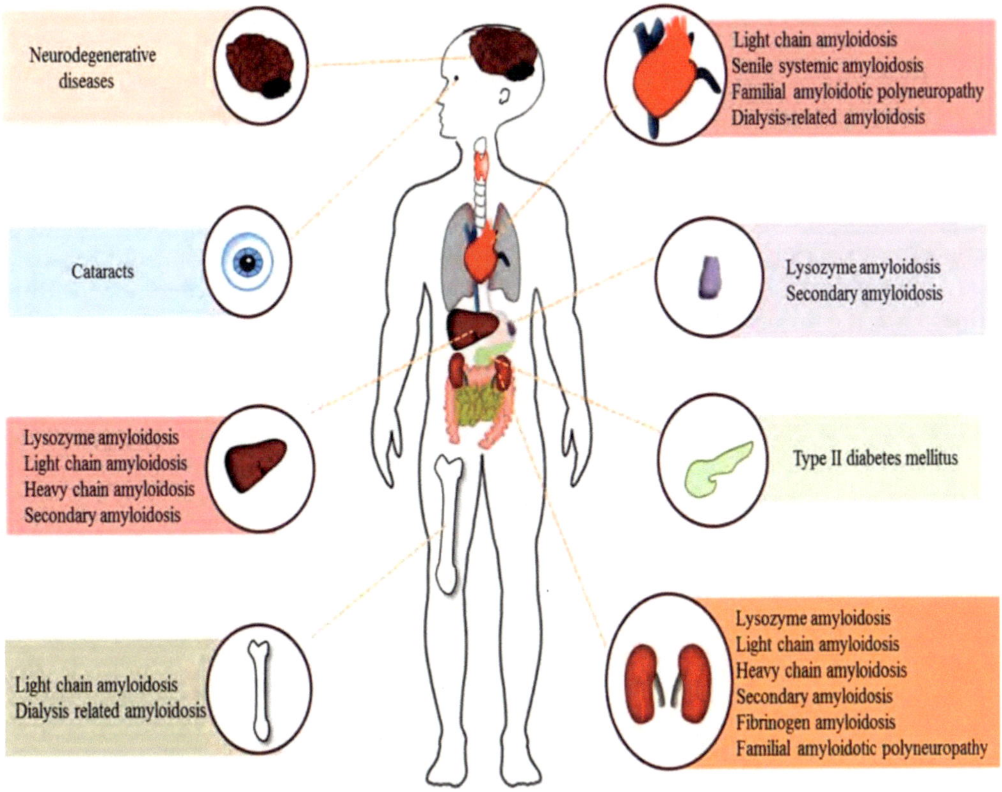

Fig. (1). Diagrammatic illustration of affected organs of the human body by various Neuropathic and non-neuropathic diseases.

Protein Folding, Misfolding and Aggregation

Proteins and peptides are the key macromolecules that perform a vast array of functions and are involved in the maintenance of life processes. For all the proteins to gain a proper structure and function, folding is essential, that is characterized by persistent and well-defined secondary and tertiary structure [16]. This is defined as a native state that is a folded state where a protein is in general highly soluble and stable. This folded state is a three dimensional structure that is a functionally active state. At this state, the propensity for undergoing aberrant aggregation is least since mostly hydrophobic moieties and most of the backbone portion is sequestered inside the protein [17]. Despite all this, there is a propensity for proteins to congregate resulting from the misfolding process. The self-association of several identical misfolded monomers of peptides or proteins into less-soluble non-native structures results in protein aggregation [18].

The proposal of energy landscape was given by Joseph Bryngelson and José N. Onuchic who gave a unique folding funnel with all the intermediate states/transition states. This narrows down to a lesser number of conformational states and lower free energy that merges to global minima corresponding to native conformations of protein (Fig. **2**) [19]. The overall folding process is very rapid and highly efficient. In contrast, partially folded or partially unfolded states also known as misfolded states tend to aggregate depending on the concentration. These are unstable and thermodynamically unfavourable states that tend to have lower energy and show more stability. Similar to the intramolecular folding, mainly hydrophobic forces drive aggregation and thus primarily result in amorphous structures whereas fibrillar aggregates known as amyloid could form that possess β-strands running perpendicular to the fibrillar axis and are characterized as the cross-β sheet rich structure [20]. Importantly, the aggregated fibrils are formed by the soluble oligomers that are less ordered and can be differentiated with the intermediates that are kinetically trapped in the folding funnel [21].

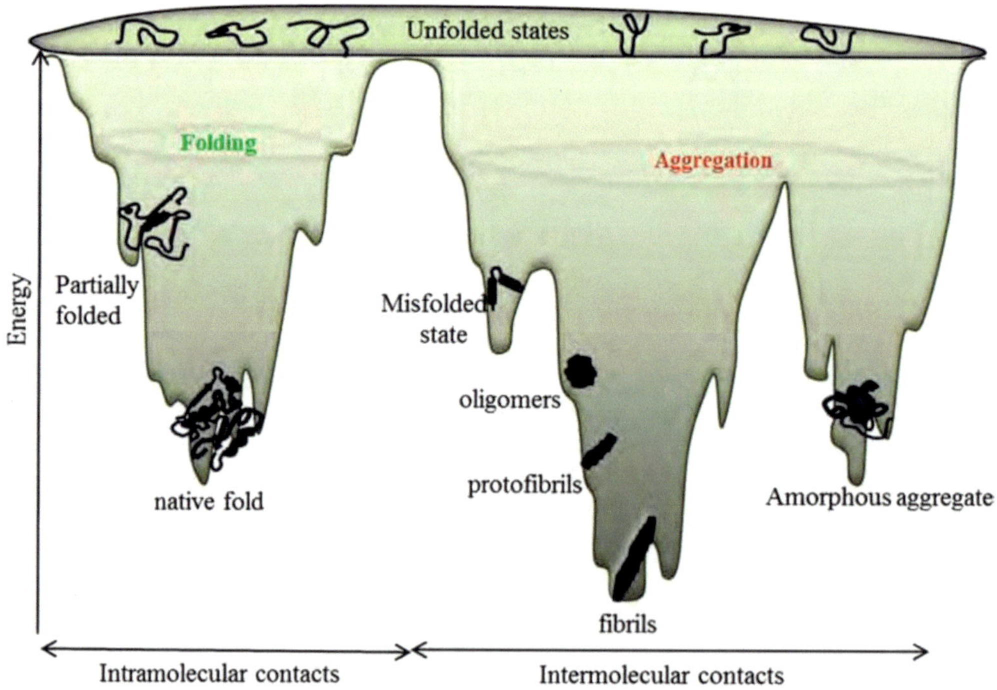

Fig. (2). Combined Energy landscape of protein folding and aggregation pathways depicting different conformational states involved.

Causative Agents of PMDs and Cellular Mechanism of Toxicity

So far we have discussed that the protein that becomes misfolded after the conformational changes results in its diminished physiological function and eventually causes pathological events in PMDs [21]. Although it is known that misfolded proteins are hazardous, there remains a debate over the specific characteristics of misfolded proteins that make them detrimental. It is largely believed that protein deposits which are highly ordered are the main reason for the clinical signs of the disease since protein aggregates and fibrils were found in individuals with protein misfolding diseases [22]. Recent research, however, points to protofibrils, micelles or β-amyloid generated diffusible ligands as the highly effective mediators of cellular harm and neurotoxicity rather than fibrils [23]. Moreover, these soluble oligomers are temporally unstable and thus can change into more developed fibrillar forms very quickly. This course of action is reinforced by the discovery that the level of small oligomeric aggregates, not the big fibrillar species, correlates with the degree of cognitive impairment in protein misfolding illnesses [24].

Inside a cell, protein aggregation may occur due to several reasons. It may result from hyper phosphorylation where several phosphate groups are added to the protein. Alternatively, a self-catalytic conformational change in protein or some mutations may take place rendering the protein unstable [25]. Aging is correlated with aggregated protein accumulation. An abnormal or uncontrolled rise in the intracellular concentration of several proteins can also lead to aggregate formation. Such protein concentration imbalances may result from mutations like amyloidogenic gene duplications or alterations in the amino acid sequence of the protein. Deficiencies in the proteasome system and the cellular mechanism responsible for degrading aged proteins can also result in imbalances [83]. In addition, toxic aggregates present outside or inside of cells can affect a variety of cellular processes. This results in impairment or the blockage of the protein degradation machinery severely affecting the protein quality control system [26, 27]. Also, the reduced expression of chaperones leads to the build-up of hazardous aggregates in cells [28]. Besides having direct harmful effects, misfolded proteins can also trigger inflammatory reactions involving a cascade of events. This leads to the activation of an inflammatory process and may even cause cell death [29]. Neuroinflammation in Alzheimer's disease patients' brains is characterised by the stimulation of local complement system, acute-phase reactions, activation of inducible nitric oxide synthase and elevated C-reactive protein expression [30, 31]. The production of a number of proinflammatory mediators, such as complement factors, cytokines, nitric oxide, secretory products, ROS and free radical species by amyloid-activated microglia cells play key roles in chronic inflammation and neuronal cell death [32, 33]. Different

PMDs especially neurodegenerative diseases are known to have an impaired system of autophagy. In all these processes, perturbed cell membrane permeability, impairment in mitochondrial function, generation of reactive oxygen species, inflammation and disruption of homeostasis take place [34]. Moreover, the misfolded aggregated proteins expose hydrophobic surfaces that are 'sticky' due to their aberrant interactions with other proteins. This results in many normal functional proteins sequestration and loss of their function [35]. Fig. (**3**) summarizes the comparison of the overall protein quality control system in a healthy cell with imbalanced proteasome in an aged cell.

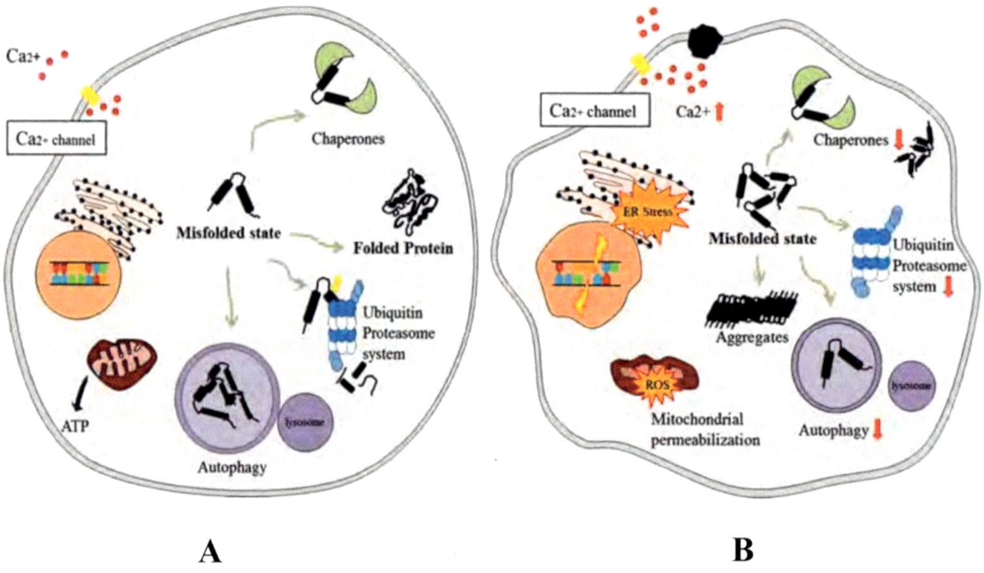

Fig. (3). Comparison of a young healthy cell (A) with an aging cell (B). The Protein Quality Control System protects the cell against misfolded protein aggregation. During ageing, the overload of protein quality control system occurs affecting the important cellular processes.

Recent studies indicate that the cellular impairment caused by aggregates of disease-associated polypeptides is typically the result of earlier disruptions to normal cellular processes. Several studies have shown that changes to the intracellular redox potential and free Ca^{2+} levels exposed to toxic aggregates play a crucial role [36]. Such cells have altered the intracellular redox status, which is accompanied by a sudden rise in reactive oxygen species (ROS). This is similar to the burst that leukocytes use to phagocytose and eliminate foreign invaders. Reactive nitrogen species, protein nitrosylation, lipid peroxidation, NO metabolism and heme oxygenase-1 (a particular indicator of oxidative stress), have also been found in cells affected by the aggregates [37, 38]. Additionally, it has been demonstrated that anti-oxidants such as tocopherol, lipoic acid, and reduced glutathione can shield cells from cumulative damage [39 - 42]. Regarding this, a fascinating study on prion-infected mice was conducted that showed that the damage to the brain is caused by an enhancement in free radical production, which is accompanied by decreased mitochondrial anti-oxidant defences, which cause the prion disease development [43]. Additionally, protein misfolding illnesses have been linked to the mitogen-activated protein kinase (MAPK) pathway activation [44]. Under stressful situations, like oxidative stress and heat shock, cell responds by activating the MAPK pathway that hampers subsequent normal reactions.

In the majority of biological systems, protein misfolding and aggregation are the inherent side effects of the conformational shifts necessary for the organism's proper operation. The development of aggregates is typically prevented by molecular chaperones and protease degradation mechanisms [127]. However, in some cases, these aggregation processes can elude the natural safeguards and result in no degradation of the proteins. The relationship between proteostasis and protein folding energetics suggests that chemical and biological agents can target the proteostasis network to stop the production and build-up of amyloid.

Under environmental stress conditions, higher amounts of proteases and chaperones may be produced in the cell which will improve the removal of hazardous aggregates [45]. Chaperones like clusterin, α2-macroglobulin and haptoglobin act on a range of aggregating proteins by different mechanisms [46, 47]. All human tissues including the brain, express a stress-related molecular chaperone-clusterin. In at least 11 diseases, clusterin co-localizes with extracellular amyloid deposits. *In vitro* tests have demonstrated that clusterin binds to prefibrillar aggregates to stop further aggregation and the development of amyloid [48]. By hydrolysing ATP, molecular chaperones that are ATP-dependent including Hsp60, Hsp70, Hsp90, and Hsp100 facilitate protein folding [49]. Other non-ATP-dependent intracellular chaperones, such as Hsp27 and αB-crystallin of the small Hsp family, also function to buffer aggregation and amyloid formation [50, 51]. For instance, it is well known that Hsp27 may prevent fibril formation of Aβ42, and that αB-crystallin can prevent the formation of amyloid of both Aβ42 and α-synuclein [52, 53].

Structural Features of Amyloid Fibrils and Oligomers

It is known that the association of misfolded proteins in an abnormal way leads to the aggregates formation. Under physiological conditions, it is possible that aggregates of small proteins may remain soluble. However, precipitation of larger protein aggregates takes place out of the solution. Morphologically aggregates can be differentiated into amorphous aggregates and amyloid fibrils [54]. When imaged by electron microscopy, amorphous aggregates appear to be granular consisting mostly of disordered polypeptide chains whereas all polypeptides adopt a common amyloid fibrillar structure that appears to be highly ordered and repetitive in structure [55, 56]. Previously, the understanding of the molecular detailing of amyloid fibrils has been quite challenging because of being low in solubility and large in size along with the non-crystalline nature. However, the discovery of solid state NMR has led to the progression in understanding the detailed structures of amyloid fibrils [57]. Amyloid fibrils display thread like aggregates composed typically of multiple twisted proto-filaments having a diameter of approx. ~10 nm [58]. Amyloid fibrils of each protein possess the same structural cross-β motif where the β-sheets runs parallel and β-strands orient perpendicular to the fibril axis [59]. The separation between β-strands and its layers is ~0.48 nm and ~ 1.0–1.3 nm, respectively [60].

The fibril forming monomers or subunits have a defined cross-array, which gives an amyloid fibril its tertiary structure [61]. These monomers or subunits subsequently self-assemble into an amyloid fibril with a quaternary structure [62]. A normal fibril includes two to six protofilaments at its core [63]. A probable structure consists of a densely packed arrangement, in which the protofilaments wound around one another in a rope-like way to produce a super coiled structure similar to a rope [64]. According to a research using AFM technology, the fibrillar protofilaments can also create a ribbon-like lateral-packing configuration, in which monomers individually form a ribbon of width of up to five monomers [65]. The monomers first create protofibrils lining to form a fibril that finally generates the fibrils by twisting at a regular interval [66].

A series of consecutive steps are involved here that initiates with the monomer and reaches a point where no further polymerization takes place. It is obvious that the growth of oligomer is accompanied by the loss of monomer as depicted in Fig. (**4**). A wide variety of sizes and shapes of soluble oligomers, huge spherical aggregates or fibril-like aggregates such as protofibrils or even annular aggregates, can occur on or off the path to amyloid [67]. The production of fibril seeds is necessary for the transformation into fibrils with a regular cross-secondary structure (nucleation) [68]. From the molecular perspective, this is still a puzzling process, however, evidence points to a coordinated conformational shift of peptides in oligomers or protofibrils that enlarge and entangle to create mature fibril.

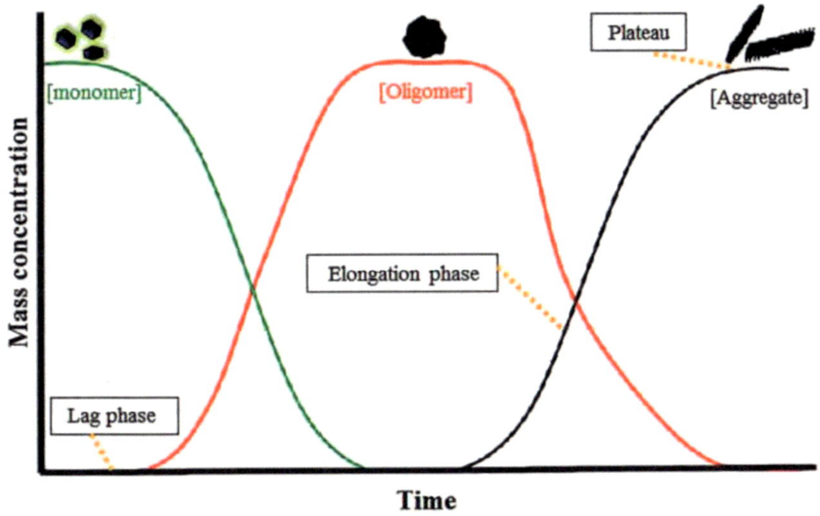

Fig. (4). Time profile depicting the loss of monomer linked with the growth of oligomer/aggregates. A series of consecutive steps that start with the native monomer followed by oligomers and eventually aggregates formation (mature fibrils or amorphous aggregates).

In both *in vitro* and *in vivo* settings, amyloid aggregates are regarded as ordered and amorphous aggregates as the disordered ones are based mainly on their shape. Inclusion bodies, which are referred to as amorphous aggregates, are discovered under *in vivo* conditions [69]. It is connected to age-related disorders, such as cataracts connected to patients' α-crystallin aggregation. Additionally, amorphous aggregates more often are discovered during the production and purification of proteins. Also, protein denaturation leads to the emergence of unfolded conformations with exposed hydrophobic surfaces, which have a higher aggregation propensity [70].

Mechanism of Amyloid Formation

The amyloid aggregates are formed and accumulated by following the seeding nucleation model. In this case, the rate-limiting step is the generation of small soluble misfolded proteins that act as nuclei/seeds accelerating the misfolding process by recruiting more native proteins [71]. After a critical concentration is attained, the misfolded proteins are thus formed to generate oligomers resulting in the protofibrils formation that eventually terminates to mature fibrils as shown in Fig. (**5**). Oligomers (dimer, hexamer, dodecamer, or higher order structure) appear in intermediate stages that are small aggregates exhibiting lower growth rate when compared to fibrils and are structurally highly variable [72]. Based on their direct or indirect participation in the fibrillation, they are classified as on-pathway oligomers and off-pathway oligomers, respectively [73] [67].

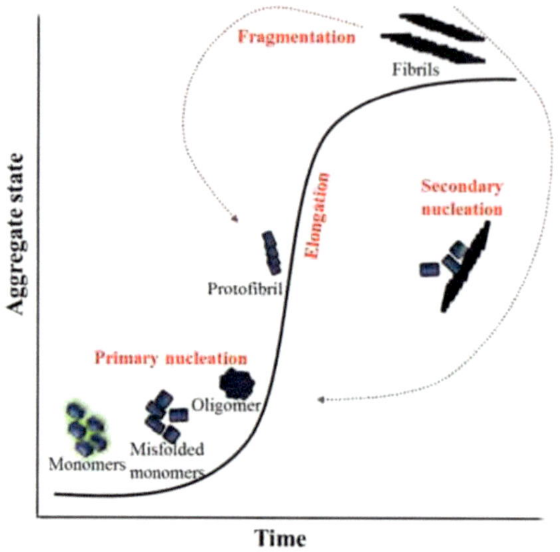

Fig. (5). Schematic representation of different intermediate species involved in the process of amyloid fibrillation.

In the nucleation model, during the lag phase, misfolded seeds are produced which nucleate the same protein aggregation (homologous seeding) or aggregation with another protein that is amyloidogenic (heterologous seeding or also known as cross-seeding) [74]. This phase is thermodynamically unfavourable and rate-limiting because a conformational change in correctly folded proteins to unstable misfolded intermediates takes place in this step [75]. This transition in the conformation happens due to stabilization brought about by oligomerization. The misfolded oligomers then enter the exponential or polymerization phase, where the recruitment of native proteins takes place with their simultaneous rapid misfolding. Certainly, these aggregates thus develop into large as well as insoluble proteolytically-resistant moiety resilient to clearance by cellular machinery. In general, amyloid formation takes place *via* nucleation-dependent oligomerization. Therefore the above mentioned mechanism is highly convincing to illustrate the protein aggregation phenomenon. In addition, upon introducing a preformed seed, we can further lead to the acceleration of the reaction by the nucleation phase attenuation [76]. Also, preformed fibrils may fragment or may provide the surface to catalyse new fibrils' formation thereby accelerating the polymerisation reaction. Along with providing accessible surface areas, few fibrils also possess the ability to generate new fibrillar ends that involve secondary nucleation reactions affecting the overall kinetics of amyloid fibrillation. Therefore, it should be noted that even though mature fibrils are considered as end-point structures, there is an involvement of continuous association and dissociation events that result in amyloid fibrils molecular recycling.

Functional Amyloids

Amyloids are usually linked to illnesses but they have several useful properties [77]. Bacteria are particularly helpful for "amyloid hunting" due to their relatively accessible cellular organisation, both as single-species colonies on agar plates and as multispecies biofilm communities. Table **2** enlists the functional amyloid proteins with their functional roles [78].

Table 2. Naturally occurring functional amyloid with their specific functions.

Serial Number	Proteins	Species	Functions	Reference
1	Chaplins	*Streptomyces coelicolor* (bacterium)	Allow aerial hypha development and lower down the surface tension of water.	[79]
2	Curlin	*Escherichia coli* (bacterium)	Mediates binding to host proteins, inert surfaces colonization.	[80]
3	Ure2p (prion)	*Saccharomyces cerevisiae* (yeast)	Promotion of poor nitrogen sources uptake ([URE3]).	[81]
4	Sup35p (prion)	*Saccharomyces cerevisiae* (yeast)	Facilitates the read through of stop codons on mRNA and conferment of new phenotypes ([PSI+]).	[82]
5	HET-s (prion)	*Podospora anserina* (fungus)	Triggers a complex programmed cell death phenomenon.	[83]
6	Hydrophobin	*Neurospora crassa* (fungus)	Allows aerial hypha development and lowers down the surface tension of water.	[84]
7	Spidroin	*Nephila edulis* (spider)	Formation of silk fibers of web.	[85]
89	Proteins of the chorion of the eggshell	*Bombyx mori* (silkworm)	Protection of the oocytes and the development of embryo from environmental hazards.	[86]
9	Intralumenal domain of Pmel17	*Homo sapiens* (humans)	Formation of inside melanosomes, fibrous striations upon which melanin granules form.	[87]

Because Amyloids maintain their nature, they offer a structural template for reproduction, which enables growth that resembles an 1D crystal or a prion mechanism that spreads as tiny fibril fragments to cause infection [88]. Close spacing of similar side chains inside the cross β-structure can produce a unique binding specificity not present in the monomeric form. A single amphipathic β-strand, for instance, could have lower affinity to bind a membrane, whereas an amyloid fibril composed of same peptide may bind lipids with great tenacity. A ligand may simply bounce from one binding pocket to the next on the amyloid surface, boosting the total apparent binding of a ligand and resulting in a very low dissociation rate. This is known as the cooperativity or avidity effect. In fact, it has been suggested that functional amyloid in bacterial biofilms operate as sponges or reservoirs, holding onto tiny quorum-sensing molecules inside the biofilm by offering a large repeating binding surface [89]. A bigger protein may also have amyloid regions as oligomerization domains.

Induction Factors Causing Aggregation

It has been found that under carefully designed *in vitro* condition, proteins can form β-sheet-rich amyloid fibrils irrespective of their native structures that led to the consensus that 'polypeptides have a generic property of amyloid formation' [90]. Assembly and organization of fibril, the kinetics of fibrillation as well as the overall stability of the fibrils are significantly influenced by the sequence of amino acid of proteins and their environmental conditions [91]. Various factors involved in amyloid fibril formation include the protein's native conformation destabilization induced by changing temperature, pH, ionic strength *etc.* that results in the partially folded intermediates' formation (Fig. **6**) [92]. Such partially folded conformers may undergo conformational rearrangements by the reorganizing specific noncovalent intermolecular interactions- hydrogen bonding, electrostatic interactions and hydrophobic contacts that eventually lead to the oligomerization and thus fibril formation [93].

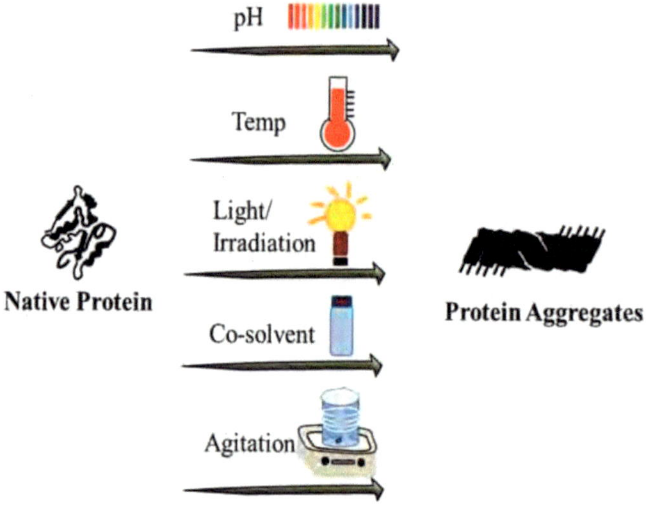

Fig. (6). Major *in vitro* factors affecting the formation of protein aggregates.

A wide variety of factors can induce protein aggregation that includes temperature, mechanical stress (vigorous shaking), freezing or thawing. It may also occur during the biopharmaceuticals manufacturing processes that include fermentation and purification followed by the formulation, then shipment and finally storage [94, 95]. Furthermore, parameters of formulation like the concentration of proteins, pH, qualitative and quantitative composition play an important role in protein aggregation [96]. This section outlines few factors that have been reported to cause the formation of protein aggregates.

A protein misfolds when once exposed to increased temperature by losing its native conformation because the higher temperature directly affects the conformation of the polypeptide chains at the level of its secondary, tertiary and quaternary structure, and the process wherein the disruption of native conformation of protein takes place is called as denaturation, that, in general, results in proteins unfolding [70]. Due to the lack of arrangement, proteins that are unfolded are unfavourably non-functional and also unstable as well. Therefore, after seeking more stability and low energy levels, unfolded proteins tend to aggregate. Also, an increased temperature results in the acceleration of chemical reactions (oxidation and deamidation) that further lead to the high levels of aggregate formation [97].

The changes in the environment of the protein solution such as pH, buffer species, ionic strength, and materials in contact may enhance the formation of protein aggregates. pH determines the electrostatic interactions *via* the distribution of charge all over the protein surface hence a changing pH strongly influences the aggregation rate [98]. Experimentalists have shown that a cleavage of protein may take place under acidic conditions whereas oxidation as well as deamidation may occur under conditions of neutral to alkaline pH. Also, the different behaviour of protein aggregation has been shown within the equivalent pH but with different buffer systems. For example, a higher aggregation rate of interferon-tau protein was observed in phosphate buffer whereas in Tris buffer solutions of equivalent pH, the aggregation process was shown to be slower. This implies that the solvent along with the excipients' quantity in the solvent impacts aggregation behaviour of proteins. Furthermore, surfactants have the ability to stabilize protein aggregation *e.g.* polysorbates (PS) that in turn depends on the ratio of protein to surfactant. In addition to this, the contact materials like glass, plastic, steel, rubbers, silicone, *etc.* may influence protein aggregation [99].

Agitation stress such as shaking or stirring has been reported to be the cause of aggregation. Shear stress is also referred to sometimes as agitation stress but shearing alone does not have the ability to cause aggregation. Agitation causes the generation of shock waves within the liquid that might be the reason for the generation of hydroxyl and hydrogen radicals thus leading to the build-up of protein aggregates [100]. However, these stress conditions do not come under real-life situation but are only applied in studies to induce aggregation.

Freezing leads to the introduction of complex physical and chemical changes in the native protein. This includes solution interfaces or new ice creation, solutes cryoconcentration, and changes in pH because of the crystallization of the components of the buffer. These effects are thus considered a probable reason for freeze-induced denaturation of protein followed by aggregation [101].

Under the condition of quiescent storage, an increased concentration of protein has been described to induce the formation of protein aggregates [102, 103]. This occurs due to the bimolecular interaction of protein molecules that are regarded as concentration-dependent event [104]. Macromolecular crowding occurs in high protein concentration that is explained as the effect of the high total volume occupancy by macromolecular solutes that potentially favour aggregation [105, 106]. In contrast, a decreased protein concentration by dilution that is in case of sample preparation, can also affect the aggregate content because the aggregates formed by weak reversible interaction may dissociate upon the decreased protein concentration [107].

Modification of a protein chemically includes oxidation, deamidation, hydrolysis and isomerization that may result in aggregation reactions [108]. Modifications in the side chains of amino acid may lead to the distortion of proteins conformation and potentially lead to self-association or aggregation [109]. Photolytic degradation of the protein on light exposure may cause photo-oxidation of the side-chains of amino acids such as Tyr, Trp, Phe, His, Met and Cys, that has been shown to enhance protein aggregation [108].

Analytical Techniques for Detection of Aggregation

A major challenge in the analysis of aggregates arises due to the diverse variety of the aggregated protein species. In order to monitor and characterize diverse types of protein aggregates, the scientific community have developed many traditional *in vitro* techniques. However, some potential drawbacks were observed in studying prefibrillar aggregates (oligomers and protofibrils). Therefore, new techniques along with traditional ones were employed to better characterize the prefibrillar aggregates and the amyloid fibrils. This section describes some of the techniques that are also listed in Table **3**.

Table 3. Techniques employed for the detection of different stages of aggregates formed in protein aggregation pathways.

Techniques	Prefibrillar Aggregates/mature Fibrils
Spectroscopy: UV, Fluoro, CD, FTIR, DLS, Mass spectroscopy Dyes: ThT, ANS, CongoRed, NileRed Separative methods: Gel Electrophoresis, Analytical ultracentrifugation, Size exclusion chromatography Solution NMR, X ray crystallography Light Scattering/Turbidity Immunoassays	Native Monomer Partially Unfolded monomer
Spectroscopy: UV, Fluoro, CD, FTIR, DLS, Mass Spectroscopy Dyes: ThT, ANS, CongoRed, NileRed Separative methods: Gel Electrophoresis, Size exclusion chromatography, Analytical ultracentrifugation Solution NMR Light Scattering/Turbidity Immunoassay	Nucleus
Spectroscopy: UV, Fluoro, CD, FTIR, DLS, Mass Spectroscopy Dyes: ThT, ANS, CongoRed, NileRed Separative methods: Gel Electrophoresis, Size exclusion chromatography, Analytical ultracentrifugation Solution NMR Light Scattering/Turbidity Immunoassay	Soluble higher order Oligomers
Spectroscopy: UV, Fluoro, CD, FTIR, DLS, Mass Spectroscopy Dyes: ThT, ANS, CongoRed, NileRed Analytical ultracentrifugation Solid state NMR, Fiber Diffraction Light Scattering/Turbidity Ultrastructural imaging (AFM, EM),Immunoassay	Amyloid Fibrils/Amorphous aggregates

Spectroscopic Methods

The use of numerous sensitive techniques to examine aggregation both *in vitro* and *in vivo* makes it feasible to satisfy curiosity to know its structure and physical appearance.

The size distribution of produced oligomers and protein aggregates along with the kinetics of aggregation can be determined *in situ*, sensitively, and without the need for labels using dynamic light scattering (DLS), which is also termed quasielastic light scattering (QELS) event. DLS can detect a very broad size ranging from around 1 nm to 4000 nm [110]. A light source is used to illuminate the sample, and changes in the intensity of the dispersed light are then monitored. This fluctuation, which is a measurement of the molecular diffusion coefficient, is brought on by the molecules' Brownian movements [111]. The molecule's size and shape affect the diffusion coefficient. Small molecules' diffusion occurs more quickly than the molecules that are bigger; hence the intensity of the scattered light will vary less as a result of small molecules. By computing the autocorrelation function, the diffusion coefficient may be calculated from the fluctuations of scattering. The Stokes-Einstein equation describes how R_h and the diffusion coefficient are related to spherical molecules [112]. DLS can only determine size-distributions qualitatively. The approach is extremely sensitive to big contaminants like dust particles because DLS is not selective for any sort of particle. In order to exclude contaminants or preformed oligomers and aggregates, ultracentrifugation or filtration of the material should be used prior to detection. Also when DLS data of amyloidogenic proteins are analysed, fibril-fibril interactions may take place resulting in incorrect conclusions. Diffusion may slow down by fibril-fibril interactions, which causes an overestimation of fibril length [113].

Separation Methods

Gel electrophoresis is a widely employed technique both for qualitative and quantitative analysis of proteins and their aggregates. The separation is based mainly upon the shape and the size. The protein from the size range of 5-500 kDa can be detected by gel electrophoresis. This way, the separation of monomers and oligomers of amyloid β (Aβ) after covalent cross-linking *via* polyacrylamide gel electrophoresis (PAGE) can be achieved [114]. In case of native gel electrophoresis, aggregates are more stable as compared to SDS electrophoresis (denaturing and reducing). However, from native gel electrophoresis, oligomers of similar size-to-charge ratio are difficult to separate due to the fact that without anionic detergent, the separation is based on a mass, charge, and shape as well. Therefore, complex aggregates are in general separated using denaturing gel electrophoresis [115].

Size exclusion chromatography also referred to as gel filtration chromatography is a historic analytical technique used for the determination of the molecular weight of an uncharacterized molecule. It is a separation technique that is driven by the liquid flow and the hydrodynamic volume (that is the size and shape of the analyte) which regulates its path length which in turn determines the emergence time of the analyte at the detector [116]. The basic components of the experiment of SEC are the matrix, the elution buffer and the chromatography column. The lesser the hydrodynamic volumes, the longer will be the path length in the separation column consisting of the beads containing pores in which molecules of the smaller size can enter [117]. Several studies have analysed Aβ oligomers and have separated them with their monomers and dimers by using SEC [118].

Although, the columns of SEC are designed for different ranges of the molecular size but is not useful for separating oligomers of higher order and fibrils due to their inability to enter the column bed or entering the void volume for elution.

An alternative technique for SEC is analytical ultracentrifugation (AUC). The properties of macromolecules can be analysed by this reliable hydrodynamic technique. The experiments are designed in such a way that it measures the analyte velocity that is subjected to hundred-thousand g radial acceleration. On the basis of sedimentation coefficients (directly correlated with molecular mass and inversely proportional with the frictional coefficient), separation takes place [119]. AUC can be employed for the assessment of the distributed sizes of the aggregates. One drawback of this technique is that it is time-taking. However, no calibration of molecular weight standards are required by using this centrifugation approach thereby measurement of the analytes' molecular weight in the solutions in their native state is easy without any assumptions about the shape and conformations of the analytes [120].

Molecular Probes for Characterization of Aggregate

ThT binding assay- The fluorescent dye thioflavin T (ThT) is frequently employed for determining the presence of existing amyloid fibrils and, in particular, for *in situ* detection of kinetics of amyloid formation, since it typically has no effect on the aggregation kinetics. When bound to amyloid fibrils, ThT shows a significant increase in fluorescence, with an excitation maximum at wavelength of 440 nm and an emission maximum at around 480 nm [121]. ThT has historically been restricted to the detection of amyloid fibrils because of the distinctive sigmoidal increase in its fluorescence between the monomer state and fibril states. But it has also been discovered that ThT can bind prefibrillar aggregates that have the binding location for the β-sheet groove (prefibrillar oligomers and protofibrils) [122]. Because prefibrillar aggregates with the β-sheet structure have lesser binding sites in contrast to fibrils, they exhibit less fluorescence, yet it is still possible to see them [52]. The existence of hazardous protofibrils and fibrillar oligomers may therefore be indicated by ThT, but not by prefibrillar oligomers due to the lack of a distinct β-sheet structure [53]. Finally, due to potential spectrum interference with ThT fluorescence, care should be given while utilising ThT for monitoring aggregation when the inhibitors of aggregation are present [54].

ThT assay can be carried out in a multi-well plate reader setup, just like with turbidity assay. Although frequently believed, the ThT fluorescence intensity is not a precise indicator of the produced amyloid quantity since at high protein concentrations, a saturation effect may be seen [55]. Importantly, protein interactions with ligands which may change the structure and shape of the aggregate, such as metal ions [56] and β-sheet antagonists [57], may significantly alter the ThT fluorescence. Consequently, when the ThT test is utilised to investigate such ligands effect on protein, it should necessarily be supplemented with some other reliable technique for examination of the aggregates.

The benzylamine and benzathiole rings of ThT can readily spin around their shared carbon-carbon bond in solution due to a low energy barrier [65]. The behaviour of ThT is suggested to be that of a "molecular rotor" by a plenty of experimental evidence as well as quantum mechanical predictions [64]. Due to the quick quenching of excited states brought on by photon excitation, free ThT emits little fluorescence as a result of this rotation. The excited state is preserved when ThT is immobilised rotationally, which leads to a high quantum yield of fluorescence [65].

Nile red assay- Nile red (9-diethylamino-5H-benzo phenoxazin-5-one) is a versatile heterocyclic dye without a charge that has been used as a red fluorescent probe for the detection of amyloid formation [123]. It is soluble in organic solvents but in water, it is poorly soluble. Being a hydrophobic and a photochemically stable dye, it has varied fluorescence maxima that depend on the environment polarity [124]. Its structure has a large chain that is in the excited state dipole because of the separation of charges between the quinoid part (electron acceptor) and the diethyl amine of the molecule (electron donor) [125]. Nile red has been used as an amyloidotropic dye for monitoring characterization of amyloid fibril formation in various proteins *in vitro* [126, 127].

CR binding assay- Similar to ThT, Congo Red (CR) is another small molecule probe commonly used for amyloid fibrils detection *in vitro* or specifically for the identification of brain tissue deposits. In addition to showing a distinctive shift in the absorbance maximum from 490 to 540 nm and green birefringence with crossed polarised light, CR also shows binding with β-sheet rich structures of amyloid fibrils [128, 129]. Recent investigations have clarified the application of CR to the study of prefibrillar aggregates. Although the change in CR absorbance was less pronounced than that of amyloid fibrils, Walsh *et al.* nevertheless saw it when protofibrils were exposed to it [130]. To determine the binding affinity/dissociation constant of CR towards prefibrillar oligomers, Maezawa *et al.* used surface Plasmon resonance [128]. For prefibrillar oligomers, a change in absorbance maximum upon CR binding was not noticed. Recent investigations show that CR could be used to characterise protofibrils and fibrillar oligomers, but not prefibrillar oligomers lacking a definite stacked β-sheet structure, as was the case with ThT [131]. On a structural level, CR binds to amyloid at two locations, one parallel to the β-sheet and the other antiparallel to it. The ratio of binding may also vary depending on the type of amyloid being studied [132]. It should be noted that computational studies may suggest different ways in which CR binds to amyloids, but caution should be used because some crucial empirical factors are frequently overlooked in calculations [133].

ANS fluorescence assay- The extrinsic fluorescent probe 8-anilino-1-naphthalenesulfonic acid (ANS) is frequently used to describe proteins in a variety of states [134]. One of the main processes through which prefibrillar aggregates confer toxicity to cells in related disorders is thought to be the disruption of hydrophobic lipid membrane bilayers after the interaction step [135]. Therefore, an evaluation of the surface hydrophobicity of protein aggregates using ANS might be highly helpful in studying prefibrillar protein aggregates. This will allow to gain an insight into the potential for toxicity through hydrophobic interactions. Free ANS exhibits modest fluorescence intensity, peaking at about 540 nm. According to certain theories, the ANS's close environment's hydrophobicity and restricted mobility both considerably contribute to the fluorescence spectra's blue shift, enhanced fluorescence intensity, and longer lifetime. Viscosity, ion pairing with positively charged side chains and change in the solvent polarity all affect the ANS fluorescence.

Immunochemical Methods: Antibody Dot Blot Assay

Antibodies are employed in complex biological specimen for the quantification of specific proteins and for the monitoring the oligomeric species and other relevant conformers' that are hallmark of the neurodegenerative diseases. The development of conformation specific antibodies helped in the identification and detection of prefibrillar aggregates and fibrils. Three conformation-specific antibodies-A11 (recognizes prefibrillar oligomers), αAPF (recognizes protofibrils) and OC (recognizes fibrils, protofibrils and fibrillar oligomers that are rich in cross-stacked β-sheet structure) were developed by Glabe *et al.* [136 - 138]. The immunoassay can be used for constructing sandwich type immunoassays for amyloidogenic species detection. But *in vitro* preparation of the homogenous prefibrillar aggregates is very challenging due to their transient nature. Moreover, the chances of false positive results are also present. Many researchers have developed different antibodies due to the polymorphism in the prefibrillar aggregates [139, 140].

Monoclonal antibodies recognising prefibrillar oligomer sub-classes have been developed. This will not react with monomers and thereby only higher order oligomers will be captured and then detected. This assay has shown great promise for the isolation of protein complexes and Aβ and αSN isoforms' characterization from the cerebrospinal fluid [141, 142].

Methods for Assaying Protein Aggregate Secondary Structure

Two widely used well-established techniques for assaying the secondary structure (e.g., α-helx, and β-sheet, disordered content) of the aggregated proteins *in vitro* are circular dichroism (CD) and Fourier transform infrared spectroscopy (FTIR) [143, 144]. The measurement of the differential absorption of left and right circularly polarized light is monitored by CD spectroscopy and vibrational frequencies of the molecular bonds are analysed by FTIR spectroscopy [145, 146]. FTIR is in general used to determine parallel vs. antiparallel β-sheet structures although through CD, this resolution can also be determined [147, 148]. For the study of protein aggregates, the determination of the content of secondary structure is important since aggregation pathways possess different stages characterized by specific secondary structures. In case of Alzheimer's disease, monomers as well as oligomers of Aβ peptide comprise α-helical/unordered structures. However oligomers of the intermediate stage, protofibrils, and mature fibril conformers mainly consist of β-sheet content [149, 150]. A few research groups consider soluble prefibrillar oligomers' secondary structure to be disordered or a random coil while others disagree with this view. There are reports that these oligomeric protein species are rich in antiparallel or parallel β-sheet secondary structures [137], [151, 152]. Extensive work has been carried out by CD and FTIR for assessing protein aggregates. However, raw data generated from CD and FTIR are used for the estimation of the content of the secondary structure. This is due to the lack of a single protocol to calculate the percentages of secondary structures. Analysis is often carried out by a comparison of the expected or the control results of the CD and FTIR spectra that are then used for establishing a correlation of the changes occurred in the overall secondary structure. For an unknown sample, the spectral features like minima and maxima of the curve between 190-250 nm (CD) and 1,600-1,700 cm^{-1} (FTIR) can be used for comparison with the control sample. This is useful for assessing the features of secondary structures in a qualitative manner [153 - 155]. Alternatively, several numerical methods such as CDSSTR, K2D2/K2D3, CONTIN and SELCON are now available to estimate the samples secondary structure and percentage of the content [156, 157].

Techniques for Visualization of Aggregated Species

Even though the tissue sections that are CR-stained can be viewed under light microscopy to uncover the deposited amyloids but the high resolution ultrastructure technique is a prerequisite for visualization of the insoluble protein deposits. Methods that provide information at a subnanometer scale are electron microscopy (EM) and atomic force microscopy (AFM). The qualitative and quantitative assessment of the characteristics of the quaternary structure of protein aggregates, which include surface features, curvature, length and width, can be carried out using EM and AFM methods. For the first time, Cohen and Calkins in the year 1959 demonstrated different forms of deposited amyloids that were imaged by the electron microscope and reported fibrillar ultrastructure that were long and unbranched fibrils [158]. Thus, the morphological features of the aggregates especially the ordered ones that are prefibrillar and fibrillar species can be examined by using both EM and AFM. This way, the inhibition and disaggregation of fibrils can also be verified. However, AFM has a disadvantage of limited scanning area $\approx 10^4$ which is much higher in EM $\approx 10^6$-10^7 μm^2. Also, EM method when combined with gold particles labelled antibodies can be utilized to pinpoint epitopes of the aggregating protein. EM works by the acceleration of the focused electrons beam towards a sample in a vacuum and the interactions between the sample and the electron beam creates an image. There are two types of EM. Based on the working and the image type formed, TEM or SEM may be used. Transmission electron microscope is a classical EM that uses high-voltage electron beam passing through the vacuum towards the specimen. The scattered electrons form the image of the specimen in TEM, whereas in SEM knocked off or the reflected electrons create an image. The 2D inner structure of sample can be visualized in TEM and the 3D image of the surface of the specimen is formed by SEM. For SEM, little sample is required whereas for TEM, heavy metals, *e.g.* Uranyl acetate, are used for negative staining to improve the resolution of the samples. TEM requires a longer duration and more steps such as freezing and adsorption to mica surface. SEM can be conducted fairly quickly because it is a direct method of sample visualization with no prerequisite of crystallization [159]. However, prefibrillar smaller aggregates that are less than 20 nm in size shows a low degree of resolution. Therefore traditional EM technique is considered as the method of low-resolution for characterizing mature fibrils. An improved resolution technique cryo-EM has been recently employed for visualizing biological specimen that unlike EM allows unfixed and unstained specimen for examination. Herein, the native specimens are hydrated, frozen and preserved in non-crystalline (vitrified) water at a temperature of -180^{0}C. Cryo-EM reconstructions reveal overall dimensions and number of protofilaments and fibrils helical pitch individually along with the branching, if present [160]. It has been used for the reconstruction of about 12 differing morphology of fibrils from Aβ (1–40) samples [161].

Strategies for Halting Protein Aggregation of Therapeutic Compounds

Strategies for halting protein aggregation of therapeutic compounds involved in misfolding and their associated toxicity may appear to be enticing in the context of diseases.

This is accomplished by avoiding new aggregates' formation, reducing aggregates' toxicity and inducing amyloidogenic species clearance. The interaction of inhibitors with amyloidogenic species takes place at different stages by inhibition, blockage or impairment of self-assembly of aggregates and the clearance. A simplified view depicting the targeted pathways of amyloid inhibition strategies and respective inhibited microscopic events is illustrated in Fig. (**7**).

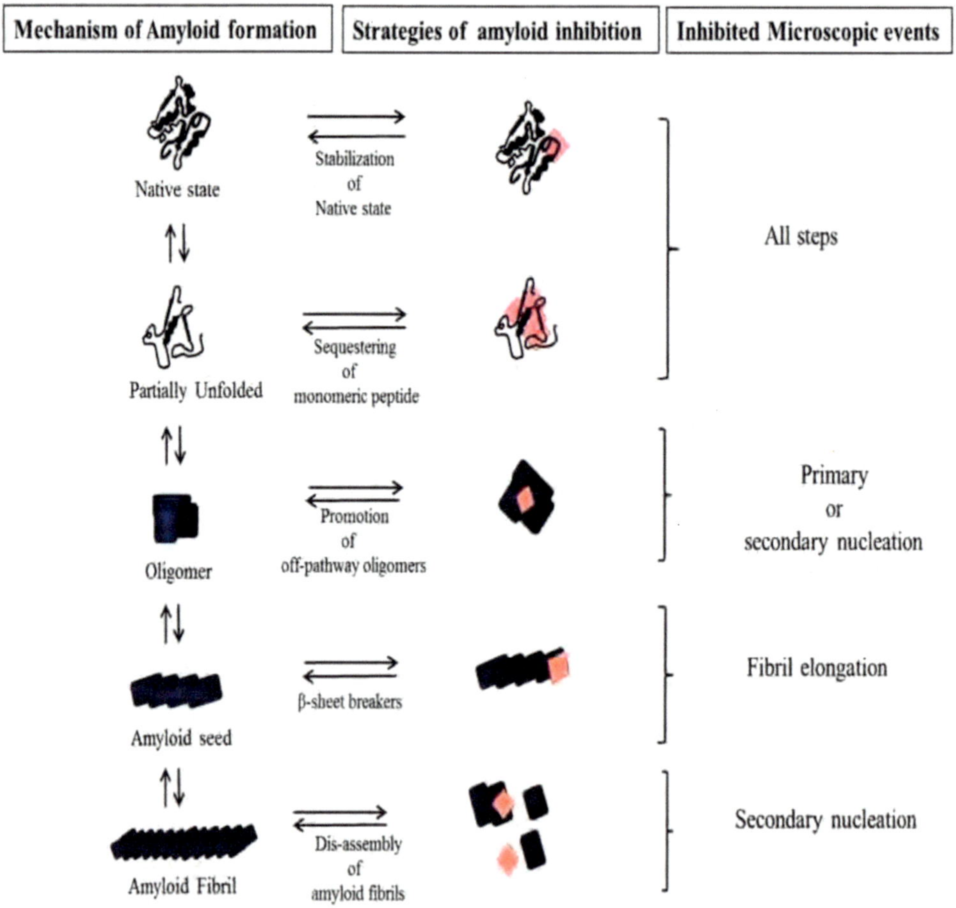

Fig. (7). Different strategies employed to combat amyloid fibril formation along with the illustration of targeted microscopic event of the amyloid fibrillation pathway.

The key event in the process of fibrillation is the conversion of native monomer conformation to β-sheet rich oligomeric species. Therefore the use of compounds that can block the aggregation process by inhibiting the conformational transition proves to be a very promising strategy since it is the first event of the cascade. An increase in the concentration of monomers may become a risk factor for developing aggregation diseases thus inhibiting the accumulation of peptide/protein monomer or hampering the misfolded aggregates production may prove to be a reliable approach. So the molecules that may reduce or inhibit the synthesis of proteins susceptible to misfolds may be the one made available during post translational modification (proteolysis, phosphorylation), could be used. This also applies to proteins that occur naturally and can aberrantly assemble under the pathological conditions (for *e.g.* β amyloid peptide). There are reports that the native monomer conformation stabilization may take place by the induction of physiological chaperones or kinetic control over the population of folded species by employing the compounds that may stabilize the functional monomeric protein. Thus, a protein's unfolding and aggregation can be prevented by proteins or tiny molecules that can bind it in its native folded shape. This can safeguard the folded population by slowing down the unfolding pace thereby blocking an early conformational transition. This may also prevent nucleation that leads to the formation of oligomeric seeds and blocking the elongation process into large amyloid fibrils. For *e.g.*, the stabilization of Aβ monomeric form into a β-hairpin conformation that inhibits its aggregation into Aβ fibrils [162].

Another strategy to halt aggregation is based on the discovery that the self-assembly of the protein molecules may be prohibited by strong binding to the regions of amyloidogenic peptides that are prone to aggregation and also by sequestering of protein. Protein engineering has discovered affinity proteins that are invaluable tools in the development of next generation therapeutics. Affibody molecules are highly soluble small three-helical bundles that have already been generated with affinities to various target proteins [163]. $Z_{a\beta3}$ is an affibody molecule that forms a complex with $A\beta_{40}$. A tunnel like large cavity is formed that sequesters Aβ aggregation-prone residues. These Aβ-sequestering affibody molecules in *in vivo* Drosophila model have demonstrated Aβ aggregation inhibition and also abolished neurotoxicity [164]. Recent studies have presented a novel approach against the pathology related to Aβ peptide using Aβ-sequestering Z_{SYM73} affibody in a transgenic mice model. With this, significant improvement in cognitive function along with a reduction in Aβ pathology was observed [165]. Thus, the approach to designing affibody to target other proteins associated with pathology is envisaged to show promising results against multiple neurodegenerative diseases.

Another strategy is to target the intermediate stage of aggregation that produces some species that do not participate directly in the aggregation process (also termed as off-pathway oligomers). Off-pathway oligomers are less toxic and less hydrophobic and may not form mature fibrils. Therefore, the compound that prevents the on-pathway conversion of misfolded polypeptides into amyloid oligomers and protofibrils rather than redirecting polypeptide molecules into an alternative pathway of aggregation would be included in this category. These substances interfere at the initial step of the cascade of amyloid formation and hence act before they become amyloidogenic. A study found curcumin to impair the aggregation of TTR through inducing its oligomerization into a characteristic homogeneous population of non-toxic small "off-pathway" aggregates.

The hindrance in the transition process of aggregation required for the amyloid fibrillation growth can be achieved by using peptide-based inhibitors that are also known as β-sheet breakers. It is cited in the literature that residues' interaction that involves 17 to 20 amino acid residues (LVFF; the core hydrophobic region) are necessary for Aβ to begin the amyloid formation process [115]. The main goal of several attempts to create Aβ aggregation inhibitors was to search β-sheet breaker peptides unfavourable for further fibril formation [116]. The peptides that target the hydrophobic core of Aβ served as the basis for the development of Aβ amyloid inhibitors and various 'β-sheet breakers'. The peptides have been designed to inhibit amyloid formation. Peptides with identical sequences and hydrophobicity, concentrating specifically on the central hydrophobic region of Aβ that contains the LVFFA motif are created. Prolines were added to the inhibitor peptides because previously they had been found to decrease the β-sheet propensity in Aβ, and charged residues were added to the peptide ends to promote solubility [117]. Also, PrP, α-synuclein, islet amyloid polypeptide (IAPP), and insulin have all been affected partially by complementary peptides' ability to prevent aggregation [120].

Promoting the elimination of misfolded aggregates by disassembling or clearing preformed aggregates is another strategy in combating amyloidoses. Therapeutics that may up regulate the degradation of amyloids or is capable of disaggregation would be pharmacologically promising to treat several disorders related to amyloidoses. Many natural product-based amyloid inhibitors have been discovered and characterised in recent years. Natural products comprise a significant class of amyloid inhibitors. Both *in vitro* investigations along with *in vivo* animal experiments have revealed the great medicinal potential of these chemicals derived from plants or microorganisms. In addition, polyphenols are a rich source of a range of distinct structural backbones that can be used in rational drug design to develop multifunctional anti-amyloid compounds. Owing to their multiple functions, such as anti-oxidant, anti-inflammatory, and metal chelating capacities, they fulfil the aspiration of precision medicine. Curcumin, epigallocatechin-3-gallate (EGCG) and resveratrol, among other polyphenols, have advanced clinical trials as amyloidoses treatments. Table **4** enlists the different classes of small molecules that have been studied to inhibit amyloid formation in various amyloidogenic proteins.

Table 4. Summary of different classes of small molecule inhibitors with the proteins studied.

-		Small Molecule Inhibitor	Protein Studied	References
-	Monolignols	Curcumin, Resveratrol, Nordihydroguaiaretic acid	Aβ_{42}, Prion, IAPP,TTR	[166][167][168]
Polyphenols	Tannic acids	Phlorotannin	Aβ,Tau	[169]
-	Naphthalene derivates	Rifampicin, 1-Naphthol, Naphthalenediol, 1,5-Naphthalenedisulfonic acid	Aβ_{40}, Insulin, αS, Lysozyme	[170][171][172][173]
-	Phenolsulfonphthalein derivitates	Phenolsulfonphthalein Diacetate, Phenolsulfonphthalein dimethyl ether	IAPP, Insulin	[174][172]
-	Flavones	Myricetin, Quercetin, Apigenin, Fisetin	Aβ_{42}, IAPP, Insulin, Lysozyme	[175][176][177] [178]
-	Flavanols	EGCG, Catechin derivatives	Aβ, IAPP, TTR, αS	[179][180][181]
Flavonoids	Isoflavonoids	Genistin, Genistein, Equol	Aβ_{25-35}, TTR	[182][183]
-	Bifalvonoids	Amentoflavone, Sumaflavone, Taiwaniaflavone,	Aβ_{42}	[184]
	Anthocyanidins	Malvidin, Meclocycline sulfosalicylate, Delphinidin	Aβ, TTR, Tau	[185][186][187]
Nitrogenous Compounds	Quinolines	Pyrroloquinoline quinone, Triazole-containing berberine derivative	Aβ_{42} ,αS	[188][189][190]
	Porphyrins	Heme, Hemin	Aβ_{42}	[191][192]
	Phthalocyanines	Cyclic tetrapyrrole phthalocyanine tetrasulfonate	αS	[193]
	Pyridines	Dihydropyridines, Thia(oxa)zolopyridines	Aβ	[194][195]
	Carbazoles	Carbazole thiazole	Aβ	[196]
	Oximes	Phenolic oximes	Aβ_{40}	[197]
	Fluoroindoles	α-Hydroxy-α-(indole-3-yl) acetic acid ethyl esters	Aβ	[198][199]
	Other indoles	Hydroxyindole derivatives	Aβ, Tau, IAPP	[200][201]
Coumarins	-	3-Benzothiazol-2-yl-7-diethylamino-4-(1H-tetrazol-5-yl)-chromen-2-one	Aβ_{40}	[202]

(Table 4) cont.....

Other Aromatic Compounds	-	Nile red, Congo red	Aβ, Tau, IAPP, Insulin	[203][204][205]
	-	Lovastatin,Tetracycline, Quinacrine, Galantamine, Minocycline	Aβ, Amyloid A	[206][207][208][209][210]
	-	Bisphenol A derivatives, Salvianic borneol ester	$A\beta_{40}$	[211][212]
Nonaromatic Compounds	-	Oleic acid, Crocetin, Docosahexaenoic acid	$A\beta_{40}$, α-Lactalbumin	[213][214][215]

CONCLUSION

Protein aggregation is a complex process influenced by various factors resulting in a wide range of debilitating disorders. This is characterized by the deposition of insoluble plaques consisting of amyloid fibrils rich in β-sheet structures [216], [121]. Many natural proteins have the ability to form amyloid fibrils and build-up of the disease-specific misfolded or aggregated proteins in the tissues associated with several human diseases. Even though traditionally amyloids have been associated with diseases, they also possess diverse advantageous properties in organisms from bacteria to human beings. We have discussed the roles of functional amyloids and also enlisted the proteins involved in protein aggregation diseases. The structural composition of aggregates and the current knowledge of the mechanism of amyloid formation have also been portrayed. Since, the important determinant to prevent pathological development of the diseases is finding the possible key factors that may control the aggregation process; therefore by targeting the microscopic events of amyloid formation, the treatment for PMDs is possible. Our present study focuses on the understanding of the protein misfolding and aggregation pathways and reliable methods of detection of diverse types of aggregates. We have contextualized therapeutic strategies to combat the process of aggregation. Still much remains to be uncovered regarding the aggregation and co-aggregation of protein molecules. It is envisaged that these information would be highly useful addressing the issues related to personalized medicine.

ACKNOWLEDGMENTS

Facilities provided by the Interdisciplinary Biotechnology Unit, Aligarh Muslim University, Aligarh, are gratefully acknowledged. S.M. is thankful to Indian Council of Medical Research, New Delhi, India, for providing financial assistance in the form of a Senior Research Fellowship.

REFERENCES

[1] Dobson CM. Protein misfolding, evolution and disease. Trends Biochem Sci 1999; 24(9): 329-32. [http://dx.doi.org/10.1016/S0968-0004(99)01445-0] [PMID: 10470028]

[2] Duran-Aniotz C, Moreno-Gonzalez I, Morales R. [Amyloid aggregates: Role in Protein Misfolding Disorders]. Rev Med Chil 2013; 141(4): 495-505. [http://dx.doi.org/10.4067/S0034-98872013000400011] [PMID: 23900371]

[3] Sweeney P. Protein misfolding in neurodegenerative diseases: Implications and strategies. Transl Neurodegener 2017; 61(1): 1-13. [http://dx.doi.org/10.1186/s40035-017-0077-5]

[4] Winklhofer KF, Tatzelt J, Haass C. The two faces of protein misfolding: Gain- and loss-of-function in neurodegenerative diseases. EMBO J 2008; 27(2): 336-49. [http://dx.doi.org/10.1038/sj.emboj.7601930] [PMID: 18216876]

[5] Shin TM, Isas JM, Hsieh CL, *et al.* Formation of soluble amyloid oligomers and amyloid fibrils by the multifunctional protein vitronectin. Mol Neurodegener 2008; 3(1): 16. [http://dx.doi.org/10.1186/1750-1326-3-16] [PMID: 18939994]

[6] Gilgun-Sherki Y, Melamed E, Offen D. Anti-inflammatory drugs in the treatment of neurodegenerative diseases: current state. Curr Pharm Des 2006; 12(27): 3509-19. [http://dx.doi.org/10.2174/138161206778343091] [PMID: 17017944]

[7] Ow SY, Dunstan DE. A brief overview of amyloids and Alzheimer's disease. Protein Sci 2014; 23(10): 1315-31. [http://dx.doi.org/10.1002/pro.2524]

[8] Li G, Han D, Wei S, Wang H, Chen L. Multiorgan involvement by amyloid light chain amyloidosis. J Int Med Res 2019; 47(4): 1778-86. [http://dx.doi.org/10.1177/0300060518814337] [PMID: 30803274]

[9] Buadi F. Localized Amyloidosis. Amyloidosis 2010; pp. 95-106. [http://dx.doi.org/10.1007/978-1-60761-631-3_7]

[10] Daniele S, Pietrobono D, Fusi J, *et al.* α-synuclein aggregated with tau and β-amyloid in human platelets from healthy subjects: Correlation with physical exercise. Front Aging Neurosci 2018; 10(JAN): 17. [http://dx.doi.org/10.3389/fnagi.2018.00017] [PMID: 29441013]

[11] Hirschfield GM. Amyloidosis: A clinico-pathophysiological synopsis. Semin Cell Dev Biol 2004; 15(1): 39-44. [http://dx.doi.org/10.1016/j.semcdb.2003.12.013] [PMID: 15036205]

[12] Przedborski S, Vila M, Jackson-Lewis V. Series Introduction: Neurodegeneration: What is it and where are we? J Clin Invest 2003; 111(1): 3-10. [http://dx.doi.org/10.1172/JCI200317522] [PMID: 12511579]

[13] Hardy J, Gwinn-Hardy K. Genetic classification of primary neurodegenerative disease. Science 1998; 282(5391): 1075-9. [http://dx.doi.org/10.1126/science.282.5391.1075] [PMID: 9804538]

[14] Chiti F, Dobson CM. Protein misfolding, functional amyloid, and human disease. Annu Rev Biochem 2006; 75(1): 333-66. [http://dx.doi.org/10.1146/annurev.biochem.75.101304.123901] [PMID: 16756495]

[15] Malik S, Siddiqi M K, Majid N, Masroor A, Moasfar Ali S, Khan R H. Unravelling the inhibitory and cytoprotective potential of diuretics towards amyloid fibrillation. Int J Biol Macromol 2020; 150: 1258-71. [http://dx.doi.org/10.1016/j.ijbiomac.2019.10.137]

[16] Sun PD, Foster CE, Boyington JC. Overview of protein structural and functional folds. Curr Protoc

Protein Sci 2004; 35(1): 17.1.
[http://dx.doi.org/10.1002/0471140864.ps1701s35] [PMID: 18429251]

[17] Richardson JS, Richardson DC. Natural β-sheet proteins use negative design to avoid edge-to-edge aggregation. Proc Natl Acad Sci USA 2002; 99(5): 2754-9.
[http://dx.doi.org/10.1073/pnas.052706099] [PMID: 11880627]

[18] Chiti F, Dobson CM. Protein misfolding, amyloid formation, and human disease: A summary of progress over the last decade. Annu Rev Biochem 2017; 86(1): 27-68.
[http://dx.doi.org/10.1146/annurev-biochem-061516-045115] [PMID: 28498720]

[19] Matsuda R, Anguizola J, Joseph KS, Hage DS. Analysis of drug interactions with modified proteins by high-performance affinity chromatography: Binding of glibenclamide to normal and glycated human serum albumin. J Chromatogr A 2012; 1265: 114-22.
[http://dx.doi.org/10.1016/j.chroma.2012.09.091] [PMID: 23092871]

[20] Siddiqi MK, Malik S, Majid N, Alam P, Khan RH. Cytotoxic species in amyloid-associated diseases: Oligomers or mature fibrils. Elsevier Ltd 2019; 118.
[http://dx.doi.org/10.1016/bs.apcsb.2019.06.001]

[21] Herczenik E, Gebbink MFBG. Molecular and cellular aspects of protein misfolding and disease. FASEB J 2008; 22(7): 2115-33.
[http://dx.doi.org/10.1096/fj.07-099671] [PMID: 18303094]

[22] Knowles TPJ, Vendruscolo M, Dobson CM. The physical basis of protein misfolding disorders. Phys Today 2015; 68(3): 36-41.
[http://dx.doi.org/10.1063/PT.3.2719]

[23] Kayed R, Head E, Thompson JL, *et al.* Common structure of soluble amyloid oligomers implies common mechanism of pathogenesis. Science 2003; 300(5618): 486-9.
[http://dx.doi.org/10.1126/science.1079469] [PMID: 12702875]

[24] Taneja V, Verma M, Vats A. Toxic species in amyloid disorders: Oligomers or mature fibrils. Ann Indian Acad Neurol 2015; 18(2): 138-45.
[http://dx.doi.org/10.4103/0972-2327.144284] [PMID: 26019408]

[25] Dobson C M. Protein-misfolding diseases: Getting out of shape. Nat 2002; 418(6899): 729-30.
[http://dx.doi.org/10.1038/418729a]

[26] Stroo E, Koopman M, Nollen EAA, Mata-Cabana A. Cellular regulation of amyloid formation in aging and disease. Front Neurosci 2017; 11(FEB): 64.
[http://dx.doi.org/10.3389/fnins.2017.00064] [PMID: 28261044]

[27] Naiki H, Nagai Y. Molecular pathogenesis of protein misfolding diseases: Pathological molecular environments versus quality control systems against misfolded proteins. J Biochem 2009; 146(6): 751-6.
[http://dx.doi.org/10.1093/jb/mvp119] [PMID: 19643812]

[28] Ben-Zvi AP, Goloubinoff P. Review: mechanisms of disaggregation and refolding of stable protein aggregates by molecular chaperones. J Struct Biol 2001; 135(2): 84-93.
[http://dx.doi.org/10.1006/jsbi.2001.4352] [PMID: 11580258]

[29] Mahul-Mellier A-L, Vercruysse F, Maco B, *et al.* Fibril growth and seeding capacity play key roles in α-synuclein-mediated apoptotic cell death. Cell Death Differ 2015; 22(12): 2107-22.
[http://dx.doi.org/10.1038/cdd.2015.79] [PMID: 26138444]

[30] Finch C, Morgan T. Systemic inflammation, infection, ApoE alleles, and Alzheimer disease: a position paper. Curr Alzheimer Res 2007; 4(2): 185-9.
[http://dx.doi.org/10.2174/156720507780362254] [PMID: 17430245]

[31] Serpente M, Bonsi R, Scarpini E, Galimberti D. Innate immune system and inflammation in Alzheimer's disease: From pathogenesis to treatment. Neuroimmunomodulation 2014; 21(2-3): 79-87.
[http://dx.doi.org/10.1159/000356529] [PMID: 24557039]

[32] Heneka M, Obanion M. Inflammatory processes in Alzheimer's disease. J Neuroimmunol 2007; 184(1-2): 69-91.
[http://dx.doi.org/10.1016/j.jneuroim.2006.11.017] [PMID: 17222916]

[33] Wang W-Y, Tan M-S, Yu J-T, Tan L. Role of pro-inflammatory cytokines released from microglia in Alzheimer's disease. Ann Transl Med 2015; 3(10): 136.
[http://dx.doi.org/10.3978/j.issn.2305-5839.2015.03.49] [PMID: 26207229]

[34] Guo C, Sun L, Chen X, Zhang D. Oxidative stress, mitochondrial damage and neurodegenerative diseases. Neural Regen Res 2013; 8(21): 2003-14.
[http://dx.doi.org/10.3969/J.ISSN.1673-5374.2013.21.009] [PMID: 25206509]

[35] Münch C, Bertolotti A. Exposure of hydrophobic surfaces initiates aggregation of diverse ALS-causing superoxide dismutase-1 mutants. J Mol Biol 2010; 399(3–3): 512.
[http://dx.doi.org/10.1016/j.jmb.2010.04.019]

[36] Kourie JI, Culverson AL, Farrelly PV, Henry CL, Laohachai KN. Heterogeneous amyloid-formed ion channels as a common cytotoxic mechanism: implications for therapeutic strategies against amyloidosis. Cell Biochem Biophys 2002; 36(2-3): 191-207.
[http://dx.doi.org/10.1385/CBB:36:2-3:191] [PMID: 12139405]

[37] Choi YG, Kim JI, Lee HP, *et al.* Induction of heme oxygenase-1 in the brains of scrapie-infected mice. Neurosci Lett 2000; 289(3): 173-6.
[http://dx.doi.org/10.1016/S0304-3940(00)01277-5] [PMID: 10961657]

[38] Hyun DH, Lee M, Hattori N, *et al.* Effect of wild-type or mutant Parkin on oxidative damage, nitric oxide, antioxidant defenses, and the proteasome. J Biol Chem 2002; 277(32): 28572-7.
[http://dx.doi.org/10.1074/jbc.M200666200] [PMID: 12034719]

[39] Zhang L, Xing G, Barker JL, *et al.* α-lipoic acid protects rat cortical neurons against cell death induced by amyloid and hydrogen peroxide through the Akt signalling pathway. Neurosci Lett 2001; 312(3): 125-8.
[http://dx.doi.org/10.1016/S0304-3940(01)02205-4] [PMID: 11602326]

[40] Yang S, Wang W, Ling T, *et al.* α-tocopherol quinone inhibits β-amyloid aggregation and cytotoxicity, disaggregates preformed fibrils and decreases the production of reactive oxygen species, NO and inflammatory cytokines. Neurochem Int 2010; 57(8): 914-22.
[http://dx.doi.org/10.1016/j.neuint.2010.09.011] [PMID: 20933033]

[41] Picone P, Nuzzo D, Di Carlo M. Ferulic acid: A natural antioxidant against oxidative stress induced by oligomeric A-beta on sea urchin embryo. Biol Bull 2013; 224(1): 18-28.
[http://dx.doi.org/10.1086/BBLv224n1p18] [PMID: 23493505]

[42] Sultana R, Ravagna A, Mohmmad-Abdul H, Calabrese V, Butterfield DA. Ferulic acid ethyl ester protects neurons against amyloid β- peptide(1–42)-induced oxidative stress and neurotoxicity: Relationship to antioxidant activity. J Neurochem 2005; 92(4): 749-58.
[http://dx.doi.org/10.1111/j.1471-4159.2004.02899.x] [PMID: 15686476]

[43] Prasad KN, Bondy SC. Oxidative and inflammatory events in prion Diseases: Can they be therapeutic targets? Curr Aging Sci 2019; 11(4): 216-25.
[http://dx.doi.org/10.2174/1874609812666190111100205] [PMID: 30636622]

[44] Kim EK, Choi EJ. Pathological roles of MAPK signaling pathways in human diseases. Biochim Biophys Acta Mol Basis Dis 2010; 1802(4): 396-405.
[http://dx.doi.org/10.1016/j.bbadis.2009.12.009] [PMID: 20079433]

[45] Goloubinoff P, Ben-Zvi AP. Mechanisms of active solubilization of stable protein aggregates by molecular chaperones. Protein Reviews 2007; 4(Nov): 165-74.
[http://dx.doi.org/10.1007/0-387-25919-8_9]

[46] Li X, Ma Y, Wei X, *et al.* Clusterin in Alzheimer's disease: A player in the biological behavior of amyloid-beta. Neurosci Bull 2014; 30(1): 162-8.

[http://dx.doi.org/10.1007/s12264-013-1391-2] [PMID: 24353014]

[47] Yerbury JJ, Kumita JR, Meehan S, Dobson CM, Wilson MR. α2-Macroglobulin and haptoglobin suppress amyloid formation by interacting with prefibrillar protein species. J Biol Chem 2009; 284(7): 4246-54.
[http://dx.doi.org/10.1074/jbc.M807242200] [PMID: 19074141]

[48] Yerbury JJ, Poon S, Meehan S, *et al.* The extracellular chaperone clusterin influences amyloid formation and toxicity by interacting with prefibrillar structures. FASEB J 2007; 21(10): 2312-22.
[http://dx.doi.org/10.1096/fj.06-7986com] [PMID: 17412999]

[49] Saibil H. Chaperone machines for protein folding, unfolding and disaggregation. Nat Rev Mol Cell Biol 2013; 14(10): 630-42.
[http://dx.doi.org/10.1038/nrm3658] [PMID: 24026055]

[50] Kostenko S, Moens U. Heat shock protein 27 phosphorylation: Kinases, phosphatases, functions and pathology. Cell Mol Life Sci 2009; 66(20): 3289-307.
[http://dx.doi.org/10.1007/s00018-009-0086-3] [PMID: 19593530]

[51] Marini I, Moschini R, Corso AD, Mura U. Alpha-crystallin: An ATP-independent complete molecular chaperone toward sorbitol dehydrogenase. Cell Mol Life Sci 2005; 62(5): 599-605.
[http://dx.doi.org/10.1007/s00018-005-4474-z] [PMID: 15747064]

[52] Cox D, Whiten DR, Brown JWP, *et al.* The small heat shock protein Hsp27 binds α-synuclein fibrils, preventing elongation and cytotoxicity. J Biol Chem 2018; 293(12): 4486-97.
[http://dx.doi.org/10.1074/jbc.M117.813865] [PMID: 29382725]

[53] Waudby CA, Knowles TPJ, Devlin GL, *et al.* The interaction of alphaB-crystallin with mature alpha-synuclein amyloid fibrils inhibits their elongation. Biophys J 2010; 98(5): 843-51.
[http://dx.doi.org/10.1016/j.bpj.2009.10.056] [PMID: 20197038]

[54] Dobson CM. Protein folding and misfolding. Nat 2003; 426(6968): 884-90.
[http://dx.doi.org/10.1038/nature02261]

[55] Khan AN, Hassan MN, Khan RH. Gallic acid: A naturally occurring bifunctional inhibitor of amyloid and metal induced aggregation with possible implication in metal-based therapy. J Mol Liq 2019; 285: 27-37.
[http://dx.doi.org/10.1016/j.molliq.2019.04.059]

[56] Siddiqi MK, Alam P, Chaturvedi SK, *et al.* Capreomycin inhibits the initiation of amyloid fibrillation and suppresses amyloid induced cell toxicity. Biochim Biophys Acta Proteins Proteomics 2018; 1866(4): 549-57.
[http://dx.doi.org/10.1016/j.bbapap.2018.02.005] [PMID: 29496560]

[57] Tycko R. Solid-state NMR studies of amyloid fibril structure. Annu Rev Phys Chem 2011; 62(1): 279-99.
[http://dx.doi.org/10.1146/annurev-physchem-032210-103539] [PMID: 21219138]

[58] Eisenberg D, Jucker M. The amyloid state of proteins in human diseases. Cell 2012; 148(6): 1188-203.
[http://dx.doi.org/10.1016/j.cell.2012.02.022] [PMID: 22424229]

[59] Otzen D. Amyloid Fibrils and Prefibrillar Aggregates: Molecular and Biological Properties. Wiley-VCH Verlag GmbH & Co. KGaA 2013.
[http://dx.doi.org/10.1002/9783527654185]

[60] Makin OS, Serpell LC. Structures for amyloid fibrils. FEBS J 2005; 272(23): 5950-61.
[http://dx.doi.org/10.1111/j.1742-4658.2005.05025.x] [PMID: 16302960]

[61] Fändrich M. On the structural definition of amyloid fibrils and other polypeptide aggregates. Cell Mol Life Sci 2007; 64(16): 2066-78.
[http://dx.doi.org/10.1007/s00018-007-7110-2] [PMID: 17530168]

[62] Adamcik J, Mezzenga R. Proteins fibrils from a polymer physics perspective. Macromolecules 2012;

45(3): 1137-50.
[http://dx.doi.org/10.1021/ma202157h]

[63] Eanes ED, Glenner GG. X-ray diffraction studies on amyloid filaments. J Histochem Cytochem 1968; 16(11): 673-7.
[http://dx.doi.org/10.1177/16.11.673] [PMID: 5723775]

[64] Lashuel HA, LaBrenz SR, Woo L, Serpell LC, Kelly JW. Protofilaments, filaments, ribbons, and fibrils from peptidomimetic self-assembly: implications for amyloid fibril formation and materials science. J Am Chem Soc 2000; 122(22): 5262-77.
[http://dx.doi.org/10.1021/ja9937831] [PMID: 22339465]

[65] Khurana R, Ionescu-Zanetti C, Pope M, *et al.* A general model for amyloid fibril assembly based on morphological studies using atomic force microscopy. Biophys J 2003; 85(2): 1135-44.
[http://dx.doi.org/10.1016/S0006-3495(03)74550-0] [PMID: 12885658]

[66] Segers-Nolten I, van Raaij M, Subramaniam V. Biophysical analysis of amyloid formation. Compr Biomater 2011; 2: 347-59.
[http://dx.doi.org/10.1016/B978-0-08-055294-1.00086-6]

[67] Dear AJ, Meisl G, Šarić A, *et al.* Identification of on- and off-pathway oligomers in amyloid fibril formation. Chem Sci 2020; 11(24): 6236-47.
[http://dx.doi.org/10.1039/C9SC06501F] [PMID: 32953019]

[68] Greenwald J, Riek R. Biology of amyloid: Structure, function, and regulation. Structure 2010; 18(10): 1244-60.
[http://dx.doi.org/10.1016/j.str.2010.08.009] [PMID: 20947013]

[69] Morell M, Bravo R, Espargaró A, *et al.* Inclusion bodies: Specificity in their aggregation process and amyloid-like structure. Biochim Biophys Acta Mol Cell Res 2008; 1783(10): 1815-25.
[http://dx.doi.org/10.1016/j.bbamcr.2008.06.007] [PMID: 18619498]

[70] Lapidus LJ. Protein unfolding mechanisms and their effects on folding experiments. F1000 Res 2017; 6: 1723.
[http://dx.doi.org/10.12688/f1000research.12070.1] [PMID: 29034084]

[71] Yamamoto N, Tsuhara S, Tamura A, Chatani E. A specific form of prefibrillar aggregates that functions as a precursor of amyloid nucleation. Sci Rep 2018; 8(1): 62.
[http://dx.doi.org/10.1038/s41598-017-18390-y] [PMID: 29311640]

[72] Fändrich M. Oligomeric intermediates in amyloid formation: structure determination and mechanisms of toxicity. J Mol Biol 2012; 421(4-5): 427-40.
[http://dx.doi.org/10.1016/j.jmb.2012.01.006] [PMID: 22248587]

[73] Dear AJ, Michaels TCT, Meisl G, *et al.* Kinetic diversity of amyloid oligomers. Proc Natl Acad Sci 2020; 117(22): 12087-94.
[http://dx.doi.org/10.1073/pnas.1922267117] [PMID: 32414930]

[74] Auer S. Nucleation of polymorphic amyloid fibrils. Biophys J 2015; 108(5): 1176-86.
[http://dx.doi.org/10.1016/j.bpj.2015.01.013] [PMID: 25762329]

[75] Horwich A. Protein aggregation in disease: A role for folding intermediates forming specific multimeric interactions. J Clin Invest 2002; 110(9): 1221-32.
[http://dx.doi.org/10.1172/JCI0216781] [PMID: 12417558]

[76] Törnquist M, Michaels TCT, Sanagavarapu K, *et al.* Secondary nucleation in amyloid formation. Chem Commun 2018; 54(63): 8667-84.
[http://dx.doi.org/10.1039/C8CC02204F] [PMID: 29978862]

[77] Otzen D, Riek R. Functional Amyloids. Cold Spring Harb Perspect Biol 2019; 11(12): a033860.
[http://dx.doi.org/10.1101/cshperspect.a033860] [PMID: 31088827]

[78] Larsen P, Nielsen JL, Dueholm MS, Wetzel R, Otzen D, Nielsen PH. Amyloid adhesins are abundant

in natural biofilms. Environ Microbiol 2007; 9(12): 3077-90.
[http://dx.doi.org/10.1111/j.1462-2920.2007.01418.x] [PMID: 17991035]

[79] Gebbink MFBG, Claessen D, Bouma B, Dijkhuizen L, Wösten HAB. Amyloids — a functional coat for microorganisms. Nat Rev Microbiol 2005; 3(4): 333-41.
[http://dx.doi.org/10.1038/nrmicro1127] [PMID: 15806095]

[80] Barnhart MM, Chapman MR. Curli biogenesis and function. Annu Rev Microbiol 2006; 60(1): 131-47.
[http://dx.doi.org/10.1146/annurev.micro.60.080805.142106] [PMID: 16704339]

[81] Chien P, Weissman JS, DePace AH. Emerging principles of conformation-based prion inheritance. Annu Rev Biochem 2004; 73(1): 617-56.
[http://dx.doi.org/10.1146/annurev.biochem.72.121801.161837] [PMID: 15189155]

[82] Kushnirov VV, Kochneva-Pervukhova NV, Chechenova MB, Frolova NS, Ter-Avanesyan MD. Prion properties of the Sup35 protein of yeast Pichia methanolica. EMBO J 2000; 19(3): 324-31.
[http://dx.doi.org/10.1093/emboj/19.3.324] [PMID: 10654931]

[83] Saupe SJ. Molecular genetics of heterokaryon incompatibility in filamentous ascomycetes. Microbiol Mol Biol Rev 2000; 64(3): 489-502.
[http://dx.doi.org/10.1128/MMBR.64.3.489-502.2000] [PMID: 10974123]

[84] de Vries OMH, Fekkes MP, Wösten HAB, Wessels JGH. Insoluble hydrophobin complexes in the walls of Schizophyllum commune and other filamentous fungi. Arch Microbiol 1993; 159(4): 330-5.
[http://dx.doi.org/10.1007/BF00290915]

[85] Kenney JM, Knight D, Wise MJ, Vollrath F. Amyloidogenic nature of spider silk. Eur J Biochem 2002; 269(16): 4159-63.
[http://dx.doi.org/10.1046/j.1432-1033.2002.03112.x] [PMID: 12180993]

[86] Li JS, Li J. Major chorion proteins and their crosslinking during chorion hardening in Aedes aegypti mosquitoes. Insect Biochem Mol Biol 2006; 36(12): 954-64.
[http://dx.doi.org/10.1016/j.ibmb.2006.09.006] [PMID: 17098170]

[87] Berson JF, Theos AC, Harper DC, Tenza D, Raposo G, Marks MS. Proprotein convertase cleavage liberates a fibrillogenic fragment of a resident glycoprotein to initiate melanosome biogenesis. J Cell Biol 2003; 161(3): 521-33.
[http://dx.doi.org/10.1083/jcb.200302072] [PMID: 12732614]

[88] Alper T, Cramp WA, Haig DA, Clarke MC. Does the agent of scrapie replicate without nucleic acid? Nature 1967; 214(5090): 764-6.
[http://dx.doi.org/10.1038/214764a0] [PMID: 4963878]

[89] Seviour T, Hansen SH, Yang L, *et al.* Functional amyloids keep quorum-sensing molecules in check. J Biol Chem 2015; 290(10): 6457-69.
[http://dx.doi.org/10.1074/jbc.M114.613810] [PMID: 25586180]

[90] Masroor A, Zaidi N, Chandel TI, Aqueel Z, Malik S, Khan RH. Probing the nongeneralized amyloid inhibitory mechanism of hydrophobic chaperone. ACS Chem Neurosci 2020; 11(3): 373-84.
[http://dx.doi.org/10.1021/acschemneuro.9b00593] [PMID: 31935057]

[91] Adler J, Scheidt HA, Krüger M, Thomas L, Huster D. Local interactions influence the fibrillation kinetics, structure and dynamics of Aβ(1–40) but leave the general fibril structure unchanged. Phys Chem Chem Phys 2014; 16(16): 7461-71.
[http://dx.doi.org/10.1039/C3CP54501F] [PMID: 24626742]

[92] Wang W, Li N, Speaker S. External factors affecting protein aggregation. Aggreg Ther Proteins 2010; (Aug): 119-204.
[http://dx.doi.org/10.1002/9780470769829.ch4]

[93] Wang W, Nema S, Teagarden D. Protein aggregation—pathways and influencing factors. Int J Pharm 2010; 390(2): 89-99.

[http://dx.doi.org/10.1016/j.ijpharm.2010.02.025] [PMID: 20188160]

[94] Vázquez-Rey M, Lang DA. Aggregates in monoclonal antibody manufacturing processes. Biotechnol Bioeng 2011; 108(7): 1494-508.
[http://dx.doi.org/10.1002/bit.23155] [PMID: 21480193]

[95] Hamrang Z, Rattray NJW, Pluen A. Proteins behaving badly: Emerging technologies in profiling biopharmaceutical aggregation. Trends Biotechnol 2013; 31(8): 448-58.
[http://dx.doi.org/10.1016/j.tibtech.2013.05.004] [PMID: 23769716]

[96] Sahin E, Grillo AO, Perkins MD, Roberts CJ. Comparative effects of pH and ionic strength on protein-protein interactions, unfolding, and aggregation for IgG1 antibodies. J Pharm Sci 2010; 99(12): 4830-48.
[http://dx.doi.org/10.1002/jps.22198] [PMID: 20821389]

[97] Brange J, Havelund S, Hougaard P. Chemical stability of insulin. 2. Formation of higher molecular weight transformation products during storage of pharmaceutical preparations. Pharm Res 1992; 9(6): 727-34.
[http://dx.doi.org/10.1023/A:1015887001987] [PMID: 1409352]

[98] Chi EY, Krishnan S, Randolph TW, Carpenter JF. Physical stability of proteins in aqueous solution: Mechanism and driving forces in nonnative protein aggregation. Pharm Res 2003; 20(9): 1325-36.
[http://dx.doi.org/10.1023/A:1025771421906] [PMID: 14567625]

[99] Sacha GA, Saffell-Clemmer W, Abram K, Akers MJ. Practical fundamentals of glass, rubber, and plastic sterile packaging systems. Pharm Dev Technol 2010; 15(1): 6-34.
[http://dx.doi.org/10.3109/10837450903511178] [PMID: 20088708]

[100] Siska C, Harber P, Kerwin BA. Shocking data on parcel shipments of protein solutions. J Pharm Sci 2020; 109(1): 690-5.
[http://dx.doi.org/10.1016/j.xphs.2019.10.064] [PMID: 31689428]

[101] Cao E, Chen Y, Cui Z, Foster PR. Effect of freezing and thawing rates on denaturation of proteins in aqueous solutions. Biotechnol Bioeng 2003; 82(6): 684-90.
[http://dx.doi.org/10.1002/bit.10612] [PMID: 12673768]

[102] Shire SJ, Shahrokh Z, Liu J. Challenges in the development of high protein concentration formulations. J Pharm Sci 2004; 93(6): 1390-402.
[http://dx.doi.org/10.1002/jps.20079] [PMID: 15124199]

[103] Alford JR, Kendrick BS, Carpenter JF, Randolph TW. High concentration formulations of recombinant human interleukin-1 receptor antagonist: II. Aggregation kinetics. J Pharm Sci 2008; 97(8): 3005-21.
[http://dx.doi.org/10.1002/jps.21205] [PMID: 17924426]

[104] Treuheit MJ, Kosky AA, Brems DN. Inverse relationship of protein concentration and aggregation. Pharm Res 2002; 19(4): 511-6.
[http://dx.doi.org/10.1023/A:1015108115452] [PMID: 12033388]

[105] Ellis RJ, Minton AP. Protein aggregation in crowded environments. Biol Chem 2006; 387(5): 485-97.
[http://dx.doi.org/10.1515/BC.2006.064] [PMID: 16740119]

[106] van den Berg B, Ellis RJ, Dobson CM. Effects of macromolecular crowding on protein folding and aggregation. EMBO J 1999; 18(24): 6927-33.
[http://dx.doi.org/10.1093/emboj/18.24.6927] [PMID: 10601015]

[107] Liu J, Andya JD, Shire SJ. A critical review of analytical ultracentrifugation and field flow fractionation methods for measuring protein aggregation. AAPS J 2006; 8(3): E580-9.
[http://dx.doi.org/10.1208/aapsj080367] [PMID: 17025276]

[108] Li S, Schöneich C, Borchardt RT. Chemical instability of protein pharmaceuticals: Mechanisms of oxidation and strategies for stabilization. Biotechnol Bioeng 1995; 48(5): 490-500.
[http://dx.doi.org/10.1002/bit.260480511] [PMID: 18623513]

[109] Zapadka KL, Becher FJ, Gomes dos Santos AL, Jackson SE. Factors affecting the physical stability (aggregation) of peptide therapeutics. Interface Focus 2017; 7(6): 20170030. [http://dx.doi.org/10.1098/rsfs.2017.0030] [PMID: 29147559]

[110] Carpenter DK. Dynamic light scattering with applications to chemistry, biology, and physics (Berne, Bruce J.; Pecora, Robert). J Chem Educ 1977; 54(10): A430. [http://dx.doi.org/10.1021/ed054pA430.1]

[111] Lomakin A, Teplow DB. Quasielastic light scattering study of amyloid β-protein fibrillogenesis. Methods Mol Biol 2012; 849: 69-83. [http://dx.doi.org/10.1007/978-1-61779-551-0_6] [PMID: 22528084]

[112] Amin S, Barnett GV, Pathak JA, Roberts CJ, Sarangapani PS. Protein aggregation, particle formation, characterization & rheology. Curr Opin Colloid Interface Sci 2014; 19(5): 438-49. [http://dx.doi.org/10.1016/j.cocis.2014.10.002]

[113] Shen CL, Scott GL, Merchant F, Murphy RM. Light scattering analysis of fibril growth from the amino-terminal fragment beta(1–28) of beta-amyloid peptide. Biophys J 1993; 65(6): 2383-95. [http://dx.doi.org/10.1016/S0006-3495(93)81312-2] [PMID: 8312477]

[114] Khan RH. Mechanisms of protein aggregation and inhibition. Front Biosci 2017; 9(1): 1-20. [http://dx.doi.org/10.2741/e781]

[115] Coalier KA, Paranjape GS, Karki S, Nichols MR. Stability of early-stage amyloid-β(1–42) aggregation species. Biochim Biophys Acta Proteins Proteomics 2013; 1834(1): 65-70. [http://dx.doi.org/10.1016/j.bbapap.2012.08.017] [PMID: 22944394]

[116] Fekete S, Beck A, Veuthey JL, Guillarme D. Theory and practice of size exclusion chromatography for the analysis of protein aggregates. J Pharm Biomed Anal 2014; 101: 161-73. [http://dx.doi.org/10.1016/j.jpba.2014.04.011] [PMID: 24816223]

[117] Arakawa T, Ejima D, Li T, Philo JS. The critical role of mobile phase composition in size exclusion chromatography of protein pharmaceuticals. J Pharm Sci 2010; 99(4): 1674-92. [http://dx.doi.org/10.1002/jps.21974] [PMID: 19894271]

[118] Walsh DM, Tseng BP, Rydel RE, Podlisny MB, Selkoe DJ. The oligomerization of amyloid β-protein begins intracellularly in cells derived from human brain. Biochemistry 2000; 39(35): 10831-9. [http://dx.doi.org/10.1021/bi001048s] [PMID: 10978169]

[119] Brown PH, Balbo A, Schuck P. Characterizing protein-protein interactions by sedimentation velocity analytical ultracentrifugation. Curr Protoc Immunol 2008. [http://dx.doi.org/10.1002/0471142735.im1815s81]

[120] Balbo A, Schuck P. Analytical ultracentrifugation in the study of protein self-association and heterogeneous protein-protein interactions. Protein-Protein Interact Golemis 2005; 301: 253-77.

[121] Malik S, Zaidi N, Siddiqi MK, *et al.* Mechanistic insight into inhibition of amyloid fibrillation of human serum albumin by Vildagliptin. Colloids Surf B Biointerfaces 2022; 216(March): 112563. [http://dx.doi.org/10.1016/j.colsurfb.2022.112563] [PMID: 35588684]

[122] Biancalana M, Koide S. Molecular mechanism of Thioflavin-T binding to amyloid fibrils. Biochim Biophys Acta Proteins Proteomics 2010; 1804(7): 1405-12. [http://dx.doi.org/10.1016/j.bbapap.2010.04.001] [PMID: 20399286]

[123] Greenspan P, Mayer EP, Fowler SD. Nile red: A selective fluorescent stain for intracellular lipid droplets. J Cell Biol 1985; 100(3): 965-73. [http://dx.doi.org/10.1083/jcb.100.3.965] [PMID: 3972906]

[124] Ghoneim N. Photophysics of Nile red in solution. Spectrochim Acta A Mol Biomol Spectrosc 2000; 56(5): 1003-10. [http://dx.doi.org/10.1016/S1386-1425(99)00199-7] [PMID: 10809076]

[125] Sackett DL, Wolff J. Nile red as a polarity-sensitive fluorescent probe of hydrophobic protein surfaces.

Anal Biochem 1987; 167(2): 228-34.
[http://dx.doi.org/10.1016/0003-2697(87)90157-6] [PMID: 3442318]

[126] Masroor A, Chandel TI, Malik S, Mateen QN, Uversky VN, Khan RH. Evaluation of ThT augmentation and RLS inner filter effect caused by highly fluorescent coumarin derivative and establishing it as true inhibitor of amyloid fibrillation. Arch Biochem Biophys 2021; 709(February): 108981.
[http://dx.doi.org/10.1016/j.abb.2021.108981] [PMID: 34214556]

[127] Mishra R, Sjölander D, Hammarström P. Spectroscopic characterization of diverse amyloid fibrils *in vitro* by the fluorescent dye Nile red. Mol Biosyst 2011; 7(4): 1232-40.
[http://dx.doi.org/10.1039/c0mb00236d] [PMID: 21279219]

[128] Maezawa I, Hong HS, Liu R, *et al.* Congo red and thioflavin-T analogs detect Aβ oligomers. J Neurochem 2008; 104(2): 457-68.
[http://dx.doi.org/10.1111/j.1471-4159.2007.04972.x] [PMID: 17953662]

[129] Hatters DM, Griffin MDW. Diagnostics for amyloid fibril formation: where to begin? Methods Mol Biol 2011; 752: 121-36.
[http://dx.doi.org/10.1007/978-1-60327-223-0_8] [PMID: 21713634]

[130] Gregoire S, Irwin J, Kwon I. Techniques for monitoring protein misfolding and aggregation *in vitro* and in living cells. Korean J Chem Eng 2012; 29(6): 693-702.
[http://dx.doi.org/10.1007/s11814-012-0060-x] [PMID: 23565019]

[131] Chimon S, Shaibat MA, Jones CR, Calero DC, Aizezi B, Ishii Y. Evidence of fibril-like β-sheet structures in a neurotoxic amyloid intermediate of Alzheimer's β-amyloid. Nat Struct Mol Biol 2007; 14(12): 1157-64.
[http://dx.doi.org/10.1038/nsmb1345] [PMID: 18059284]

[132] Klunk WE, Pettegrew JW, Abraham DJ. Quantitative evaluation of congo red binding to amyloid-like proteins with a beta-pleated sheet conformation. J Histochem Cytochem 1989; 37(8): 1273-81.
[http://dx.doi.org/10.1177/37.8.2666510] [PMID: 2666510]

[133] Wang CC, Huang H, Tsay HJ, *et al.* Characterization of Aβ aggregation mechanism probed by congo red. J Biomol Struct Dyn 2012; 30(2): 160-9.
[http://dx.doi.org/10.1080/07391102.2012.677767] [PMID: 22702727]

[134] Hawe A, Sutter M, Jiskoot W. Extrinsic fluorescent dyes as tools for protein characterization. Pharm Res 2008; 25(7): 1487-99.
[http://dx.doi.org/10.1007/s11095-007-9516-9] [PMID: 18172579]

[135] Glabe CG. Amyloid Oligomer Structures and Toxicity. Open Biol J 2009; 2: 222-7.
[http://dx.doi.org/10.2174/1874196700902010222]

[136] Glabe CG. Structural classification of toxic amyloid oligomers. J Biol Chem 2008; 283(44): 29639-43.
[http://dx.doi.org/10.1074/jbc.R800016200] [PMID: 18723507]

[137] Kayed R, Pensalfini A, Margol L, *et al.* Annular protofibrils are a structurally and functionally distinct type of amyloid oligomer. J Biol Chem 2009; 284(7): 4230-7.
[http://dx.doi.org/10.1074/jbc.M808591200] [PMID: 19098006]

[138] Kayed R, Head E, Sarsoza F, *et al.* Fibril specific, conformation dependent antibodies recognize a generic epitope common to amyloid fibrils and fibrillar oligomers that is absent in prefibrillar oligomers. Mol Neurodegener 2007; 2(1): 18.
[http://dx.doi.org/10.1186/1750-1326-2-18] [PMID: 17897471]

[139] Kayed R, Canto I, Breydo L, *et al.* Conformation dependent monoclonal antibodies distinguish different replicating strains or conformers of prefibrillar Aβ oligomers. Mol Neurodegener 2010; 5(1): 57.
[http://dx.doi.org/10.1186/1750-1326-5-57] [PMID: 21144050]

[140] Kayed R, Head E, Thompson JL, *et al.* Common structure of soluble amyloid oligomers implies

common mechanism of pathogenesis. Science 2003; 300(5618): 486-9.
[http://dx.doi.org/10.1126/science.1079469] [PMID: 12702875]

[141] Öhrfelt A, Zetterberg H, Andersson K, *et al.* Identification of novel α-synuclein isoforms in human brain tissue by using an online nanoLC-ESI-FTICR-MS method. Neurochem Res 2011; 36(11): 2029-42.
[http://dx.doi.org/10.1007/s11064-011-0527-x] [PMID: 21674238]

[142] Öhrfelt A, Dumurgier J, Zetterberg H, *et al.* Full-length and C-terminal neurogranin in Alzheimer's disease cerebrospinal fluid analyzed by novel ultrasensitive immunoassays. Alzheimers Res Ther 2020; 12(1): 168.
[http://dx.doi.org/10.1186/s13195-020-00748-6] [PMID: 33353563]

[143] Benjwal S, Verma S, Röhm KH, Gursky O, Gursky O. Monitoring protein aggregation during thermal unfolding in circular dichroism experiments. Protein Sci 2006; 15(3): 635-9.
[http://dx.doi.org/10.1110/ps.051917406] [PMID: 16452626]

[144] Byler DM, Susi H. Examination of the secondary structure of proteins by deconvolved FTIR spectra. Biopolymers 1986; 25(3): 469-87.
[http://dx.doi.org/10.1002/bip.360250307] [PMID: 3697478]

[145] Breydo L, Reddy KD, Piai A, Felli IC, Pierattelli R, Uversky VN. The crowd you're in with: Effects of different types of crowding agents on protein aggregation. Biochim Biophys Acta Proteins Proteomics 2014; 1844(2): 346-57.
[http://dx.doi.org/10.1016/j.bbapap.2013.11.004] [PMID: 24252314]

[146] Poureshghi F, Ghandforoushan P, Safarnejad A, Soltani S. Interaction of an antiepileptic drug, lamotrigine with human serum albumin (HSA): Application of spectroscopic techniques and molecular modeling methods. J Photochem Photobiol B 2017; 166: 187-92.
[http://dx.doi.org/10.1016/j.jphotobiol.2016.09.046] [PMID: 27951518]

[147] Perczel A, Park K, Fasman GD. Deconvolution of the circular dichroism spectra of proteins: The circular dichroism spectra of the antiparallel β-sheet in proteins. Proteins 1992; 13(1): 57-69.
[http://dx.doi.org/10.1002/prot.340130106] [PMID: 1594578]

[148] Whitmore L, Wallace BA. Protein secondary structure analyses from circular dichroism spectroscopy: Methods and reference databases. Biopolymers 2008; 89(5): 392-400.
[http://dx.doi.org/10.1002/bip.20853] [PMID: 17896349]

[149] Harry L, Lary CW. Molecular polymorphism of Aβ in Alzheimer's disease Neurobiol Aging 2010; 31(4): 542-8.

[150] Lee S, Fernandez EJ, Good TA. Role of aggregation conditions in structure, stability, and toxicity of intermediates in the Aβ fibril formation pathway. Protein Sci 2007; 16(4): 723-32.
[http://dx.doi.org/10.1110/ps.062514807] [PMID: 17327396]

[151] Arosio P, Cukalevski R, Frohm B, Knowles TPJ, Linse S. Quantification of the concentration of Aβ42 propagons during the lag phase by an amyloid chain reaction assay. J Am Chem Soc 2014; 136(1): 219-25.
[http://dx.doi.org/10.1021/ja408765u] [PMID: 24313551]

[152] Ahmed M, Davis J, Aucoin D, *et al.* Structural conversion of neurotoxic amyloid-β1–42 oligomers to fibrils. Nat Struct Mol Biol 2010; 17(5): 561-7.
[http://dx.doi.org/10.1038/nsmb.1799] [PMID: 20383142]

[153] Sood A, Abid M, Sauer C, *et al.* Disassembly of preformed amyloid beta fibrils by small organofluorine molecules. Bioorg Med Chem Lett 2011; 21(7): 2044-7.
[http://dx.doi.org/10.1016/j.bmcl.2011.02.012] [PMID: 21354796]

[154] Siddiqi MK, Alam P, Malik S, *et al.* Stabilizing proteins to prevent conformational changes required for amyloid fibril formation. J Cell Biochem 2019; 120(2): 2642-56.
[http://dx.doi.org/10.1002/jcb.27576] [PMID: 30242891]

[155] Arunkumar R, Drummond CJ, Greaves TL. FTIR spectroscopic study of the secondary structure of globular proteins in aqueous protic ionic liquids. Front Chem 2019; 7(FEB): 74. [http://dx.doi.org/10.3389/fchem.2019.00074] [PMID: 30815435]

[156] Greenfield NJ. Using circular dichroism spectra to estimate protein secondary structure. Nat Protoc 2007; 1(6): 2876-90. [http://dx.doi.org/10.1038/nprot.2006.202]

[157] Gregoire S, Irwin J, Kwon I. Techniques for monitoring protein misfolding and aggregation *in vitro* and in living cells. Korean J Chem Eng 2012; 29(6): 693-702. [http://dx.doi.org/10.1007/s11814-012-0060-x] [PMID: 23565019]

[158] Cohen AS, Calkins E. Electron microscopic observations on a fibrous component in amyloid of diverse origins. Nature 1959; 183(4669): 1202-3. [http://dx.doi.org/10.1038/1831202a0] [PMID: 13657054]

[159] Gras SL, Waddington LJ, Goldie KN. Transmission electron microscopy of amyloid fibrils. Methods Mol Biol 2011; 752: 197-214. [http://dx.doi.org/10.1007/978-1-60327-223-0_13] [PMID: 21713639]

[160] Langkilde AE, Vestergaard B. Methods for structural characterization of prefibrillar intermediates and amyloid fibrils. FEBS Lett 2009; 583(16): 2600-9. [http://dx.doi.org/10.1016/j.febslet.2009.05.040] [PMID: 19481541]

[161] Meinhardt J, Sachse C, Hortschansky P, Grigorieff N, Fändrich M. Abeta(1-40) fibril polymorphism implies diverse interaction patterns in amyloid fibrils. J Mol Biol 2009; 386(3): 869-77. [http://dx.doi.org/10.1016/j.jmb.2008.11.005] [PMID: 19038266]

[162] Hoyer W, Grönwall C, Jonsson A, Ståhl S, Härd T. Stabilization of a β-hairpin in monomeric Alzheimer's amyloid-β peptide inhibits amyloid formation. Proc Natl Acad Sci USA 2008; 105(13): 5099-104. [http://dx.doi.org/10.1073/pnas.0711731105] [PMID: 18375754]

[163] Ståhl S, Gräslund T, Eriksson Karlström A, Frejd FY, Nygren PÅ, Löfblom J. Affibody Molecules in Biotechnological and Medical Applications. Trends Biotechnol 2017; 35(8): 691-712. [http://dx.doi.org/10.1016/j.tibtech.2017.04.007] [PMID: 28514998]

[164] Luheshi LM, Hoyer W, de Barros TP, *et al.* Sequestration of the Abeta peptide prevents toxicity and promotes degradation in vivo. PLoS Biol 2010; 8(3): e1000334. [http://dx.doi.org/10.1371/journal.pbio.1000334] [PMID: 20305716]

[165] Boutajangout A, Lindberg H, Awwad A, *et al.* Affibody-mediated sequestration of amyloid β demonstrates preventive efficacy in a transgenic alzheimer's disease mouse model. Front Aging Neurosci 2019; 11: 64. [http://dx.doi.org/10.3389/fnagi.2019.00064] [PMID: 30967771]

[166] Hafner-Bratkovič I, Gašperšič J, Šmid LM, Bresjanac M, Jerala R. Curcumin binds to the α-helical intermediate and to the amyloid form of prion protein – a new mechanism for the inhibition of PrP^{Sc} accumulation. J Neurochem 2008; 104(6): 1553-64. [http://dx.doi.org/10.1111/j.1471-4159.2007.05105.x] [PMID: 17996023]

[167] Jiang P, Li W, Shea JE, Mu Y. Resveratrol inhibits the formation of multiple-layered β-sheet oligomers of the human islet amyloid polypeptide segment 22-27. Biophys J 2011; 100(6): 1550-8. [http://dx.doi.org/10.1016/j.bpj.2011.02.010] [PMID: 21402038]

[168] Li B, Zhong H, Scheuer T, Catterall WA. Nordihydroguaiaretic acid does not disaggregate beta-amyloid(1-40) protofibrils but does inhibit growth arising from direct protofibril association. Mol Pharmacol 2004; 66(3): 761-9. [http://dx.doi.org/10.1124/MOL.66.3] [PMID: 15322269]

[169] Kang IJ, Jeon YE, Yin XF, *et al.* Butanol extract of Ecklonia cava prevents production and aggregation of beta-amyloid, and reduces beta-amyloid mediated neuronal death. Food Chem Toxicol

2011; 49(9): 2252-9.
[http://dx.doi.org/10.1016/j.fct.2011.06.023] [PMID: 21693162]

[170] Umar T, Gusain S, Raza MK, *et al.* Naphthalene-triazolopyrimidine hybrid compounds as potential multifunctional anti-Alzheimer's agents. Bioorg Med Chem 2019; 27(14): 3156-66.
[http://dx.doi.org/10.1016/j.bmc.2019.06.004] [PMID: 31176571]

[171] Li J, Zhu M, Rajamani S, Uversky VN, Fink AL. Rifampicin inhibits alpha-synuclein fibrillation and disaggregates fibrils. Chem Biol 2004; 11(11): 1513-21.

[172] Levy-Sakin M, Shreberk M, Daniel Y, Gazit E. Targeting insulin amyloid assembly by small aromatic molecules: Toward rational design of aggregation inhibitors. Islets 2009; 1(3): 210-5.
[http://dx.doi.org/10.4161/isl.1.3.9609] [PMID: 21099274]

[173] Lieu VH, Wu JW, Wang SSS, Wu CH. Inhibition of amyloid fibrillization of hen egg-white lysozymes by rifampicin and p-benzoquinone. Biotechnol Prog 2007; 23(3): 698-706.
[http://dx.doi.org/10.1021/bp060353n] [PMID: 17492832]

[174] Levy M, Porat Y, Bacharach E, Shalev DE, Gazit E. Phenolsulfonphthalein, but not phenolphthalein, inhibits amyloid fibril formation: implications for the modulation of amyloid self-assembly. Biochemistry 2008; 47(22): 5896-904.
[http://dx.doi.org/10.1021/bi800043d] [PMID: 18457421]

[175] Kim H, Park BS, Lee KG, *et al.* Effects of naturally occurring compounds on fibril formation and oxidative stress of beta-amyloid. J Agric Food Chem 2005; 53(22): 8537-41.
[http://dx.doi.org/10.1021/jf051985c] [PMID: 16248550]

[176] Zelus C, Fox A, Calciano A, Faridian BS, Nogaj LA, Moffet DA. Myricetin inhibits islet amyloid polypeptide (IAPP) aggregation and rescues living mammalian cells from IAPP toxicity. Open Biochem J 2012; 6(1): 66-70.
[http://dx.doi.org/10.2174/1874091X01206010066] [PMID: 22792130]

[177] Prajapati KP, Singh AP, Dubey K, *et al.* Myricetin inhibits amyloid fibril formation of globular proteins by stabilizing the native structures. Colloids Surf B Biointerfaces 2020; 186: 110640.
[http://dx.doi.org/10.1016/j.colsurfb.2019.110640] [PMID: 31835184]

[178] Akaishi T, Morimoto T, Shibao M, *et al.* Structural requirements for the flavonoid fisetin in inhibiting fibril formation of amyloid β protein. Neurosci Lett 2008; 444(3): 280-5.
[http://dx.doi.org/10.1016/j.neulet.2008.08.052] [PMID: 18761054]

[179] Ferreira N, Saraiva MJ, Almeida MR. Natural polyphenols inhibit different steps of the process of transthyretin (TTR) amyloid fibril formation. FEBS Lett 2011; 585(15): 2424-30.
[http://dx.doi.org/10.1016/j.febslet.2011.06.030] [PMID: 21740906]

[180] Khalatbary AR, Khademi E. The green tea polyphenolic catechin epigallocatechin gallate and neuroprotection. Nutr Neurosci 2018; 23(4): 281-94.
[http://dx.doi.org/10.1080/1028415X.2018.1500124]

[181] Martinez Pomier K, Ahmed R, Melacini G. Catechins as Tools to Understand the Molecular Basis of Neurodegeneration. Molecules 2020; 25(16): 3571.
[http://dx.doi.org/10.3390/molecules25163571] [PMID: 32781559]

[182] Green NS, Foss TR, Kelly JW. Genistein, a natural product from soy, is a potent inhibitor of transthyretin amyloidosis. Proc Natl Acad Sci 2005; 102(41): 14545-50.
[http://dx.doi.org/10.1073/pnas.0501609102] [PMID: 16195386]

[183] Alhazmi MA, Khalifa FK, Zeyadi MA. Effect of soy isoflavones on the performance of cerebral neurotransmitter systems in adult and aged male rats. Biosci Biotechnol Res Commun 2020; 13(15): 54-60.
[http://dx.doi.org/10.21786/bbrc/13.15/11]

[184] Thapa A, Woo ER, Chi EY, *et al.* Biflavonoids are superior to monoflavonoids in inhibiting amyloid-β toxicity and fibrillogenesis via accumulation of nontoxic oligomer-like structures. Biochemistry 2011;

50(13): 2445-55.
[http://dx.doi.org/10.1021/bi101731d] [PMID: 21322641]

[185] Yamakawa MY, Uchino K, Watanabe Y, *et al.* Anthocyanin suppresses the toxicity of Aβ deposits through diversion of molecular forms in *in vitro* and *in vivo* models of Alzheimer's disease. Nutr Neurosci 2016; 19(1): 32-42.
[http://dx.doi.org/10.1179/1476830515Y.0000000042] [PMID: 26304685]

[186] Rivière C, Richard T, Vitrac X, Mérillon JM, Valls J, Monti JP. New polyphenols active on β-amyloid aggregation. Bioorg Med Chem Lett 2008; 18(2): 828-31.
[http://dx.doi.org/10.1016/j.bmcl.2007.11.028] [PMID: 18042380]

[187] Salehi B, Sharifi-Rad J, Cappellini F, *et al.* The therapeutic potential of anthocyanins: Current approaches based on their molecular mechanism of action. Front Pharmacol 2020; 11: 1300.
[http://dx.doi.org/10.3389/fphar.2020.01300] [PMID: 32982731]

[188] Umar T, Shalini S, Raza MK, *et al.* New amyloid beta-disaggregating agents: synthesis, pharmacological evaluation, crystal structure and molecular docking of *N* -(4-((7-chloroquinol-n-4-yl)oxy)-3-ethoxybenzyl)amines. MedChemComm 2018; 9(11): 1891-904.
[http://dx.doi.org/10.1039/C8MD00312B] [PMID: 30568757]

[189] Jones MR, Dyrager C, Hoarau M, *et al.* Multifunctional quinoline-triazole derivatives as potential modulators of amyloid-β peptide aggregation. J Inorg Biochem 2016; 158: 131-8.
[http://dx.doi.org/10.1016/j.jinorgbio.2016.04.022] [PMID: 27133802]

[190] Kim J, Harada R, Kobayashi M, Kobayashi N, Sode K. The inhibitory effect of pyrroloquinoline quinone on the amyloid formation and cytotoxicity of truncated alpha-synuclein. Mol Neurodegener 2010; 5(1): 20.
[http://dx.doi.org/10.1186/1750-1326-5-20] [PMID: 20482893]

[191] Atamna H, Frey WH II. A role for heme in Alzheimer's disease: Heme binds amyloid β and has altered metabolism. Proc Natl Acad Sci 2004; 101(30): 11153-8.
[http://dx.doi.org/10.1073/pnas.0404349101] [PMID: 15263070]

[192] Howlett D, Cutler P, Heales S, Camilleri P. Hemin and related porphyrins inhibit β-amyloid aggregation. FEBS Lett 1997; 417(2): 249-51.
[http://dx.doi.org/10.1016/S0014-5793(97)01290-8] [PMID: 9395306]

[193] Lamberto GR, Torres-Monserrat V, Bertoncini CW, *et al.* Toward the discovery of effective polycyclic inhibitors of alpha-synuclein amyloid assembly. J Biol Chem 2011; 286(37): 32036-44.
[http://dx.doi.org/10.1074/jbc.M111.242958] [PMID: 21795682]

[194] Pandolfi F, De Vita D, Bortolami M, *et al.* New pyridine derivatives as inhibitors of acetylcholinesterase and amyloid aggregation. Eur J Med Chem 2017; 141: 197-210.
[http://dx.doi.org/10.1016/j.ejmech.2017.09.022] [PMID: 29031067]

[195] Jones MR, Service EL, Thompson JR, *et al.* Dual-function triazole–pyridine derivatives as inhibitors of metal-induced amyloid-β aggregation. Metallomics 2012; 4(9): 910-20.
[http://dx.doi.org/10.1039/c2mt20113e] [PMID: 22825244]

[196] Saengkhae C, Salerno M, Adès D, *et al.* Ability of carbazole salts, inhibitors of Alzheimer β-amyloid fibril formation, to cross cellular membranes. Eur J Pharmacol 2007; 559(2-3): 124-31.
[http://dx.doi.org/10.1016/j.ejphar.2007.01.005] [PMID: 17291491]

[197] Dolphin GT, Renaudet O, Ouberai M, Dumy P, Garcia J, Reymond JL. Phenolic oxime oligomers inhibit Alzheimer's amyloid fibril formation and disaggregate fibrils *in vitro*. ChemBioChem 2009; 10(8): 1325-9.
[http://dx.doi.org/10.1002/cbic.200900044] [PMID: 19415707]

[198] Török M, Abid M, Mhadgut SC, Török B. Organofluorine inhibitors of amyloid fibrillogenesis. Biochemistry 2006; 45(16): 5377-83.
[http://dx.doi.org/10.1021/bi0601104] [PMID: 16618127]

[199] Török B. Structure-Activity Relationships of Organofluorine Inhibitors of β-Amyloid Self-Assembly 2012. Available from: https://www.academia.edu/81490344/Structure_Activity_Relationships_of_Organofluorine_Inhibitors_of_

[200] Cohen T, Frydman-Marom A, Rechter M, Gazit E. Inhibition of amyloid fibril formation and cytotoxicity by hydroxyindole derivatives. Biochemistry 2006; 45(15): 4727-35. [http://dx.doi.org/10.1021/bi051525c] [PMID: 16605241]

[201] Morshedi D, Rezaei-Ghaleh N, Ebrahim-Habibi A, Ahmadian S, Nemat-Gorgani M. Inhibition of amyloid fibrillation of lysozyme by indole derivatives – possible mechanism of action. FEBS J 2007; 274(24): 6415-25. [http://dx.doi.org/10.1111/j.1742-4658.2007.06158.x] [PMID: 18028426]

[202] Soto-Ortega DD, Murphy BP, Gonzalez-Velasquez FJ, *et al.* Inhibition of amyloid-β aggregation by coumarin analogs can be manipulated by functionalization of the aromatic center. Bioorg Med Chem 2011; 19(8): 2596-602. [http://dx.doi.org/10.1016/j.bmc.2011.03.010] [PMID: 21458277]

[203] Heller GT, Aprile FA, Michaels TCT, *et al.* Small-molecule sequestration of amyloid-β as a drug discovery strategy for Alzheimer's disease. Sci Adv 2020; 6(45): eabb5924. [http://dx.doi.org/10.1126/sciadv.abb5924] [PMID: 33148639]

[204] Frid P, Anisimov SV, Popovic N. Congo red and protein aggregation in neurodegenerative diseases. Brain Res Brain Res Rev 2007; 53(1): 135-60. [http://dx.doi.org/10.1016/j.brainresrev.2006.08.001] [PMID: 16959325]

[205] Lorenzo A, Yankner BA. Beta-amyloid neurotoxicity requires fibril formation and is inhibited by congo red. Proc Natl Acad Sci USA 1994; 91(25): 12243-7. [http://dx.doi.org/10.1073/pnas.91.25.12243] [PMID: 7991613]

[206] van der Hilst JCH, Kluve-Beckerman B, Bodar EJ, van der Meer JWM, Drenth JPH, Simon A. Lovastatin inhibits formation of AA amyloid. J Leukoc Biol 2008; 83(5): 1295-9. [http://dx.doi.org/10.1189/jlb.1107723] [PMID: 18285405]

[207] Malmo C, Vilasi S, Iannuzzi C, *et al.* Tetracycline inhibits W7FW14F apomyoglobin fibril extension and keeps the amyloid protein in a prefibrillar, highly cytotoxic state. FASEB J 2006; 20(2): 346-7. [http://dx.doi.org/10.1096/fj.05-4652fje] [PMID: 16317065]

[208] Dolphin GT, Chierici S, Ouberai M, Dumy P, Garcia J. A multimeric quinacrine conjugate as a potential inhibitor of Alzheimer's β-amyloid fibril formation. ChemBioChem 2008; 9(6): 952-63. [http://dx.doi.org/10.1002/cbic.200700602] [PMID: 18330854]

[209] Matharu B, Gibson G, Parsons R, *et al.* Galantamine inhibits β-amyloid aggregation and cytotoxicity. J Neurol Sci 2009; 280(1-2): 49-58. [http://dx.doi.org/10.1016/j.jns.2009.01.024] [PMID: 19249060]

[210] Familian A, Boshuizen RS, Eikelenboom P, Veerhuis R. Inhibitory effect of minocycline on amyloid β fibril formation and human microglial activation. Glia 2006; 53(3): 233-40. [http://dx.doi.org/10.1002/glia.20268] [PMID: 16220550]

[211] Zhou Y, Jiang C, Zhang Y, *et al.* Structural optimization and biological evaluation of substituted bisphenol A derivatives as beta-amyloid peptide aggregation inhibitors. J Med Chem 2010; 53(15): 5449-66. [http://dx.doi.org/10.1021/jm1000584] [PMID: 20684593]

[212] Han M, Liu Y, Zhang B, *et al.* Salvianic borneol ester reduces β-amyloid oligomers and prevents cytotoxicity. Pharm Biol 2011; 49(10): 1008-13. [http://dx.doi.org/10.3109/13880209.2011.559585] [PMID: 21936627]

[213] Yang F Jr, Zhang M, Zhou BR, Chen J, Liang Y. Oleic acid inhibits amyloid formation of the intermediate of alpha-lactalbumin at moderately acidic pH. J Mol Biol 2006; 362(4): 821-34. [http://dx.doi.org/10.1016/j.jmb.2006.07.059] [PMID: 16935298]

[214] Ahn JH, Hu Y, Hernandez M, Kim JR. Crocetin inhibits beta-amyloid fibrillization and stabilizes beta-amyloid oligomers. Biochem Biophys Res Commun 2011; 414(1): 79-83. [http://dx.doi.org/10.1016/j.bbrc.2011.09.025] [PMID: 21945434]

[215] Hashimoto M, Shahdat HM, Yamashita S, *et al.* Docosahexaenoic acid disrupts *in vitro* amyloid β_{1-40} fibrillation and concomitantly inhibits amyloid levels in cerebral cortex of Alzheimer's disease model rats. J Neurochem 2008; 107(6): 1634-46. [http://dx.doi.org/10.1111/j.1471-4159.2008.05731.x] [PMID: 19014387]

[216] Uversky V. The triple power of D^3: Protein intrinsic disorder in degenerative diseases. Front Biosci 2014; 19(2): 181-258. [http://dx.doi.org/10.2741/4204] [PMID: 24389181]

CHAPTER 5

Resiliency of Protein Dictates Human Health

Tajalli Ilm Chandel[1], **Ifrah Fareed**[1] and **Rizwan Hasan Khan**[1,*]

[1] *Interdisciplinary Biotechnology Unit, Aligarh Muslim University, Aligarh 202002, India*

Abstract: Proteins are functional in their three-dimensional form; any type of modification in the conformation of the protein affects its functions. Thus, the role of the proteins in the body depicts the functional ability and ensures health of an organism. Besides its presence in the body, proteins are consumed by the body in the form of dietary uptake. The free amino group of the protein in the body when interacting with the carbonyl group of the reducing sugar follows the Maillard reaction to produce hazardous by-products which is an advanced glycation end products (AGEs). The process of AGEs formation routes towards the aggregation process. Different studies have shown different aggregation pathways, some restricting the partial unfolding of the protein and the other oligomerization leading to fibril formation depending upon the conditions of the study. It is noteworthy that in *in-vivo* cases, glycation and aggregation are the two sides of the same coin because it is obvious that we have seen the diseased condition due to AGEs formation that also shows aggregation or *vice versa*. Hence, the two causative agents depend upon each other.

Keywords: Advanced glycation end products (AGEs), amyloid fibrils, human diseases, oligomer, protein.

INTRODUCTION

Proteins are the most adaptable macromolecules in living systems and are essential to practically all biological processes. The term "protein" coined from the Greek word "proteios", means primary. This term is quite dependable in nourishment because of its fundamental role in the tissues of animals and humans. They act as catalysts, carry and store molecules such as oxygen, offer immunological protection, mechanical support, produce movement, conduct nerve impulses, and regulate the growth and differentiation of the cells. To support this wide variety of proteins' functions, they are constituted by varied permutations and combinations of the 20 amino acids; the highest for any biomolecule. These amino acids are connected by peptide bonds [1].

* **Corresponding author Rizwan Hasan Khan:** Interdisciplinary Biotechnology Unit, Aligarh-202002, India; Tel: 99977786691; E-mail: rizwanhkhan1@gmal.com

Farzana Mahdi & Abbas Ali Mahdi (Eds.)

DIETARY PROTEINS

Non-essential amino acids and essential amino acids both are synthesized by our body from the abundance of food. Unless they are digested by peptidases and proteases to simpler amino acids in the lumen of the small intestine, these proteins have no nutritional value. The combination of amino acids can have an impact on health, "pure" protein, sourced from plant and animal nutrition, and has equal impacts on health. There are certain "complete proteins" in food, which means they have all the twenty types of amino acids, required by the body. Apart from the complete proteins, others lack one or more necessary amino acids, which our bodies cannot synthesise on their own or even from other amino acids. Edibles from plants frequently lack one or more important amino acids, but foods derived from animals typically provide a complete protein (Fig. **1**) [2, 3].

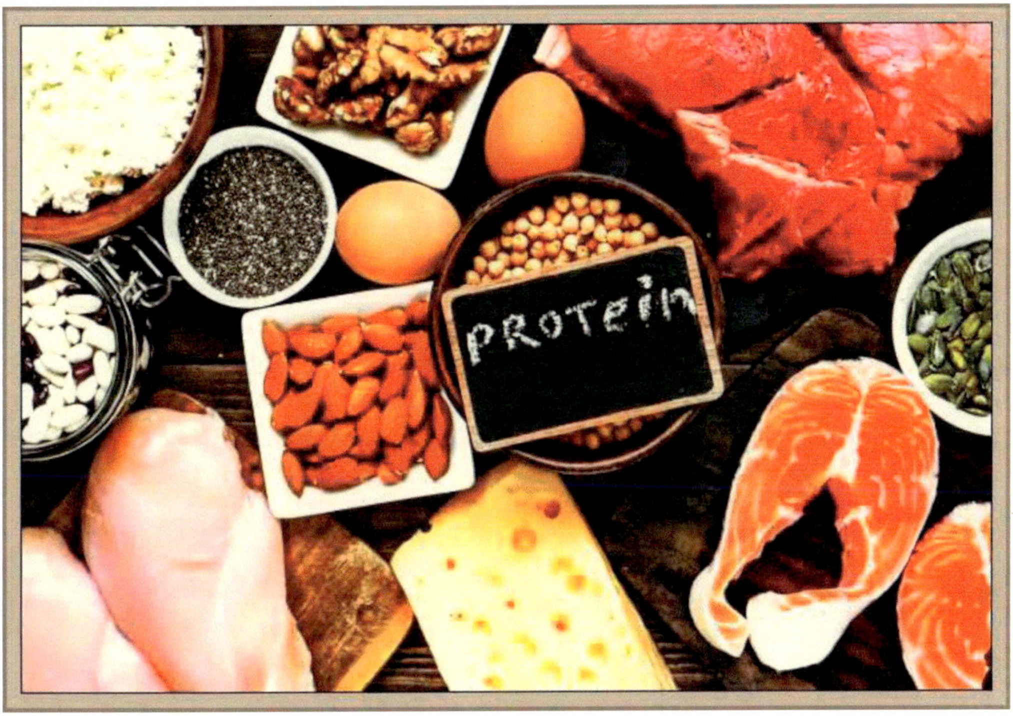

Fig. (1). Pictorial representation of dietary proteins. Source: Internet.

The oxidation of amino acids is enhanced following the substrate-enzyme relationship of Michaelis-Menton kinetics. Thus, this should be taken into account when determining the human diet's needs for amino acids and proteins. Overabundant amino acids are oxidised to carbon dioxide (CO_2), water (H_2O), and urea, except glutamine in the skeletal muscle. There is very little amino acid oxidation when the intake of protein is at the perfect level for protein synthesis The oxidation of amino acids is decreased to spare amino acids for protein synthesis when the animal's nutritional requirements for protein or amino acids are not met. This is because the enzymes responsible for the synthesis of proteins, such as tRNA-amino acid synthases, have substantially lower K_M values and thus, a higher affinity for amino acid substrates than the enzymes responsible for amino acid degradation. Amino acids are largely directed to the pathway of protein synthesis compared to amino acid catabolism. Hence, only a little amount of dietary amino acids are accessible for oxidation in animals nourished with a balanced diet.

The quantity of the protein required by the human diet can be ascertained using a variety of approaches. These methods include nitrogen balancing studies, which examine the relationship between nitrogen intake from food and nitrogen excretion in various forms; factorial analysis, which examines the amount of nitrogen excreted in the urine and faeces in response to a diet low in protein (maintenance); amino acid deposits in the body; and amino acid excreted as animal products (such as milk and foetal growth); and tracer studies, which use the direct and indirect oxidation of the amino acids to detect specific amino acids.

Protein and amino acid requirements are influenced by dietary factors, such as amino acid content, its proportions, the presence of other substances in the food, energy intake; physiological characteristics of the individual, such as genotypic and phenotypic traits, enzymes, hormones, pregnancy, lactation, and physical activity; pathological conditions, such as infection, trauma, diabetes, obesity, cardiovascular disease, and foetal growth restriction; and environmental factors *e.g.*, temperatures, air pollution, sanitation, and personal hygiene, toxic agents and dietary habits [4].

Role of Dietary Proteins

Chemically, the human body is made up of proteins, lipids, minerals, and water. The metabolism of the body is predominantly influenced by the protein component, which is frequently measured as Lean Body Mass (LBM). Protein content in the diet is metabolically significant because it supplies the amino acids needed for the body to synthesize new proteins. They are essential to body metabolism as well as a source of non-communicable or self-styled diseases commonly as diabetes, hypertension, and cardiovascular disease that are ultimately related to disturbances in body metabolism. Dietary protein is necessary for the body's growth and LBM maintenance. It also plays a crucial role in the maintenance of overall health, muscle mass, and strength [2].

Neither sulphur nor nitrogen is produced by the body; amino acids are the only source of these critical components for organisms. No other nutrients, including carbohydrates and lipids, can substitute for amino acids. Amino acids are crucial building blocks of proteins, peptides, and low-molecular-weight compounds with major physiological roles, such as glutathione, creatine, nitric oxide, dopamine, serotonin, RNA, and DNA. In the fed state, the mammalian small intestine uses dietary glutamate, glutamine, and aspartate as significant metabolic fuels, whereas, in the post-absorptive state, glutamine in the arterial blood serves as the organ's nearly exclusive source of energy. Glutamine supplies 50% and 35% of ATP in lymphocytes and macrophages, respectively to support immunological responses. Amino acids are necessary for an organism's survival, reproduction, growth, development, and lactation [4].

PROTEINS IN THE BODY

The condensation process between amino acids results in the production of a peptide bond that needs energy to form the main structure of the protein. Once the main structure has been formed, it is quite likely that some of the amino acid residues, such as glycine and leucine, will have hydrophobic nonpolar side chains, while others, such as serine and glutamine, would have hydrophilic polar and charged side chains. The hydrophilic side chains actively interact with water present in the aqueous environment of the cell through hydrogen bonding, but the hydrophobic side groups fold into one another to reduce interaction with water, resulting in the formation of a compact structure. The side group of the amino acids in the peptide backbone containing the amide (NH) and carbonyl groups (C=O), is brought into the hydrophobic core as a result of the hydrophobic side groups infolding. Hence, the peptide backbone is forced to interact with itself by forming hydrogen bonds, which results in the formation of distinct structural components known as secondary structures. The α-helix and β-pleated sheets are the two secondary structures that are formed most frequently. The α-turn and β-loop are additional ones.

The α-helix and the β-sheet are the primary and secondary-structural moieties in globular proteins. The other secondary structures such as π-helix (pi helix), 310-helix, β-turn, and Ω-loop (omega loop) are also present, along with some areas of the protein whose secondary structure is uncategorized. This is called random coil, more precisely stated to be unstructured regions [5]. 310-helix is the fourth most common type of secondary structure. 3_{10} helices are present at the N and C-terminal of the α-helix which constitute approximately 15-20% of the total α-helix of the protein. Thus it can be said that 3_{10}-helices comprises 03-05 residues relative to an average of ten to twelve residues for α-helices in the protein [6]. This entity has been proposed to be intermediate in the folding/unfolding of α-helices [6]. Hence it can be stated that 310-helices may have a key role in oligomerization.

The solid tertiary structure is made up of the components of the secondary structure. The ensuing tertiary structure, which is stabilized by weak interactions between polar and nonpolar groups, is created when the protein folds upon itself. The spatial arrangement of subunits and the type of interactions between them are referred to as the quaternary structure stabilized by non-covalent interactions as well as disulfide linkages [7].

According to the "framework" theory, the emergence of an intermediate stage known as the molten globule is the result of the collapse, arrangement, and interaction of well-defined local secondary structures, leading to the formation of the tertiary element with the hydrophobic core. The "hydrophobic collapse" theory states that the hydrophobic side chains collapse first during protein folding, which is then followed by the development of different secondary structures. Combining the aforementioned ideas, the "nucleation condensation" hypothesis postulates that the hydrophobic groups coalesce as the secondary structures take shape [7].

Its Functions

The basic function of the protein is based on its fundamental structure mentioned in Fig. (**2**).

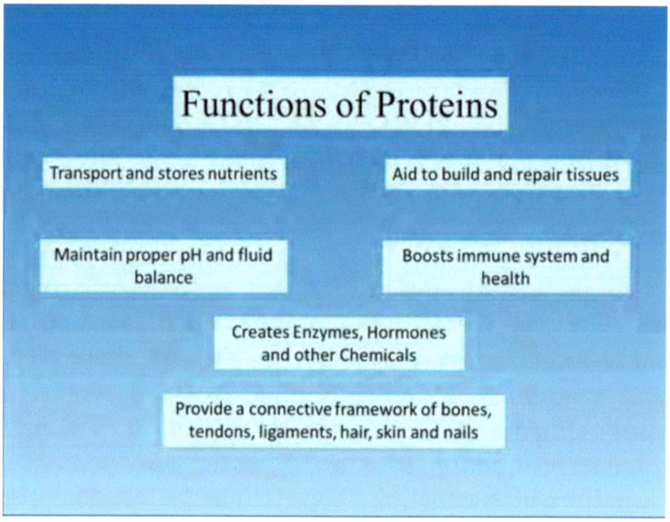

Fig. (2). Basic function of the proteins.

The fundamental structure of the peptide chain itself contains all the information required to fold the protein into its natural tertiary structure. Chaperones occasionally help the cellular process of protein folding. These chaperones are not required for the unfolding and refolding of proteins in the diluted solution. The proteins can be divided into three main groups according to their structural makeup: fibrous, globular, and intermediate.

Fibrous Proteins: In fibrous proteins, polypeptide chains are organized parallel along a single axis, resulting in long thread like fibres. These proteins provide mechanical strength and resistance to water solubilization resulting in exhibiting a structural role in nature. The β-keratin, collagen, elastin, and fibrin are a few examples of fibrous proteins [8].

Globular Protein: The most prevalent proteins in nature are globular proteins, which get their name from how roughly spherical they are. There is a huge range of three-dimensional configurations that globular proteins can take. Nearly all globular proteins have significant amounts of folded α-helices and β-sheets that are stabilized by both polar and nonpolar interactions. The formation of the globular three-dimensional structure of the protein is caused because of the interactions between the side chains of the amino acids. Globular proteins are frequently soluble in aqueous solutions. The functions carried out by the globular proteins, including binding, catalysis, regulation, transport, immunity, and cellular signalling, is reflected in the diversity of protein shapes. Troponin, haemoglobin, albumin, lysozyme, insulin, as well as innumerable antibodies, hormones, and enzymes, are examples of globular proteins [8].

Human Serum Albumin (HSA): The liver produces HSA, a protein with a molecular weight of 66.5 kDa. It has 585 amino acids residues, cysteine residues, and various negatively-charged amino acids. Albumin makes up the majority of plasma proteins (~ 60%), and maintenance of the plasma's colloid osmotic pressure is the main function of albumin protein. Thyroxine, hemin, bilirubin, as well as both saturated and unsaturated fatty acids, are among the many metabolites that HSA transports and aids in the removal. Albumin binds a range of exogenous cationic and anionic hydrophobic ligands in addition to fatty acids, which are its primary physiological ligands. Three helical domains in HSA have a similar structural makeup [9]. Each subdomain's stability is supported by a large number of disulfide bonds. On both domains, 2 and 3, there is a pocket that is mainly composed of hydrophobic and positively charged residues, and it may accommodate a remarkably varied spectrum of molecules [10, 11].

Human Lysozyme (HL): A ubiquitous, cationic enzyme with a molecular weight of 14 kDa, breaks the β-glycosidic bond between the C_1 and C_4 of N-acetyl muramate (NAM) and N-acetyl glucosamine (NAG). The lone polypeptide chain in the HL structure is made up of seven helices and a single three stranded β-sheet. The physiological isoelectric point of lysozyme is 9.28. The native state of enzyme has four random coils, two antiparallel beta-pleated sheets, and four alpha helices. The primary focus of lysozyme is on peptidoglycan, a glycosidic polymer and structural composition of the bacterial cell wall that imparts shape and structure of the cells and osmotic resistance. Lysozyme is found in high concentrations in mammalian milk, tears, granulocytes, macrophages, and respiratory secretions. Human granulocytes' phagocytic and secretory granules contain large amounts of lysozyme, the primary protein produced by macrophages. The structure, function, folding and unfolding of the lysozyme have all been the subject of intense studies. The main cause of the uncommon but fatal disorder known as hereditary non-neuropathic systemic amyloidosis is the accumulation of massive amounts of amyloid deposits in the spleen, kidneys and liver of the affected individuals [12, 13].

Human Insulin (HI): The islets of Langerhans' beta-cells secrete the hormone insulin. It is a 6000 Da polypeptide made up of amino acid chains A and B that are connected by two-disulfide-bridges. Preproinsulin which is a precursor insulin is produced by pancreatic cells. It has 31-residue C-peptide (residues 57-84] that connects the A-chains and B-chains (residues 90-110, and 25-54 respectively). The 110-residue-long preprohormone is cleaved into three segments by proteolytic enzymes during the maturation of insulin. This results in the elimination of the C-chain and the attachment of the A and B chains by disulphide bonds, resulting in a final length of 51 residues. Insulin's crucial job is to make it easier for glucose to enter body cells. Insulin primarily affects the liver, adipose tissue, and skeletal muscle all at once. Insulin molecules in their hexameric shape are found in the secretory granules of the pancreatic beta-cells. The conversion of insulin from a hexamer to a monomer has very little effect on the protein's structural makeup [1]. However, insulin undergoes a partial but noteworthy unfolding process under amyloidogenic conditions (high temperatures, ionic strength, insulin concentration, *etc*.), leading to the formation of amyloid fibrils made up of insoluble insulin deposits close to the site of its application, particularly in connection with the insulin pump used for diabetes therapy. Amyloidosis from an injection is the pathological disease in question [14].

Intrinsically disordered proteins (IDPs): It was believed from a very long time that a protein's 3D structure and function were inextricably linked. For this reason, a lot of study on the subject of proteins has been and continues to be centred on figuring out protein structures. Many eukaryotic gene sequences encode complete proteins or substantial portions of proteins without a three-dimensional fold. All organisms frequently contain IDPs and IDPRs, or functional proteins and protein regions lacking distinctive structures. They typically have a low percentage of bulk hydrophobic side chains and a high percentage of polar and charged amino acid residues. IDPs/IDRs come in a wide range of structural subtypes, from compact, disorder-restricted states to highly disordered, extended conformational ensembles. IDPs frequently play key roles in controlling signalling pathways and putting together molecular machinery. They frequently serve as hubs in protein interaction networks. IDRs (intrinsically disordered regions) can be divided into two categories: those that fold when bound or when the environment changes and those that remains largely unfolded. The capacity of IDRs to assume non-native states of globular proteins, such as the molten globule or the coiled-coil state, adds another layer of diversity exhibiting weak and fleeting interactions and being metastable. IDRs' structural changes over time may fluctuate between several low energetic levels. IDPs/IDPRs are known to have distinctive amino acid sequences that are known to be enriched in disorder-promoting residues (Arg, Pro, Gln, Gly, Glu, Ser, Ala, and Lys) and depleted in order-promoting residues (Trp, Cys, Tyr, Ile, Phe, Phe, Val, Asn, and Leu). IDPs are enriched in proteins that are linked to cancer, diabetes, cardiovascular disease, and neurological diseases. Cancer-related proteins, such as the oncogene c-Myc and the cancer suppressor gene p53, frequently contain disordered regions, and the fluctuating abundance of these proteins aids in the growth of cancer. In addition, mutations in several disordered proteins, including α-synuclein and amyloid β-peptide (Aβ), can encourage aggregation and causes neurodegenerative disorders [15 - 17].

Amyloid-β (Aβ) peptide: The bigger amyloid precursor protein (APP), a single-pass transmembrane protein, is converted into the intrinsically disordered protein (IDP) Aβ, which has a length of 39 to 43 amino acids. A segment of Aβ is present in the C-terminal region of the APP, inserted into the cytoplasmic membrane and forms a hydrophobic transmembrane area there. The Aβ- and Aβ-secretases sequentially cleave APP to create the A-peptides. According to the amyloid Aβ cascade hypothesis, cleavage products from the APP are neurotoxic and eventually lead to the production of neurofibrillary tangles, which results in cell death [18].

α-Synuclein (αS): Parkinson's disease (PD) is one of the synucleopathies, a group of conditions characterized by Lewy bodies (LBs) or other types of α-synuclein (αS) deposits. It belongs to a family of three proteins that includes α-synuclein, β-synuclein, and γ-synuclein in humans. An N-terminal domain (residues 1-65], a non-amyloid component of plaques (NAC) domain (residues 66-95], and a C-terminal domain (residues 96-140] make up the 140 amino acid residues of this disordered protein. Studies revealed that this disease is brought on by the misfolding and accumulation of mutant-type αS. The N-terminal region of αS is home to all known clinical mutations, highlighting the importance of this region in sunuclein pathophysiology. The NAC domain, has a stretch of 12 amino acids, is in charge of the aggregation qualities by preventing its breakdown and encouraging its fibrillation [18].

The kinase-inducible transcriptional-activation domain (KID) of CREB is one of the best-studied dynamic IDPs. When the KID polypeptide binds to its target domain in CBP41, despite being intrinsically disordered it folds and generate a pair of orthogonal helices, both as an isolated peptide and in full-length CREB39. Interestingly, the intrinsic disorder of the KID and a natural tendency of helices in the region that experiences the coupled folding and binding transition may both be accurately anticipated from the amino-acid sequence [19].

GLYCATION

Many external influences, such as temperature, pH, chemical species, agitation, and oxidising species, cause instability of the protein. This in turn disrupts the native structure of the protein, resulting in denaturation, ultimately leading to protein dysfunction. As a result, the proteins overcome the energy barrier for unfolding and become unfolded. The conformational and functional destruction of macromolecules, followed by cellular malfunction and death, is a result of several mechanisms, including both by oxidative and carbonyl stresses. Furthermore, glycation, is an attachment of reducing to bio-macromolecules, plays a role in a number of degenerative diseases and certain other chronic disorders, including cardiac dysfunction, diabetes mellitus, vascular disorders, visual disorders, nephropathy, and diabetic atherosclerosis. Protein glycation is a non-enzymatic process that differs greatly from glycosylation, which involves an enzyme-catalyzed process and the addition of carbohydrate molecules at specified sites. Glycation is a complicated network reaction that takes place as a result of covalent condensation between the carbonyl group of acyclic carbohydrates and a nucleophilic reaction, also known as the oxidative Maillard reaction. For most cells, glucose serves as a vital macronutrient and a source of energy and carbons for growth and survival. However, due to its natural propensity to react with free amines in proteins, especially in long-lived proteins, glucose also has a harmful effect. All reducing sugars can initiate glycation, although d-ribose has the highest activity. The principal intracellular glycation agent, methylglyoxal, is much more reactive than d-glucose, which has the lowest reactivity and the smallest intracellular concentration [20].

End products produced at various glycation stages come in a variety of forms. The condensation of free amino groups from proteins and carbonyl groups form the reducing sugars in stage A. A reversible product with aldimine linkage as a Schiff base carbon-nitrogen double bond structure and useful electrophilic characteristics is produced in this process. This reaction occurs within an hour depending upon the concentration of the sugar. Stage B is an intramolecular rearrangement that occurs as keto-enol tautomerism occurs in Schiff bases to Amadori products (over the course of days) with a rather stable keto-mine bond but the reaction is still reversible. In stage C of the glycation process, the accumulated Amadori products, will undergo complicated chemical rearrangements (oxidations, reductions, and hydrations) and form cross-linked proteins. This process undertakes weeks or months and it is irreversible. The final brownish products are called AGEs (Fig. **3**).

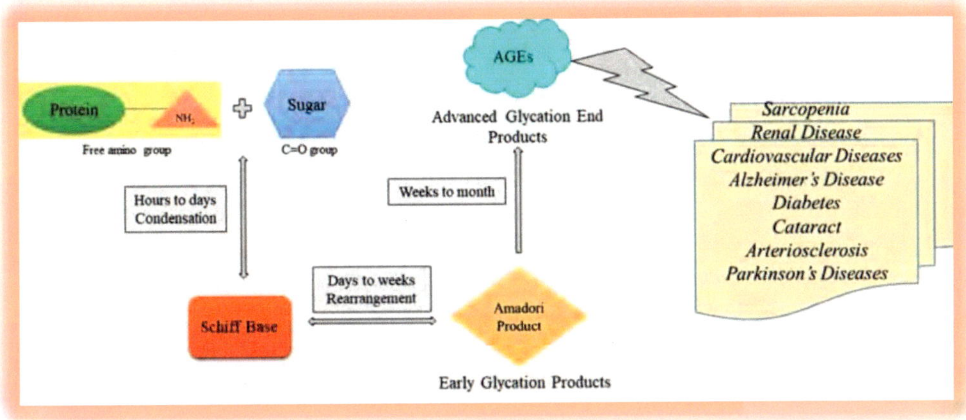

Fig. (3). AGEs formation: Reducing sugar and free amino group of protein produce schiff base and undergo rearrangement to form Amadori products, finally converted to AGEs.

Among the most widely studied AGEs are pentosidine, carboxymethyl-lysine (CML) and pyrraline (Fig. **4**). Out of these pentosidine is a fluorescent protein crosslink while others are not fluorescent and not cross-linked AGEs. They are very stable, and accumulate endogenously and exogenously that interfere with protein function.

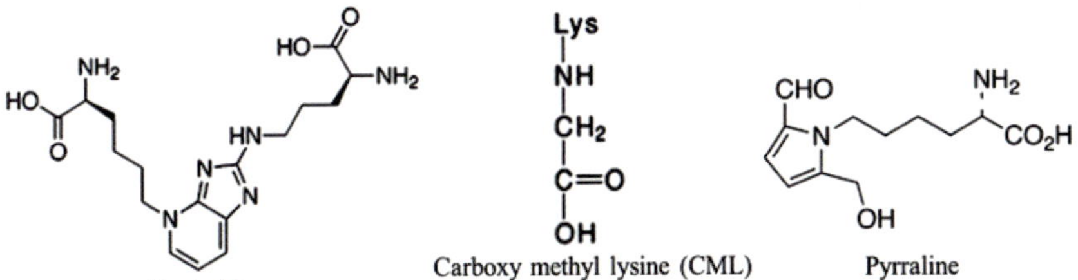

Fig. (4). Chemical structure of most widely studied advanced glycation end products (AGEs).

Glycation leads to the formation of aggregates or induction or promotion of aggregation process, which is a known causal factor in the emergence of degenerative illnesses. Heterogeneous reactive glycol-toxins with an oxidative and aggressive nature dominate the glycation products.

a. Schiff base is an unstable compound. The microenvironment of the target point is altered by the formation of covalent bonds between reducing sugar and free amino group in lysine and arginine residues, which causes the polypeptide to partially unfold and further exposes residues for additional interactions like intra and intermolecular cross-linking. For instance, due to its particular reducing agents, the Schiff base is directly engaged in the glycation of lens crystallins and the production of high molecular weight aggregates (HMW) in ascorbylated calf lens water-soluble proteins (CLP).

b. Glycation, rearrange the Schiff base and produce the *Amadori products*. The rearrangement and dehydration of Amadori products, results in aggregation of protein and advanced glycated ends products formation which are the sources of the cross-links between adjacent proteins. Amadori products, which are early glycation products, play the largest role in the complexity of diabetes.

c. The Amadori product degradation initiates the middle stage of the Maillard reaction, which is then followed by the creation of very small intermediates known as reactive carbonyl species (RCS), which serve as precursors to the AGE products. The primary intracellular reactive carbonyl intermediate is methylglyoxal. The Maillard process, its hazardous by-products, and protein inter- and intra-cross linking can all be enhanced by these chemicals' re-interaction with protein-free amino groups.

d. Amadori products undergo a complicated process that results in heterogeneous covalent adducts as *AGE products*, including condensation, dehydration, rearrangement, oxidation, and possible fragmentation. The diseases of long-term consequences of diabetes and the general ageing process are both directly impacted by AGE product accumulation. By creating intra or intermolecular cross-links that cause a local or global unfolding, AGE products are regarded as denaturants and mechanical stress inducers on the polypeptide. These are the two basic ways that AGEs cause tissue destruction: (a) cross-linking mechanism; (b) activation of numerous inflammatory signalling pathways because the creation of reactive species like ROS occurs simultaneously with the development of AGEs [20].

Several studies have been conducted on diverse proteins to learn more about the glycation-induced aggregation mechanisms and dynamics. On different AGE derived-peptides, various *in-vitro* experiments have been conducted. The substantial effects of lysine residue glycation on oligomer stability, secondary structure content, structural disorder, and inter-peptide salt bridge propensities have been demonstrated. The glycated peptide produced an assembly that was stiffer and had a higher beta-sheet component, which suggests that glycation changes the conformational constitution of important self-assembling components, making them more prone to aggregation [21, 22].

MALADIES

The intimate connection between protein glycation and amyloidosis illnesses is strongly underscored by the presence of glycated proteins in amyloid plaques.

The most prevalent serum protein, human serum albumin (HSA), which has many uses both *in-vivo* and *in-vitro* includes 83 possible glycation sites. This has been utilized extensively as a model for understanding the structural implications of glycation (59 lysine and 23 arginine residues, N terminus) [23]. Although, HSA is a highly soluble protein that is mostly structured in α-helical form, it has been linked to several issues of diabetes due to its ability to produce amyloid fibrils through partial tertiary structure unfolding and secondary structure conformational changes. Several glycating agents, including glucose, D-ribose, (methylglyoxal), MGO, and GO, can effectively glycate this protein *in-vitro*, and effects on the amyloid tendency have been seen with all of them. By lowering the number of helices and boosting the creation of a β-structure, which quickly transforms into the production of amyloid aggregates, glycation increases amyloid aggregation in HSA. In addition to boosting amyloid formation, glycation of albumin carried out in the presence of D-ribose has been demonstrated to stabilise the partially folded oligomeric species that cause substantial cytotoxicity in neuronal cells. It has been demonstrated that preservatives like potassium sorbate which causes the Maillard reaction, increases β-structure elements, and hydrophobicity. This causes human serum albumin to lose some of its native structure and encourage the formation of toxic intermediates like molten globules. According to a study, glycation distorts the helix and transforms it near the site of glycation into a 3_{10}-helical structure in a di-lysine motif obtained from human serum albumin used as a model helical peptide system. *In-vitro* glycation of HSA has been reported to be inhibited by a number of medications and organic substances. For instance, rosmarinic acid, which is present in a variety of plants from the Lamiaceae (the mint) family, is significant because it can suppress AGEs and early glycation products such as fructosamine [24]. Additionally, it has been found that, in a dose-dependent manner, garlic extract inhibits the development of AGEs, carbonyl compounds, and ketoamine, which are products of the glycation reaction [25]. HSA glycation is also prevented by vitamin B_3 [26].

Advanced glycation end-products (AGEs) and α-Syn are co-localized in the brains of individuals with Parkinson's disease in both the early and advanced phases, suggesting that glycation plays a significant role in the aggregation of α-Syn. It has been demonstrated that glycation of -Syn in the presence of D-ribose, MGO, and GO as glycating agents significantly stabilises the N-terminal domain and prevents the development of amyloid fibrils. Glycation encourages the development of persistent cross-linked oligomeric species, able to cause oxidative stress and significant cytotoxicity, despite inhibiting fibril formation. Additionally, individuals with diabetes mellitus (DM) may be more susceptible to the deposition of AGEs on LBs, which may help to explain why PD is more common in DM patients. Additionally, glycated α-Syn causes lipid peroxidation *in vivo* and cell damage. These factors suggest that glycation may be crucial in the amyloid aggregation of α-Syn associated with the development of Lewy bodies in PD [21].

Another well known protein Insulin, is connected to glycemia and is vulnerable to *in vivo* glycation by glucose and other highly reactive carbonyls, particularly in diabetic environments. According to studies, glycation can influence insulin's structure, stability, and amyloid aggregation, and different glycated species have distinct structural characteristics depending on the experimental setup. While glycation greatly suppresses amyloid formation in non-reducing settings in a manner proportional to the degree of glycation, it enhances insulin oligomerization in reducing conditions, which speeds up amyloid aggregation. The production of AGE can be prevented by pharmaceuticals including metformin, angiotensin receptor antagonists, aminoguanidine, angiotensin-converting enzyme inhibitors, and other hypoglycemic medicines [21].

Amylin is also secreted along with insulin. The cleavage of islet amyloid polypeptide (hIAPP) results in the formation of amylin. hIAPP, the 37-residue natively unstructured polypeptide is known to aggregate into amyloid fibrils, which results in islet cell mass loss, cell death, and pancreatic cell dysfunction. Therefore, it is believed that one of the main reasons for type-2 Diabetes Mellitus is the accumulation of hIAPP. It has been demonstrated that *in vitro* glycation of IAPP with glucose encourages the development of protein aggregates with higher cytotoxicity and better seeding efficiency than freshly dissolved IAPP. Similar data were recently obtained on the chemically synthesized AGE-IAPP by modification of Lys-1, the only Lys residue, with carboxymethyl-lysine (CML) AGE. This CML-modified IAPP was forming amyloid aggregates faster than non-modified IAPP, and higher molecular weight AGE-IAPP oligomers were also observed in the early stage of aggregation [21].

Polysaccharides like Auricularia or Astragalus; Polyphenols like caffeic acid, ferulic acid, syringic acid, and others; Common natural substances like vitamins A, C, E, and B_6 have been demonstrated to reduce protein glycation. Despite having several side effects, synthetic drugs like ibuprofen, warfarin, and diclofcnac which do inhibit glycation, have become more and more popular over time [22].

AGGREGATION

The self-assembly of proteins into supra-molecular structures, such as dimers or intricately structured amyloid fibrils, is known as protein aggregation. The capacity to aggregate is a characteristic of polypeptide chains more generally rather than merely being unique to uncommon or disease-related proteins. Intrinsically disordered proteins, such as α-synuclein, are frequently found in proteins involved in aggregation-related disorders (IDP). Through hydrophobic interactions, two or more improperly folded protein intermediates join together to create either amorphous aggregates with a granular appearance or highly organised fibrillar aggregates known as amyloid, which has the β-sheet secondary structure. An organism's life is greatly impacted by the aggregation of proteins, both in desired and undesirable ways. Our bodies exhibit two main types of protein aggregation:

Innate productive aggregation. For instance, the management of the shape and motility of the cells depends on the fibrillation of G-actin to F-actin.

Unwanted aggregation in biology: Aggregation of α-synuclein, amyloid, polyglutamine, and prions, respectively, is linked to neurodegenerative illnesses like Parkinson's, Alzheimer's, Huntington's, and Prion disease.

In addition to these two types of protein aggregation that occur naturally in our bodies, the biotechnology sector also experiences protein aggregation during production and purification of the biopharmaceuticals. In other cases, beneficial protein aggregation products are created explicitly, such as protein nanofibers that are exploited in drug administration [27].

On Pathway Aggregation

While off-pathway oligomers are stable and unable to further seed the aggregation, on-pathway oligomers are distinguished by their capacity to further integrate the monomers. Depending on the protein concentration, the aggregation kinetics for on-pathway oligomers in amyloidogenic proteins can be either nucleation-dependent or an independent process.

Nucleation Dependent Mechanism

The creation of nuclei is required for the emergence of higher-ordered structures including oligomers, protofibrils, and fibrils, which is how the majority of amyloid fibrils normally form. Since the nucleus is the species in the aggregation route with the highest energy level, the nucleation process is a lengthy and rate-determining step. Pre-nuclear aggregation formation is not favourable because the energy gain from the bond formation is outweighed by the loss of rotational and translational entropy. The amyloid production process through nucleated polymerization exhibits concentration-dependent behaviour. A concentration exists below which aggregation formation does not occur. Critical concentration is the term used to describe this focus. The monomer and oligomer/aggregate are in equilibrium at this concentration.

The three steps, sigmoidal curve that characterizes the nucleation-dependent mechanism of amyloid production includes a nucleation phase, an elongation phase, and a saturation phase (Fig. **5**). The creation of the crucial nuclei is represented by the nucleation phase. Nuclei are sluggish to develop and transform into larger aggregates fairly quickly due to the downhill dynamic character of their growth. The interaction of the nucleus/oligomer and monomers during the elongation phase results in prefibrillar structures, which quickly develop into protofibrils, an organised fibrillar structure. Once the nucleus is established, the addition of monomers proceeds quickly, which may be caused by cluster stabilisation brought on by interactions between monomers. Typically, during the saturation phase, protofibrils associate with mature amyloid fibrils. By introducing fibrillar species or pre-formed aggregates known as seeds, the nucleation phase can be speeded up or completely avoided (Fig. **6**).

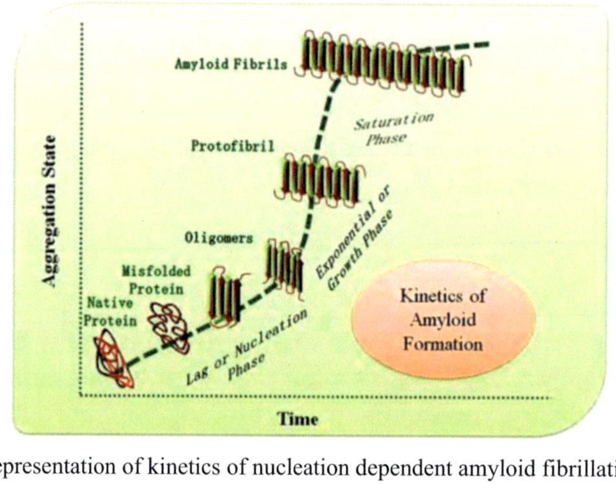

Fig. (5). Schematic representation of kinetics of nucleation dependent amyloid fibrillation.

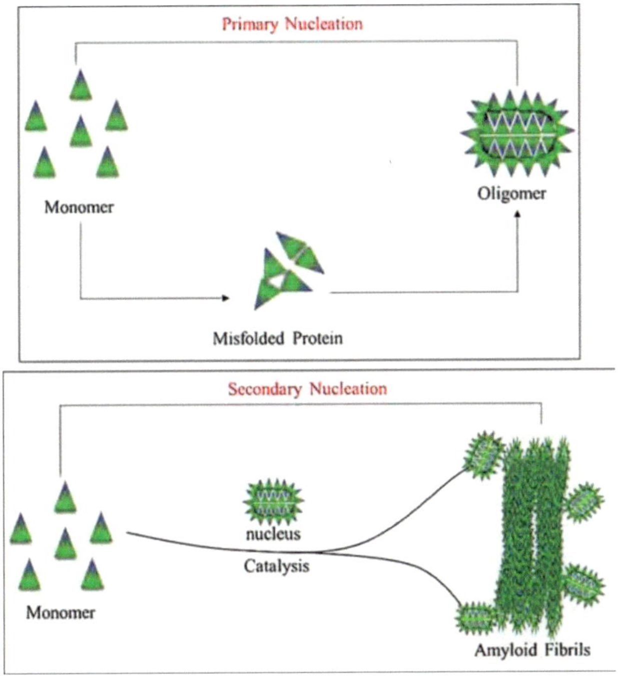

Fig. (6). Schematic representation of mechanisms of nucleation dependent amyloid fibril formation. Upper panel: Primary nucleation. Lower panel: Secondary nucleation mechanism of aggregation.

Primary nucleation: It is the process of producing amyloidogenic nuclei without the aid of seeds or oligomers that have already been created. Both homogeneous and heterogeneous primary nucleation is possible. While heterogeneous primary nucleation involves the interaction of monomers on the surface of a distinct object, such as phospholipid bilayers at the air-water interface, homogeneous primary nucleation involves the formation of monomer aggregates in bulk solution.

Secondary nucleation: Contrary to the heterogeneous primary nucleation, where new aggregates are created on an external surface, fibril-catalyzed secondary nucleation expressly forms new aggregates on the surface of pre-existing fibrils. Secondary processes for fibril formation rely on the population of pre-existing aggregates, whereas primary processes only consider the concentration of free monomers. One of the crucial secondary nucleation processes that accelerate the production of amyloid fibrils is thought to be fibril fragmentation. The fragmentation of fibrils caused by mechanical processes like agitation or sonication boosts the proportion of growth-competent fibril ends and quickens the process of turning monomers into fibrils. Branching is a different secondary pathway that increases the number of aggregates. In contrast to heterogeneous nucleation, branching does not establish a nucleus; instead, new aggregates form on top of older aggregates. In contrast to heterogeneous nucleation, branching does not have a free energy barrier [27, 28].

Aggregates

Abnormal association of protein into larger insoluble moieties, under stressed condition is called as aggregates. *e.g.* amyloid fibrils, oligomers, amorphous aggregates, and inclusion bodies.

Amyloid Fibres

The recurring substructure of amyloid fibrils is made up of β-strands that run parallel to the fibril axis. These β-strands exclusively form intermolecular β-sheets that run the entire length of the fibril rather than the intramolecular ß-sheets that would typically occur in globular proteins. They exhibit helical symmetry, with each repeating unit having a twist and rise. The twist in amyloids is typically gradual, only a few degrees per subunit. Two proto filaments, which are often symmetric, make up the majority of amyloid fibrils. There are two distinct layouts for the symmetry between the protofilaments: (a) an approximate 21-screw symmetry, where the layer in one protofilament is in between layers of the opposing protofilaments. (b) The C2 symmetry, where two corresponding layers in the opposing filaments are precisely on the same height along the fibril axis.

Oligomer

Depending on their capacity to develop into fibrils, oligomers may be classified as "on-pathway" or "off-pathway" oligomers. Off pathway aggregation process restricts the growth of oligomers to fibril formation.

The term "polymorphism" describes the presence of various fibril folds made from the same amino acid sequence. The various folds, or "morphs," can vary in the polypeptide chain segments that make up the β-strands or how they are arranged in the protofilament, each of which results in a distinct protofilament conformation. The relative arrangement of protofilaments to one another can also vary between forms. Small, soluble, easily diffusible protein complexes that are more globular in form than fibrils are sometimes referred to as oligomers. Some oligomers have undergone structural investigation, producing heterogeneous structures with high-sheet content [29].

Multiple approaches allow amyloidogenic proteins to aggregate into various assembly configurations. To grow into mature fibrils and attract additional similar building blocks, monomers can create growth-competent fibrillary oligomers. The recruitment of non-identical building blocks is made possible *via* cross-seeding. Fibril-induced fibril production has been used to describe secondary nucleation. Most oligomers have been shown to aggregate into curvilinear protofibrils even though they are off-pathway and cannot develop into fibrils [30].

Amorphous Aggregates

These are the aggregates that, when viewed under an ultra-microscope, appear to lack organised intermolecular connections. However, many of them exhibit local β–structure. A protein loses its function when present in concentrations greater than its solubility and aggregates, most frequently as amorphous aggregates. However, unlike ß-sheeted fibrillar aggregates called amyloidogenic aggregates, which are frequently linked to neurological disorders, proteins aggregate and oligomerize in amorphous aggregates without forming a particular high-order structures. Amorphous aggregates are more than just clumps of improperly folded proteins that cling to one another *via* random hydrophobic interactions. Instead, they are frequently abundant in cross-β structure, and their tendency to form structures correlates with charge as well as secondary structure propensity (Fig. **7**) and hydrophobicity, pointing to a particular method of production. We know very little about the dynamics of the production of amorphous aggregates, in contrast to the kinetics of the creation of amyloid fibrils. It is not quite obvious how nucleation affects amorphous aggregation [31, 32].

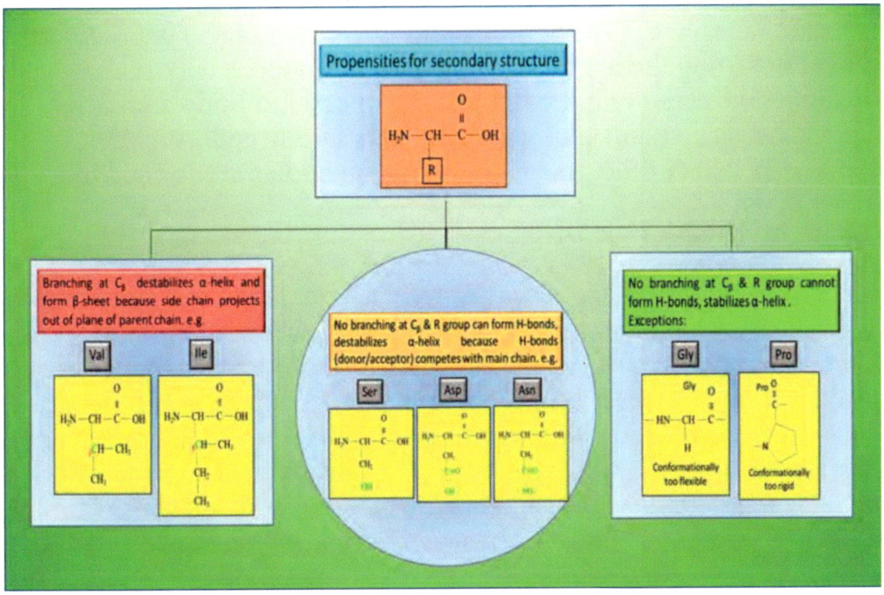

Fig. (7). Secondary structural propensity to form cross-β sheet structure.

Inclusion Bodies

Inclusion Bodies are thought to be disordered aggregates that are produced by both heterologous and homologous overexpression of proteins in both prokaryotes and eukaryotes. This stresses that the aggregation is caused by the overexpression itself. Lewy Bodies, which are inclusion bodies in the human, are discovered during the pathophysiology of Parkinson's disease. Lewy bodies (LBs) are cytoplasmic proteinaceous α-synuclein (α-syn) and lipid-rich aggregates. To date, immunohistochemistry investigations have identified more than 100 additional proteins within LBs. The Lewy body was formed of an exterior zone made up of radially aligned filaments and an interior core that looked to be relatively dense. Initial research identified cytoskeletal proteins as well as proteins present in pathological inclusions linked to other disorders (for example, neurofilaments, tubulin, and tau-paired helical filaments). Many inclusion bodies, which are typically found at the poles or cell bodies of neuronal cells, are refractile in phase contrast microscopy and show up as electron-dense deposits in transmission electron micrographs. Classical inclusion bodies are somewhat resistant to solubilization, whereas some insoluble material is morphologically distinct and much more easily dissolved in denaturant. High local protein concentration, a reducing environment in the cytoplasm, a lack of post-translational modifications, improper interactions with chaperones and other enzymes involved *in vivo* folding, and intermolecular disulfide crosslinking have all been proposed as causes of inclusion body formation (although inclusion bodies can form from proteins lacking cysteine). The aggregation of native proteins with low solubility, the unfolded state, and the aggregation of intermediate partially folded states have all been suggested as potential pathways for inclusion body formation. Despite technological advancements and improvements in our understanding of amyloid dynamics, we still don't fully grasp how inclusion bodies are formed [33, 34].

NEURODEGENERATIVE DISEASES

The term "neurodegenerative disease" refers to a broad category of illnesses (progressive loss of neuronal structure or function) that predominantly impact the brain's neurons and result in their death. Neuronal circuitry can exhibit neurodegeneration at several levels, from the molecular to the systemic. Protein aggregates and misfolded proteins build up in the brain in a variety of neurodegenerative illnesses, including prion, Alzheimer's, Parkinson's, Creutzfeldt-Jacob, Huntington's, and amyotrophic lateral sclerosis. More than 20 polypeptides have been found to go through misfolding transitions linked to a variety of human ailments, including prion diseases, amyloidosis, type 2 diabetes, and the diseases Alzheimer's and Parkinson's. Misfolded prion aggregates can disseminate their particular conformations and pathogenic states among cells and tissues. A large body of research indicates that various aggregation-prone proteins may possess prion-like structural variances that are linked to unique disease symptoms and that self-replicate through seeding. Aging is the biggest risk factor for neurological disorders. Many of these diseases have a late onset, which means that each disease has a different cause that varies as a person ages. One characteristic that is continuous across all diseases is the progressive loss of neuronal function as the condition worsens with age. Progressive spinal muscular atrophies, hereditary sensory motor neuropathies, and Alzheimer's disease are just a few of the clinical entities that result from progressive neural loss. Other less common clinical entities include amyotrophic lateral sclerosis (ALS), progressive spinal muscular atrophies, and Parkinson's disease. In terms of prevalence and socioeconomic impact, Alzheimer's type dementia and Parkinson's disease are the most prevalent in the category. Below, a few prevalent neurodegenerative conditions are mentioned [35, 36].

Causes and Remedies

Alzheimer's Disease (AD)

The most prevalent type of progressive dementia, AD is marked by cognitive decline, memory loss, and aberrant behaviour. Amyloid peptide misfolding and tau aggregation, which result in the formation of amyloid plaques and neurofibrillary tangles, respectively, are the main contributors to this protein misfolding condition. The 42-residue product known as Aβ is the result of two sequential cleavages of the transmembrane protein known as the amyloid precursor protein (APP), which has no known function. A major intracellular repository of cytotoxic peptides, autophagosomes, and other forms of autophagic vacuoles are particularly abundant in damaged neurons in AD brains. Senile neurons that have an excessive build-up of immature autophagic vacuoles have increased its core component synthesis, retrograde trafficking of autophagosomes, and poor fusion with lysosomes, all of which contribute to the build-up of pathogenic Aβ. Neurofibrillary tangles, which are predominantly made of phosphorylated tau, are another characteristic of AD. Although neurofibrillary tangles were once believed to be one of the main factors in the aetiology of AD, recent research suggests that a pathologically modified monomeric form of tau and its soluble oligomers may be more harmful [35].

AD has been researched for more than a century, the only medications licenced for managing it are acetyl cholinesterase inhibitors (Tacrine, Donepezil, Rivastigmine, and Galantamine), along with memantine. These medications primarily alleviate symptoms; they do little to alter the course of the disease. Lecanemab, a humanised IgG1 monoclonal antibody that binds with high affinity to soluble protofibrils, has shown some promise in recent clinical trials for reducing amyloid symptoms in early Alzheimer's disease. This resulted in a moderately slower decline in measures of cognition and function than placebo at 18 months, but it also caused adverse effects [37].

Parkinson's Disease (PD)

Reduced motor function and the death of dopaminergic neurons in the substantia nigra pars compacta are the defining features of PD. A mutant version of the presynaptic nerve terminal protein α-synuclein is the main pathogenic factor in Parkinson's disease (PD). Point mutations that make α-synuclein more susceptible to misfolding and aggregation, such as A53T, A30P, and E46K, are linked to the activity of mutant α-synuclein as an autosomal dominant cause of Parkinson's disease (PD). Lewy bodies (LBs), which are the primary markers of both sporadic and familial PD, are formed as a result of the accumulation of aggregated mutant α-synuclein [35]. The two drugs that are most frequently administered for Parkinson's are levodopa and carbidopa. Parkinson's patients' brains lack sufficient dopamine to regulate their movements. Levodopa functions by converting to dopamine in the brain tissue. Levodopa works better when combined with carbidopa, which also lessens its negative effects. Other drugs available either work as dopamine agonists such as pramipexole, rotigotine, and ropinirole, or by increasing the dopamine levels in the brain *via* synthesis or reduced breakdown [38].

Although research on neurodegeneration has gained momentum over the past 25 years, there are still no effective treatments that can reverse the disease, necessitating the need for novel interventional methods. Perhaps, herbal based medicine may be evaluated systematically based on our ancient literature to uncover a formulation fit to arrest neurological degeneration.

Huntington's Disease

The neurodegenerative disorder Huntington's disease (HD) is autosomal dominant. People who are affected experience increasing physical and cognitive deficits that are linked to loss of self-awareness and spatial awareness, depression, dementia, and elevated anxiety. Aggregation of mutant huntingtin (mHTT) proteins is the primary cause of this neurological disease that progresses. A section of glutamine residue known as the polyQ tract can be found in the wild-type huntingtin protein (HTT). A defensive mechanism to sequester small oligomeric forms of mHTT, which are extremely toxic to neurons, may result in polyQ inclusion. It has been suggested that mHTT may function as an infectious agent through a mechanism seen in prion illnesses because extracellular polyQ aggregates can be absorbed by cells to start a new round of polyQ aggregation.

Several studies have demonstrated that mHTT inhibits the machinery that produces proteins, frequently during the process of its turnover. As opposed to being a direct outcome of proteasomal inhibition, it has been proposed that the build-up of mHTT inclusion is caused by the egregious breakdown of protein quality control mechanisms in conjunction with the sequestration of molecular chaperones. Intranuclear inclusions and perinuclear cytoplasmic aggregates build up in the neurons of HD patients are the result of the inability to break down mHTT [35].

Prion Disease

Known as "proteinaceous infectious particles," prions are a class of neuro-degenerative disorders that affect the nervous system. The prion protein, also called PrP, is the culprit behind prion disorders. The most common names for the human prion diseases include Kuru and Variably Protease-Sensitive Prionsopathy, as well as Creutzfeldt-Jakob disease (CJD), Fatal Familial Insomnia (FFI), Gertsmann Straussler-Scheinker Syndrome (GSS), and (VPSPr). All of these diseases are called prion disease because they are all caused by only slightly different forms of the same protein. Each disease is triggered by the prion protein (PrP), which when folded incorrectly forms a prion and prompts additional PrP molecules to follow suit. Then, for years, prions can "silently" proliferate throughout a person's brain without manifesting any symptoms. When symptoms appear, prions eventually begin to destroy neurons, causing quick deterioration of cognitive function. There are three possible causes of prion diseases: acquired, genetic, or sporadic. Acquired refers to a condition when a person contacts the diease after being exposed to prions. Infection is the least likely way to cause prion disease, although prions are frightening and difficult to catch. Familial forms of Prion illnesses may potentially be inherited following autosomal dominance. Everybody possesses the gene PRNP, which produces the protein PrP, and the majority of the time, this protein is completely healthy and normal. Some individuals develop mutant variants of PrP as a result of DNA mutations in their PRNP gene. Most individuals with PRNP mutations live a normal life for many years despite having these mutant forms, which take time to develop into prions. However, the likelihood that mutant forms of PrP may fold improperly and produce prions increases with age. The fact that the prion protein can fold up in so many distinct hazardous and disease-causing ways is one of the remarkable characteristics of this protein. Human prion disease comes in a bewildering array of variations. Over 40 genetic alterations contribute to the development of over 6 different sporadic prion disease strains. In a recent study, quinacrine was found to be a strong inhibitor of prion disease in cultured neuroblastoma cells, along with lysosomotropic drugs and cysteine protease inhibitors. Quinacrine suppresses PrPSc accumulation, but due to its toxicity, it is not a good option for therapeutic purposes. Acridine, phenothiazine, and other tricyclic chemicals, such as quinacrine, and their analogues attach to PrPC with certain amino acid residues. Nearly all research on the functions of phenothiazines, acridines, and quinolines has been done on substances with aliphatic side chains [35].

CROSS-TALK BETWEEN MISFOLDED PROTEINS

Traditionally, it has been assumed that each neurodegenerative condition has a unique pathogenic mechanism and is caused by the misfolding and aggregation of a specific protein. However, there is growing data showing that there is significant overlap across many neurodegenerative disorders. First, it was discovered that dementias are associated with Alzheimer's disease, and tau and α-synuclein are the result of co-deposition (ADRD). For instance, misfolded α-synuclein aggregates were discovered in more than 50% of patients with familial AD, Down's syndrome, and AD. Patients with Parkinson's disease dementia were also shown to have tau aggregates, and there is a strong correlation between the number of tau aggregates and cognitive deterioration. The synergistic interactions between the two pathogenic proteins may make ADRD pathogenesis worse, as it has already been demonstrated that tau and α-synuclein can increase each other's aggregation. It was demonstrated in particular that different misfolded α-synuclein aggregates (strains) variably trigger the production of different tau strains *in vivo*. These findings highlight the complexity of ADRD pathogenesis by showing a large overlap between AD and PD pathology, which is caused by synergistic interactions between tau and α-synuclein. Additionally, type-2 diabetes develops in around 80% of Alzheimer's patients, raising the possibility that type-2 diabetes and AD are related. It was also demonstrated that misfolded IAPP could initiate aggregation, both *in vitro* and *in vivo* [36].

TECHNIQUES FOR INVESTIGATION

To understand the overall protein dynamics and its varying biological functions, different techniques are employed depending upon the type of studies, its conditions, objectives, and sub-objectives. It may be noted that total number of diverse proteins across the species is not known. Further, it would perhaps never be known because every genome tends to mutate thus adding constantly the heterogeneity resulting constantly in newer form of proteins.

Non-clinical Studies (*in vitro*)

In Eppendorf (Small Tube)

Understanding the mechanism of protein aggregation and developing new treatments for amyloid-associated disease depends on the ability to characterize protein aggregates using a variety of analytical techniques. Here, we explain the key characteristics of some of the popular techniques for characterising protein aggregates, such as amyloid fibrils, as well as the underlying theories and specific methodology.

Turbidity Measurements

Turbidity is the cloudiness or haziness that individual particles of different sizes induce to appear in liquids. Turbidity rises over time during protein aggregation, indicating the process. The recorded optical density at max, which refers to the wavelength at which maximum absorption occurs and corresponds to the particle size in the solution, can be used to assess the turbidity spectrophotometrically [39].

Rayleigh Scattering Measurements

According to Rayleigh's theory of light scattering, light can be scattered by particles whose diameter is less than the light's wavelength. By establishing identical excitation and emission wavelengths, typically at 350 nm, a fluorescence spectrophotometer can measure light scattering, which is mostly utilized in the study of protein aggregation. Utilizing this technique, one may determine when protein aggregates occur [9].

Circular Dichroism Spectroscopy

A secondary and tertiary structure in the protein can be found using circular dichroism (CD) spectroscopy. Far-ultraviolet (UV) CD [190-250 nm) and near-UV CD [250-320 nm) are used, respectively, to determine the secondary and tertiary structure of proteins and peptides. The production of a β-sheet conformation occurs concurrently with the assembly of proteins into protofibrils and amyloid fibrils, and this conformation produces the distinctive minima at 215-218 nm in the far-UV CD area [32].

Steady-state Fluorescence Measurements

As a result of their high sensitivity to changes in the structural dynamics and polarity of protein chromophores like Trp and Tyr, intrinsic fluorescence metrics like fluorescence intensity (FI) and emission maxima (λ_{max}) can be utilized to analyse protein folding and assembly [40].

Dye Binding Assays

For the identification and detection of protein aggregates, fluorescence microscopy is a crucial tool. Different substances or colours can bind to hydrophobic residues or the cross β-sheet structure and are consequently used to characterize the aggregates that are generated. Thioflavin T, Congo red, and ANS are the most often used dyes Fig. (**8**).

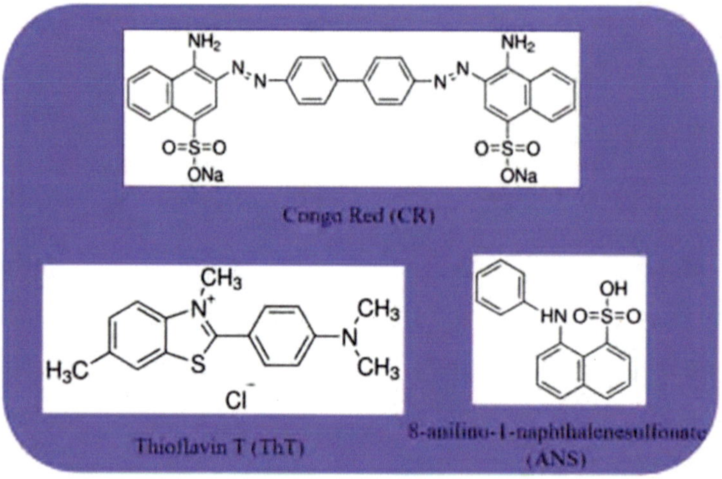

Fig. (8). Molecular structure of various dyes for probing conformational alteration of the proteins.

Thioflavin T (ThT): A benzothiazole dye binds to cross β-sheet-rich structures like amyloid fibrils and exhibits increased fluorescence as well as a distinctive blue shift in the emission spectrum from around 510 nm in the free-state to 480 nm when linked to amyloid fibrils. Typically, the experiment's excitation wavelength is set at 440 nm, and spectra between 450 and 600 nm are measured. ThT interacts very specifically with amyloid fibrils in protein-only solutions. The fluorescence of ThT is not enhanced by amorphous aggregates or soluble proteins that are folded, unfolded, or partially folded [41, 42].

Congo red (CR): A symmetrical azo dye with both nonpolar and polar moieties is another dye that has long been employed as the amyloid marker. The absorption shows maximum shifts from 490nm to 540nm when CR is associated with amyloid assemblies, producing a distinctive green-yellow birefringence under the polarised light. The alignment of the CR molecule within the grooves along the fibril axis is favoured by dye-protein interactions that are ionic and hydrophobic [9].

8-aniline-1-naphthalene sulphate (ANS): It is highly helpful for examining protein conformational changes in the solution. This probe specifies the creation and dissolution of structured hydrophobic patches and clefts as well as the orientation of aromatic side chains. The creation of the beta sheet-rich structure of fibrils is greatly influenced by the exposure of a hydrophobic amino acid residue to an external environment or by hydrophobic contact. An ANS fluorescent test is used to track changes in surface hydrophobicity during aggregation. ANS displayed negligible fluorescence in an aqueous solution, but when it interacted with the hydrophobic moiety, the dye's fluorescence emission intensified and its maximum emission wavelength shifted to blue [3].

Transmission Electron Microscopy (TEM)

High-resolution microscopic methods like transmission electron microscopy have made it possible to directly observe how proteins self-assemble into oligomers, protofibrils, and mature fibrils. It offers qualitative data on the aggregates [43].

Atomic Force Microscopy (AFM)

The potential of AFM to provide extremely high-resolution 3D structural information of multiple protein-based samples or fibrils has been utilized by the biological sciences. It works based on scanning the tip over the samples while the laser beam looks for deflection. It can be used to examine the supra-molecular architecture of living cells and amyloid fibril development. AFM gives length, breadth, and surface properties of protein aggregation as well as other qualitative and quantitative information at the nanoscale scale.

In Cell Lines

Within cell lines, it is feasible to research the mechanisms of a potential detrimental or protective role of individual molecules and compounds, as well as the function of isolated cells of one particular kind in an environment that simulates the disease. Second, they have facilitated screening for possible medication effects. In this way, *in vitro* cell models of neurodegenerative processes have been employed to shed light on the disease's causes and possible pharmaceutical targets. To investigate these potential disease pathways, many cell culture techniques have been used. The HEK293 cell line (human embryonic kidney 293) is a frequently utilized human cell line in research on AD and PD. The kinetics of α-Syn aggregation was examined in one article concerning aggregation formation. It has been demonstrated that increased expression of wild-type α-Syn causes the development of cytoplasmic aggregates. The SH-SY5Y cell line, which is generated from human neuroblastoma cells, is another cell line that is frequently utilized in the field of neurological research. Numerous studies on the mechanisms of neurodegeneration use these cells. These cell lines can be used to transfect tau, amyloid-precursor proteins, or their mutant variants. Currently utilized human cell lines include NT2, and hNT, which are primarily produced from embryonic teratocarcinoma and can be used to create post-mitotic neuronal phenotypes. The oligomerization of intracellular α-Syn has been investigated by fluorescent lifetime imaging (FLIM) for the first time using the human H4 neuroglioma cell line. Lund human mesencephalic (LUHMES) cell line and another recent cell line, has been extensively employed to research dopamine-related cell death pathways. Primary cortical and hippocampal cultures, in addition to cell lines, are important resources in the study of AD. Neuronal cells can be used to study a variety of HD pathogenic traits, such as the function of the mHtt protein. These cells include the human SH-SY5Y, the mouse Neuro2a (N2a), and the rat pheochromocytoma (PC-12). Different PolyQ-expanded huntingtin constructs can be transfected into PC-12 cells [44, 45].

Identification of the origin, purity, and characteristics of cell lines depends on their characterization. The following are common methods for characterising protein aggregation in cell lines:

Immunocytochemistry

Antibody-based immunocytochemistry (ICC) uses cell labelling to ascertain population homogeneity and molecular composition. This technique analyses the distribution of molecular markers in the cell culture and visualises individual cells. Cell morphology is revealed by immunocytochemistry, which also reveals the subcellular location of a specific antigen. To determine staining appropriateness, the experiment should include a negative control (one without the main antibody) and a positive control (one with a cell known to express a certain antigen). In immunocytochemistry, the primary antibody attached to an epitope on the target molecule is frequently made evident by fluorescently labelled secondary antibodies. The heavy chain of the original antibody can be found by a secondary antibody. To identify certain antigens in specimens, IHC uses monoclonal and polyclonal antibodies. IHC uses four different types of specimen preparations: paraffin-embedded, frozen, free-floating, and cytological ones. The paraffin-embedded method is the one that is most frequently utilized in these formats. IHC is one of the most used methods for analysing the characteristics of cells, such as the presence of particular protein aggregates or the overexpression of proteins in cancer [46].

Western Blotting

Proteins can be separated and identified using the western blot (WB) technique. During electrophoresis, a combination of proteins, aggregates, and amyloids are initially separated. The combination is then transferred to the membrane, where it is exposed to certain antibodies. Following incubation, the unbounded antibody is rinsed. Antibodies that have attached themselves to proteins are found and seen on the membrane. Each band's thickness varies according to the protein content.

Confocal Microscope

For evaluations of cells and tissues, a confocal fluorescent microscope is an excellent instrument. Although it is achievable to create a 3D dataset using a sequence of confocal images, just one image known as a slice, is required for quantification. Reconstruction and measurement of the entire sample volume are made possible by the 3D model. When determining the localization of molecules from diverse cellular compartments, fluorescent compounds are used.

CLINICAL STUDIES (*IN VIVO*)

While genetics-based models of neurodegenerative illnesses do not always mimic sporadic disease, they are usually effective surrogates and provide intrinsic validity to them. It could be argued that no animal model of AD, PD, FTD, or ALS is there mimicking the phenocopies of human disease completely. Several simulations reproduce the original proteinopathy or other problematic aspects of the human condition. Some models also produce a more thorough neurodegenerative cascade, although it's still unclear if they accurately represent the entire chain of pathophysiologic occurrences that characterize the human disease. Understanding the molecular and cellular pathways of brain cell malfunction and degeneration has improved owing to the use of animal models. The discipline has been able to create, test, and improve targeted medicines because of such animal models.

Types of the Studied Model

For the research of neurodegeneration, three different kinds of animal models can be used. Spontaneous mutants are strains that have been developed to maintain phenotypic traits brought about by unintentional genetic mutations. They are employed in the research of the illness due to spontaneous mutation. The *genetically modified* or “Knock-in”/”Knock-out” mutants, or strains whose genes have been turned on or off, are a different type. They are employed while trying to determine the effects of particular genes. Transgenic strains are those whose genomes have been altered to include a gene from an unrelated species used in research projects that call for a toxicological and illness model based on an authentic microenvironment. Mice and rats are the most popular animal species in neuroscience research because their brains are complex enough to be comparable to humans and provide a clear picture of how the human brain works [47].

Three pathologies *i.e.* senile plaques, neurofibrillary tangles, and hippocampal & cortical neurodegeneration define AD. Amyloid deposition in senile plaques and, in some cases, cerebrovascular amyloid is modelled in transgenic animals that promote Aβ aggregation and accumulation. The mouse model closely resembles how AD-associated human mutations in APP, PSEN1, and PSEN2 function. APP mutations either produce more total Aβ or, more frequently produce more of the aggregation-prone Aß42 relative to total Aβ. PSEN1/2 mutations change the way that mouse APP is processed naturally, but they don't cause amyloid build-up. By raising the generation of Aß42, the co-expression of PSEN1/2 mutants with an APP transgene speeds up the amyloid phenotype. Furthermore, it is not even certain that the FTD-linked P301L or P301S MAPT mutations are indicative of tau dysfunction in all forms of FTD-MAPT, though these mutations are the basis for the two most commonly utilized tau transgenic animals. The human bacterial artificial chromosome (BAC) hTau mice, which produces all human tau (wild-type) isoforms on a mouse MAPT-knockout background, shows minimal tau pathology and mild age-dependent neurodegenerative alterations that may be more pertinent to AD Tauopathy in the human system. Injecting aggregated Aβ into a tau transgenic mouse and co-expressing mutant human tau protein and mutant APP both accelerate tau disease. Though conceptually appealing, the usefulness of animals carrying human mutant tau, mutant APP, and occasionally mutant PSEN1/2 is still debatable because it is unclear if these models reflect synergistic interactions between the two diseases [47 - 49].

Dopamine (DA) neurons in the substantia nigra par compacta (SN) are gradually lost in Parkinson's disease (PD), which is also characterized by the presence of misfolded α-synuclein in Lewy bodies and neurites. In the past, successful PD symptomatic therapy was developed using drug-induced models. The 6-hydroxydopamine [6-OHDA) and 1-methyl-4-phenyl-1,2,3,6-tetrahydropyridine (MPTP) models have been utilized extensively to improve the medicines used to treat PD symptoms. Autosomal dominant PD with distinctive Lewy body pathology is brought on by α-synuclein mutations. Using a variety of different promoters that constitutively overexpress various familial-PD-associated mutant forms of synuclein (A53T, A30P, and E46K), diverse models of synuclein-induced degeneration show varying degrees of neurodegeneration and develop many clinical and biochemical features of PD, LBD, and MSA, including the formation of oligomeric and fibrillary α-synuclein Some people consider the absence of a loss of DA neurons to be a critical flaw in these models, although several mutants of α-synuclein transgenic mice demonstrate significant neurodegeneration. Germline LRRK2 transgenic mice based on the overexpression of the G2019S or R1441C/G mutations have variable degrees of DA anomalies but don't show any evidence of age-dependent DA neuron degradation [47, 49].

The organisms utilized to model these illnesses are not limited to rodents. Understanding the pathological toxicity of proteins associated with various neurodegenerative illnesses has been achieved using several species, including yeast *Caenorhabditis elegans*, *Danio rerio*, and *Drosophila*. There are just a few naturally occurring, non-rodent animal models, like the SOD1 mutations that cause canine amyotrophic lateral sclerosis (ALS). Aß does collect in the form of plaque-like structures in old non-human primates, which has led to substantial research on them as possible AD models. Even the seeding of AD brain lysate into these mice has not resulted in tau pathology and neurodegeneration [50].

Human Model

There is a critical need for timely and accurate neurodegenerative disease diagnosis in clinical practice. This need includes giving patients access to clinical trial possibilities, optimising treatment plans, providing the right support and care, and providing patients with diagnostic and prognostic information about their diseases. Even at specialised dementia clinics, studies comparing clinical and postmortem diagnoses show that roughly 25–30% of patients with a clinical diagnosis of AD are misdiagnosed. Numerous possible anti-A, anti-tau, or anti-synuclein treatments are now being developed or tested in clinical studies. If pathology-specific biomarkers are not employed for screening, there is an obvious danger of including patients without the pathology of interest in studies due to the limited accuracy of clinical diagnosis to predict the underlying brain disorders. Today, participation in many AD trials requires biomarker confirmation of a disease. However, because elderly people frequently have multiple ailments, it is crucial to identify the underlying cause of each symptom. Therapies will probably be more effective in the early pre-symptomatic or prodromal disease stages before apparent and permanent neurodegeneration has taken place when addressing upstream pathologies, such as Aβ in AD and α-synuclein in PD.

The following techniques are used for *in-vivo* imaging: positron emission tomography (PET), single-photon emission computed tomography (SPECT), voxel-based morphometry (VBM), magnetic resonance imaging (MRI), magnetic resonance perfusion imaging (MRPI), functional magnetic resonance imaging (fMRI), diffusion and perfusion imaging, diffusion-weighted imaging (DWI), and magnetic resonance spectroscopy [51]. While other brain imaging methods were created to assess the structure or function of the brain, PET and SPECT were specifically created to diagnose AD by identifying amyloid plaques. These techniques use data interpretation to indirectly diagnose AD [42].

FUTURE PERSPECTIVE

In this book chapter, we've talked about proteins, as the fundamental macromolecules, their role in our diets, and the ways in which protein degradation affects human health. In this section, we reviewed the importance of proteins, different model proteins, their misfolding and Glycation, the associated diseases, and the most popular approaches for examining the general aspects of protein aggregation, characterization of biophysical and structural changes, as well as the kinetic process. The *ex-vivo* and *in-vivo* protein aggregation have been discussed in this chapter. Protein conformational alterations are thought to be the main factor contributing to aggregation. These conformational changes expose compellingly amyloidogenic amino acid sequences to the environment that would normally be hidden inside the protein molecule's core. Our comprehension of the molecular foundation for various molecular conformations would be considerably improved by additional structural investigations of filamentous aggregates cross-seeded by other misfolded proteins and *in vivo* filaments recovered from patients themselves. A more in-depth understanding of the structure-function link of the conformationally varied misfolded strains would also come through an investigation of their biological activities, such as toxicity and cross-seeding capacity. As they are at the frontiers of protein biochemistry and clinical medicine, protein aggregation and glycation are intriguing areas of protein chemistry and are of clinical significance since AGEs and protein aggregates are linked to pathophysiological situations. The molecular architectures of natural compounds serve as important beginning points for drug development. Numerous studies have demonstrated that a wide range of natural substances, including polyphenols, polysaccharides, terpenoids, osmolytes [52], vitamins, and alkaloids, are promising candidates for the development of novel medications to prevent aggregation and AGEs formation. Effective techniques are required for the analysis of the pathogenesis of neurodegenerative pathologies as well as their diagnosis. One or more of the aforementioned strategies can be coupled with one another or contrasted depending on the research question(s). Methods for examining the biophysical properties, such as amyloid-specific dye binding and morphological conformational alteration, can be used to determine the forms of protein aggregates. Although protein aggregation has been studied in great detail, many questions remain thus, it is essential to comprehend protein aggregation to combat disorders associated with amyloid. Major obstacles in understanding protein aggregation include the process' complexity and dynamic nature, the issue of creating homogeneous samples due to aggregation's polymorphic character, and more. Additionally, due to the complexity of the structure and conformational alteration of protein, *in-vitro* and *in-vivo* investigations don't always yield the same results. There are many approaches utilized nowadays to comprehend neurodegenerative diseases, but they all have some drawbacks. For conceptualising therapeutic targets that could be used in future drug development, primary neuronal cultures are essential. As many medicines for neurodegenerative disorders have failed only at the very end of clinical trials, the present cell models of neurodegeneration have demonstrated poor prognostic utility. This emphasises the necessity of thorough and coordinated scientific efforts to improve cell models. Considering the complexity of the CNS, a feasible model would require the integration of both the architecture of brain tissue and our present understanding of the molecular pathways underlying neurodegenerative disorders. Microfluidic technology mixed with 3D cell models, or organ-on-a-chip systems, is still in their infancy and has a lot of space for development. Major proteinopathies in humans can be studied using animal models, although they do not accurately mimic all human diseases. A process occurring in humans must be reflected in the downstream events for them to be suitable models for exploring some features of downstream occurrences. We need to know which aspects of the human disease they accurately and inaccurately reproduce. Increasing our knowledge of all these important subjects should help with the development of true drug.

CONCLUDING REMARKS

This chapter has been prepared to apprise the reader about the various forms of proteins, their involvement both as disease causing agents and protector of the genome. The human immune system cannot function without proteins. The muscles in the human body cannot be formed and brain would remain bereft of the much vital molecules for its function. Keeping in view the details of the protein and their overall functioning, it would be prudent to develop precision medicine so that the same has no side effect but proves to be a magic bullet. Other chapters in this book would add additional health dimension to make the story less insipid. Finally, it is envisaged that the information presented here would pave the path to pursue research in the area of precision medicine in a more focused manner.

ACKNOWLEDGEMENTS

Tajalli Ilm Chandel acknowledges Indian Council of Medical Research (ICMR) New Delhi, Govt. of India, for the award of Research Associate (2020-6821/ PROTEOMICS-BMS). The authors would like to acknowledge support to Interdisciplinary Biotechnology Unit, Aligarh Muslim University, Aligarh.

REFERENCES

[1] Seiya Asai JM. Lenka žáková, irena selicharová, romana hadravová, andrzej marek brzozowski, jiří nováček andjiří jiráček, characterization of insulin crystalline form in isolated î²-cell secretory granules. Open Biol 2022; 12(12): 220322.
[PMID: 36541100]

[2] Moughan PJ. Protein: Digestion, absorption and metabolism.Encyclopedia of Food and Health. Elsevier 2015; pp. 524-9.

[3] Siddiqi MK, Alam P, Chaturvedi SK, *et al.* Capreomycin inhibits the initiation of amyloid fibrillation and suppresses amyloid induced cell toxicity. Biochim Biophys Acta Proteins Proteomics 2018; 1866(4): 549-57.

[http://dx.doi.org/10.1016/j.bbapap.2018.02.005] [PMID: 29496560]

[4] Wu G. Dietary protein intake and human health. Food Funct 2016; 1251-65.

[5] Choudhuri S. Bioinformatics for beginners: Genes, genomes, molecular evolution, databases and analytical tools. Elsevier 2014.

[6] Armen R, Alonso DOV, Daggett V. The role of α-, 3_{10} -, and π-helix in helix→coil transitions. Protein Sci 2003; 12(6): 1145-57.
[http://dx.doi.org/10.1110/ps.0240103] [PMID: 12761385]

[7] Murray JE, Laurieri N, Delgoda R. Proteins: Pharmacognosy: Fundamentals, applications and strategy.Pharmacognosy: Fundamentals, Applications and Strategy. Elsevier 2017; pp. 477-94.
[http://dx.doi.org/10.1016/B978-0-12-802104-0.00024-X]

[8] Shen C-H. Gene expression: Translation of the genetic code.Diagnostic Molecular Biology. Elsevier 2019; pp. 87-116.
[http://dx.doi.org/10.1016/B978-0-12-802823-0.00004-3]

[9] Chandel TI, Zaidi N, Zaman M, *et al.* A multiparametric analysis of the synergistic impact of anti-Parkinson's drugs on the fibrillation of human serum albumin. Biochim Biophys Acta Proteins Proteomics 2019; 1867(3): 275-85.
[http://dx.doi.org/10.1016/j.bbapap.2018.10.003] [PMID: 30312771]

[10] Pappa T, Refetoff S. Thyroid hormone transport proteins: Thyroxine-binding globulin, transthyretin, and albumin.The Curated Reference Collection in Neuroscience and Biobehavioral Psychology. Elsevier 2016; pp. 483-90.

[11] Ezra A. Multifunctional effects of human serum albumin toward neuroprotection in alzheimer disease. Neuroprotection in Alzheimer's Disease. Elsevier 2017.

[12] Ahn M, Hagan CL, Bernardo-Gancedo A, *et al.* The significance of the location of mutations for the native-state dynamics of human lysozyme. Biophys J 2016; 111(11): 2358-67.
[http://dx.doi.org/10.1016/j.bpj.2016.10.028] [PMID: 27926837]

[13] Alam MT, Rizvi A, Rauf MA, Owais M, Naeem A. Thermal unfolding of human lysozyme induces aggregation: Recognition of the aggregates by antisera against the native protein. Int J Biol Macromol 2018; 113: 976-82.
[http://dx.doi.org/10.1016/j.ijbiomac.2018.02.095] [PMID: 29462680]

[14] Naik SR, Kokil GR. Development and discovery avenues in bioactive natural products for glycemic novel therapeutics.Studies in Natural Products Chemistry. Elsevier 2013; pp. 431-66.

[15] Ruan H. Targeting intrinsically disordered proteins at the edge of chaos.Drug Discovery Today. Elsevier 2019; pp. 217-27.
[http://dx.doi.org/10.1016/j.drudis.2018.09.017]

[16] Uversky VN. Intrinsically disordered proteins and their "Mysterious" (meta)physics. Front Phys 2019; 2019

[17] Strodel B. Energy landscapes of protein aggregation and conformation switching in intrinsically disordered proteins: Energy landscapes of IDPS and protein aggregation. J Mol Biol 2021.

[18] Coskuner O, Uversky VN. Intrinsically disordered proteins in various hypotheses on the pathogenesis of Alzheimer's and Parkinson's diseases. Progress in Molecular Biology and Translational Science. Elsevier 2019; pp. 145-223.

[19] Dyson HJ, Wright PE. Intrinsically unstructured proteins and their functions. Nat Rev Mol Cell Biol 2005; 6(3): 197-208.
[http://dx.doi.org/10.1038/nrm1589] [PMID: 15738986]

[20] Taghavi F. The status of glycation in protein aggregation. Int J Biol Macromol 2017; 67-74.
[http://dx.doi.org/10.1016/j.ijbiomac.2015.12.085]

[21] Sirangelo I, Iannuzzi C. Understanding the role of protein glycation in the amyloid aggregation process. Int J Mol Sci 2021; 2021: 22126609.
[http://dx.doi.org/10.3390/ijms22126609]

[22] Song Q. Novel advances in inhibiting advanced glycation end product formation using natural compounds. Biomedicine and Pharmacotherapy. Elsevier 2021.

[23] Bouma B, Kroon-Batenburg LMJ, Wu YP, *et al.* Glycation induces formation of amyloid cross-beta structure in albumin. J Biol Chem 2003; 278(43): 41810-9.
[http://dx.doi.org/10.1074/jbc.M303925200] [PMID: 12909637]

[24] Shamsi A, Ahmed A, Khan MS, Husain FM, Bano B. Rosmarinic acid restrains protein glycation and aggregation in human serum albumin: Multi spectroscopic and microscopic insight - Possible Therapeutics Targeting Diseases. Int J Biol Macromol 2020; 161: 187-93.
[http://dx.doi.org/10.1016/j.ijbiomac.2020.06.048] [PMID: 32526295]

[25] Khan MWA. Garlic extract: Inhibition of biochemical and biophysical changes in glycated hsa. Appl Sci 2021; 11(22) .

[26] Abdullah KM, Qais FA, Ahmad I, Naseem I. Inhibitory effect of vitamin B_3 against glycation and reactive oxygen species production in HSA: An *in vitro* approach. Arch Biochem Biophys 2017; 627: 21-9.
[http://dx.doi.org/10.1016/j.abb.2017.06.009] [PMID: 28624351]

[27] Sharma S. Kinetics theories to understand the mechanism of aggregation of a protein and to design strategies for its inhibition.Biophysical Chemistry. Elsevier 2021.

[28] Nguyen PH. Amyloid oligomers: A joint experimental/computational perspective on Alzheimer's disease, Parkinson's disease, type II diabetes, and amyotrophic lateral sclerosis. Chem Rev 2021; 2545-647.
[http://dx.doi.org/10.1021/acs.chemrev.0c01122]

[29] Willbold D. Amyloid-type Protein Aggregation and Prion-like Properties of Amyloids.Chem Rev 2021; 8285-307.
[http://dx.doi.org/10.1021/acs.chemrev.1c00196]

[30] Candelise N. Protein aggregation landscape in neurodegenerative diseases: Clinical relevance and future applications.Int J Mol Sci 2021; 22(11): 6016.
[http://dx.doi.org/10.3390/ijms22116016]

[31] Kuroda Y. Biophysical studies of protein solubility and amorphous aggregation by systematic mutational analysis and a helical polymerization model. Biophys Rev 2018; 473-80.
[http://dx.doi.org/10.1007/s12551-017-0342-y]

[32] Housmans JAJ. A guide to studying protein aggregation. John Wiley and Sons Inc. 2021.

[33] Mitraki A. Protein aggregation: From inclusion bodies to amyloid and biomaterials.Advances in Protein Chemistry and Structural Biology. Academic Press Inc. 2010; pp. 89-125.
[http://dx.doi.org/10.1016/S1876-1623(10)79003-9]

[34] Lashuel HA. Do Lewy bodies contain alpha-synuclein fibrils? and Does it matter? A brief history and critical analysis of recent reports.Neurobiology of Disease. Academic Press Inc. 2020.

[35] Khanam H, Ali A, Asif M, Shamsuzzaman . Neurodegenerative diseases linked to misfolded proteins and their therapeutic approaches: A review. Eur J Med Chem 2016; 124: 1121-41.
[http://dx.doi.org/10.1016/j.ejmech.2016.08.006] [PMID: 27597727]

[36] Lim KH. Diverse misfolded conformational strains and cross-seeding of misfolded proteins implicated in neurodegenerative diseases.Frontiers in Molecular Neuroscience. Frontiers Media S.A. 2019.
[http://dx.doi.org/10.3389/fnmol.2019.00158]

[37] Anand R, Gill KD, Mahdi AA. Therapeutics of Alzheimer's disease: Past, present and future. Neuropharmacology 2014; 76(Pt A): 27-50.

[http://dx.doi.org/10.1016/j.neuropharm.2013.07.004] [PMID: 23891641]

[38] Stoker TB, Barker RA. Recent developments in the treatment of Parkinson's Disease. F1000 Res 2020; 9: 862.
[http://dx.doi.org/10.12688/f1000research.25634.1] [PMID: 32789002]

[39] Chandel TI, Afghani M, Masroor A, *et al.* An insight into the inhibition of fibrillation process verses disaggregation of preformed fibrils of bovine serum albumin by isoprenaline hydrochloride. Int J Biol Macromol 2020; 154: 1448-59.
[http://dx.doi.org/10.1016/j.ijbiomac.2019.11.026] [PMID: 31778695]

[40] Chandel TI, Rabbani G, Khan M, *et al.* Binding of anti-cardiovascular drug to serum albumin: An insight in the light of spectroscopic and computational approaches. J Biomol Struct Dyn 2018; 36(1): 54-67.
[http://dx.doi.org/10.1080/07391102.2016.1266968] [PMID: 27910732]

[41] Gade Malmos K. ThT 101: A primer on the use of thioflavin T to investigate amyloid formation.Amyloid. Taylor and Francis Ltd. 2017; pp. 1-16.
[http://dx.doi.org/10.1080/13506129.2017.1304905]

[42] Tiwari V, Solanki V, Tiwari M. In-vivo and in-vitro techniques used to investigate Alzheimer's disease.Frontiers in Life Science. Taylor and Francis Ltd. 2015; pp. 332-47.

[43] Chandel TI, Masroor A, Siddiqi MK, *et al.* Molecular basis of the inhibition and disaggregation of thermally-induced amyloid fibrils of human serum albumin by an anti-Parkinson's drug, benserazide hydrochloride. J Mol Liq 2019; 278: 553-67.
[http://dx.doi.org/10.1016/j.molliq.2018.12.127]

[44] Cetin S. Cell models for Alzheimer's and Parkinson's disease: At the interface of biology and drug discovery. Biomedicine and Pharmacotherapy. Elsevier 2013.

[45] Schlachetzki JCM, Saliba SW, de Oliveira ACP. Studying neurodegenerative diseases in culture models. Brazil J Psych 2013; 35(S2): 92-100.
[http://dx.doi.org/10.1590/1516-4446-2013-1159]

[46] Olsson TT, Klementieva O, Gouras GK. Prion-like seeding and nucleation of intracellular amyloid-β. Neurobiol Dis 2018; 113: 1-10.
[http://dx.doi.org/10.1016/j.nbd.2018.01.015] [PMID: 29414379]

[47] Dawson TM, Golde TE, Lagier-Tourenne C. Animal models of neurodegenerative diseases.Nature Neuroscience. Nature Publishing Group 2018; pp. 1370-9.

[48] Myers A, McGonigle P. Overview of Transgenic Mouse Models for Alzheimer's Disease. Current Protocols in Neuroscience. Blackwell Publishing Inc. 2018.

[49] Hansson O. Biomarkers for neurodegenerative diseases.Nature Medicine. Nature Research 2021; pp. 954-63.

[50] Hickman DL. Commonly Used Animal Models. Principles of Animal Research for Graduate and Undergraduate Students. Elsevier 2017.

[51] Geerts H, Bergeler S, Walker M, van der Graaf PH, Courade JP. Analysis of clinical failure of anti-tau and anti-synuclein antibodies in neurodegeneration using a quantitative systems pharmacology model. Sci Rep 2023; 13(1): 14342.
[http://dx.doi.org/10.1038/s41598-023-41382-0] [PMID: 37658103]

[52] Chandel TI, Khan MV, Khan RH. Impact of osmolytes in conformational modulation of protein and its applications in biotechnology.Cellular Osmolytes. Springer 2017; pp. 143-60.
[http://dx.doi.org/10.1007/978-981-10-3707-8_7]

CHAPTER 6

Status of *Helicobacter pylori* in Gut Microbiome and Precision Medicine

Navin Kumar[1,*]

[1] *School of Biotechnology, Gautam Buddha University, Greater Noida, Uttar Pradesh 201310 UP, India*

Abstract: *Helicobacter pylori* (*H. pylori*) is a Gram-negative, slow-growing microaerobic bacterium that infects over 50% of the global population. Around 58,000 years ago, *H. pylori* and humans co-evolved and migrated from East Africa, the original birthplace of *Homo sapiens*. Its distinct characteristics, such as urease, helical structure, and motile flagella, allow it to survive in the human stomach under stressful conditions. The occurrence of *H. pylori* in the stomach can be beneficial or detrimental to human health, depending on the host's genetic vulnerability, immunity, and environmental factors. Although most of the *H. pylori*-infected patients are asymptomatic, about 20% develop stomach illnesses such as peptic ulcer (10-15%), gastric adenocarcinoma (1-3%), and mucosa-associated lymphoid tissue (MALT) lymphoma that is common to aged people. People who do not have *H. pylori* infection, on the other hand, are predisposed to a variety of diseases, including gastric esophageal disease (GERD), oesophageal cancer, diabetes mellitus, and asthma. Clinical symptoms in infected patients vary significantly geographically due to the high level of genetic variation in the bacterial genome and the presence of numerous virulence factors. The entire sickness is treated by eradicating *H. pylori* with antibiotics and proton pump inhibitors. However, the rise in antibiotic resistance and a lack of effective vaccinations make it tough to combat the infection. This chapter aims to shed light on host-pathogen interactions by analysing the bacterium's persistence and pathogenesis in the context of human health and precision medicine.

Keywords: CagA, Gastric ulcer, Gastric cancer, Gut microbiota, *Helicobacter pylori*, Standard triple therapy, Virulence factors.

INTRODUCTION

H. pylori is one of the most successful colonizing bacteria in the human stomach which is found in over 50% of the global population. Bizzorero first time in 1893 emphasized the existence of spiral-shaped microbes in biopsy samples of mammalian stomachs [1] (Fig. **1**). Almost a century later, in 1984, Barry Marshall

[*] **Corresponding author Navin Kumar:** School of Biotechnology, Gautam Buddha University, Greater Noida, Uttar Pradesh 201310 UP, India; Tel: 91 8800335687; Email: navinkumar@gbu.ac.in

and Robin Warren isolated a spiral-shaped bacterium from the gastric biopsy of a human stomach and proved its role in the development of gastritis after the ingestion of microbial culture. In 2005, Warren R. and Marshall B. got a Nobel Prize in Physiology or medicine for the discovery of *Helicobacter pylori* and its association with gastric disease. Initially, it was named "C*ampylobacter pylori*" and latter following its thorough characterization renamed as *Helicobacter pylori* [2]. Human is the only host for *H. pylori*; however, other *Helicobacter* species have also been reported in cattle (*Helicobacter bovis*), pigs (*Helicobacter suis*), cats (*Helicobacter felis*), and dogs (*Helicobacter canis*) as well as for many other mammalian species which are mostly asymptomatic.

Scientific classification

Kingdom:	Bacteria
Phylum:	Proteobacteria
Class:	Epsilon Proteobacteria
Order:	Campylobacterales
Family:	Helicobacteraceae
Genus:	*Helicobacter*
Species:	*pylori*

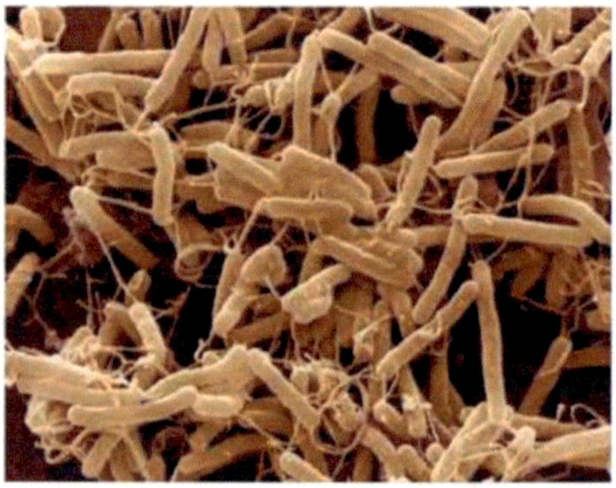

Fig. (1). Scanning micrograph shows several *H. pylori* (Adapted from: Meridian Bioscience: Europe website).

H. pylori transmits during childhood or early adolescence and persists throughout the life span of the host. *H. pylori* remains largely asymptomatic in infected people even after decades of infection or throughout the lifetime. However, about 20% of the infected people become symptomatic, including most of them as elder people who are above 40 years old. Long-term infection of *H. pylori* is responsible for chronic inflammation that leads to the development of gastritis, gastric ulcer, gastric adenocarcinoma, and gastric mucosal-associated lymphoid tissue (MALT) lymphoma. In 1994, the International Agency for Research on Cancer (IARC), a unit of the World Health Organization (WHO) classified *H. pylori* strain as a class I carcinogen [3]. *H. pylori* strain encodes cagA (cytotoxin-associated gene A), also known as an 'oncogene', which is predominantly responsible for the occurrence of chronic inflammation and subsequent gastric cancer.

Around 58,000 years ago, geographical analysis revealed that *H. pylori* moved from East Africa to Western Europe, Eastern Asia, and Southern Africa. It is believed that modern human was already infected with this bacterium before leaving East Africa as both have similar migration history. The bacterium is well-transformed and adapted accordingly to survive in the gastric mucus during the course of co-evolution. It is evident that people without *H. pylori* infections are more at risk for other diseases like Gastroesophageal reflux disease (GERD), esophagus carcinoma, gastric atrophy, diabetes, and asthma. This association hints towards the symbiotic behaviour of the bacterium with humans. The frequency and/or severity of disease outcomes with *H. pylori* infection is variable geographically among humans depends on multiple factors including bacterial genetics and virulence factors, host epigenetics as well as environmental factors. *H. pylori* infection is identified using various tests and successfully treated with one or more medicines. Unfortunately, the rise in antibiotic resistance and the lack of vaccine development are the key impediments to creating more effective medicines for this common but deadly pathogen. This chapter will cover disease diagnosis and treatment methods as well as the persistence and pathophysiology of *H. pylori* with respect to human health.

BACTERIOLOGY

H. pylori is a Gram-negative, spiral-shaped, small (3.5µm x 0.5 µm), micro-aerophilic, and non-spore-forming bacteria. It is able to survive in a high acidic environment (~pH 2) of the gastric lumen [4] and can grow at pH 6-8. It is a slow-growing bacterium with a generation time of 4–6 hours and requires low oxygen environmental conditions (*i.e.*, 5% O_2, 10% CO_2, 85% N_2, and high humidity) and 37°C for optimal growth [5]. There is no requirement for H_2, although it is not detrimental to bacterial growth. The organism has 2-6 sheathed flagella at one end that allow rapid movement in a highly viscous condition across the gastric mucus layer [6]. Typically, bacterial colonies are quite visible and grow well on blood or serum containing solid agar media like Columbia blood or Brain heart infusion (BHI) media with specific growth supplements. *H. pylori* is spiral-shaped and appears as a rod under normal physiological conditions, however, it transforms from spiral to coccoid form during prolonged *in vitro* culture or under stressed conditions like antibiotic treatment and/or the presence of high oxygen level [7]. The coccoid form of the organism is viable but non-culturable [8, 9]. *In vitro*, the coccoid form can attach to and colonise stomach epithelial cells [10 - 12].

GENOME AND GENETIC DIVERSITY

The genome sequences of several strains including *Helicobacter pylori* 26695, J99, HPAG1, and G27 are annotated. The genome size varies among different strains of the organism like the size of the *H. Pylori* 26695 genome is ~1.7 Mb, however, it is 24 kb larger than the J99 strain and about 71 kb larger than HPAG1

[13 - 15]. Its genome contains 35-40% GC content and two copies of 16S rRNA, 23S rRNA, and 5S rRNA genes. *H. pylori* 26695 has about 1,590 open reading frames (ORFs), which share 91% of the chromosome [13]. Among the 1,590 ORFs, 1,091 are present in other organisms, allowing putative biological functions that are assigned to them, although not all ORFs are orthologous with a similar function. These bacteria uptake naked DNA more frequently within their external environment during natural transformation in comparison to any other naturally competent bacterial species which is evidence of the high rate of horizontal gene transfer among *H. pylori* strains. *H. pylori's* genomes display a high degree of sequence diversity due to genetic plasticity, DNA rearrangement, and high rate of transformation and recombination frequency. This microevolution is a driving force of genetic diversity among the bacterial strains. Compared to the 36 two-component regulatory systems found in Escherichia coli K-12, its genome only contains 4 complete regulatory systems [16]. Many bacterial strains are diverse and contain one or more cryptic plasmids, which lack functional genes for virulence or antibiotic resistance [17]. *H. pylori* strains isolated from unrelated individuals of different ethnic groups and geographic areas reveal a high degree of genetic diversity [18 - 20]. The gene content of isolated strains has 3% and 22% genetic variability from the same [21] and unrelated individuals, respectively [18]. This genetic diversity is helpful for the successful adaptation of organisms under constant exposure to environmental stresses and distinct patterns of immunological stress into the new host [22, 23]. The genetic heterogeneity makes the organism more flexible and competitive for persistent colonization [24]. Sequence variability in several virulence genes like cag-PAI (cag-Pathogenicity Island), vacA, outer membrane protein-encoding genes (sabA, sabB, hopZ, and oipA), *etc.* display different degrees of clinical outcomes in infected individuals of the same or different ethnic and geographical regions.

BACTERIAL COLONIZATION AND ADHERENCE TO HOST CELL

The persistence of microorganisms in the gastric mucosa depends upon several parameters like physiological environmental conditions, nutrient availability, immune response, oxygen tension, *etc.* Usually, the stomach is considered a sterile place for microbial growth because of its highly acidic pH (pH 1.5 to 2.5), a condition that is lethal to microbes. However, *H. pylori* is able to neutralize acidic pH for a short period that is sufficient to cross the acidic gastric lumen to a higher pH (pH 4.5 6.5) in the gastric mucus layer where it resides successfully [25]. *H. pylori* requires at least four basic properties for persistent colonization and establishment of infection in gastric mucosa: high amount of urease, highly motile flagella, helical shape, and surface adhesins. The organism produces a large number of ureases that are decorated on the outer surface. Acidic pH and the presence of ammonia in the gastric lumen induce the expression of urease in bacteria [26]. Urease hydrolyses urea into carbonic acid and ammonia. The released ammonia is eventually converted into ammonium hydroxide in the aqueous gastric lumen and thereby, neutralizes local acidic pH in the gastric lumen enabling bacteria to survive. Urease-defective bacterial mutants cannot survive in the human stomach [27]. Several other microbes like *Proteus mirabilis, Yersinia, Staphylococcus saprophyticus,* and some yeast also express urease but are unable to colonize in the stomach. This is because *H. pylori* urease is different in size and structure. It is a relatively high molecular weight protein (300-600kDa) which is broken down into two smaller subunits: UraA, 26.5 kDa and UraB, 61.5 kDa [28]. Both UraA and UraB help to neutralize acidic pH inside (bacterial periplasm) and outside the bacteria in the stomach. The presence of urease is critical for the survival of the bacterium. The migration of bacteria in the gastric lumen is directed by chemotactic factors including urea, ammonia, and bicarbonate ions [29]. *H. pylori* has chemotaxis-signalling regulators (*i.e.*, CheW, CheA, and CheY) that sense chemotactic factors and direct them to the specific site in gastric mucosa. Unipolar sheathed flagella and specialized shapes of bacterium enable predominant colonization in gastric mucin, a regular web of high molecular weight glycoproteins [30]. *H. pylori* is a "good swimmer" that possesses 2-6 sheathed flagella present at one pole. Highly motile flagella and helicoidal shape make the bacterium bore through the viscous mucin web that guards the gastric epithelium layer [27, 31]. *H. pylori* encodes over fifty proteins responsible for forming the intricate flagellar assembly, which includes a basal body, flagellar hook, and filament. Mutational analysis shows that flaA and/or flaB are absolutely essential for full motility [32] and successful colonization in the piglet model [33]. However, most of the other Campylobacter and *Helicobacter* species have distinct shapes other than *H. pylori* and are unable to colonize in the gastric mucosa like *Helicobacter heilmannii*, which is a pleomorphic cork-screw shaped, unable to penetrate the mucin layer. Moreover, *H. pylori* secrete collagenase/pronase proteases extracellularly that help to digest the mucous layer [34], which otherwise is too thick to allow the passage of the organism (Fig. **2**).

Continuous secretion of gastric juice and slimy mucin layer inhibits microbes to adhere with the gastric wall. For persistent colonization, the bacterium needs to adhere to gastric epithelium and avoid being brushed into the intestine. H. pylori is typically non-invasive which swims freely within the mucus layer and adheres superficially to the gastric epithelium, where immune responses are minimum [35]. *H. pylori* encodes more than 30 outer membrane proteins and helps to adhere to gastric epithelial cells (Fig. **2**). Many of them are classified as adhesins that have variable modes of attachment to the various sites of the host cell. These adhesins interact with the gastric epithelium primarily *via* fucosylated glycoproteins and sialylated glycolipids as extracellular receptors [36, 37]. For example, BabA and SabA interact with the blood group Antigen-Lewis b/ and sialyl-Lewis x, respectively [36, 38]. Other adhesins are AlpA and AlpB, HopZ, HopH (OipA), AhpC, UreA, CagA, CagI, and CagL, which enable the bacterium to adhere to gastric mucosa at different physiological conditions [39, 40]. This organism is able to deal with unstable physiological conditions like mild to string acidity, inconsistent nutrient and oxygen availability, and distinct patterns of immunological responses of the host. Despite these conditions, *H. pylori* is a successful organism that is consistently proliferating in the host stomach over thousands of years.

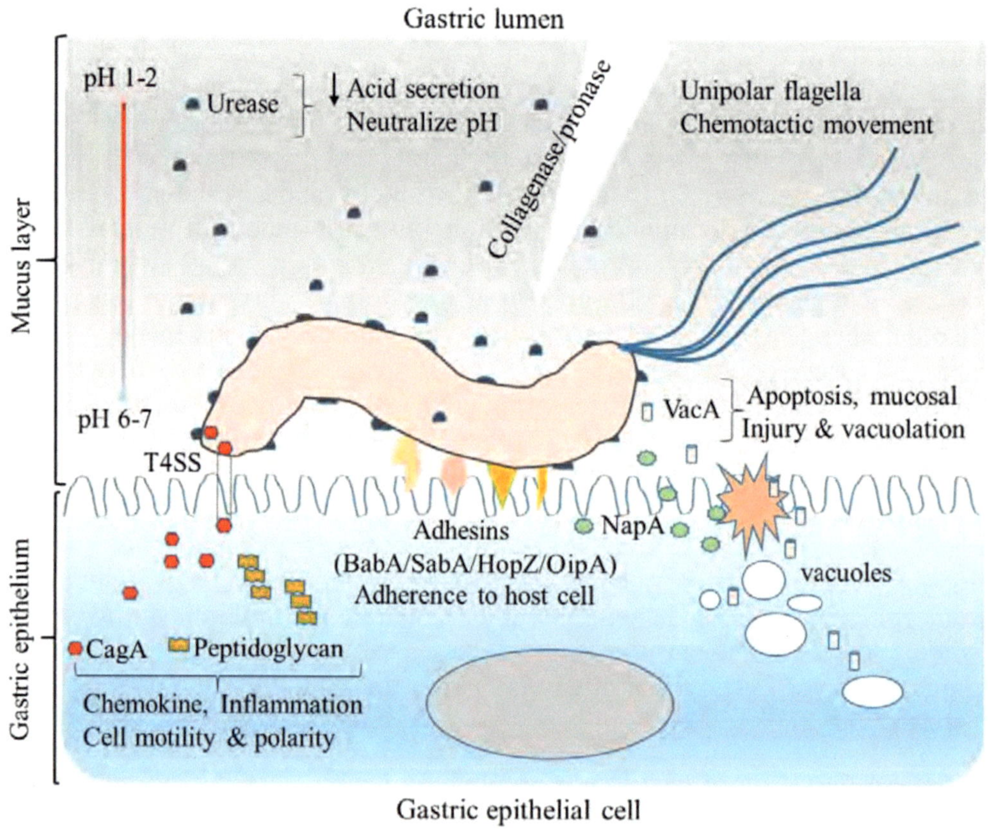

Fig. (2). Stepwise representation of major factors involved in *H. pylori* adherence and colonization in gastric mucosa. The figure shows that urease neutralises pH and regulates acid secretion, flagella require for motility, collagenase/pronase are used to digest the mucin layer, adhesins help to adhere with specific gastric epithelial receptors, and virulence factors like CagA are involved in the induction of chemokines alters cell motility and polarity, peptidoglycan, and NapA induce inflammation, and VacA involved in apoptosis, vacuolation, and mucosal injury.

VIRULENCE FACTORS

H. pylori encodes several virulence factors like CagA (cytotoxin associated gene A) and VecA (vacuolating cytotoxin A), NapA (neutrophil activating factor A), OipA (outer inflammatory protein A), DupA (duodenal ulcer promoting gene A), Urease, and lipopolysaccharide (LPS) that contribute to the onset of gastric diseases. The expression of virulence genes is variable due to high genetic diversity among *H. pylori* strains. Therefore, the degree of clinical outcomes greatly varies among infected individuals. Based on the varying expressions of virulence genes, *H. pylori* strains are categorised as Type I and Type II strains. Type I strains are more virulent strains that consist of two primary antigens, CagA and VecA. While Type II strains are devoid of both of these antigens and are considered as non-virulent strains. The following key virulence factors are cited in the persistence and pathogenesis of *H. pylori* infection.

CagA: It is an immunogenic antigen that is encoded by cag-Pathogenicity Island (cag-PAI), a ~37kbp genomic region that consists of 27 Cag proteins including CagA, a secretory toxin. Cag-PAI constitutes a type IV secretion system (T4SS) that transfers CagA into the host cell in the contact-dependent manner [41]. CagA contacts with the surface exposed to phospholipid phosphatidylserine (PS) to initiate its translocation into the host cell [42]. Once CagA translocates into the host cell, it undergoes phosphorylation by Src-family kinases (*e.g.* cSrc, Fyn, and Lyn) and c-Abl kinases and hijacks host cell signaling pathways [43 - 46]. Both phosphorylated and unphosphorylated forms of CagA equally contribute to altering gastric epithelial cells. Phosphorylated CagA directly interacts with SHP-2, Grb2, Csk, cMet, and phospholipase Cy (PLCy) and alters downstream MEK-ERK kinases, thereby inducing cell elongation, membrane polarity, and pro-inflammatory responses. CagA also promotes the degradation of tumor suppressor factors like RUNX3 and P^{53} [47 - 49]. It also induces the expression of MCL1, an anti-apoptotic protein, and alongside; deregulates the Wnt/β-catenin pathway that eventually results in the development of gastritis, intestinal metaplasia, and/or resistance to apoptosis [50]. Unphosphorylated CagA physically interacts with multiple host proteins like ZO1, JAM (junctional adhesion molecule), E-Cadherin, and all forms of PAR1, which activate phosphatidylinositol 3-kinase (PI3K)/Akt pathway, NF-kB signalling, and Wnt/β-catenin pathway [50 - 52] that result in the disruption of the apical junction and induction of mitogenic responses. CagA/PAR1 and CagA/SHP2 interactions alter cell polarity and induce inflammatory responses, respectively [53, 54]. Moreover, CagA compromises dendritic cells causing impaired activation and reduces the induction of inflammatory cytokines and Th1 immune responses [55]. However, the actual frequency of CagA interaction with host proteins and further modulation of cellular responses into pathogenesis are yet to be comprehensively investigated.

VacA: VacA is a pore-forming toxin that contributes to the colonization of bacteria in gastric mucosa [56]. *H. pylori* releases VacA near the apical region of the plasma membrane in gastric mucosa. VacA creates pores in gastric epithelial cell membranes including intracellular organelles and creates pores after oligomerization [57, 58]. It also increases the cell membrane permeability and thus releases urea, nutrients, and various other solutes like bicarbonates, chloride, and calcium out of the host cell [59 - 61]. VacA reduces acid secretion from the parietal cell which helps bacteria to survive in gastric mucosa [62]. VacA binds with host cell receptors primarily with EGFR (epidermal growth factor receptor), sphingomyelin, LRP1 (low-density lipoprotein receptor-related protein-1), and RPTP (receptor protein tyrosine phosphatases) and modulates multiple cellular responses like the inhibition of endosomal maturation, promotes vacuolation, induction of autophagy and apoptosis, and avoids host immune responses. All these VacA-mediated cellular functions potentiate bacterial colonization and survival in extreme stress conditions in gastric mucosa.

NAP: NapA is a potent immunomodulatory molecule that induces the accumulation of neutrophils and monocytes at the site of infection [63]. Adhesion of neutrophils at gastric epithelial cells promotes the induction of reactive oxygen species (ROS) which results in mucosal injury and the release of nutrients for bacterial growth [64]. Thereby, it helps in the initial colonization and development of chronic gastritis in infected patients. Several studies show that VacA activates monocytes and dendritic cells which release IL12 and IL23 and trigger the differentiation of specific T cells towards Th1 responses and subsequently inhibit Th2 immune responses, thereby inhibiting allergic responses [65, 66]. Stimulated Th1 eventually releases various inflammatory molecules, hence it is considered a potential vaccine candidate to protect against gastric maladies and allergic responses in infected patients.

DupA: DupA is encoded by a combination of two continuous covering genes jhp0917 and jhp0918. Clinical studies show variable disease outcomes in dupA-positive bacterial strains in infected individuals. *In vivo* studies show that dupA triggers IL8 induction and infiltration of inflammatory cells in gastric antrum that can lead to the development of duodenal ulcers [67 - 69]. However, other epidemiological studies show discrepancies in clinical outcomes in different dupA-positive individuals [70, 71]. dupA is present in the plasticity region of the bacterial genome, which has a high degree of genetic variability among different populations [72]. Consequently, *H. pylori* strains consist of different lengths of dupA, which are distinctly related to variable disease outcomes. The exact role of

DupA in gastric maladies needs to be investigated further in geographically different populations.

OipA: OipA serves as an adhesion molecule to the host cell. It is also known as an inflammation-inducing antigen. It induces the expression of several pro-inflammatory cytokines like IL-1, IL-8, IL-17, and TNF-α that increase the risk of chronic gastritis and cancer adenocarcinoma [73]. However, oipA is present in all *H. pylori* strains and usually expressed together with other antigens like CagA, therefore further study is required to understand the actual role of individual protein *in vitro* or in infected animal modules [74]. OipA mutant *H. pylori* strain inhibits translocation of β-Catenin into the nucleus thus dampening the risk of gastric tumorigenesis in animals.

EPIDEMIOLOGY

Transmission and Prevalence

Sequence analysis reveals genetically similar *H. pylori* population in the closely related family members that underlines vertical transmission of the organism from parents to child. *H. pylori* is transmitted by fecal-oral or oral-oral routes mostly in early childhood as it is identified in saliva, vomitus, gastric refluxate, and feces [75 - 77]. Other possible transmission factors could be pickings of food as this organism can survive longer on refrigerated food [78]. *H. pylori* is one of the most common infectious agents in the human stomach worldwide. The prevalence of *H. pylori* is distantly related to different geographic regions. Hooi *et al.*, recently published a meta-analysis of 62 countries showing that in the last four decades (1970-2016) its prevalence greatly varies from high to low-to industrialized countries. Till 2016, the highest prevalence was found in Africa (70.1), South America (69.4%), and Western Asia (66.6%); whereas the lowest prevalence was in Oceania (24.4%), Western Europe (34.43%), and Northern America (37.1%). In 2015, 4.4 billion people (60.3% of the global population) were infected with this organism. Likewise, the prevalence markedly varies among human races, ethnic, and indigenous populations within the same region. For example, three racial communities in the United States: non-Hispanic whites, non-whites, and the Alaskan Natives have variable prevalence as high as 26.2%, 61.6%, and 75% respectively. In Australia, the average prevalence in the general population is 24.6%, while it is 76% in the indigenous community of rural Western Australia. The prevalence is almost similar in males (46.3%) and females (42.7%). In the 21st century, the prevalence has rapidly decreased in developed or highly industrialized countries, however, there is almost no change in developing and growing industrialized countries [79]. Higher prevalence in developing and low-income countries is related to low socioeconomic status, poor hygiene and sanitation, polluted water, and local population density.

Clinical Outcomes of *H. pylori* Infection

Once *H. pylori* infects an individual, it remains in the stomach throughout his lifetime until treated *H. pylori* is asymptomatic in a large proportion of the colonized population. About 15-20% of *H. pylori*-infected people show clinical outcomes even that are mostly restricted to older age people. The pathological effects of the organism greatly vary among infected individuals worldwide depending on the intensity of virulence factors, duration of exposure, physiological conditions of habitat, bacterial strain, and host genetic susceptibility. *H. pylori* infection is primarily associated with the development of chronic gastritis, peptic ulcer (*i.e.*, gastric and duodenum ulcers), gastric cancer, and MALT lymphoma. *H. pylori* is associated with 80% peptic ulcer disease (PUD) and 90% non-cardia gastric cancer in infected patients. Besides, chronic infection is also having a causal relationship with a wide range of diseases like iron deficient anemia, non-ulcer dyspepsia, immune thrombocytopenic and vitamin B12 deficiency, Non-alcoholic fatty acid disease (NAFLD), insulin resistance and diabetes mellitus. On the other hand, *H. pylori* is considered to have a friendly relationship with humans and protects against colonization of other bacterial pathogens and diseases like esophageal cancer, allergy, asthma, inflammatory bowel disease, celiac disease multiple sclerosis, rhinitis and gastroesophageal reflux disease (GERD). *H. pylori* has both deleterious and protective links that are based on correlative rather than direct involvement. Here, the negative correlation of *H. pylori* infection in human health is well studied and are as follows.

Acute and Chronic Gastritis

Gastric colonization of *H. pylori* and the development of gastritis is well documented. Once *H. pylori* inter gastric mucosa it prefers to localize at no or less acid producing region *i.e.*, the antrum, lower part of the stomach. During compromised condition, *H. pylori* reduces acid secretion in gastric mucosa [80] and establishes an active infection that leads to gastritis, a phase of inflammation that leads to mucosal injury in the stomach. Histologic studies show a limited active inflammation with a smaller number of bacterial cells which is defined as an antrum-predominant gastritis. Most of the *H. pylori* colonized individuals develop histologic gastritis with age worldwide. Acute gastritis may resolve spontaneously in most of the infected cases. During acute gastritis, bacteria invade deeper into the gastric carpus, inhibiting acid secretion further results in the establishment of more active chronic inflammation *i.e.*, defined as carpus-dominant chronic gastritis. Over time it leads to infiltration of both gastric antrum and carpus with neutrophils, monocytes, lymphocytes, *etc*., and consequently, acute gastritis turns into atrophic gastritis. Inflamed gastric mucosa induces secretion of cytokine including IL-1β, a potent inhibiter of parietal cells, that further supresses acid secretion and facilitates persistent infection in the gastric pits of the carpus region and advances the severity of atrophic gastritis.

Peptic Ulcer Disease

Peptic ulcer is strongly related to gastric colonization of *H. pylori*. More than 90% of duodenum ulcers and about 80% of gastric ulcers have *H. pylori* infection. Clinical evidence reveal that *H. pylori*-positive individuals have a 2-to-4-fold higher risk of developing peptic ulcer than *H. pylori*-negative individuals [81]. About 50% of the ulcer patients suffered recurrence of the disease in infected patients. Chronic inflammation and *H. pylori* persistence lead to the destruction of the thick mucus layer resulting in the development of peptic ulcers that extend from the stomach to the lower esophagus and duodenum. Peptic ulcer includes both gastric ulcer and/or duodenum ulcer. A gastric ulcer occurs in gastric mucosa mostly in between the antrum and carpus, however, a duodenum ulcer occurs primarily in the duodenum bulb which is mostly exposed to gastric acid. About 15% of *H. pylori* colonized individuals develop peptic ulcers in their lifetime. Several *in vitro* and *in vivo* studies reveal the association of *H. pylori* antigens primarily VacA, CagA, and DupA with the development of peptic ulcers. VacA increases the permeability of the gastric membrane and also inhibits acid secretion in the stomach. CagA is an immunodominant antigen that induces pro-inflammatory responses in gastric mucosa. In Western countries, the incidence rate of duodenal ulcers is fourfold higher than others. Other than *H. pylori* infection, long-term medication of aspirin and Non-steroidal anti-inflammatory drugs (NSAIDs) [82], stress, and spicy and salted food significantly contribute to the development of a peptic ulcer. Eradication of *H. pylori* infection completely cures ulcers and also reduces 3-4 times recurrence rate in infected patients in comparison to placebo [83, 84].

Intestinal Metaplasia and Gastric Cancer

Chronic *H. pylori*-mediated inflammation finally results in mucosal lining destruction, gastric gland loss, and replacement by fibrous tissue and intestinal metaplastic cells (Fig. **3**). Over time, the area of mucosal destruction and intestinal metaplasia extend multifocally. Chronic *H. pylori* infection induces the expression of various cytokines *e.g*. IL-1B, IL-6, IL-8, IL-12, TNF-α, and cyclooxygenase-2 (COX-2) in gastric mucosa [85, 86]. Prolonged inflammation eventually leads to the accumulation of mitotic errors, resulting in gastric epithelial dysplasia, and abnormal changes in gastric lining. Gastric mucosa destruction and intestinal metaplasia raise the risk of gastric cancer by 5 to 90-fold, depending on the severity of atrophy [87, 88]. Clinical studies reveal that about 90% of the non-cardia cancer is associated with *H. pylori* infection [89]. However, 1-3% of the *H. pylori*-positive individuals develop gastric adenocarcinoma. The prevalence of gastric cancer greatly varies among different countries worldwide. The incidence rate of gastric cancer is 4 to 6-fold higher in developed or industrialized countries than in developing or low-income countries. Subsequently, the occurrence of *H. pylori* is distinctly decreased in developed countries than in poor countries. Almost 50% of gastric cancers are reported in East Asia *i.e.*, Korea, Mongolia, Japan, and China. Eradication therapy sharply decreases the incidence of gastric cancer in *H. pylori*-infected patients in comparison to placebo. A high incidence rate of gastric cancer in developed and East Asian countries is expected due to changes in lifestyle and food habits.

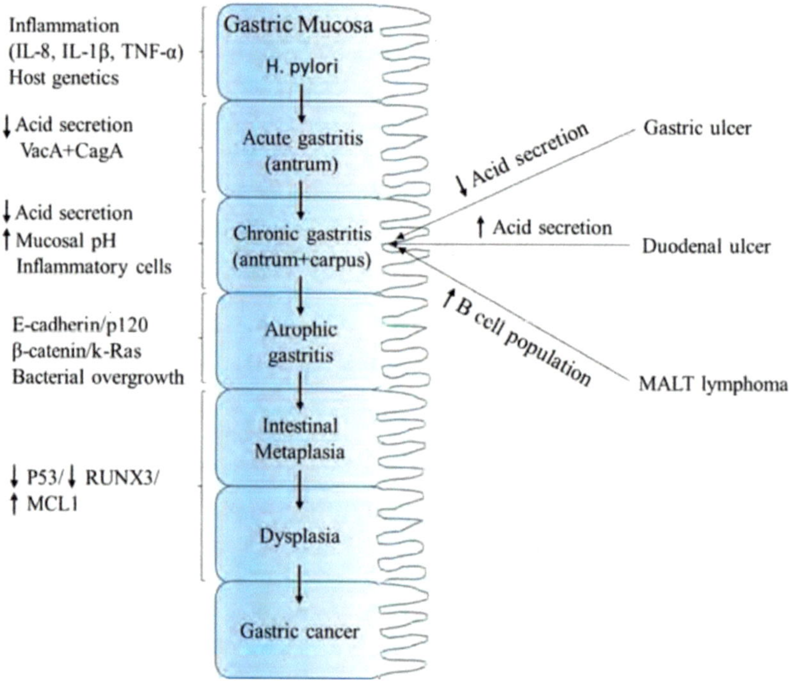

Fig. (3). Stepwise progression of peptic ulcer (gastric and duodenum), MALT lymphoma, and gastric cancer in *H. pylori*-infected gastric mucosa. Colonized *H. pylori* and released virulence factors primarily CagA and VacA, induce inflammation and reduce acid secretion in gastric mucosa and result in antrum gastritis. Infiltration of inflammatory cells like neutrophils, and macrophages extend antrum gastritis to chronic carpus gastritis and is associated with the development of peptic ulcer. Proliferation and accumulation of altered B cells in gastric mucosa results in MALT lymphoma. Prolonged inflammation and atrophic gastritis successively result in deregulation of host cell signalling that eventually develops gastric adenocarcinoma.

Adherence of *H. pylori* with gastric epithelial cells has direct effects on genetic and epigenetic changes, and loss of membrane polarity that leads to altered cell behaviour and malignant transformation. In 1994, the International Agency for Research on Cancer (IARC), WHO defined *H. pylori* infection as a "group I carcinogen". *In vivo* studies in animals showed that *H. pylori* infection is directly associated with the development of gastric adenocarcinoma [90]. Several studies reveal that CagA-positive *H. pylori* strains are associated with the development of precancerous gastric lesions and cancer progression in infected subjects. *H. pylori* translocates CagA along with peptidoglycan directly into the host cell and alters several signalling pathways including mitogen-activated protein kinase (MAPK), phosphoinositide-3 kinase (PI3K-AKT) and Wnt/β-catenin. Translocated CagA induces nuclear accumulation of β-catenin and subsequently reduces expression of tumor suppressors like Runx3, trefoil, and p53. Moreover, VacA promotes Th1 phenotype response and induces apoptosis and autophagy *via* induction of pro-inflammatory cytokine and membrane permeability [91]. A meta-analysis reveals that Cag-positive strains induce the risk of non-cardia cancer by 2-3-fold in comparison to CagA-negative strains.

Gastric MALT Lymphoma

Normally, gastric mucosa is devoid of lymphoid tissues, however, all the patients with gastric MALT lymphoma have *H. pylori* infection [92]. About 1% population of *H. pylori*-infected patients develop MALT lymphoma. During prolonged *H. pylori* infection, a population of B cells arises in gastric mucosa and initiates to proliferate which eventually raises MALT lymphoma. *H. pylori* colonized individuals have a higher risk of developing MALT lymphoma than uninfected individuals.

H. PYLORI AND GUT MICROBIOME

Blaser stated in 1998 that *H. pylori* might be thought of as indigenous or 'normal' flora, which the majority of people acquire during their early childhood and thereafter carry for the rest of their lives [93]. *H. pylori* is thought to have coevolved in the human stomach and travelled with humans from Africa to the Middle East between 58,000 and 150,000 years ago. *H. pylori* successfully colonize and adapt to the gut environment over the course of evolution and stays as a silent companion. It is well known that *H. pylori* interact favourably with the biology of the human stomach, the gut microbiota, and immune reactions. Several recent studies found that gastric Actinobacteria decrease after *H. pylori* removal, Proteobacteria increase during short-term follow-up and then reduce to baseline levels, and Enterobacteriaceae and Enterococcus increase during short-term and interim follow-up. Following *H. pylori* eradication from the human gut, various gastric mucosal pro-inflammatory bacteria, including Actinomyces, Granulicatella, Bacteroides ovatus, Parvimonas, Peptostreptococcus, Sphingomonas, Prevotella, Rothia, Fusobacterium varium, Streptococcus, and Lactobacillus rise and may contribute to unfavourable gastric consequences such as precancerous lesions. A study that evaluated the effects of gastric cancer revealed that Proteobacteria, Firmicutes (genera Veilonella and Streptococcus), and species from the Bifidobacterium/Lactobacillus group were more frequent [94]. Moreover, contrary to other pathogenic/opportunistic bacteria, T helper type 2 immunity promotes *H. pylori* colonization of newborns/infants and results in the maturation of immunological tolerance [95]. Due to the bacteria's millennia of co-evolution with the human host, the host's immune system most likely regards *H. pylori* as a commensal symbiont rather than a pathogenic organism. Early *H. pylori* colonization can benefit the host in a number of ways, including by regulating the hormones leptin and ghrelin, defence against a number of autoimmune and allergy illnesses (such as asthma), as well as protection against inflammatory bowel disease (IBD) [95, 96]. According to the data, eradication cannot be recommended in every case of *H. pylori* infection because, in the vast majority of cases, *H. pylori* behaves as a commensal and can be advantageous in mutualistic contact with the host [93, 97]. Most individuals with undifferentiated dyspepsia are advised to use a "test-and-treat" approach. Patients are subjected to a non-invasive test for *H. pylori* infection in this method, and if positive, eradication medication is administered.

DIAGNOSIS AND TREATMENT

The presence of urease, unique antigens, and immunoglobulin are used for the identification of *H. pylori* by using various diagnostic samples like biopsies of the gastric antrum and corpus, saliva, blood, dental plaque, stool, and faeces in infected individuals. Several invasive and non-invasive diagnostic tests are employed for the diagnosis of *H. pylori* in infected patients that are listed in Table **1**. Invasive tests are based on endoscopic biopsy samples including culture, rapid urease test, histology, and various other molecular-based methods. Fecal antigen tests and urease breath tests are routinely used in hospitals as non-invasive tests. A serological test is commonly used to screen and epidemiological analysis. Computed tomography (CT) scan which uses powerful X-ray, and magnetic resonance imaging (MRI) are commonly used to take detailed visualisation of the gastric mucosa.

Table 1. ***H. pylori*** **diagnostic testing.**

Diagnostic test	Type of sample	Sensitivity	Specificity
Invasive methods			
Microbial Culture	gastric biopsy	>70	>90
PCR	gastric biopsy	>95	>95
Rapid urease test	antrum biopsy	>95	>99
Histology	gastric biopsy	>95	>99
Non-invasive methods			
Urease breath test	isotope carbon in exhaled breath	>95	>95
Fecal antigen test	stool	>95	>95
Serology (ELISA IgG)	blood	>75	>90
Culture	saliva, faces and dental plaque	>70	>99

When *H. pylori* infection is determined in patients with active infection, the standard therapy is to remove it and allow the ulcer to heal on its own. There is no regimen available to eradicate 100% *H. pylori* infection. There are few regimens which have more than a 90% cure rate. Dual therapies consisting of proton pump inhibitor (PPI) and amoxicillin are used in some countries, but it is now almost replaced *via* triple therapies. The conventional first-line therapy is clarithromycin triple therapy, which comprises a PPI such as omeprazole and two antibiotics, clarithromycin, and amoxicillin or metronidazole, for 14 days [98]. In the last decade, *H. pylori* resistance to clarithromycin has been widely reported. So, clarithromycin is not recommended in the area where its resistance is more than 15%. Bismuth quadruple therapy is also considered first-line therapy and is commonly preferred to avoid use at location where clarithromycin resistance is high. This therapy consists of bismuth, a protective gastric lining, a PPI, tetracycline, and nitroimidazole for 10-14 days. Another therapeutic option for *H. pylori* strains that are resistant to clarithromycin is levofloxacin triple therapy. Numerous variations of the triple therapy have been created over time with the addition of various PPI, such as pantoprazole or rabeprazole, or switching out amoxicillin for metronidazole in the case of penicillin allergies [99]. These treatments have completely changed how *H. pylori* infections are handled, and they have also made it feasible to cure the condition. The selected regimen is usually a combination of antibiotics, acid inhibitors, and gastric lining protectors as listed below.

• Antibiotics: to kill bacteria such as metronidazole, clarithromycin, and amoxicillin. Tetracycline or tinidazole,

• H_2-blockers: to reduce acid secretion such as cimetidine, ranitidine, famotidine, and nizatidine.

• Proton pump inhibitors: esomeprazole, lansoprazole, omeprazole, pantapzole.

Stomach-lining protector: bismuth subsalicylate. Successful two-week triple therapy eradicates the bacteria, reduces symptoms, and prevents the recurrence rate of *H. pylori* infection in more than 90 percent of medical cases. Even in regions with a high frequency of antibiotic resistance, the quadruple therapy regimen (proton pump inhibitor, tetracycline, metronidazole, and a bismuth salt) is quite effective and could be used as an alternate first-line therapy. Peptic ulcer disease,dyspepsia, and contagious diarrhoea have all long been treated with bismuth. An increasing number of antibiotic-resistant bacteria is a matter of concern and require urgent need to develop alternative treatment strategies. However, some research has begun to concentrate on probiotics as a therapeutic strategy due to the rise in antibiotic resistance. The term "probiotics" refers to a class of living microorganisms that may have antioxidant and anti-inflammatory properties that may benefit intestinal microbiology and overall health [100]. Live bacteria known as probiotics can help the host's health when given in sufficient doses. Lactobacillus and Bifidobacterium are the two most popular probiotic microorganisms [101]. Probiotics may help with *H. pylori* eradication and minimise the negative effects of treatment. The use of probiotics to combat *H. pylori* will be a key component of this upgrade.

CONCLUDING REMARKS

The gut of half of the world's population is home to *H. pylori*. Only 15% of those who are infected, however, exhibit clinical signs. The infection prevalence and severity of diseases are not limited to a particular region or country but greatly vary geographically. Several studies showed lifestyle choices, dietary patterns, and bacterial strains have a greater impact on clinical outcomes than *H. pylori* alone. Moreover, the severity of the disease against the infection depends on a number of variables, such as age, bacterial strain, genetic susceptibility of the host, and local environmental irritants. For the treatment of *H. pylori* infection, a proton pump inhibitor (PPI), clarithromycin, and amoxicillin were chosen as the standard triple therapy. However, since eradication rates have dropped to unsafely low levels in recent years, the efficacy of standard triple therapy has been drastically altered in many parts of the world. Patient compliance, bacterial virulence, overweight, smoking, subsequent infection, over-activation of drug transporters, and genetic polymorphisms in CYP2C19 may all be significant contributors to this reduction. However, antibiotic resistance may be critical in the decreased global success in eradicating *H. pylori* infection. Additionally, even within the same nation, the rates of eradication vary by region. One study in South Korea showed that first-line therapy eradication rates fell from 81.3% to 77.5% between 2001 and 2007 [102], while the other study found no conclusive evidence that the rate changed significantly between 2000 and 2010 [103]. The "universal eradication" of *H. pylori* may be harmful to people who are already infected, claim Miller and Williams [104]. To lessen the harmful effects of eradication, probiotics, prebiotics, and microbial metabolites (for instance, butyrate + inulin) [105] should be added. This is because antibiotics and PPIs can have substantial side effects and/or long-term dysbiotic alterations in the gastrointestinal flora. To boost eradication rates and reduce antibiotic resistance, novel therapeutic procedures must be developed.

ACKNOWLEDGEMENTS

The author extends the appreciation to the central instrumental facility of the School of Biotechnology, Gautam Buddha University. Special thanks to Professor Sher Ali for reviewing and editing the manuscript and making relevant suggestions.

REFERENCES

[1] Bizzozero G. Uber die schlauchformingen drusen des magendarmkanals und die beziehung ihres epithels zu dem oberflachenepithel de schleimhaut. Arch Mikr Anat 1893; 42: 82-152. [http://dx.doi.org/10.1007/BF02975307]

[2] Goodwin CS, Armstrong JA, Chilvers T, *et al.* Transfer of *Campylobacter pylori* and campylobacter mustelae to Helicobacter gen. nov. as *Helicobacter pylori* comb. nov. and *Helicobacter mustelae* comb. nov., Respectively. Int J Syst Bacteriol 1989; 39(4): 397-405. [http://dx.doi.org/10.1099/00207713-39-4-397]

[3] Schistosomes, liver flukes and *Helicobacter pylori*. IARC Monogr Eval Carcinog Risks Hum 1994; 61: 1-241. [PMID: 7715068]

[4] Meyer-Rosberg K, Scott DR, Rex D, Melchers K, Sachs G. The effect of environmental pH on the proton motive force of *Helicobacter pylori*. Gastroenterology 1996; 111(4): 886-900. [http://dx.doi.org/10.1016/S0016-5085(96)70056-2] [PMID: 8831583]

[5] Marshall B, Warren JR. Unidentified curved bacilli in the stomach of patients with gastritis and peptic ulceration. Lancet 1984; 323(8390): 1311-5. [http://dx.doi.org/10.1016/S0140-6736(84)91816-6] [PMID: 6145023]

[6] O'Toole PW, Lane MC, Porwollik S. *Helicobacter pylori* motility. Microbes Infect 2000; 2(10): 1207-14. [http://dx.doi.org/10.1016/S1286-4579(00)01274-0] [PMID: 11008110]

[7] Kusters JG, Gerrits MM, Van Strijp JA, Vandenbroucke-Grauls CM. Coccoid forms of *Helicobacter pylori* are the morphologic manifestation of cell death. Infect Immun 1997; 65(9): 3672-9. [http://dx.doi.org/10.1128/iai.65.9.3672-3679.1997] [PMID: 9284136]

[8] Bode G, Mauch F, Malfertheiner P. The coccoid forms of *Helicobacter pylori*. Criteria for their

viability. Epidemiol Infect 1993; 111(3): 483-90.
[http://dx.doi.org/10.1017/S0950268800057216] [PMID: 8270008]

[9] Cellini L, Allocati N, Angelucci D, *et al.* Coccoid *Helicobacter pylori* not culturable *in vitro* reverts in mice. Microbiol Immunol 1994; 38(11): 843-50.
[http://dx.doi.org/10.1111/j.1348-0421.1994.tb02136.x] [PMID: 7898382]

[10] Cellini L. Coccoid forms of *Helicobacter pylori*. J Infect Dis 1996; 173(5): 1288-9.
[http://dx.doi.org/10.1093/infdis/173.5.1288] [PMID: 8627089]

[11] Chan WY, Hui PK, Leung KM, Chow J, Kwok F, Ng CS. Coccoid forms of *Helicobacter pylori* in the human stomach. Am J Clin Pathol 1994; 102(4): 503-7.
[http://dx.doi.org/10.1093/ajcp/102.4.503] [PMID: 7524304]

[12] Sörberg M, Nilsson M, Hanberger H, Nilsson LE. Morphologic conversion of *Helicobacter pylori* from bacillary to coccoid form. Eur J Clin Microbiol Infect Dis 1996; 15(3): 216-9.
[http://dx.doi.org/10.1007/BF01591357] [PMID: 8740856]

[13] Tomb JF, White O, Kerlavage AR, *et al.* The complete genome sequence of the gastric pathogen *Helicobacter pylori*. Nature 1997; 388(6642): 539-47.
[http://dx.doi.org/10.1038/41483] [PMID: 9252185]

[14] Alm RA, Ling LSL, Moir DT, *et al.* Genomic-sequence comparison of two unrelated isolates of the human gastric pathogen *Helicobacter pylori*. Nature 1999; 397(6715): 176-80.
[http://dx.doi.org/10.1038/16495] [PMID: 9923682]

[15] Oh JD, Kling-Bäckhed H, Giannakis M, *et al.* The complete genome sequence of a chronic atrophic gastritis *Helicobacter pylori* strain: Evolution during disease progression. Proc Natl Acad Sci 2006; 103(26): 9999-10004.
[http://dx.doi.org/10.1073/pnas.0603784103] [PMID: 16788065]

[16] Oshima T, Aiba H, Masuda Y, *et al.* Transcriptome analysis of all two-component regulatory system mutants of *Escherichia coli* K-12. Mol Microbiol 2002; 46(1): 281-91.
[http://dx.doi.org/10.1046/j.1365-2958.2002.03170.x] [PMID: 12366850]

[17] Heuermann D, Haas R. Genetic organization of a small cryptic plasmid of *Helicobacter pylori*. Gene 1995; 165(1): 17-24.
[http://dx.doi.org/10.1016/0378-1119(95)00469-M] [PMID: 7489910]

[18] Salama N, Guillemin K, McDaniel TK, Sherlock G, Tompkins L, Falkow S. A whole-genome microarray reveals genetic diversity among *Helicobacter pylori* strains. Proc Natl Acad Sci 2000; 97(26): 14668-73.
[http://dx.doi.org/10.1073/pnas.97.26.14668] [PMID: 11121067]

[19] Blaser MJ, Berg DE. *Helicobacter pylori* genetic diversity and risk of human disease. J Clin Invest 2001; 107(7): 767-73.
[http://dx.doi.org/10.1172/JCI12672] [PMID: 11285290]

[20] Suerbaum S, Josenhans C. *Helicobacter pylori* evolution and phenotypic diversification in a changing host. Nat Rev Microbiol 2007; 5(6): 441-52.
[http://dx.doi.org/10.1038/nrmicro1658] [PMID: 17505524]

[21] Israel BA, Lichtenstein R, Lantz P, *et al.* The detroit community-academic urban research center: Development, implementation, and evaluation. J Public Health Manag Pract 2001; 7(5): 1-19.
[http://dx.doi.org/10.1097/00124784-200107050-00003] [PMID: 11680026]

[22] Baltrus DA, Guillemin K, Phillips PC. Natural transformation increases the rate of adaptation in the human pathogen *Helicobacter pylori*. Evolution 2008; 62(1): 39-49.
[http://dx.doi.org/10.1111/j.1558-5646.2007.00271.x] [PMID: 17976191]

[23] Robinson K, Loughlin MF, Potter R, Jenks PJ. Host adaptation and immune modulation are mediated by homologous recombination in *Helicobacter pylori*. J Infect Dis 2005; 191(4): 579-87.
[http://dx.doi.org/10.1086/427657] [PMID: 15655782]

[24] Dorer MS, Talarico S, Salama NR. Helicobacter pylori's unconventional role in health and disease. PLoS Pathog 2009; 5(10): e1000544. [http://dx.doi.org/10.1371/journal.ppat.1000544] [PMID: 19855816]

[25] Suerbaum S, Josenhans C. Virulence factors of *Helicobacter pylori*: Implications for vaccine development. Mol Med Today 1999; 5(1): 32-9. [http://dx.doi.org/10.1016/S1357-4310(98)01390-2] [PMID: 10088130]

[26] Skouloubris S, Labigne A, De Reuse H. Identification and characterization of an aliphatic amidase in *Helicobacter pylori*. Mol Microbiol 1997; 25(5): 989-98. [http://dx.doi.org/10.1111/j.1365-2958.1997.mmi536.x] [PMID: 9364923]

[27] Eaton KA, Morgan DR, Krakowka S. Motility as a factor in the colonisation of gnotobiotic piglets by *Helicobacter pylori*. J Med Microbiol 1992; 37(2): 123-7. [http://dx.doi.org/10.1099/00222615-37-2-123] [PMID: 1629897]

[28] Ha NC, Oh ST, Sung JY, Cha KA, Lee MH, Oh BH. Supramolecular assembly and acid resistance of *Helicobacter pylori* urease. Nat Struct Biol 2001; 8(6): 505-9. [http://dx.doi.org/10.1038/88563] [PMID: 11373617]

[29] Yoshiyama H, Nakamura H, Kimoto M, Okita K, Nakazawa T. Chemotaxis and motility of *Helicobacter pylori* in a viscous environment. J Gastroenterol 1999; 34(S11): 18-23. [PMID: 10616760]

[30] Kavermann H, Burns BP, Angermüller K, *et al.* Identification and characterization of *Helicobacter pylori* genes essential for gastric colonization. J Exp Med 2003; 197(7): 813-22. [http://dx.doi.org/10.1084/jem.20021531] [PMID: 12668646]

[31] Slomiany BL, Murty VLN, Piotrowski J, Liau YH, Sundaram P, Slomiany A. Glycosulfatase activity of *Helicobacter pylori* toward gastric mucin. Biochem Biophys Res Commun 1992; 183(2): 506-13. [http://dx.doi.org/10.1016/0006-291X(92)90511-I] [PMID: 1372502]

[32] Josenhans C, Labigne A, Suerbaum S. Comparative ultrastructural and functional studies of *Helicobacter pylori* and *Helicobacter mustelae* flagellin mutants: Both flagellin subunits, FlaA and FlaB, are necessary for full motility in *Helicobacter* species. J Bacteriol 1995; 177(11): 3010-20. [http://dx.doi.org/10.1128/jb.177.11.3010-3020.1995] [PMID: 7768796]

[33] Eaton KA, Suerbaum S, Josenhans C, Krakowka S. Colonization of gnotobiotic piglets by *Helicobacter pylori* deficient in two flagellin genes. Infect Immun 1996; 64(7): 2445-8. [http://dx.doi.org/10.1128/iai.64.7.2445-2448.1996] [PMID: 8698465]

[34] Beil W, Birkholz C, Wagner S, Sewing KF. Interaction of *Helicobacter pylori* and its fatty acids with parietal cells and gastric H+/K(+)-ATPase. Gut 1994; 35(9): 1176-80. [http://dx.doi.org/10.1136/gut.35.9.1176] [PMID: 7959221]

[35] Datta De D, Roychoudhury S. To be or not to be: The host genetic factor and beyond in *Helicobacter pylori* mediated gastro-duodenal diseases. World J Gastroenterol 2015; 21(10): 2883-95. [http://dx.doi.org/10.3748/wjg.v21.i10.2883] [PMID: 25780285]

[36] Mahdavi J, Sondén B, Hurtig M, *et al. Helicobacter pylori* SabA adhesin in persistent infection and chronic inflammation. Science 2002; 297(5581): 573-8. [http://dx.doi.org/10.1126/science.1069076] [PMID: 12142529]

[37] Borén T, Falk P, Roth KA, Larson G, Normark S. Attachment of *Helicobacter pylori* to human gastric epithelium mediated by blood group antigens. Science 1993; 262(5141): 1892-5. [http://dx.doi.org/10.1126/science.8018146] [PMID: 8018146]

[38] Ilver D, Arnqvist A, Ögren J, *et al. Helicobacter pylori* adhesin binding fucosylated histo-blood group antigens revealed by retagging. Science 1998; 279(5349): 373-7. [http://dx.doi.org/10.1126/science.279.5349.373] [PMID: 9430586]

[39] Kwok T, Zabler D, Urman S, *et al.* Helicobacter exploits integrin for type IV secretion and kinase

activation. Nature 2007; 449(7164): 862-6.
[http://dx.doi.org/10.1038/nature06187] [PMID: 17943123]

[40] Bugaytsova JA, Björnham O, Chernov YA, *et al.* *Helicobacter pylori* adapts to chronic infection and gastric disease via ph-responsive BabA-mediated adherence. Cell Host Microbe 2017; 21(3): 376-89. [http://dx.doi.org/10.1016/j.chom.2017.02.013] [PMID: 28279347]

[41] Fischer W. Assembly and molecular mode of action of the *Helicobacter pylori* Cag type IV secretion apparatus. FEBS J 2011; 278(8): 1203-12. [http://dx.doi.org/10.1111/j.1742-4658.2011.08036.x] [PMID: 21352490]

[42] Murata-Kamiya N, Kikuchi K, Hayashi T, Higashi H, Hatakeyama M. *Helicobacter pylori* exploits host membrane phosphatidylserine for delivery, localization, and pathophysiological action of the CagA oncoprotein. Cell Host Microbe 2010; 7(5): 399-411. [http://dx.doi.org/10.1016/j.chom.2010.04.005] [PMID: 20478541]

[43] Poppe M, Feller SM, Römer G, Wessler S. Phosphorylation of *Helicobacter pylori* CagA by c-Abl leads to cell motility. Oncogene 2007; 26(24): 3462-72. [http://dx.doi.org/10.1038/sj.onc.1210139] [PMID: 17160020]

[44] Tammer I, Brandt S, Hartig R, König W, Backert S. Activation of Abl by *Helicobacter pylori*: A novel kinase for CagA and crucial mediator of host cell scattering. Gastroenterology 2007; 132(4): 1309-19. [http://dx.doi.org/10.1053/j.gastro.2007.01.050] [PMID: 17408661]

[45] Ohnishi N, Yuasa H, Tanaka S, *et al.* Transgenic expression of *Helicobacter pylori* CagA induces gastrointestinal and hematopoietic neoplasms in mouse. Proc Natl Acad Sci 2008; 105(3): 1003-8. [http://dx.doi.org/10.1073/pnas.0711183105] [PMID: 18192401]

[46] Mueller D, Tegtmeyer N, Brandt S, *et al.* c-Src and c-Abl kinases control hierarchic phosphorylation and function of the CagA effector protein in Western and East Asian *Helicobacter pylori* strains. J Clin Invest 2012; 122(4): 1553-66. [http://dx.doi.org/10.1172/JCI61143] [PMID: 22378042]

[47] Tsang YH, Lamb A, Romero-Gallo J, *et al.* *Helicobacter pylori* CagA targets gastric tumor suppressor RUNX3 for proteasome-mediated degradation. Oncogene 2010; 29(41): 5643-50. [http://dx.doi.org/10.1038/onc.2010.304] [PMID: 20676134]

[48] Buti L, Spooner E, Van der Veen AG, Rappuoli R, Covacci A, Ploegh HL. *Helicobacter pylori* cytotoxin-associated gene A (CagA) subverts the apoptosis-stimulating protein of p53 (ASPP2) tumor suppressor pathway of the host. Proc Natl Acad Sci 2011; 108(22): 9238-43. [http://dx.doi.org/10.1073/pnas.1106200108] [PMID: 21562218]

[49] Wei J, Noto JM, Zaika E, *et al.* Bacterial CagA protein induces degradation of p53 protein in a p14ARF-dependent manner. Gut 2015; 64(7): 1040-8. [http://dx.doi.org/10.1136/gutjnl-2014-307295] [PMID: 25080447]

[50] Mimuro H, Suzuki T, Nagai S, *et al.* *Helicobacter pylori* dampens gut epithelial self-renewal by inhibiting apoptosis, a bacterial strategy to enhance colonization of the stomach. Cell Host Microbe 2007; 2(4): 250-63. [http://dx.doi.org/10.1016/j.chom.2007.09.005] [PMID: 18005743]

[51] Zeaiter Z, Cohen D, Müsch A, Bagnoli F, Covacci A, Stein M. Analysis of detergent-resistant membranes of *Helicobacter pylori* infected gastric adenocarcinoma cells reveals a role for MARK2/Par1b in CagA-mediated disruption of cellular polarity. Cell Microbiol 2008; 10(3): 781-94. [http://dx.doi.org/10.1111/j.1462-5822.2007.01084.x] [PMID: 18005242]

[52] Suzuki M, Mimuro H, Kiga K, *et al.* *Helicobacter pylori* CagA phosphorylation-independent function in epithelial proliferation and inflammation. Cell Host Microbe 2009; 5(1): 23-34. [http://dx.doi.org/10.1016/j.chom.2008.11.010] [PMID: 19154985]

[53] Saadat I, Higashi H, Obuse C, *et al.* *Helicobacter pylori* CagA targets PAR1/MARK kinase to disrupt epithelial cell polarity. Nature 2007; 447(7142): 330-3.

[http://dx.doi.org/10.1038/nature05765] [PMID: 17507984]

[54] Goldstein B, Macara IG. The PAR proteins: Fundamental players in animal cell polarization. Dev Cell 2007; 13(5): 609-22.
[http://dx.doi.org/10.1016/j.devcel.2007.10.007] [PMID: 17981131]

[55] Tanaka H, Yoshida M, Nishiumi S, *et al.* The CagA protein of *Helicobacter pylori* suppresses the functions of dendritic cell in mice. Arch Biochem Biophys 2010; 498(1): 35-42.
[http://dx.doi.org/10.1016/j.abb.2010.03.021] [PMID: 20363211]

[56] Salama NR, Otto G, Tompkins L, Falkow S. Vacuolating cytotoxin of *Helicobacter pylori* plays a role during colonization in a mouse model of infection. Infect Immun 2001; 69(2): 730-6.
[http://dx.doi.org/10.1128/IAI.69.2.730-736.2001] [PMID: 11159961]

[57] Tombola F, Carlesso C, Szabò I, *et al. Helicobacter pylori* vacuolating toxin forms anion-selective channels in planar lipid bilayers: Possible implications for the mechanism of cellular vacuolation. Biophys J 1999; 76(3): 1401-9.
[http://dx.doi.org/10.1016/S0006-3495(99)77301-7] [PMID: 10049322]

[58] Czajkowsky DM, Iwamoto H, Cover TL, Shao Z. The vacuolating toxin from *Helicobacter pylori* forms hexameric pores in lipid bilayers at low pH. Proc Natl Acad Sci 1999; 96(5): 2001-6.
[http://dx.doi.org/10.1073/pnas.96.5.2001] [PMID: 10051584]

[59] Papini E, Satin B, Norais N, *et al.* Selective increase of the permeability of polarized epithelial cell monolayers by *Helicobacter pylori* vacuolating toxin. J Clin Invest 1998; 102(4): 813-20.
[http://dx.doi.org/10.1172/JCI2764] [PMID: 9710450]

[60] Tombola F, Morbiato L, Del Giudice G, Rappuoli R, Zoratti M, Papini E. The *Helicobacter pylori* VacA toxin is a urea permease that promotes urea diffusion across epithelia. J Clin Invest 2001; 108(6): 929-37.
[http://dx.doi.org/10.1172/JCI13045] [PMID: 11560962]

[61] Akazawa Y, Isomoto H, Matsushima K. Endoplasmic reticulum stress contributes to *Helicobacter pylori* VacA-induced apoptosis. PLoS One 2013; 8(12): e82322.
[http://dx.doi.org/10.1371/journal.pone.0082322]

[62] Kobayashi H, Kamiya S, Suzuki T, *et al.* The effect of *Helicobacter pylori* on gastric acid secretion by isolated parietal cells from a guinea pig. Association with production of vacuolating toxin by H. pylori. Scand J Gastroenterol 1996; 31(5): 428-33.
[http://dx.doi.org/10.3109/00365529609006760] [PMID: 8734337]

[63] Satin B, Del Giudice G, Della Bianca V, *et al.* The neutrophil-activating protein (HP-NAP) of *Helicobacter pylori* is a protective antigen and a major virulence factor. J Exp Med 2000; 191(9): 1467-76.
[http://dx.doi.org/10.1084/jem.191.9.1467] [PMID: 10790422]

[64] Montecucco C, de Bernard M. Molecular and cellular mechanisms of action of the vacuolating cytotoxin (VacA) and neutrophil-activating protein (HP-NAP) virulence factors of *Helicobacter pylori*. Microbes Infect 2003; 5(8): 715-21.
[http://dx.doi.org/10.1016/S1286-4579(03)00124-2] [PMID: 12814772]

[65] Amedei A, Bergman MP, Appelmelk BJ, *et al.* Molecular mimicry between *Helicobacter pylori* antigens and H+, K+ --adenosine triphosphatase in human gastric autoimmunity. J Exp Med 2003; 198(8): 1147-56.
[http://dx.doi.org/10.1084/jem.20030530] [PMID: 14568977]

[66] Codolo G, Mazzi P, Amedei A, *et al.* The neutrophil-activating protein of *Helicobacter pylori* down-modulates Th2 inflammation in ovalbumin-induced allergic asthma. Cell Microbiol 2008; 10(11): 2355-63.
[http://dx.doi.org/10.1111/j.1462-5822.2008.01217.x] [PMID: 18671823]

[67] Hussein NR, Abdullah SM, Salih AM, Assafi MA. dupA1 is associated with duodenal ulcer and high

interleukin-8 secretion from the gastric mucosa. Infect Immun 2012; 80(8): 2971-2. [http://dx.doi.org/10.1128/IAI.00076-12] [PMID: 22811495]

[68] Shiota S, Nguyen LT, Murakami K, *et al.* Association of *Helicobacter pylori* dupA with the failure of primary eradication. J Clin Gastroenterol 2012; 46(4): 297-301. [http://dx.doi.org/10.1097/MCG.0b013e318243201c] [PMID: 22298090]

[69] Takahashi A, Shiota S, Matsunari O, *et al.* Intact long-type dupA as a marker for gastroduodenal diseases in Okinawan subpopulation, Japan. Helicobacter 2013; 18(1): 66-72. [http://dx.doi.org/10.1111/j.1523-5378.2012.00994.x] [PMID: 23067336]

[70] Imagawa S, Ito M, Yoshihara M, Eguchi H, Tanaka S, Chayama K. *Helicobacter pylori* dupA and gastric acid secretion are negatively associated with gastric cancer development. J Med Microbiol 2010; 59(12): 1484-9. [http://dx.doi.org/10.1099/jmm.0.021816-0] [PMID: 20829397]

[71] Nguyen LT, Uchida T, Tsukamoto Y, *et al. Helicobacter pylori* dupA gene is not associated with clinical outcomes in the Japanese population. Clin Microbiol Infect 2010; 16(8): 1264-9. [http://dx.doi.org/10.1111/j.1469-0691.2009.03081.x] [PMID: 19832706]

[72] Queiroz DMM, Rocha GA, Rocha AMC, *et al.* dupA polymorphisms and risk of *Helicobacter pylori*-associated diseases. Int J Med Microbiol 2011; 301(3): 225-8. [http://dx.doi.org/10.1016/j.ijmm.2010.08.019] [PMID: 21050811]

[73] Yamaoka Y, Kwon DH, Graham DY. A M_r 34,000 pro-inflammatory outer membrane protein (*oipA*) of *Helicobacter pylori*. Proc Natl Acad Sci 2000; 97(13): 7533-8. [http://dx.doi.org/10.1073/pnas.130079797] [PMID: 10852959]

[74] Yamaoka Y. Mechanisms of disease: *Helicobacter pylori* virulence factors. Nat Rev Gastroenterol Hepatol 2010; 7(11): 629-41. [http://dx.doi.org/10.1038/nrgastro.2010.154] [PMID: 20938460]

[75] Leung WK, Siu KLK, Kwok CKL, Chan SY, Sung R, Sung JJY. Isolation of *Helicobacter pylori* from vomitus in children and its implication in gastro-oral transmission. Am J Gastroenterol 1999; 94(10): 2881-4. [http://dx.doi.org/10.1111/j.1572-0241.1999.01431.x] [PMID: 10520837]

[76] Allaker RP, Young KA, Hardie JM, Domizio P, Meadows NJ. Prevalence of *Helicobacter pylori* at oral and gastrointestinal sites in children: evidence for possible oral-to-oral transmission. J Med Microbiol 2002; 51(4): 312-7. [http://dx.doi.org/10.1099/0022-1317-51-4-312] [PMID: 11926736]

[77] Kabir S. Detection of *Helicobacter pylori* DNA in feces and saliva by polymerase chain reaction: a review. Helicobacter 2004; 9(2): 115-23. [http://dx.doi.org/10.1111/j.1083-4389.2004.00207.x] [PMID: 15068412]

[78] Poms RE, Tatini SR. Survival of *Helicobacter pylori* in ready-to-eat foods at 4°C. Int J Food Microbiol 2001; 63(3): 281-6. [http://dx.doi.org/10.1016/S0168-1605(00)00441-4] [PMID: 11246912]

[79] Hooi JKY, Lai WY, Ng WK, *et al.* Global prevalence of *Helicobacter pylori* infection: Systematic review and meta-analysis. Gastroenterology 2017; 153(2): 420-9. [http://dx.doi.org/10.1053/j.gastro.2017.04.022] [PMID: 28456631]

[80] Ramsey EJ, Carey KV, Peterson WL, *et al.* Epidemic gastritis with hypochlorhydria. Gastroenterology 1979; 76(6): 1449-57. [http://dx.doi.org/10.1016/0016-5085(79)90415-3] [PMID: 437444]

[81] Nomura A, Stemmermann GN, Chyou PH, Perez-Perez GI, Blaser MJ. *Helicobacter pylori* infection and the risk for duodenal and gastric ulceration. Ann Intern Med 1994; 120(12): 977-81. [http://dx.doi.org/10.7326/0003-4819-120-12-199406150-00001] [PMID: 7741826]

[82] Huang JQ, Sridhar S, Hunt RH. Role of *Helicobacter pylori* infection and non-steroidal anti-

inflammatory drugs in peptic-ulcer disease: A meta-analysis. Lancet 2002; 359(9300): 14-22. [http://dx.doi.org/10.1016/S0140-6736(02)07273-2] [PMID: 11809181]

[83] Rauws EAJ, Tytgat GNJ. Cure of duodenal ulcer associated with eradication of *Helicobacter pylori*. Lancet 1990; 335(8700): 1233-5. [http://dx.doi.org/10.1016/0140-6736(90)91301-P] [PMID: 1971318]

[84] Ford AC, Delaney BC, Forman D, Moayyedi P. Eradication therapy for peptic ulcer disease in *Helicobacter pylori*-positive people. Cochrane Database Syst Rev 2006; 4(4): CD003840. [http://dx.doi.org/10.1002/14651858.CD003840.pub4]

[85] Lindholm C, Quiding-Järbrink M, Lönroth H, Hamlet A, Svennerholm AM. Local cytokine response in *Helicobacter pylori*-infected subjects. Infect Immun 1998; 66(12): 5964-71. [http://dx.doi.org/10.1128/IAI.66.12.5964-5971.1998] [PMID: 9826379]

[86] Chan FKL, To KF, Ng YP, *et al.* Expression and cellular localization of COX-1 and -2 in *Helicobacter pylori* gastritis. Aliment Pharmacol Ther 2001; 15(2): 187-93. [http://dx.doi.org/10.1046/j.1365-2036.2001.00918.x] [PMID: 11148436]

[87] Slpponen P, Kekki M, Haapakoski J, Ihamäki T, Siurala M. Gastric cancer risk in chronic atrophic gastritis: Statistical calculations of cross-sectional data. Int J Cancer 1985; 35(2): 173-7. [http://dx.doi.org/10.1002/ijc.2910350206] [PMID: 3871738]

[88] Kusters JG, van Vliet AHM, Kuipers EJ. Pathogenesis of *Helicobacter pylori* infection. Clin Microbiol Rev 2006; 19(3): 449-90. [http://dx.doi.org/10.1128/CMR.00054-05] [PMID: 16847081]

[89] Plummer M, Franceschi S, Vignat J, Forman D, de Martel C. Global burden of gastric cancer attributable to *Helicobacter pylori*. Int J Cancer 2015; 136(2): 487-90. [http://dx.doi.org/10.1002/ijc.28999] [PMID: 24889903]

[90] Watanabe T, Tada M, Nagai H, Sasaki S, Nakao M. *Helicobacter pylori* infection induces gastric cancer in Mongolian gerbils. Gastroenterology 1998; 115(3): 642-8. [http://dx.doi.org/10.1016/S0016-5085(98)70143-X] [PMID: 9721161]

[91] Cover TL, Blanke SR. *Helicobacter pylori* VacA, a paradigm for toxin multifunctionality. Nat Rev Microbiol 2005; 3(4): 320-32. [http://dx.doi.org/10.1038/nrmicro1095] [PMID: 15759043]

[92] Eidt S, Stolte M, Fischer R. *Helicobacter pylori* gastritis and primary gastric non-Hodgkin's lymphomas. J Clin Pathol 1994; 47(5): 436-9. [http://dx.doi.org/10.1136/jcp.47.5.436] [PMID: 8027397]

[93] Blaser MJ. Science, medicine, and the future: *Helicobacter pylori* and gastric diseases. BMJ 1998; 316(7143): 1507-10. [http://dx.doi.org/10.1136/bmj.316.7143.1507] [PMID: 9582144]

[94] Sjöstedt S, Heimdahl A, Kager L, Nord CE. Microbial colonization of the oropharynx, esophagus and stomach in patients with gastric diseases. Eur J Clin Microbiol 1985; 4(1): 49-51. [http://dx.doi.org/10.1007/BF02148660] [PMID: 3987678]

[95] Kononova S, Litvinova E, Vakhitov T, Skalinskaya M, Sitkin S. Acceptive immunity: The role of fucosylated glycans in human host-microbiome interactions. Int J Mol Sci 2021; 22(8): 3854. [http://dx.doi.org/10.3390/ijms22083854]

[96] Bravo D, Hoare A, Soto C, Valenzuela MA, Quest AFG. *Helicobacter pylori* in human health and disease: Mechanisms for local gastric and systemic effects. World J Gastroenterol 2018; 24(28): 3071-89. [http://dx.doi.org/10.3748/wjg.v24.i28.3071] [PMID: 30065554]

[97] Reshetnyak VI, Burmistrov AI, Maev IV. *Helicobacter pylori* : Commensal, symbiont or pathogen? World J Gastroenterol 2021; 27(7): 545-60. [http://dx.doi.org/10.3748/wjg.v27.i7.545] [PMID: 33642828]

[98] Mirbagheri SA, Hasibi M, Abouzari M, Rashidi A. Triple, standard quadruple and ampicillin-sulbactam-based quadruple therapies for *H pylori* eradication: A comparative three-armed randomized clinical trial. World J Gastroenterol 2006; 12(30): 4888-91. [http://dx.doi.org/10.3748/wjg.v12.i30.4888] [PMID: 16937475]

[99] Malfertheiner P, Megraud F, O'Morain C, *et al.* Current concepts in the management of *Helicobacter pylori* infection: the Maastricht III Consensus Report. Gut 2007; 56(6): 772-81. [http://dx.doi.org/10.1136/gut.2006.101634] [PMID: 17170018]

[100] Lu C, Sang J, He H, *et al.* Probiotic supplementation does not improve eradication rate of *Helicobacter pylori* infection compared to placebo based on standard therapy: A meta-analysis. Sci Rep 2016; 6: 23522. [http://dx.doi.org/10.1038/srep23522]

[101] Ruggiero P. Use of probiotics in the fight against *Helicobacter pylori*. World J Gastrointest Pathophysiol 2014; 5(4): 384-91. [http://dx.doi.org/10.4291/wjgp.v5.i4.384] [PMID: 25400981]

[102] Chung JW, Lee GH, Han JH, *et al.* The trends of one-week first-line and second-line eradication therapy for *Helicobacter pylori* infection in Korea. Hepatogastroenterology 2011; 58(105): 246-50. [PMID: 21510323]

[103] Yoon JH, Baik GH, Sohn KM, *et al.* Trends in the eradication rates of *Helicobacter pylori* infection for eleven years. World J Gastroenterol 2012; 18(45): 6628-34. [http://dx.doi.org/10.3748/wjg.v18.i45.6628] [PMID: 23236238]

[104] Miller AK, Williams SM. *Helicobacter pylori* infection causes both protective and deleterious effects in human health and disease. Genes Immun 2021; 22(4): 218-26. [http://dx.doi.org/10.1038/s41435-021-00146-4] [PMID: 34244666]

[105] Butorova LI, Ardatskaya MD, Osadchuk MA, *et al.* [Comparison of clinical-metabolic efficacy of pre- and probiotics in the conducted optimized protocols of eradication therapy of *Helicobacter pylori* infection]. Ter Arkh 2020; 92(4): 64-9. [http://dx.doi.org/10.26442/00403660.2020.04.000647]

CHAPTER 7

Prevalence of Triple Negative Breast Cancer and its Therapeutic Challenges

Mir Shahid Maqbool[1], **Loveleena Kour Anand**[1] and **Fayaz Malik**[1,*]

[1] *Indian Institute of Integrative Medicine, Sanat Nagar, JK 190005, India*

Abstract: Breast cancer (BC) is the most common among females. The current status of BC worldwide shows that more than 1 million women are affected and ~400 000 die every year. Partial success has been achieved by mammography coupled with adjuvant treatment. However, its incidence and mortality both are increasing. Several sub-categories of BC have been reported; of which, one is triple-negative breast cancer (TNBC). This is defined by a lack of expression of oestrogen and progesterone receptors and human epidermal growth factor receptor 2 (HER-2). Several approaches have been used for speedy and accurate diagnosis and precise treatment of BC. In this context, precision medicine approach is of great relevance in ameliorating the suffering of the patient's from the menace of BC. The present chapter aims to provide background information, different types of BC and its sub-types and molecular mechanisms for therapeutic intervention required for precision medicine.

Keywords: Breast cancer, Human epidermal growth factor receoptor-2 (HER-2), Triple-negative breast cancer, Therapeutic intervention.

INTRODUCTION

Abnormal cell growth and multiplication are referred to as cancer. Normal cells divide and multiply in a regular manner but cancer cells do not follow the regular process instead they ignore signalling and molecular events which control the abnormal growth. After heart-related issues, cancer ranks as the second most common cause of death worldwide (WHO report). Globally, 20 million incidences of cancer were reported in 2020 resulting in 1 million deaths. Thus, one in every six fatalities was caused due to the cancer [Globocan report 2020]. Despite recent major advances in the field of cancer biology, metastasis continues to pose a challenge because it is the leading cause of mortality for both the sexes globally.

* **Corresponding author Fayaz Malik:** Indian Institute of Integrative Medicine, Sanat Nagar, JK 190005, India
Tel: 9419187187; E-mail: fmalik@iiim.ac.in

Farzana Mahdi & Abbas Ali Mahdi (Eds.)

In metastasis, cancer cells leave the primary tumour site and invade other parts of the body proliferating to develop secondary tumours. Metastasis accounts for about 90 percent of cancer-related mortality [1]. With time, these metastatic cells experience many molecular modifications that alter the characteristics of such cancerous cells [1]. There are currently ten known features of cancer that tumour cells use to continue their unchecked multiplication and progress while evading increasing inhibition signals [2].

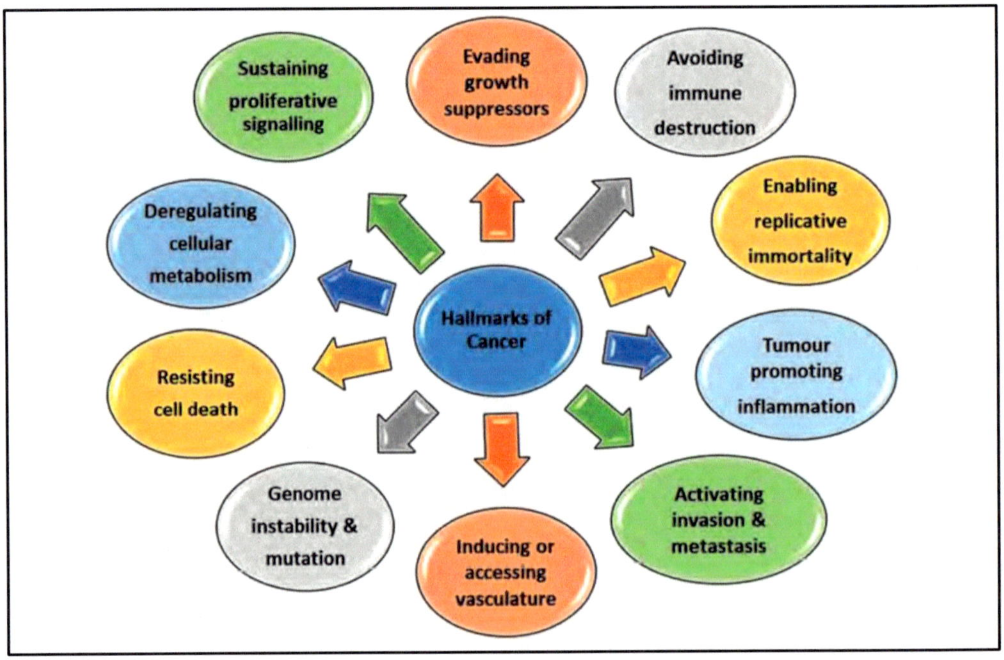

Fig. (1). Hallmarks of the cancer include several aspects in a well-orchestrated manner.

BREAST CANCER (BC)

The most aggressive form of tumour across the globe in females is breast cancer. About 2.6% women that is 1 in every 38 will develop breast cancer in their lifespan. In America, 12% women that are 1 in 8 may develop aggressive breast cancer. BC is an aggressive tumour that can originate from cells in the breast lobule or glandular milk duct. The degree to which a tumour has started to grow within the luminal surface determines if it is aggressive or non-aggressive. Lobular carcinomas are those breast cancers that originate from the lobules of mammary gland whereas ductal carcinomas originate from epithelial cell of the duct of the breasts. Tumorous cells in non-metastatic (non-invasive) breast cancer are confined to the milk ducts or lobules, whereas in metastatic breast cancer (invasive), the altered cells spread to the surrounding tissues and metastasis to the liver, lungs, brain, and bones [3]. Breast cancer is a complex disease consisting of many functionally diverse components with specific medical and therapeutic ramifications [4]. According to studies, breast cancer with different anatomical and biological features exhibit distinct characteristics that lead to different clinical results and thus warrant to be treated with a wide range of therapies [5]. With the aim of maximising clinical results, it is crucial to classify breast carcinoma into therapeutically relevant groups. Using cancer immune-histochemical and gene expression analyses, the following subgroups of BC have been classified [6].

INCIDENCE AND MORTALITY

World-wide Status of Breast Cancer

BC continues to be one of the main causes of death in women, accounting for an estimated 2.3 million new cases diagnosed and 684996 mortalities reported globally in 2020. In terms of global death, BC is the sixth worldwide cause and the second among women in developed nations. GLOBOCAN 2020 database shows all types of cancers, with the incidence of BC in females being the highest that is 47.8/100000 with the highest mortality rate of 13.6/100000. In 2020, France had the highest incidence (99.1/100000 females) and mortality rate (15.6/100000) followed by New Zealand with 93/100000 incidence and 14.1/100000 mortality (Globocan 2020).

National Status of Breast Cancer

BC has the highest incidence and fatality rates among all the females in India. The expected rate of new incidences in India is 3465951 out of 14388382 cases. This represents 24.1% of all female cancer cases, and the expected number of fatalities is 11214132 out of 7302147 cases, representing 15.4% of all cancer-related deaths (Globocan-2020). Hyderabad has India's highest incidence of breast cancer (48.0 per 100000 women), Chennai (42.2), followed by Bangalore (40.5) and Delhi (38.6) according to the National Cancer Registry Programme (NCRP). During the last 5 years, BC mortality all over the world has reached the highest among all the other cancer types. Thus, BC is the world's most common cancer as 7.8 million females are diagnosed with this type of malignancy. More than 90% of the developed countries have better survival rates of BC (at least five years) after diagnosis compared to India and South Africa having survival rates of 66% and 40%, respectively (Globocan-2020). In developed nations with advanced diagnostics, early assessment and treatment have proven more successful than in poor countries. Age-standardized mortality rates for BC reduced by 40% in high-income countries between the 1980s and 2020. In women under the age of 70, a 2.5% annual mortality reduction would result in a reduction of 25% by 2030 and 40% by 2040, preventing roughly 2.5 million BC-related deaths between 2020 and 2040 (WHO report, 2021). Environmental, dietary, cultural, hereditary, and chronological background variables all contribute to varying number of BC cases and mortality. Moreover, there are more factors listed by Globocan-2012 and the WHO. These factors are involved in the progress and development of BC (WHO report 2021).

SUBTYPES OF BC

Luminal – A

It is a common subgroup, accounting for about 30 and 70% of all subgroups of BC and is distinguished by ER or PR positive expression and reduced expression of KI67 and other genes linked to cell proliferation. This subtype has a better prognosis, limited mitotic activity, and unique histological characteristics compared to other subtypes of BC [7, 8]. Patients with these types of tumours undergo hormonal therapy-based regimens, which show lower recurrence and better survival rates. The chance of metastases in the lung, liver, and neurological system is lower than 10% if there is a recurrence of this subgroup of BC [9].

Luminal-B

This subtype of BC, according to immunohistochemical analysis, is estrogen receptor and HER-2 positive with high level of expression of Ki67 [7]. This subtype has a more aggressive phenotype with a worse prognosis, a stronger histological grade, and a higher proliferative index. Ki67 index levels clinically describes the faster growth of tumor cells which differentiates it from the Luminal A subtype [7, 8]. This subtype has worse post-relapse survival rates and a higher recurrence rate than the luminal-A subtype. The overall life expectancy for luminal-B breast malignancies if untreated would be equivalent to other sub groups such as basal-like and HER2-positive malignancies and both are regarded as high-risk ones. For patients with Luminal B, hormone-therapy is less effective. On the other hand, neo-adjuvant chemotherapy has a better effect on luminal-B malignancy than it does on luminal-A subtype [9].

HER 2 Enrichment

This subtype makes up 15% to 20% of all subgroups of BC. This cancer subgroup is related to a higher degree of aggression in both biological and therapeutic behaviour. These tumors express the HER2 protein related to its regulation. These subgroups of malignancy have a p53 gene mutation. This results in poor prognosis, high proliferation, and high histological grade [8, 9]. These subgroups are more susceptible to some cytotoxic agents like doxorubicin, less responsive to hormone therapy, and often likely to spread to the brain and visceral organs.

Humanised monoclonal antibody, Trastuzumab is the primary choice given to these individuals. However, Trastuzumab as a single agent is not so effective but is given in combination with different chemotherapies and shows more desired results [11].

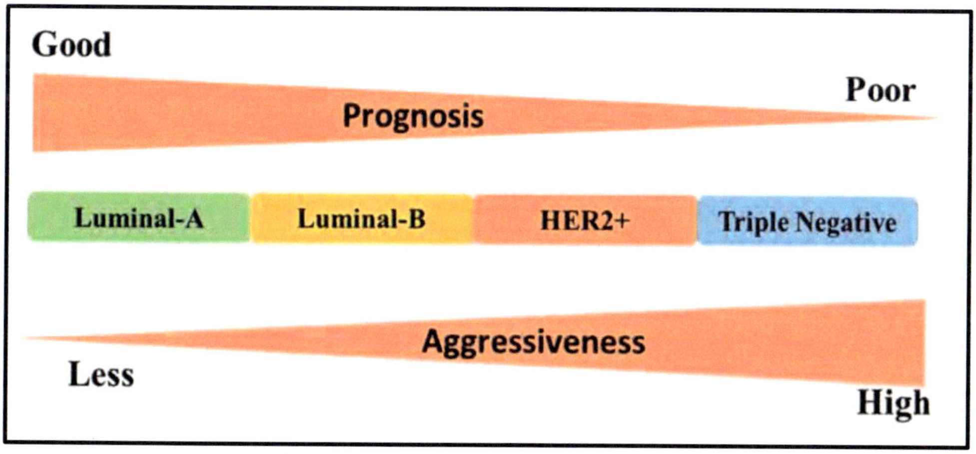

Fig. (2). Breast cancer showing subgroups with trends in prognosis and aggressiveness.

Triple Negative Breast Cancer (TNBC)

TNBC accounts for about 10 to 15% of all breast tumours. This sub-group lacks the expression of PR, ER and HER2 receptors as mentioned earlier compared to other subgroups of BC. TNBC is the highly aggressive metastatic subgroup [12 - 14]. At the time of assessment, TNBC tumours have greater mean tumour sizes, tumour grades, and proliferation indices [15, 16]. Even after optimizing for tumour phase, age, histological grade, race, and receipt of adjuvant treatment, TNBC offers the worst prognostic value than other subgroups with 78.5% of 5-year overall survival (OS) incidence [14, 16 - 18]. One in three patients suffering from TNBC will encounter a tumour relapse depending on how well they responded to the first therapy cycle. This is likely to happen within the initial three years of the first assessment. One in five individuals suffering from TNBC will typically die naturally in less than five years as a result of their aggressive metastatic nature [19, 20]. The five-year life expectancies for confined TNBC are 91%, 65% for regional TNBC and 11% for metastatic one. Given the dismal outlook of high-risk, rapidly progressing, invasive, and aggressive, a higher rate of survival in this subgroup is thought to be significant. Another reason for poor outcome for the TNBC subtype is the absence of a specific target and potent regimens, that are frequently used to address the ER, PR, and HER2-positive subgroups of breast malignancy [18, 19, 21, 22]. As the TNBC lacks the expression of HER2, PR, and ER proteins, hormonal therapies such as specific "oestrogen receptor modulators" (SERMs), aromatase blockers, or HER2-based humanised monoclonal antibodies like Trastuzumab are inefficient [17]. Therefore, the mainstay of standard therapies for TNBC continues to be standard cytotoxic chemotherapy [22, 12].

VARIATION IN DIAGNOSTIC AND THERAPEUTIC INTERVENTIONS IN TNBC

Even though there is a significant relationship between pathologic responses, "pathologic complete response" (pCR), "pathologic incomplete response" (pIR), residual cancer burden (RCB) and diagnostic results, the prognosis of individuals suffering from TNBC with pIR tumours can vary substantially. Differentiating between pIR patients who will have a disease-free state and those who will experience a relapse after receiving SOC chemotherapy is an unmet need. Multiple TNBC individuals with the same clinico-pathological characteristics may vary substantially in their responses to conventional chemotherapeutics [26, 28, 29]. As a result, clinical oncology still has challenges with precisely diagnosing and forecasting what number will experience a relapse and which ones will maintain their remission after NACT. Individual pIR patient's tumour recurrence and metastatic potential cannot be accurately predicted using current imaging techniques or RCB classifications. Identifying and classifying RCB tumours with high risk after NACT is crucial but still troubling. This is because it is difficult to distinguish between those tumor clones that are resistant to chemotherapies especially those at outlying locations growing continuously compared to remaining resistant tumours that have ceased growth after NACT [29]. Contemporary, accurate, and highly efficient diagnostic biochemical markers are therefore needed to categorise and identify high and low-risk residues of TNBC malignancies post-NACT.

New diagnostic and prognostic biological markers are required to help clinicians choose and steer second-line regimens with the goal of curing chemo-resistant TNBC malignancies [29 - 31]. These markers ought to provide measurable and relevant real feedback about these malignancies. Such biomarkers could potentially serve as new diagnostic targets for future complementary remedies [31]. If complete eradication of resistant malignant clones was not achieved by initial and second line regimens, they are subjected to chemo-therapies, radio-therapies and directed therapies given to these patients to achieve complete eradication [29, 32]. Most pIR individuals with remaining malignancies undergo quality, targeted, and effective therapeutic interventions at combat sites to control and clear resistant metastatic malignancies, regardless of the RCB classification post-NACT. Patients given neo-adjuvant or adjuvant chemotherapy have equal survival benefits when receiving concurrent or sequential chemotherapies for high-risk TNBC [33]. Patients suffering from TNBC receiving adjuvant treatment may have enhanced anxiety since it is unclear whether recommended post-operative medication has entirely eliminated all the undetectable dispersed tumour cells or not. The prevailing consensus is that TNBC relapse, either confined or widespread, might never be treatable despite all the current therapeutic protocols and approaches. Conversely, NACT provides different clinical and pathological benefits by evaluating the cancer responses of each single individual suffering from TNBC malignancy in a matched way prior to and following NACT. Additionally, based on their first response to conventional chemotherapy, adjuvant-treated TNBC patients are denied the chance to receive further proof-based therapies proven to enhance the possibility of survival. It would be helpful to those individuals suffering from TNBC to measure the efficacy of chemotherapies, forecast initial recurrence, and predict possible survivability of the patient using such platform which is qualitative, interactive, comparative, and precision-driven. Early detection and detailed examination of the residual and disseminated tumour cells resistant to chemotherapies that cause early tumour recurrence and local metastases post-NACT have a clear advantage. NACT presents positive information based on scientific observation and quantified platform of genuine TNBC tumour reactions. This is a necessary step toward precise genetic and biological prediction of tumour recurrence, prognosis, and possible survival in the clinic [26, 34, 35].

Based on changing tumour reactions and substantial tumour susceptibility shown immediately, it offers opportunities to create novel exploitable goals and innovative therapeutics. These can be implemented in order to diminish resistant and aggressive surviving cancer cells post-NACT. During the past 30 years, there has been little improvement in the life expectancy for patients with drug resistance, and recurrent, and aggressive TNBC [36]. Advanced TNBC tumours have significant heterogeneity, which results in multi-drug resistant, recurrent, and aggressive conditions. Multi-drug resistance of TNBC has limited the capacity to produce more potent drugs to serve individuals suffering from advanced and progressive illness [26, 37 - 39]. In the end, it is important to identify the main vulnerabilities in TNBC, focusing entirely on the preserved and important signalling mechanisms that drive TNBC to multi drug resistant and create revolutionary, novel strategies to address and cure chemo-resistant, recurred, final stage TNBC [24, 40, 41].

CURRENT THERAPEUTIC APPROACHES FOR TNBC

TNBC patients' clinical management can be difficult because these tumours are a molecularly heterogeneous group and could respond to treatment very differently. Although the optimum regimens and order of treatment for metastatic cancer are still unknown, chemotherapy still plays a significant role in treatment. Because these patients have a higher risk of recurrence, the existence of residual illness after neo-adjuvant chemotherapy is a poor prognostic indication. Additionally, optimising treatment in this situation is still a big unmet need as mentioned earlier [23]. There are several factors to consider while choosing the desirable treatment and drug combinations for curing low risk and initial-stage TNBC. Without a doubt inadequate therapies can result in an early recurrence and a poor outcome, while excess therapies can cause chemo-toxicity. For high-risk and advanced metastatic TNBC, intensive interventions with a wide range of chemotherapeutic regimens and therapeutic variations are required. Since chemotherapy with cytotoxicity is the only option available for treating this subset of breast cancer to minimise and avoid tumour recurrence and local metastasis. Patients suffering from TNBC have high-risk and aggressive malignancies that are typically required to undergo standard chemotherapies [19, 20, 23, 24]. Several initiatives to increase therapeutic choices have been made in the last few years as a result of the absence of specific therapies for TNBC. Recent research has focused on the treatment of drugs which are the inhibitors of PARP, immune check points like PD-1 and PD-L1 antibodies. Current studies focus on the development of criteria that could help them identify some novel therapies for patients suffering from invasive and metastatic TNBC. Similarly, novel targetable pathways and drugs are also being investigated. Chemotherapy that is ineffective or toxic adds to the treatment burden and usually has worse side effects and it prolongs adverse health effects that decrease the patient's standard of life [23]. About 35-45% of TNBC patients responded favourably to conventional neo-adjuvant chemotherapy in 2020 [11]. Additionally, most of the patients who responded to conventional treatments could only be found at the non-metastatic stage. Nonetheless, the conventional treatments did not appreciably affect the total survival rate. Thus, emphasis is given to genetic evaluation of therapy resistance [23, 25]. It may be noted that more than 90% of the people who survived this kind of malignancy had changed signalling pathways. This could be addressed by the development of focused strategies.

Five important pathways or functional changes were found in this molecular profiling study. This includes a change in the "cell cycle", "PI3K/AKT/mTOR", "phosphatase and tensin-homolog" (PTEN), "growth factor receptor overexpression", "RAS/mitogen-activated protein kinase" (MAPK), and "DNA repair".

The clinical alternatives for targeted intervention owing to this molecular profiling include DNA damage response; inhibition of angiogenesis and "MAPK" and "PI3K" pathway down regulation [23, 26]. Based on the molecular analysis, Table **1** highlights the details of "phase II to IV" clinical trials.

Table 1. Different sub-groups of BC, their biomarkers and prevalence in terms of percentages.

Subgroup	Biomarkers	Percentage
Luminal A	ER^{+},PR^{+},$HER2^{-}$ KI67 low	30-70%
Luminal B	ER^{+},$PR^{+/-}$,$HER2^{+/-}$ KI67 High	10-20%
HER-2 enriched	ER^{-},PR^{-},$HER2^{+}$ KI67 low	15-20%

Systemic chemotherapy is the main recommended course of medication for TNBC patients with a tumour size more than 1 cm, regardless of the presence of lymph node (LN) metastases. TNBC patients usually get anthracyclines, alkylators, and taxanes in addition to conventional chemotherapy regimens [23, 27]. Furthermore, it has been discovered that taxane and anthracycline therapy enhance the diagnosis of patients suffering from TNBC. Chemotherapy could be given as a neo-adjuvant and/or adjuvant treatment as there is not much difference in the life expectancy of the two groups between the patients who have high risk and initial stage TNBC treated with adjuvant and neo-adjuvant regimens [26, 25]. At this point, aesthetic surgeons and genomic counsellors may be consulted before surgery is conducted to evaluate tumour behaviour, outcome, and the chance for recurrence [26].

FOCUSED THERAPY FOR TNBC RECENTLY GRANTED BY THE FDA

Therapies that Block Immune Check Points

Immune barrier blockers that address the "PD-1/PD-L1" proteins in permutation with conventional chemotherapies have shown some promise in the diagnosis of progressed and aggressive TNBC [26, 42 - 46]. In TNBC patients, PDL1 is mostly found on infiltrating immune cells while TILs, and T cells express PD-1. When PD-L1 binds to PD-1, it yields the antagonistic signals which lead to the suppression of T cells [47 - 49]. In TNBC, tumour cells and some immune cells that have invaded the tissue, mainly express PD-L1 [47, 50, 51]. A better prognosis, enhanced tumour immunity and the identification of prospective patients for immune check point blockade therapy are typically related to higher or tightly packed TIL or the development of "PD-L1/PD-1", which is primarily responsible for immune inhibitory functions [47, 52, 53]. Compared to non-TNBC tumors, PD-L1 is present in about 40% of tumor cells and related stromal and invading immune cells in the TME of TNBC [58]. Thus, PD-L1 has become a potential novel diagnostic strategy due to its high occurrence and high expression in aggressive and mTNBC [44, 45] cases.

In the "phase 3 IMpassion130 trial (NCT02425891)", 902 mTNBC individuals were grouped into 451 patients for each therapy group. The study examined the advantages of combining atezolizumab, an anti-PD-L1 mAb with paclitaxel chemotherapeutic as a first-line strategy. Based on the outcome of the IMpassion130 study, FDA approved the licensing of atezolizumab (Tecentriq) for the diagnosis of PD-L1-positive recurring, progressed, and mTNBC. This protocol involves the use of Tecentriq in conjunction with nab-paclitaxel (Abraxane) [42, 43]. The "phase III KEYNOTE-522 trial (NCT03036488)" explored the introduction of pembrolizumab (Keytruda), an antagonist PD-1 MAb to NAC and on-going AC in 1174 unattended phase II or III TNBC patient populations. 784 individuals received pembrolizumab therapy, and 390 received a placebo chemotherapy. The rate of progression-free survival (pCR) was 64.8% (95% CI, 59.9-69.5) in the pembrolizumab therapy -cohort and 51.2% (95% CI, 44.1-58.3) in the placebo-cohort [54, 55]. Despite these developments, encouraging potency, and swift FDA approval of immuno-chemotherapy in combination with the treatment of relapsed, locally progressed, chronic, and mTNBC, the progress of atezolizumab/ pembrolizumab is even now marginal as measured by a five-year improvement in survival. To potentiate pair up, and accelerate PD-1 blockage in TNBC, chemotherapeutic, radiation, and specific therapy may all be administered.

Poly ADP-ribose Polymerase (PARP) Inhibitors

It is established that the loss-of-function in the tumour suppressor genes BRCA1/2 is associated with early breast cancer initiation, increased family transmission, random prevalence, tumour aggressiveness, and poor prognosis [56 - 59]. Inhibitors of PARP that have been recently developed using synthesized lethal testing were therapeutically investigated and quickly awarded FDA approval [60 - 64]. BRCA1/2-mutant breast tumours, which make up about 19.5% of TNBC, are currently being treated with anti-PARP targeted drugs. With the aid of other protein associates, such as PARP enzymes, normal BRCA1/2 proteins are able to fix identical double-stranded dsDNA. The most common PARP enzymes, PARP1 or PARP2, when inhibited, result in the formation of irreparable single and double-stranded DNA breaches as well as cytotoxic PARP-DNA complexes [60, 62, 64, 65]. TNBC tumours that have BRCA or related mutations to the DNA repair machinery are consequently sensitive to the PARP inhibitor intervention [25, 58, 66, 67].

In the phase 3 randomised OlympiAD trial (NCT02000622), patients with distant metastasis, germ-line BRCA-mutated, breast cancer who are HER2-negative and have undergone more than two lines of chemotherapeutic drugs or other treatments will be evaluated for the effectiveness of olaparib, a PARP1 inhibitor.

The trial findings demonstrated a notable advantage of olaparib monotherapy over conventional chemotherapy, with the ones receiving olaparib living 2.8 months longer and experiencing a 42% lesser probability of death or disease advancement in comparison to those getting capecitabine, eribulin, or vinorelbine as standard treatment [68 - 70]. With few side effects and low toxicity, olaparib was well-tolerated. However, there was no substantial difference in OS between olaparib and traditional therapies in this group. This group of invasive breast tumor lacks the HER2 receptor with the BRCA variant, including a subgroup with TNBC and an effective PFS was shown in this OlympiAD study [68 - 70]. The EMBRACA study evaluated the effectiveness of one more PARP antagonist talazopari on patients with aggressive breast malignancy who had undergone chemotherapy in the past and who had Germline BRCA1/2 mutations. Additionally, this trial discovered that talazoparib patients had a greater PFS contrasted to those who have undergone single-agent chemotherapy [24]. In the hope of enhancing the clinical output and standard of life of TNBC patients with Germline alterations in different genes like "BRCA1, BRCA2, PALB2, RAD51, p53, and CHEK2", PARP antagonists are generally well accepted drugs that can be combined with chemotherapy drugs to treat breast tumours.

Anti-Trop2 Antibody Drug Conjugate Therapy in TNBC

A glycoprotein called "Trophoblast Cell-Surface Antigen" (Trop-2) is overexpressed as a growth-promoting signal in various tumors [71]. "Anti-Trop-2 antibody sacituzumab govitecan-hziy" is coupled with a potent irinotecan substrate (SN-38) [72, 73]. This antibody therapeutic combo prevents double-strand DNA breaks, decreases DNA replication, and inhibits topoisomerase function and DNA binding in cancer cells [71, 72]. It also prevents the repair of broken DNA strands and induces cell death. Patients with severely medicated mTNBC have been studied for the outcomes of sacituzumab govitecan-hziy [73 - 76]. Contrary to standard chemotherapeutic (10-15% and 2-3 months), "sacituzumab govitecan-hziy" is well resisted and has a greater reaction rate and mean PFS (33.3% and 5.5 months) [75]. The aim of the study of 3 ASCENT phase (NCT02574455), which is a clinical investigation, was to confirm the efficacy and safety outcomes of sacituzumab govitecan that had been reported earlier in a stage 2 research of individuals with aggressive TNBC who had received intensive pre-treatment [75]. In the progressed mTNBC population, "sacituzumab govitecan" showed a good enhancement in PFS compared to the recommended treatment ("HR, 0.41; 95% CI, 0.32-0.52"). PFS for individuals with mTNBC who underwent "sacituzumab govitecan-hziy" was 5.6 months (95% CI, 4.3-6.3), in contrast to 1.7 months (95% CI, 1.5-2.6) for those who followed oncologist -recommended chemotherapies ($p<0.0001$) [75]. "Sacituzumab govitecan-hziy" (Trodelvy) earned FDA permission for severely treated and progressive mTNBC in April 2020 on such encouraging and intriguing outcomes [74, 75]. The first antibody-drug conjugate Trodelvy®, was authorized for individuals with recurrent or resistant mTNBC who had already experienced two chemotherapeutic failures.

Given their clinical efficacy, PD-L1/PD-1, PARP blockers, and anti-Trop-2 antibody drug conjugates have obtained FDA permission and are now accepted for curing specific subgroups of TNBC individuals with the above mentioned diagnostic purposes. A significant pre-treatment and progressive mTNBC group treated with trodelvy had significant clinical importance. In order to see whether they fit the criteria for one of the novel aimed therapies, mTNBC individuals are also being examined for PD-L1 expression in TILs Germline BRCA1/2 alterations. Given the promising outcomes of the "IMpassion130 and KEYNOTE-355" studies, Pembrolizumab and atezolizumab, PD-L1 inhibitors are being investigated for treatment in frontline circumstances to treat progressed, relapsing, and aggressive TNBC [42, 43, 24].

FUTURE THERAPEUTIC APPROACHES FOR TRIPLE NEGATIVE BREAST CANCER

TNBC's tumor-driving signalling pathways are being targeted by a variety of therapeutic approaches and repurposed medications. These include PI3K/AKT/mTOR blockers, androgen receptor (AR) antagonists, (EGFR/HER1) antibodies, and oestrogen receptor beta (ER) agonists [22, 76 - 78]. Standard of care (SOC) therapy does not include these medications since they are still undergoing clinical trials with modest or inconsistent results.

Targeting Epidermal Growth Factor Receptor (EGFR)

In 25-50% of TNBC individuals, EGFR stimulation or overexpression has been documented [78, 79]. Experimentally, EGFR-driven TNBC should respond well to anti-EGFR mAb like Cetuximab and EGFR small molecule antagonists. Unfortunately, Cetuximab has not been proven to be an effective treatment for TNBC in different clinical trials. For example, the TBCRC 001 study examined the outcomes of the "Cetuximab alone and Cetuximab plus carboplatin" regimen in stage IV TNBC patients whose tumours had spread and sustained despite receiving several chemotherapy treatments. Only 6% and 16% of patients were observed to respond to "Cetuximab alone or Cetuximab plus carboplatin" [22, 80]. After taking "Cetuximab alone or Cetuximab with carboplatin", only a small percentage of TNBC patients who underwent repeated biopsies revealed little EGFR pathway suppression. A robust signalling pathway activity downstream of the EGFR receptor is most likely the reason why Cetuximab was shown to be greatly ineffective in suppressing EGFR signalling in TNBC. By signalling heterogeneity, tumor network interplay, and remedial pathway stimulation, the activation of the EGFR signal was retained rather than diminished. This is because there are several interlinked critical cellular signalling networks that are closely controlled by effective EGFR signals [80]. Due to these disappointing results, Cetuximab is not presently used as a prescribed treatment for TNBC patients having EGFR amplification [24].

Table 2. On-going phase II–IV studies related to different molecular targets.

Target	Drugs	Design	Register ID	Phase	Status
Cell cycle	Trilaciclib	Trilaciclib with gemcitabine and carboplatin	NCT02978716	II	Active
		Trilaciclib	NCT04799249	III	Recruiting
	Etoposide	Etoposide plus anlotinib	NCT04452370	II	Recruiting
	PF-06873600	PF-06873600 plus endocrine therapy	NCT03519178	II	Recruiting
	Abemaciclib	Abemaciclib	NCT03979508	II	Recruiting
	Prexasertib	Prexasertib plus samotolisib	NCT04032080	II	Recruiting
		Prexasertib	NCT02203513	II	Active
Microtubule dynamics	Eribulin mesylate	Eribulin mesylate	NCT04502680	II	Not yet recruiting
		Eribulin mesylate, apatinib, and camrelizumab	NCT04303741	II	Recruiting

(Table 2) cont.....

Target	Drugs	Design	Register ID	Phase	Status
VEGF/VEGFR	Anlotinib	Anlotinib plus etoposide	NCT04452370	II	Recruiting
		Anlotinib and penpulimab plus chemotherapy	NCT04877821	II	Not yet recruiting
	Apatinib	Apatinib combined with paclitaxel and carboplatin	NCT03735082	II	Unknown
		Apatinib plus capecitabine versus capecitabine	NCT03775928	II	Recruiting
		Apatinib combined with paclitaxel	NCT03348098	II	Unknown
		Apatinib combined with albumin paclitaxel, and carboplatin	NCT03650738	II	Unknown
		Apatinib with camrelizumab, and eribulin mesylate	NCT04303741	II	Recruiting
		Vinorelbine with or without apatinib mesylate	NCT03932526	II	Not yet recruiting
	Afatinib	Afatinib with paclitaxel	NCT02511847	II	Unknown
	Lenvatinib	Lenvatinib plus pembrolizumab	NCT03797326	II	Recruiting
	Erlotinib	Erlotinib with neoadjuvant chemotherapy	NCT00491816	II	Unknown
	Famitinib	Famitinib with camrelizumab and nab-paclitaxel	NCT04395989	II	Recruiting
	Pyrotinib	Pyrotinib with capecitabine			
	Bevacizumab	Bevacizumab and nab-paclitaxel			
		Bevacizumab	NCT03577743	II	Completed
		Bevacizumab	NCT00528567	III	Completed
		Bevacizumab with taxane	NCT01094184	IV	Completed
		Bevacizumab, abraxane, and carboplatin	NCT00479674	II	Completed
		Bevacizumab with nab-paclitaxel followed by bevacizumab and erlotinib	NCT00733408	II	Completed
		Bevacizumab together with docetaxel, and carboplatin	NCT01208480	II	Completed
		Bevacizumab, pegylated liposomal doxorubicin, and everolimus	NCT02456857	II	Active, not recruiting
	Bintrafusp alfa	Bintrafusp alfa (M7824)	NCT04489940	II	Recruiting

(Table 2) cont.....

Target	Drugs	Design	Register ID	Phase	Status
EGFR	Dasatinib	Dasatinib	NCT02720185	II	Active
	Gefitinib	Gefitinib	NCT01732276	II	Unknown
	Sorafenib	Sorafenib and pemetrexed	NCT02624700	II	Terminated
	Nimotuzumab	Nimotuzumab plus docetaxel, and capecitabine	NCT01939054	II	Unknown
	Panitumumab	Panitumumab, carboplatin, and paclitaxel	NCT02593175	II	Recruiting
			NCT02876107	II	Recruiting
	SCT200	SCT200	NCT03692689	II	Unknown
PI3K/AKT/mTOR	Alpelisib	Alpelisib and nab-paclitaxel	NCT04216472	II	Recruiting
		Alpelisib with nab-paclitaxel	NCT04251533	III	Recruiting
	Buparlisib	Buparlisib plus capecitabine	NCT02000882	II	Completed
	Eganelisib	Eganelisib with front-line regimens	NCT03961698	II	Recruiting
	Sapanisertib	TAK-228 and TAK-117 followed by cisplatin and nab-paclitaxel	NCT03193853	II	Active, not recruiting
	Samotolisib	Samotolisib and prexasertib	NCT04032080	II	Recruiting
	Ipatasertib	Ipatasertib with nontaxane chemotherapy agents	NCT04464174	II	Recruiting
		Ipatasertib with paclitaxel versus placebo with paclitaxel	NCT03337724	III	Active
		Ipatasertib with atezolizumab, and paclitaxel	NCT04177108	III	Active
	Uprosertib	Uprosertib with trametinib	NCT01964924	II	Completed
	Capivasertib	Capivasertib plus paclitaxel or paclitaxel plus placebo	NCT02423603	II	Active, not recruiting
		Capivasertib with paclitaxel versus placebo with paclitaxel	NCT03997123	III	Recruiting
	Everolimus	Everolimus plus cisplatin	NCT01931163	II	Has results
		Everolimus plus carboplatin compared with carboplatin	NCT02531932	II	Recruiting
HDAC	Entinostat	Entinostat with atezolizumab	NCT02708680	II	Unknown
	Chidamide	Chidamide with Cisplatin	NCT04192903	II	Not yet recruiting
Endocrinotherapy	Estradiol	Estradiol	NCT03941730	II	Recruiting
			NCT01083641	II	Terminated
	Crizotinib	Fulvestrant and crizotinib	NCT03620643	II	Recruiting

(Table 2) cont.....

Target	Drugs	Design	Register ID	Phase	Status
	Goserelin	Additional goserelin to the neoadjuvant chemotherapy	NCT03444025	II	Not yet recruiting
	Mifepristone	Nab-paclitaxel with or without mifepristone	NCT02788981	II	Recruiting
	Neratinib	Paclitaxel and carboplatin plus neratinib	NCT03812393	II	Recruiting
	Anastrozole	Anastrozole and entinostat	NCT01234532	II	Terminated
		Anastrozole/toremifene	NCT02089854	IV	Unknown
Other targets					
γ-secretase	AL101	AL101	NCT04461600	II	Recruiting
	PF-03084014	PF-03084014	NCT02299635	II	Terminated
AXL kinase	Bemcentinib	Bemcentinib in combination with pembrolizumab	NCT03184558	II	Terminated
Hedgehog pathway	Vismodegib	Additional vismodegib to neoadjuvant chemotherapy	NCT02694224	II	Unknown

Table Adapted from: Li et al. Journal of Hematology & Oncology (2022) 15:121.

Targeting Vascular Endothelial Growth Factor (VEGF)

VEGF, a key angiogenesis factor in breast cancer promotes both the development of new blood vessels and the multiplication of cancer cells. No matter the tumour size, nodal state, or histopathology, greater VEGF expression is linked to poor prognosis in TNBC more regularly than in non-TNBC [81]. Bevacizumab, an anti-VEGF antibody, improved PFS but not OS in TNBC individual clinical tests. In the BEATRICE trial, TNBC individual's outcomes were evaluated between chemotherapy alone and adjuvant bevacizumab treatment [82]. Bevacizumab treatment did not significantly enhance three-year IDFS or OS relative to chemotherapeutic only (83.7% against 82.7%) [24]. One more study looked at the advantages of using bevacizumab in conjunction with therapy as the initial form of care for individuals with advanced breast tumor who were tested negative for the HER2 gene. Patients receiving bevacizumab with chemotherapy resulted in increased mean PFS relative to only chemotherapy (8.1 months against 5.4 months) and a slightly enhanced mean OS (18.9 months vs. 17.5 months). One more study in the neo-adjuvant establishment demonstrated that adding bevacizumab to chemotherapy boosted the pCR rate for TNBC. However, a different study revealed that the enhancement in pCR was attained with the inclusion of bevacizumab which was restricted to other groups of breast cancer except TNBC [83]. Nevertheless, no study discovered a significant increase in TNBC patients' five-year survivability, which is comparable with a number of other neoadjuvant trial [83 - 85]. Finally, given its less anticancer potential and negligible impact on patient survivability, bevacizumab is not recommended as the first choice drug to treat aggressive TNBC.

Targeting PI3K/AKT/mTOR Signalling Pathway

TNBC may benefit from targeting AKT and phosphoinositide-3 kinase (PI3K) signalling as a possible future therapeutic target. In primary TNBC, about 25% of patients have activating alterations in several signal transductions such as PIK3CA and AKT1 [85 - 87]. Additionally, TNBC patients in stage II–III with PIK3CA abnormalities had shown some encouraging results when treated with PI3K antagonists [85, 76, 88]. A phase II trial combining alpelisib and paclitaxel was carried out in TNBC, which are anthracycline-resistant with alterations in PTEN or PI3K as a result of alpelisib's success in extending PFS for HR-positive breast tumor patients [85, 89 - 91]. Individuals with stage II/III TNBC were shown to have advantages from the permutation of paclitaxel and cisplatin along the mTOR antagonist everolimus. Temisirolimus or everolimus have also been tested in the integration of bevacizumab with liposomal doxorubicin as this mesenchymal subgroup of TNBC is typically linked to aberrant PI3K/mTOR pathway activation. In patients with metaplastic TNBC whose TNBC malignancies displayed increased PI3K pathway activity, the addition of mTOR inhibitor significantly improved the patients' response rate (31% vs. 0%; $p = 0.04$) but did not increase the diagnostic response rate (44% vs. 45%; $p > 0.99$).

Individuals with high TNBC may benefit from using AKT inhibitors like capivasertib and ipatasertib, which have demonstrated good results in this regard [92, 76]. Untreated, locally advanced, or aggressive TNBC individuals with no prior treatment were enrolled in the study (NCT02162719), LOTUS a phase II randomised double-blinded study was conducted. To receive paclitaxel with ipatasertib or a placebo, individuals in the trial were randomly allocated (1:1). According to the research, individuals from metastatic TNBC who underwent ipatasertib had a longer average PFS compared to those who took a placebo (6.2 against 4.9 months; p, 0.037). One more subgroup of aggressive TNBC individuals with PI3K/ PTEN alterations, who have received ipatasertib, had an average PFS of 5.3 months as opposed to 3.7 months in the placebo cohort (p,0.36) [93]. The inclusion of capivasertib slightly increased mean OS and PFS compared to the paclitaxel alone "(5.9 against 4.2 months) (19.1 months vs. 12.6 months)". With a mean PFS of 9.3 months versus the mean PFS of 3.7 months, participants were treated with paclitaxel and placebo. The advantages of capivasertib were much more prominent than TNBC individuals with PTEN/PIK3CA variants ($n = 28$) 94.

Targeting Androgen Receptor (AR)

About 10-40% of individuals suffering from TNBC express steroid hormone androgen receptor (AR), which is present in the nucleus [88, 87, 95]. There are still questions and concerns about the relations between AR expression and outcome in TNBC individuals [96]. Certain populations in Nigeria and the United States have shown significant outcomes when androgen receptor expression is present in these patients suffering from malignancies. In contrast, patients in certain places, like Norway and India, have a worse prognosis when AR expression is present [97]. A couple of phase 2 clinical tests for patients having androgen receptor-positive prostate tumour were conducted as a feasible therapeutic target for androgen receptor positive TNBC [98]. Bicalutamide, an androgen receptor inhibitor had a six month diagnostic improvement rate of "19% (95% CI, 7-39%) and a mean PFS of 12 weeks (95% CI, 11-22 weeks)" in the initial phase 2 study of aggressive androgen receptor positive TNBC breast tumor individuals [98]. Another AR antagonist, prednisone, combined with abiraterone acetate was administered in a separate phase 2 single trial (UCBG 12-1) to cure androgen receptor positive TNBC individuals with treatable progressed or aggressive metastatic tumors [99]. It is unclear though as the clinical advantages of androgen receptor antagonists like abiraterone, enzalutamide and bicalutamide must be related to anti androgen receptor therapeutic approaches or to successful results for the androgen receptor positive TNBC subgroup, given the uncertainty regarding the relationship between the diagnosis and AR expression in the TNBC with AR-positive. The use of AR antagonists in the medication of androgen receptor-positive metastatic TNBC will therefore demand significant investigation to determine if the AR expression offers a useful diagnostic marker and a successful clinical target in metastatic TNBC [22, 100].

Targeting Oestrogen Receptor beta (ERβ)

Healthy breast tissue has an overexpression of the oestrogen receptor beta (ER) [101 - 103]. A variety of highly invasive and metastatic breast malignancies exhibit a quick decrease or disappearance of ER expression levels during breast tumorigenesis [102 - 106]. Sustained ER expression is a well-known tumour suppressor that is linked to a lesser invasive and less metastatic as well as prolonged patient survival [107]. About 30% of TNBCs still exhibit ER, however, 70% of TNBC patients do not show oestrogen receptors [108, 109]. In ER-positive TNBC cells, activation of the canonical TGF signal pathway, hinderance of cell growth, stoppage of the EMT and restriction of the tumorigenic aggression invasion can be achieved by activating the ER receptor with oestrogen (E2) or any other ER-selective inhibitor [110 - 114]. These results suggest that ER-augmentation treatment may result in significant pharmacological benefits in a subgroup of ER-positive TNBC cancer with a promising outcome [115, 116]. One drawback is that people with ER-negative TNBC who exhibit an invasive phenotype and a worse prognosis will not benefit from anti-ER therapies.

CONCLUSION

Chemo-resistant aggressive tumours with the worst prognosis and high recurrence are a serious clinical problem in TNBC cases. The norm of treatment for females with high-risk TNBC is NACT. Either of two fates for a session of NACT is probable: pCR or pIR plus prolonged illness. Overall, pCR individuals do well, whereas pIR individuals show significantly variable diagnostic results. Novel biomarkers are required to recognize TNBC individuals who show uncertainty to react to present therapeutics considering the poor outcomes for chemo-resistant TNBC. Therefore, distinct, efficient, therapeutic response and diagnostic biomarkers are needed in patients with remnant cancer in the actual period during or after NACT. This is important to recognise individuals who are at risk of cancer relapse and to create actionable potential therapeutic interventions to stop the spread of malignant, multi drug resistance, relapsed, and un-repairable metastatic TNBC. Further investigations are required to enhance the effectiveness of currently available therapies and combat drug resistance. Although certain clinical analyses have shown that permutation therapies are more effective than single prescribed drugs. However, more research is needed to determine the best pattern and schedule for permutation therapies. The genomic complexity of TNBC, the heterogeneity of the tumour microenvironment, and the lack of therapeutic interventions in resilient, relapsing, and aggressive conditions all lead to variations in therapeutic targets. Normal TNBC treatment is only available with a few cytotoxic chemotherapy agents due to the lack of ER, PR, and HER2-neu expression. The ultimate objective is to merge this into therapeutic research to identify chemo-resistant cancer populations, identify causes of poor treatment, anticipate cancer recurrence, and evaluate the prognosis and chances of survival of the patient.

ABBREVIATIONS

AR	Androgen receptor
BRCA1/2	Breast Cancer Gene 1/2
dsDNA	Double stranded deoxyribonucleic acid
EGFR	Epidermal growth factor
EMT	Epithelial to mesenchymal transition
ERβ	Oestrogen receptor beta

HER2	Human epidermal growth factor receptor 2
IDFS	Invasive disease free survival
LN	Lymph node
MAb	Monoclonal Antibody
MAPKL	Mitogen activated protein kinase
mTNBC	Metastatic triple negative
mTOR	Mammalian target of rapamycin
NACT	Neo adjuvant chemotherapy
NCRP	National cancer registry programme
OS	Overall survival
PARP	Poly (ADP-ribose) polymerase
pCR	Pathologic complete response
PD-1	Programmed cell death 1
PD-L1	Programmed cell death ligand 1
PFS	Progression free survival
PI3K	Phosphoinositide-3 kinase
pIR	Pathologic incomplete response
PR	Progesterone receptor
PTEN	Phosphatase and tensin homolog
RCB	Residual cancer burden
SERMs	Specific oestrogen receptor modulators
SOC	Standard of care
TGF	Transforming growth factor
TILs	Tumor infiltrating lymphocytes
TNBC	Triple negative breast cancer
Trop2	Trophoblast Cell-Surface Antigen

ACKNOWLEDGEMENTS

The authors are grateful to the IIIM for support and infrastructural facilities.

REFERENCES

[1] Steeg PS. Tumor metastasis: mechanistic insights and clinical challenges. Nat Med 2006; 12(8): 895-904.
[http://dx.doi.org/10.1038/nm1469] [PMID: 16892035]

[2] Revisiting the hallmarks of cancer - PubMed. Available from: https://pubmed.ncbi.nlm.nih.gov/28560055/ (Accessed on 2023 Feb 5).

[3] Feng Y, Spezia M, Huang S, *et al.* Breast cancer development and progression: Risk factors, cancer

stem cells, signaling pathways, genomics, and molecular pathogenesis. Genes Dis 2018; 5(2): 77-106. [http://dx.doi.org/10.1016/j.gendis.2018.05.001] [PMID: 30258937]

[4] Yersal O, Barutca S. Biological subtypes of breast cancer: Prognostic and therapeutic implications. World J Clin Oncol 2014; 5(3): 412-24. [http://dx.doi.org/10.5306/wjco.v5.i3.412] [PMID: 25114856]

[5] Histological types of breast cancer: how special are they? - PubMed. Available from: https://pubmed.ncbi.nlm.nih.gov/20452298/ (Accessed on 2023 Feb 5).

[6] Molecular Subtypes and Local-Regional Control of Breast Cancer - PubMed. Available from: https://pubmed.ncbi.nlm.nih.gov/29132568/ (Accessed on 2023 Feb 5).

[7] Pathology of hereditary breast cancer - PubMed. Available from: https://pubmed.ncbi.nlm.nih.gov/21336636/ (Accessed on 2023 Feb 5).

[8] Various types and management of breast cancer: an overview - PubMed. Available from: https://pubmed.ncbi.nlm.nih.gov/22247839/ (Accessed on 2023 Feb 5).

[9] Histological, molecular and functional subtypes of breast cancers - PubMed. Available from: https://pubmed.ncbi.nlm.nih.gov/21057215/ (Accessed on 2023 Feb 5).

[10] Malhotra GK, Zhao X, Band H, Band V. Histological, molecular and functional subtypes of breast cancers. Cancer Biol Ther 2010; 10(10): 955-60. [http://dx.doi.org/10.4161/cbt.10.10.13879] [PMID: 21057215]

[11] Chromogenic in situ hybridization: A novel approach to a practical and sensitive method for the detection of HER2 oncogene in archival human breast carcinoma - PubMed. Available from: https://pubmed.ncbi.nlm.nih.gov/12177239/ (Accessed on 2023 Feb 5).

[12] Ciriello G, Gatza ML, Beck AH, *et al.* Comprehensive molecular portraits of invasive lobular breast cancer. Cell 2015; 163(2): 506-19. [http://dx.doi.org/10.1016/j.cell.2015.09.033] [PMID: 26451490]

[13] Vici P, Pizzuti L, Natoli C, *et al.* Triple positive breast cancer: A distinct subtype? Cancer Treat Rev 2015; 41(2): 69-76. [http://dx.doi.org/10.1016/j.ctrv.2014.12.005] [PMID: 25554445]

[14] Risk factors for triple-negative breast cancer in women under the age of 45 years - PubMed. Available from: https://pubmed.ncbi.nlm.nih.gov/19336554/ (Accessed on 2023 Feb 5).

[15] Comprehensive molecular portraits of human breast tumours. Nature 2012; 490(7418): 61-70. [http://dx.doi.org/10.1038/nature11412] [PMID: 23000897]

[16] Triple negative breast cancer: the kiss of death - PubMed. Available from: https://pubmed.ncbi.nlm.nih.gov/28445140/(Accessed on 2023 Feb 5).

[17] Triple negative breast cancer: unmet medical needs - PubMed. Available from: https://pubmed.ncbi.nlm.nih.gov/21161370/(Accessed on 2023 Feb 5).

[18] Bianchini G, Balko JM, Mayer IA, Sanders ME, Gianni L. Triple-negative breast cancer: Challenges and opportunities of a heterogeneous disease. Nat Rev Clin Oncol 2016; 13(11): 674-90. [http://dx.doi.org/10.1038/nrclinonc.2016.66] [PMID: 27184417]

[19] Triple-negative breast cancer - PubMed. Available from: https://pubmed.ncbi.nlm.nih.gov/21067385/ (Accessed on 2023 Feb 5).

[20] Triple-negative breast cancer: challenges and opportunities of a heterogeneous disease - PubMed. Available from: https://pubmed.ncbi.nlm.nih.gov/27184417/ (Accessed on 2023 Feb 5).

[21] Triple-negative breast cancer: disease entity or title of convenience? - PubMed. Available from: https://pubmed.ncbi.nlm.nih.gov/20877296/Accessed on 2023 Feb 5).

[22] Vagia E, Mahalingam D, Cristofanilli M. The Landscape of Targeted Therapies in TNBC. Cancers (Basel) 2020; 12(4): 916.

[http://dx.doi.org/10.3390/cancers12040916] [PMID: 32276534]

[23] Advances in Therapeutic Approaches for Triple-Negative Breast Cancer - PubMed. Available from: https://pubmed.ncbi.nlm.nih.gov/33781662/ (Accessed on 2023 Feb 5).

[24] Perspectives on Triple-Negative Breast Cancer: Current Treatment Strategies, Unmet Needs, and Potential Targets for Future Therapies - PubMed Available from: https://pubmed.ncbi.nlm.nih.gov/32846967/ (Accessed on 2023 Feb 5).

[25] Neoadjuvant Treatment for Triple Negative Breast Cancer: Recent Progresses and Challenges - PubMed. Available from: https://pubmed.ncbi.nlm.nih.gov/32486021/ (Accessed on 2023 Feb 5).

[26] Garrido-Castro AC, Lin NU, Polyak K. Insights into molecular classifications of triple-negative breast cancer: Improving patient selection for treatment. Cancer Discov 2019; 9(2): 176-98. [http://dx.doi.org/10.1158/2159-8290.CD-18-1177] [PMID: 30679171]

[27] Blum JL, Flynn PJ, Yothers G, *et al.* Anthracyclines in Early Breast Cancer: The ABC Trials—USOR 06-090, NSABP B-46-I/USOR 07132, and NSABP B-49 (NRG Oncology). J Clin Oncol 2017; 35(23): 2647-55. [http://dx.doi.org/10.1200/JCO.2016.71.4147] [PMID: 28398846]

[28] Haddad TC, Goetz MP. Landscape of neoadjuvant therapy for breast cancer. Ann Surg Oncol 2015; 22(5): 1408-15. [http://dx.doi.org/10.1245/s10434-015-4405-7] [PMID: 25727557]

[29] Li Y, Zhang H, Merkher Y, *et al.* Recent advances in therapeutic strategies for triple-negative breast cancer. J Hematol Oncol 2022; 15(1): 121. [http://dx.doi.org/10.1186/s13045-022-01341-0] [PMID: 36038913]

[30] Association of circulating tumor dna and circulating tumor cells after neoadjuvant chemotherapy with disease recurrence in patients with triple-negative breast cancer preplanned secondary analysis of the bre12-158 randomized clinical trial - pubmed . Available from: https://pubmed.ncbi.nlm.nih.gov/32644110/ (Accessed on 2023 Feb 5).

[31] Madic J, Kiialainen A, Bidard FC, *et al.* Circulating tumor DNA and circulating tumor cells in metastatic triple negative breast cancer patients. Int J Cancer 2015; 136(9): 2158-65. [http://dx.doi.org/10.1002/ijc.29265] [PMID: 25307450]

[32] Prat A, Fan C, Fernández A, *et al.* Response and survival of breast cancer intrinsic subtypes following multi-agent neoadjuvant chemotherapy. BMC Med 2015; 13(1): 303. [http://dx.doi.org/10.1186/s12916-015-0540-z] [PMID: 26684470]

[33] Xia LY, Hu QL, Zhang J, Xu WY, Li XS. Survival outcomes of neoadjuvant versus adjuvant chemotherapy in triple-negative breast cancer: a meta-analysis of 36,480 cases. World J Surg Oncol 2020; 18(1): 129. [http://dx.doi.org/10.1186/s12957-020-01907-7] [PMID: 32539858]

[34] Current approaches and challenges in monitoring treatment responses in breast cancer - PubMed. Available from: https://pubmed.ncbi.nlm.nih.gov/24396498/ (Accessed on 2023 Feb 5).

[35] I-SPY 2--Toward more rapid progress in breast cancer treatment - PubMed Available from: https://pubmed.ncbi.nlm.nih.gov/27406352/ (Accessed on 2023 Feb 5).

[36] Survival in patients with metastatic recurrent breast cancer after adjuvant chemotherapy: little evidence of improvement over the past 30 years - PubMed. Available from: https://pubmed.ncbi.nlm.nih.gov/23065954/ (Accessed on 2023 Feb 5).

[37] Almendro V, Marusyk A, Polyak K. Cellular heterogeneity and molecular evolution in cancer. Annu Rev Pathol 2013; 8(1): 277-302. [http://dx.doi.org/10.1146/annurev-pathol-020712-163923] [PMID: 23092187]

[38] Yap TA, Gerlinger M, Futreal PA, Pusztai L, Swanton C. Intratumor heterogeneity: Seeing the wood for the trees. Sci Transl Med 2012; 4(127): 127ps10.

[http://dx.doi.org/10.1126/scitranslmed.3003854] [PMID: 22461637]

[39] Paoletti C, Li Y, Muñiz MC, *et al.* Significance of circulating tumor cells in metastatic triple-negative breast cancer patients within a randomized, phase II Trial: TBCRC 019. Clin Cancer Res 2015; 21(12): 2771-9.
[http://dx.doi.org/10.1158/1078-0432.CCR-14-2781] [PMID: 25779948]

[40] Progress in the treatment of breast cancer. reply - pubmed. Available from: https://pubmed.ncbi.nlm.nih.gov/31914254/(Accessed on 2023 Feb 5).

[41] Van Sciver R, Lee M, Lee C, *et al.* A New Strategy to Control and Eradicate "Undruggable" Oncogenic K-RAS-Driven Pancreatic Cancer: Molecular Insights and Core Principles Learned from Developmental and Evolutionary Biology. Cancers (Basel) 2018; 10(5): 142.
[http://dx.doi.org/10.3390/cancers10050142] [PMID: 29757973]

[42] Schmid P, Rugo HS, Adams S, *et al.* IMpassion130 Investigators. Atezolizumab plus nab-paclitaxel as first-line treatment for unresectable, locally advanced or metastatic triple-negative breast cancer (IMpassion130): updated efficacy results from a randomised, double-blind, placebo-controlled, phase 3 trial. Lancet Oncol 2020; 21(1): 44-59.
[http://dx.doi.org/10.1016/S1470-2045(19)30689-8] [PMID: 31786121]

[43] Adams S, Diéras V, Barrios CH, *et al.* Patient-reported outcomes from the phase III IMpassion130 trial of atezolizumab plus nab-paclitaxel in metastatic triple-negative breast cancer. Ann Oncol 2020; 31(5): 582-9.
[http://dx.doi.org/10.1016/j.annonc.2020.02.003] [PMID: 32178964]

[44] Building momentum for subsets of patients with advanced triple-negative breast cancer - PubMed. Available from: https://pubmed.ncbi.nlm.nih.gov/31786122/(Accessed on 2023 Feb 5).

[45] Killock D. Chemotherapy as a TONIC to invigorate PD-1 inhibition in TNBC. Nat Rev Clin Oncol 2019; 16(8): 464.
[http://dx.doi.org/10.1038/s41571-019-0232-2] [PMID: 31114036]

[46] Romero D. Benefit in patients with PD-L1-positive TNBC. Nat Rev Clin Oncol 2019; 16(1): 6.
[PMID: 30401935]

[47] Tomioka N, Azuma M, Ikarashi M, *et al.* The therapeutic candidate for immune check point inhibitors elucidated by the status of tumor-infiltrating lymphocytes (TILs) and programmed death ligand 1 (PD-L1) expression in triple negative breast cancer (TNBC). Breast Cancer 2018; 25(1): 34-42.
[http://dx.doi.org/10.1007/s12282-017-0781-0] [PMID: 28488168]

[48] Marra A, Viale G, Curigliano G. Recent advances in triple negative breast cancer: The immunotherapy era. BMC Med 2019; 17(1): 90.
[http://dx.doi.org/10.1186/s12916-019-1326-5] [PMID: 31068190]

[49] Karn T, Denkert C, Weber KE, *et al.* Tumor mutational burden and immune infiltration as independent predictors of response to neoadjuvant immune check point inhibition in early TNBC in GeparNuevo. Ann Oncol 2020; 31(9): 1216-22.
[http://dx.doi.org/10.1016/j.annonc.2020.05.015] [PMID: 32461104]

[50] Mittendorf EA, Philips AV, Meric-Bernstam F, *et al.* PD-L1 expression in triple-negative breast cancer. Cancer Immunol Res 2014; 2(4): 361-70.
[http://dx.doi.org/10.1158/2326-6066.CIR-13-0127] [PMID: 24764583]

[51] Beckers RK, Selinger CI, Vilain R, *et al.* Programmed death ligand 1 expression in triple-negative breast cancer is associated with tumour-infiltrating lymphocytes and improved outcome. Histopathology 2016; 69(1): 25-34.
[http://dx.doi.org/10.1111/his.12904] [PMID: 26588661]

[52] Prognostic Role and Clinical Association of Tumor-Infiltrating Lymphocyte, Programmed Death Ligand-1 Expression with Neutrophil-Lymphocyte Ratio in Locally Advanced Triple-Negative Breast Cancer - PubMed. Available from: https://pubmed.ncbi.nlm.nih.gov/30064200/ (Accessed on 2023

Feb 5).

[53] Cimino-Mathews A, Thompson E, Taube JM, *et al.* PD-L1 (B7-H1) expression and the immune tumor microenvironment in primary and metastatic breast carcinomas. Hum Pathol 2016; 47(1): 52-63. [http://dx.doi.org/10.1016/j.humpath.2015.09.003] [PMID: 26527522]

[54] Zhang M, Sun H, Zhao S, *et al.* Expression of PD-L1 and prognosis in breast cancer: A meta-analysis. Oncotarget 2017; 8(19): 31347-54. [http://dx.doi.org/10.18632/oncotarget.15532] [PMID: 28430626]

[55] Schmid P, Cortes J, Pusztai L, *et al.* KEYNOTE-522 Investigators. Pembrolizumab for Early Triple-Negative Breast Cancer. N Engl J Med 2020; 382(9): 810-21. [http://dx.doi.org/10.1056/NEJMoa1910549] [PMID: 32101663]

[56] Cancer susceptibility and the functions of BRCA1 and BRCA2 - PubMed. Available from: https://pubmed.ncbi.nlm.nih.gov/11832208/(Accessed on 2023 Feb 5).

[57] BRCA1 and BRCA2: 1994 and beyond - PubMed. Available from: https://pubmed.ncbi.nlm.nih.gov/15343273/(Accessed on 2023 Feb 5).

[58] Roy R, Chun J, Powell SN. BRCA1 and BRCA2: Different roles in a common pathway of genome protection. Nat Rev Cancer 2012; 12(1): 68-78. [http://dx.doi.org/10.1038/nrc3181] [PMID: 22193408]

[59] Molecular trajectory of brca1 and brca2 mutations - PubMed. Available from: https://pubmed.ncbi.nlm.nih.gov/32269964/ (Accessed on 2023 Feb 5).

[60] Lord CJ, Ashworth A. PARP inhibitors: Synthetic lethality in the clinic. Science 2017; 355(6330): 1152-8. [http://dx.doi.org/10.1126/science.aam7344] [PMID: 28302823]

[61] Guha M. PARP inhibitors stumble in breast cancer. Nat Biotechnol 2011; 29(5): 373-4. [http://dx.doi.org/10.1038/nbt0511-373] [PMID: 21552220]

[62] Underhill C, Toulmonde M, Bonnefoi H. A review of PARP inhibitors: From bench to bedside. Ann Oncol 2011; 22(2): 268-79. [http://dx.doi.org/10.1093/annonc/mdq322] [PMID: 20643861]

[63] Available from: https://pubmed.ncbi.nlm.nih.gov/31673138/ (Accessed on 2023 Feb 5).

[64] Available from: https://pubmed.ncbi.nlm.nih.gov/30116283/ (Accessed on 2023 Feb 5).

[65] Available from: https://pubmed.ncbi.nlm.nih.gov/30177435/ (Accessed on 2023 Feb 5).

[66] Available from: https://pubmed.ncbi.nlm.nih.gov/26775620/ (Accessed on 2023 Feb 5).

[67] Beniey M, Haque T, Hassan S. Translating the role of PARP inhibitors in triple-negative breast cancer. Oncoscience 2019; 6(1-2): 287-8. [http://dx.doi.org/10.18632/oncoscience.474] [PMID: 30800714]

[68] Robson M, Im SA, Senkus E, *et al.* Olaparib for metastatic breast cancer in patients with a germline *BRCA* Mutation. N Engl J Med 2017; 377(6): 523-33. [http://dx.doi.org/10.1056/NEJMoa1706450] [PMID: 28578601]

[69] OlympiAD final overall survival and tolerability results: Olaparib versus chemotherapy treatment of physician's choice in patients with a germline BRCA mutation and HER2-negative metastatic breast cancer - PubMed. Available from: https://pubmed.ncbi.nlm.nih.gov/30689707/ (Accessed on 2023 Feb 5).

[70] Patient-reported outcomes in patients with a germline BRCA mutation and HER2-negative metastatic breast cancer receiving olaparib versus chemotherapy in the OlympiAD trial - PubMed. Available from: https://pubmed.ncbi.nlm.nih.gov/31446213/ (Accessed on 2023 Feb 5).

[71] Goldenberg DM, Stein R, Sharkey RM. The emergence of trophoblast cell-surface antigen 2 (TROP-2) as a novel cancer target. Oncotarget 2018; 9(48): 28989-9006.

[http://dx.doi.org/10.18632/oncotarget.25615] [PMID: 29989029]

[72] Ocean AJ, Starodub AN, Bardia A, *et al.* Sacituzumab govitecan (IMMU-132), an anti-Trop-2-SN-38 antibody-drug conjugate for the treatment of diverse epithelial cancers: Safety and pharmacokinetics. Cancer 2017; 123(19): 3843-54.
[http://dx.doi.org/10.1002/cncr.30789] [PMID: 28558150]

[73] Rugo HS, Bardia A, Tolaney SM, *et al.* TROPiCS-02: A Phase III study investigating sacituzumab govitecan in the treatment of HR+/HER2- metastatic breast cancer. Future Oncol 2020; 16(12): 705-15.
[http://dx.doi.org/10.2217/fon-2020-0163] [PMID: 32223649]

[74] Bardia A, Mayer IA, Diamond JR, *et al.* Efficacy and Safety of Anti-Trop-2 Antibody Drug Conjugate Sacituzumab Govitecan (IMMU-132) in Heavily Pretreated Patients With Metastatic Triple-Negative Breast Cancer. J Clin Oncol 2017; 35(19): 2141-8.
[http://dx.doi.org/10.1200/JCO.2016.70.8297] [PMID: 28291390]

[75] Bardia A, Mayer IA, Vahdat LT, *et al.* Sacituzumab govitecan-hziy in refractory metastatic triple-negative breast cancer. N Engl J Med 2019; 380(8): 741-51.
[http://dx.doi.org/10.1056/NEJMoa1814213] [PMID: 30786188]

[76] Killock D. AKT inhibition improves OS in TNBC. Nat Rev Clin Oncol 2020; 17(3): 135.
[http://dx.doi.org/10.1038/s41571-019-0322-1] [PMID: 31900440]

[77] Saini KS, Loi S, de Azambuja E, *et al.* Targeting the PI3K/AKT/mTOR and Raf/MEK/ERK pathways in the treatment of breast cancer. Cancer Treat Rev 2013; 39(8): 935-46.
[http://dx.doi.org/10.1016/j.ctrv.2013.03.009] [PMID: 23643661]

[78] Herold CI, Anders CK. New targets for triple-negative breast cancer. Oncol Williston Park N 2013; 27(9): 846-54.

[79] Masuda H, Zhang D, Bartholomeusz C, Doihara H, Hortobagyi GN, Ueno NT. Role of epidermal growth factor receptor in breast cancer. Breast Cancer Res Treat 2012; 136(2): 331-45.
[http://dx.doi.org/10.1007/s10549-012-2289-9] [PMID: 23073759]

[80] Carey LA, Rugo HS, Marcom PK, *et al.* TBCRC 001: Randomized phase II study of cetuximab in combination with carboplatin in stage IV triple-negative breast cancer. J Clin Oncol 2012; 30(21): 2615-23.
[http://dx.doi.org/10.1200/JCO.2010.34.5579] [PMID: 22665533]

[81] Ribatti D, Nico B, Ruggieri S, Tamma R, Simone G, Mangia A. Angiogenesis and antiangiogenesis in triple-negative breast cancer. Transl Oncol 2016; 9(5): 453-7.
[http://dx.doi.org/10.1016/j.tranon.2016.07.002] [PMID: 27751350]

[82] Hutchinson L. BEATRICE bevacizumab trial—every cloud has a silver lining. Nat Rev Clin Oncol 2013; 10(10): 548.
[http://dx.doi.org/10.1038/nrclinonc.2013.161] [PMID: 23982522]

[83] Bear HD, Tang G, Rastogi P, *et al.* The effect on surgical complications of bevacizumab added to neoadjuvant chemotherapy for breast cancer: NRG Oncology/NSABP Protocol B-40. Ann Surg Oncol 2017; 24(7): 1853-60.
[http://dx.doi.org/10.1245/s10434-016-5662-9] [PMID: 27864694]

[84] Sikov WM, Berry DA, Perou CM, *et al.* Impact of the addition of carboplatin and/or bevacizumab to neoadjuvant once-per-week paclitaxel followed by dose-dense doxorubicin and cyclophosphamide on pathologic complete response rates in stage II to III triple-negative breast cancer: CALGB 40603 (Alliance). J Clin Oncol 2015; 33(1): 13-21.
[http://dx.doi.org/10.1200/JCO.2014.57.0572] [PMID: 25092775]

[85] Targeting the PI3-kinase pathway in triple-negative breast cancer - PubMed. Available from: https://pubmed.ncbi.nlm.nih.gov/31050709/ (Accessed on 2023 Feb 6).

[86] Costa RLB, Han HS, Gradishar WJ. Targeting the PI3K/AKT/mTOR pathway in triple-negative breast

cancer: a review. Breast Cancer Res Treat 2018; 169(3): 397-406. [http://dx.doi.org/10.1007/s10549-018-4697-y] [PMID: 29417298]

[87] Chan JJ, Tan TJY, Dent RA. Novel therapeutic avenues in triple-negative breast cancer: PI3K/AKT inhibition, androgen receptor blockade, and beyond. Ther Adv Med Oncol 2019; 11 [http://dx.doi.org/10.1177/1758835919880429] [PMID: 31636720]

[88] Jovanović B, Mayer IA, Mayer EL, *et al.* A Randomized Phase II Neoadjuvant Study of Cisplatin, Paclitaxel With or Without Everolimus in Patients with Stage II/III Triple-Negative Breast Cancer (TNBC): Responses and Long-term Outcome Correlated with Increased Frequency of DNA Damage Response Gene Mutations, TNBC Subtype, AR Status, and Ki67. Clin Cancer Res 2017; 23(15): 4035-45. [http://dx.doi.org/10.1158/1078-0432.CCR-16-3055] [PMID: 28270498]

[89] Rugo HS, André F, Yamashita T, *et al.* Time course and management of key adverse events during the randomized phase III SOLAR-1 study of PI3K inhibitor alpelisib plus fulvestrant in patients with HR-positive advanced breast cancer. Ann Oncol 2020; 31(8): 1001-10. [http://dx.doi.org/10.1016/j.annonc.2020.05.001] [PMID: 32416251]

[90] André F, Ciruelos E, Rubovszky G, *et al.* Alpelisib for *PIK3CA* -mutated, hormone receptor–positive advanced breast cancer. N Engl J Med 2019; 380(20): 1929-40. [http://dx.doi.org/10.1056/NEJMoa1813904] [PMID: 31091374]

[91] Mosele F, Stefanovska B, Lusque A, *et al.* Outcome and molecular landscape of patients with PIK3CA-mutated metastatic breast cancer. Ann Oncol 2020; 31(3): 377-86. [http://dx.doi.org/10.1016/j.annonc.2019.11.006] [PMID: 32067679]

[92] Lin J, Sampath D, Nannini MA, *et al.* Targeting activated Akt with GDC-0068, a novel selective Akt inhibitor that is efficacious in multiple tumor models. Clin Cancer Res 2013; 19(7): 1760-72. [http://dx.doi.org/10.1158/1078-0432.CCR-12-3072] [PMID: 23287563]

[93] Kim SB, Dent R, Im SA, *et al.* Ipatasertib plus paclitaxel versus placebo plus paclitaxel as first-line therapy for metastatic triple-negative breast cancer (LOTUS): a multicentre, randomised, double-blind, placebo-controlled, phase 2 trial. Lancet Oncol 2017; 18(10): 1360-72. [http://dx.doi.org/10.1016/S1470-2045(17)30450-3] [PMID: 28800861]

[94] Schmid P, Abraham J, Chan S, *et al.* Capivasertib plus paclitaxel versus placebo plus paclitaxel as first-line therapy for metastatic triple-negative breast cancer: The PAKT Trial. J Clin Oncol 2020; 38(5): 423-33. [http://dx.doi.org/10.1200/JCO.19.00368] [PMID: 31841354]

[95] Ricciardi GRR, Adamo B, Ieni A, *et al.* Androgen Receptor (AR), E-Cadherin, and Ki-67 as Emerging Targets and Novel Prognostic Markers in Triple-Negative Breast Cancer (TNBC) Patients. PLoS One 2015; 10(6): e0128368. [http://dx.doi.org/10.1371/journal.pone.0128368] [PMID: 26039245]

[96] Faurobert E, Bouin AP, Albiges-Rizo C. Microenvironment, tumor cell plasticity, and cancer. Curr Opin Oncol 2015; 27(1): 64-70. [http://dx.doi.org/10.1097/CCO.0000000000000154] [PMID: 25415136]

[97] Bhattarai S, Klimov S, Mittal K, *et al.* Prognostic role of androgen receptor in triple negative breast cancer: a multi-institutional study. Cancers 2019; 11(7): 995. [http://dx.doi.org/10.3390/cancers11070995] [PMID: 31319547]

[98] Gucalp A, Tolaney S, Isakoff SJ, *et al.* Phase II trial of bicalutamide in patients with androgen receptor-positive, estrogen receptor-negative metastatic Breast Cancer. Clin Cancer Res 2013; 19(19): 5505-12. [http://dx.doi.org/10.1158/1078-0432.CCR-12-3327] [PMID: 23965901]

[99] Shanle EK, Zhao Z, Hawse J, *et al.* Research resource: global identification of estrogen receptor β target genes in triple negative breast cancer cells. Mol Endocrinol 2013; 27(10): 1762-75. [http://dx.doi.org/10.1210/me.2013-1164] [PMID: 23979844]

[100] Enzalutamide for the treatment of androgen receptor-expressing triple-negative breast cancer - pubmed. Available from: https://pubmed.ncbi.nlm.nih.gov/29373071/ (Accessed on 2023 Feb 6).

[101] Speirs V, Skliris GP, Burdall SE, Carder PJ. Distinct expression patterns of ER and ER in normal human mammary gland. J Clin Pathol 2002; 55(5): 371-4. [http://dx.doi.org/10.1136/jcp.55.5.371] [PMID: 11986344]

[102] Zhao C, Lam EWF, Sunters A, *et al.* Expression of estrogen receptor β isoforms in normal breast epithelial cells and breast cancer: Regulation by methylation. Oncogene 2003; 22(48): 7600-6. [http://dx.doi.org/10.1038/sj.onc.1207100] [PMID: 14576822]

[103] Hieken TJ, Carter JM, Hawse JR, *et al.* ERβ expression and breast cancer risk prediction for women with atypias. Cancer Prev Res 2015; 8(11): 1084-92. [http://dx.doi.org/10.1158/1940-6207.CAPR-15-0198] [PMID: 26276747]

[104] Dotzlaw H, Leygue E, Watson PH, Murphy LC. Estrogen receptor-beta messenger RNA expression in human breast tumor biopsies: Relationship to steroid receptor status and regulation by progestins. Cancer Res 1999; 59(3): 529-32. [PMID: 9973194]

[105] Roger P, Sahla ME, Mäkelä S, Gustafsson JA, Baldet P, Rochefort H. Decreased expression of estrogen receptor beta protein in proliferative preinvasive mammary tumors. Cancer Res 2001; 61(6): 2537-41. [PMID: 11289127]

[106] Hawse JR, Carter JM, Aspros KGM, *et al.* Optimized immunohistochemical detection of estrogen receptor beta using two validated monoclonal antibodies confirms its expression in normal and malignant breast tissues. Breast Cancer Res Treat 2020; 179(1): 241-9. [http://dx.doi.org/10.1007/s10549-019-05441-3] [PMID: 31571071]

[107] Reese JM, Suman VJ, Subramaniam M, *et al.* ERβ1: characterization, prognosis, and evaluation of treatment strategies in ERα-positive and -negative breast cancer. BMC Cancer 2014; 14(1): 749. [http://dx.doi.org/10.1186/1471-2407-14-749] [PMID: 25288324]

[108] Badve SS, Gökmen-Polar Y. TP53 Status and Estrogen Receptor-Beta in Triple-Negative Breast Cancer: Company Matters. J Natl Cancer Inst 2019; 111(11): 1118-9. [http://dx.doi.org/10.1093/jnci/djz052] [PMID: 30989234]

[109] Sellitto A, D'Agostino Y, Alexandrova E, *et al.* Insights into the Role of Estrogen Receptor β in Triple-Negative Breast Cancer. Cancers 2020; 12(6): 1477. [http://dx.doi.org/10.3390/cancers12061477] [PMID: 32516978]

[110] Lazennec G, Bresson D, Lucas A, Chauveau C, Vignon F. ER beta inhibits proliferation and invasion of breast cancer cells. Endocrinology 2001; 142(9): 4120-30. [http://dx.doi.org/10.1210/endo.142.9.8395] [PMID: 11517191]

[111] Thomas C, Rajapaksa G, Nikolos F, *et al.* ERβ1 represses basal-like breast cancer epithelial to mesenchymal transition by destabilizing EGFR. Breast Cancer Res 2012; 14(6): R148. [http://dx.doi.org/10.1186/bcr3358] [PMID: 23158001]

[112] Schüler-Toprak S, Häring J, Inwald EC, Moehle C, Ortmann O, Treeck O. Agonists and knockdown of estrogen receptor β differentially affect invasion of triple-negative breast cancer cells in vitro. BMC Cancer 2016; 16(1): 951. [http://dx.doi.org/10.1186/s12885-016-2973-y] [PMID: 28003019]

[113] Reese JM, Bruinsma ES, Monroe DG, *et al.* ERβ inhibits cyclin dependent kinases 1 and 7 in triple negative breast cancer. Oncotarget 2017; 8(57): 96506-21. [http://dx.doi.org/10.18632/oncotarget.21787] [PMID: 29228549]

[114] Reese JM, Bruinsma ES, Nelson AW, *et al.* ERβ-mediated induction of cystatins results in suppression of TGFβ signaling and inhibition of triple-negative breast cancer metastasis. Proc Natl Acad Sci USA 2018; 115(41): E9580-9.

[http://dx.doi.org/10.1073/pnas.1807751115] [PMID: 30257941]

[115] Austin D, Hamilton N, Elshimali Y, Pietras R, Wu Y, Vadgama J. Estrogen receptor-beta is a potential target for triple negative breast cancer treatment. Oncotarget 2018; 9(74): 33912-30. [http://dx.doi.org/10.18632/oncotarget.26089] [PMID: 30338035]

[116] Wisinski KB, Xu W, Tevaarwerk AJ, *et al.* Targeting estrogen receptor beta in a phase 2 study of high-dose estradiol in metastatic triple-negative breast cancer: A wisconsin oncology network study. Clin Breast Cancer 2016; 16(4): 256-61. [http://dx.doi.org/10.1016/j.clbc.2016.03.005] [PMID: 27133732]

CHAPTER 8

Molecular Mechanisms Implicated with Depression and Therapeutic Intervention

Loveleena Kour Anand[1], **Mir Shahid Maqbool**[1] and **Fayaz Malik**[1,*]

[1] *Indian Institute of Integrative Medicine, Sanat Nagar, 190005, J.K. India*

Abstract: Depression is a pervasive, arduous psychological condition with profound neurological ramifications. The parameters for leveraging depression involve the diagnosis and evaluation of depression, the endorsement to implement substantiated therapies and rigorous follow-up of the patients. Many individuals suffering from depression undertake a recurring or persistent therapy that correlates to a decline in cognitive processing. The underpinnings of exact aetiology and pathogenesis of melancholy are probably the outcome of a variety of mechanisms. These include physiological, behavioural, and socio-economic variables, all playing their roles. Multiple refinements to the treatments encompassing therapies, medications and medical interventions are employed, in relation to effective approaches reassuring the brighter side. In this chapter, we discuss more integrative and multifaceted aspects of psychological health, minimizing the segmented understanding to achieve a consensus on multiple possibilities for effective interventions.

Keywords: Heterogeneous, Health disorder, Resource-based economies, Trial-and-error strategy.

INTRODUCTION

The term "depression" was coined in the 19th century to describe "mental depression," an enervating ailment that is predominantly syndromal, distressing individuals all over the globe. Depression or Major Depressive Disorder is among the most pervasive, highly heterogeneous and often disabling syndrome with relatively higher lifetime prevalence rates, yet very difficult to recognise. Depression bears modest correlations from being a neuropsychiatric disorder to its anchored biological roots, motivating interest in diagnosing depression for treatment and research purposes.

MDD is epitomized by a cluster of signs and manifestations which allude to a distinct illness with discrete aetiologies. The aphorism "No health without mental health [1]" rationalizes depression as being an illness of hindered mental well-being. Anguish, diminished motivation, protracted melancholy, suicidal ideation, and psychosocial impairment are the critical attributes of the cognitive and

* **Corresponding author Fayaz Malik:** Indian Institute of Integrative Medicine, Sanat Nagar, 190005, J.K. India; Tel: 9419187187; E-mail: fmalik@iiim.ac.in

Farzana Mahdi & Abbas Ali Mahdi (Eds.)

somatic facets of depressive episodes. Besides these, circadian rhythm disruption and hormonal imbalances, notably cortisol and melatonin release, are among other major markers of depression disorders [2].

Depression departs from regular mood swings and fleeting emotional reactions, specifically when recurrent with moderate or severe intensity. Depression has proven to be a significant drain on workforces in knowledge-based industries and resource-based economies with exceptionally high rates of debility and abridged productivity. It is prophesied that by 2030, depression will be the utmost debilitating and prevalent health disorder. An estimated 50% of depressed patients do not present any emotional variability despite manifold health care visits, and often misdiagnosed and thereby incompetently treated with available interventions. There are multiple non-invasive treatments, evidence-based psychotherapies, and antidepressant therapies for treating depressed patients, nevertheless, the therapy response rates are relatively lower [3].

Even with an ensuing recovery, several patients may necessitate a trial-and-error strategy, as there are no reliable guidelines for optimal treatments, with patients developing treatment resistance over time. This scenario stems from the heterogeneity of depression and the lack of biomarkers for subtype-specific stratification. The principles of upkeep for this condition are quite simple, relying on early detection, accurate diagnosis, appropriate therapy selection and post-intervention monitoring. Regardless of advances, a number of significant issues have emerged regarding depression diagnosis and novel therapy. To address these known challenges, this chapter aims to address the basic precepts of depression, the implicated brain circuits with molecular dysfunction, and the diagnostic parameters with accessible therapies. Taking these points into consideration, one can then chalk out the program for precision medicine, the titration of dose, and the one that has no side effects. Several drug molecules are available to treat neurological disorders. However, a great deal of additional work is required to achieve a consensus on drugs, treatment and the duration of follow-up of the patients.

EPIDEMIOLOGICAL BURDEN

Depressive malaises foray approximately 3.8% of the global population, encompassing primarily 5.0% of adolescents and individuals over the age of 60 [4]. Depression affects nearly 280 million people across the globe. Annually, around 700 000 people commit suicide, mostly amongst those who are 15 to 29 years of age, making suicide the fourth leading root of mortality. Despite the widespread availability of established, budget-friendly drugs, about 75% of people in low and middle-income nations do not receive treatment for mental health issues. Inadequate funding, unsatisfactory healthcare, a shortage of competent workers, and undeniably the stigma allied with psychological ailments are the foremost impediments in the direction of efficacious care.

Prevalence

Depression typifies one of the utmost predominant chronic conditions universally, having a detrimental impact on the emotions, thoughts, and social interaction abilities of individuals. Approximately 2-6% of people globally suffer from depression, affecting roughly 1 in every 15 adults annually and 1 in every 6 people may happen to pass through depressive episodes at some phase in their lifespan. Prior to 2020, psychological illness, precisely anxiety and depression, were the key causes of global health burden. Nevertheless, the COVID-19 predicament has fostered a scenario where frequent variables of meagre mental state have been accentuated. As a consequence, there is a heightened urge to strengthen mental health treatment by initiatives to include in the mitigation [8].

In accordance with the "Global Burden of Diseases, Injuries, and Risk Factors Study (GBD)" 2019, both depression and anxiousness are the two major incapacitating mental conditions, explicitly labelled among the top 25 major contributing factors for escalating mental health globally. This pressure was great across the spectrum, affecting both genders, in a plethora of settings [7]. Despite mounting evidence of interventions that mitigate the impact, there has been no decline in global prevalence rates since 1990. The frequency of DALYs globally due to mental diseases surged from 80.8 million in 1990 to 125.3 million in 2019, while the overall percentage of all DALYs rose from 3.1% to 4.9%. In 2019 approximately 125.3 million YLDs were ascribed to mental disorders, who were in 17361.5 YLLs attributable to eating disorders [6].

According to WHO projections, the 10 leading nations with the maximum and minimum (Table **1**) prevalence rate of depression are enlisted. However, the percentages mentioned over and under are completely substantial and relevant [7]. However, it may be noted that the real figures are apparently far larger and are heavily influenced by age and gender.

Table 1. Prevalence of depression across some leading countries of the world.

S. No.	%Highest Prevalence	%Lowest Prevalence
1	Ukraine-6.3%	Solomon Islands-2.9%
2	United States-5.9%	Papua New Guinea-3.0%
3	Estonia-5.9%	Timor-Leste-3.0%
4	Australia-5.9%	Vanuatu-3.1%

(Table 1) cont.....

S. No.	%Highest Prevalence	%Lowest Prevalence
5	Brazil-5.8%	Kiribati-3.1%
6	Greece-5.7%	Tonga-3.2%
7	Portugal-5.7%	Samoa-3.2%
8	Belarus-5.6%	Laos-3.2%
9	Finland-5.6%	Nepal-3.2%
10	Lithuania-5.6%	Philippines-3.3%

Age Standardised

The average life expectancy for the initiation of depressive episodes in the global population aged 18 to 64 years spans from 24 to 35 years, with a recent trend toward a younger onset. Approximately 40% of individuals who are depressed experience their first bout between the ages of 20 and 50, with the remaining 10% acquiring depression beyond the age of 50. Age-standardized melancholy is further segmented hereunder.

Childhood depression

Psychiatric disorders in children are recognized as substantial shifts in the way children learn behavioural and emotional attributes [12]. Childhood distress diverges from distinctive "blues" and regular symptoms known by an upsurge in somatic anomalies, aggression, and social disengagement. Children with a prior history of domestic violence, or abuse, who experience moderate or severe depressive bouts are at a greater risk for committing suicide.

Among the most prevalent psychological disorders that can be identified in children is attention deficit/hyperactivity disorder (ADHD), striking 9.8% population (approx. 6.0 million) [12]. In addition to ADHD, more frequent disorders comprise anxiety, inflicting 8.9% (nearly 5.5 million), and depression, striking 4.4% of the population (approx. 2.7 million) individuals [13].

Depressive symptoms are frequently undiagnosed and misconstrued as characteristic psychological and emotional changes, predominantly in Children exhibiting hopelessness or gloomy behaviour. The CDC undertakes a study, "The National Survey of Children's Health", to evaluate the frequency of mental ailments [14]. The study establishes the surge in ADHD, anxiousness, and depressed mood with the progression of age (Fig. **1**). Additionally, children between the ages of 6 to 11 seem to be more exposed to face behavioural issues contrary to children over or underneath the same age group.

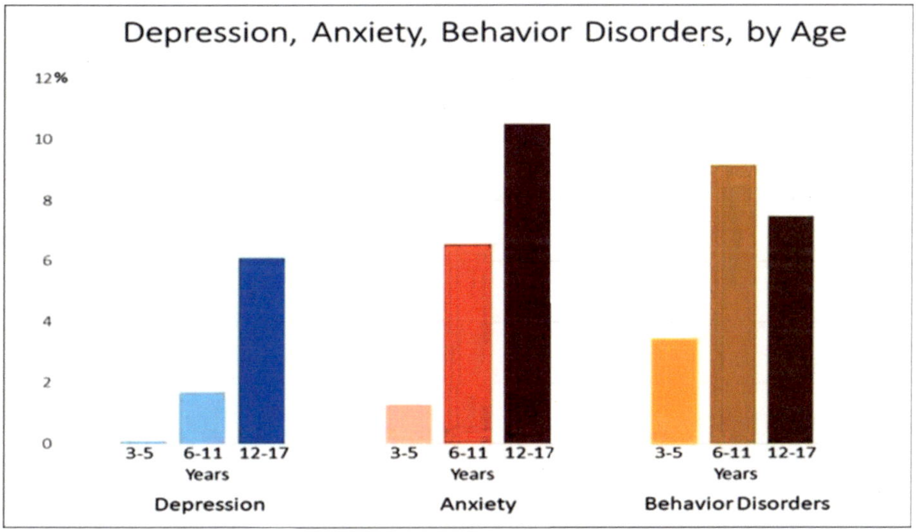

Fig. (1). Adapted: Center of disease dontrol and prevention, "Data and statistics on children's mental health," center of disease control and prevention retrieved september, vol. 13, 2022.

The foremost cautionary signs and symptoms of paediatric depression comprise:

- Irritability with persistent melancholy and despondency.
- Preconditioned to social isolation and disillusionment.
- Variations in appetite and sleeping patterns.
- Loud intonations with reduced concentration and fatigue.
- Physiological complications, resulting in a diminished sensitivity to treatments.
- Feelings of obligation coupled with suicidal or death-related thoughts.

Adolescence Depression

Adolescence is a vital stage in a person's growth, speculated as a high-risk phase for the inception of depressive episodes, with meagre functional prognosis and a high-frequency incidence [15]. Despite variations in hereditary architecture and therapeutic response spectra, the global proportion of depressive symptoms and MDD vividly upsurges during adolescence, with an early manifestation at the age of fifteen [16]. This is the time when teenagers suffer disproportionately from anxiety, substance abuse, and suicidal ideation. According to 2018–2019 surveys, 36.7% of adults have persistent depression, equated to 15.1% of adults aged 12 to 17 who have a severe bout of depression [17]. Within the initial years of the COVID-19 outburst, the prevalence of juvenile mental illness has increased significantly. While one in every five adolescents had heightened emotional experiences, roughly one in every four adults has clinically elevated depression-related manifestations [18].

Unprecedented usage of social media and other cutting-edge technology seem to be sturdily allied to an upsurge in conduct disorder, the relapse of episodic drinking and smoking, and an elevated chances of anxiety and depression [19]. In accordance with a recent study by the "Norwegian Media Authority", approximately 90% of young people spend a considerable amount of time on social media, resulting in severe consequences, prompting questions concerning juvenile mental well-being and allied specific physical issues and vegetative symptoms.

The chief indications and manifestations of depression in adolescence are [20] given hereunder.

- Appetite suppression with disordered eating practices
- Weight fluctuation and diminished concentration
- Extreme fatigue and narcolepsy
- Absence of interest and depersonalization
- Mental fogginess and hypersomnia patterns

Elderly Depression

Ageing is a universal phenomenon that entails physical degeneration and, occasionally, leads to brain anomalies. It imperils the integrity of front striatal networks, particularly the hippocampus and amygdala, leading to the medical condition known as "Late life depression" [5]. According to the International Classification of Diseases (ICD-10) and the Diagnostic and Statistical Manual of the American Psychiatric Association (DSM-IV), "Late Life Depression" is a psychiatric disorder that typically manifests over the age of 65, with the proportion of people suffering from it nearly quadrupling from 11% to 22% by 2050 [25]. As per GBD 2020 statistics, the incidence of MDD has also soared to 17%, with roughly 21.0 million persons in the United States suffering from melancholy [10], showing a substantial influence on expanding economies. However, the predicament is particularly dire in middle- and low-income nations [27].

"Late Life Depression" induces psychosocial alterations in elderly individuals that are driven by congenital elements and physiological impairment, inclining them to severe depressive episodes [22]. Elderly adults suffering from MDD recurrently perceive desolation along with some unfavourable manifestations enlisted hereunder [23, 24].

- Disturbed perception heightened by recurrent episodes of sadness.
- Cognitive impairment, loss of motivation, and suicidal tendencies.
- Long-term medical conditions that induce agitation, anxiety, or discomfort.

- A sense of inadequacy, inferiority, guilt, or melancholy.
- Lowered energy, fatigue, and sleep disturbances.
- Consuming more or fewer calories than usual frequently resulting in an unforeseen weight gain or loss.

Gender Based Standardisation

Adolescence has been identified as a transition phase predominantly susceptible to a varied array of physiological and psychological elements that can have both immediate and long-term ramifications on physical well-being, leading to gender disparities in depression. Previous epidemiological studies state that [30], women in their midlife, emerging adulthood and adolescence are more inclined towards depression, experiencing more severe complications than their male counterparts in the same age range [34]. Cognitive deficits and stressors are the significant predictors of gender disparity [29]. The odds ratio (OR) of the gender gap in depression is 1.95, which is averaged meta-analytically across all countries and age groups [32]. By the age of 12, the gender gap becomes apparent, somewhere between 5 - 13% of adolescent boys and 10-17% of young females experiencing depressive mood disorders [33].

Globally, the projected estimate of DALYs for men is 1426.5/100000 and for women, 1703.0/100000, experiencing depressive episodes [8]. According to 2020 surveys, the prevalence of MDD in individuals aged 18 or above in the US was significantly higher in females (10.5%) compared to males. (6.2%) [9]. However, the 2019 statistics depicted that 21.8% of women experience mild (13.4%), moderate (3.4%) or chronic (3.5%) depressive bouts, comparable to 9.6% mild, 3.4% moderate and 2.1% severe symptoms in male counterparts of same age groups (Fig. **2**), respectively [10].

Gender breaches in depression still remain substantiated, but their implementation into unified aetiological theories remains challenging. Additionally, age plays a crucial role because women experience more severe depression from adolescence through adulthood, as opposed to men, who predominate till puberty. The risk factors for disparities between the two sexes in psychiatric conditions are also increasing because female preponderance is not universal due to homogeneous civilizations. However, irrespective of the causative factors, depression cannot be overlooked in any gender.

DIAGNOSTIC CRITERIA

Precise understanding is vital for an effective medication of MDD; clinicians have developed strategies for recognizing the effective approach to comply MDD diagnostic standards. On the conflicting side of the spectrum, explicit symptoms coincide significantly more often than could be hypothesized. Thus, whether all possible variants should be taken into consideration for qualifying the MDD standards to eventuate the individuals needs to be carefully monitored [35]. The globally recognized classifiers for depressive episodes, as per clinician nosology, are the "Diagnostic and Statistical Manual, Fifth Edition" (DSM-5; American Psychiatric Association, 2013) and "The International Classification of Diseases", Tenth Edition (ICD-10; World Health Organization, 1992). Aside from these, clinical evaluations and Self-report inventory constitute the most predominant methods for diagnosis and treatment.

Clinical Ratings

The depression scaling scheme is a psychiatric assessment approach that employs evocative words and expressions to imitate the severity of depressive symptomatology [36]. Rating scales can be employed to appraise a person's behaviour and predict whether more assessment for a depressed episode is anticipated [35]. A multitude of valuation scales are exploited to accomplish this objective, segmented as under:

- Scales accomplished by investigators,
- Scales completed out through sufferers,
- Scales completed by sick people and researchers.

Scales Accomplished by Investigators

Numerous depressive ratings are accomplished by the psychiatrist, where they interview the patients and evaluate the symptoms to ascertain the probable responses to every question. These rating scales include the following.

- Hamilton Depression Rating Scale
- Montgomery Asberg Depression Rating Scale
- Raskin Depression Rating Scale

Hamilton Depression Rating Scale

The Hamilton Depression Rating Scale (HDRS) or HAM-D empowers the diagnosis of varied depressive states and is designed to evaluate the performance of several antidepressants in depressed subjects [49]. This scale was established by Max Hamilton in 1960 [37], and revised manifold in 1966, 1968, 1969 and 1980 [38 - 41]. However, this is still cast off extensively for clinical evaluations and aids as a bench mark for gauging recovery in depressed subjects. HAM-D is considered as gold standard for grading based on the assortment of 21 questions with 3-5 utmost probable assumptions that imitate the severity of depressive episodes [50]. According to the 17-item scoring function, normal scores range from 0-7, mild depressive states are signified by scores of 8-16, and moderate depression by scores of 17 to 23. These were severe depressive states with scores of 24 or higher. To regulate the magnitude of depression, the questionnaire appraises a person's state of mind, suicidal tendencies, emotions of guilt, sleeplessness, nervousness, hyperactivity or lethargy, body weight, and somatic manifestations.

HAM-D relies on three main psychometric characteristics scaling comprising reliability, item response, and validity. Nevertheless, one of the chief limitations of HAMD-D is the masking of (DSM-IV) diagnostic criteria, such as a sense of worthlessness and anhedonia that have been challenged for modification [50] in the following two forms shown hereunder.

1. **HAMD-7**: This is the shortest version of the original HAMD scale. The apparent variables related to the HAMD's multidimensional nature are mitigated by this abridged version centered on a one-dimensional core group of depressive signs and symptoms [53].
2. **GRID-HAMD**: The GRID-HAMD was published by the "Depression Rating Scale Standardization Team" (DRSST) in 2002 with the aim to augment the HAMD's standardisation, management, and grading flaws [52].

Montgomery Asberg Depression Rating Scale (MADRS)

This scale encompasses ten elements cast-off typically by psychologists to appraise the severity of depressive episodes [54]. This scale was designed in 1979 by Marie Asberg to be used in conjunction with the Hamilton Rating Scale for Depression (HAMD) [55]. Every question on the MADRS is dispensed as a score ranging from 0- 6; advanced score depicts severe depression (0-60) [56].

Raskin Depression Rating Scale

The Raskin Rating Scale is a brief, spectator-rated evaluation used to diagnose depressive symptoms. To determine the alterations integrated following the pharmacological intervention, RRS includes three key domains:

- Oral statement
- Subsequent indicators
- Cognitive behaviour [57]

Scales Completed by Subjects

Patients complete a few melancholy rating measures on their own, including:

- Beck Depression Rating Scale
- Geriatric Depression Rating Scale
- Zung Depression Rating Scale

Beck Depression Rating Scale (BDR)

In 1961, a psychiatrist Aaron T. Beck recognized the Beck Depression Inventory for self-appraisal entailing indications like irritation, exhaustion, and weight loss, a lack of interest, feelings of guilt, pessimism, or fear of retribution [58]. Patients fill out the scale to gauge the incidence and severity of episodes, which mollifies the DSM-IV diagnostic criteria [59].

Geriatric Depression Rating Scale (GDR)

The Geriatric Depression Scale is another self-administered valuation used for elderly patients and individuals enduring mild to moderate dementia [60]. In the assessment of a five-category system, GDS inquiries permit a “yes” or “no” response from patients for scaling purposes [61].

Zung Depression Rating Scale (ZDR)

The Zung Depression Scale, like the GDS, embraces pre-formatted responses, comprising 20-item questionnaires, 10 of which are favourable and 10 of which are stressful. The four probable responses to each question individually are evaluated on a gauge of 1-4 [61].

Scales Completed by Investigators and Subjects Together

The “Primary Care Evaluation of Mental Disorders” is accomplished by the patient and a clinician (PRIME-MD). This melancholy scoring system, which comprises a follow-up practitioner consultation and a 27-item diagnostic questionnaire, is designed to assist primary care practitioners in evaluating common psychological diseases. It was succeeded by the PHQ-9 Patient Health Questionnaire due to its lengthy duration [62].

The International Classification of Mental and Behavioural Disorders (ICD)

The International Classification of Diseases (ICD), originated in Paris in 1900, is the most extensively documented diagnostic standard used to compile morbidity and mortality figures [63]. The World Health Organization (WHO) devised the ICD primarily to designate medical illnesses, and since then, it has progressed through eleven revisions, the most current one being ICD-11. This categorisation is employed to generate authorized statistics on all patients in psychiatric care across the globe. The main features of ICD are listed as under:

- Recognised global categorisation.
- Designed for practice by all health care specialists.
- Distinct attention is devoted to primary care in impoverished and middle-income economies.
- Key apprehension in regard to therapeutic implication and abridged diagnosis.
- Provides diagnostic descriptions and suggestions instead of improving organisational parameters [64].

According to ICD-10, "mental disorder" is not a precise phase to imply the possession of a pathologically recognisable assortment of signs or behaviours allied with discomfort and impairment with social activities 65]. The ICD-10 code set was adopted in 1992, and embodies probably the most significant amendment to the manual. The orthodox distinction between psychosis and neurosis is dissolved; rather, ailments are huddled together chiefly on commonalities [66]. Among clusters, there are additional specialised subdivisions. The WHO amended ICD-10 to generate ICD-11, which was adopted by the 72nd World Health Assembly in 2019 and became effective on January 1, 2022 [67].

The WHO recently published the 11th edition of the International Classification of Diseases (ICD-11), a universal classification framework for both physical and psychological disorders. It is the enhanced version of the ICD-10 and is approximately five times more comprehensive [68], incorporating more diagnostic codes and modifications, ensuring a superior level of precision. The ICD-11 provides a clear description of disorders rather than operational criteria [69].

Diagnostic and Statistical Manual of Mental Disorders (DSM)

The DSM, foremost presented in 1952 to diagnose mental disorders and behavioural issues, is still the authoritative organization for clinical diagnosis across the globe. The "American Psychiatric Association" established the utmost recent iteration of the Diagnostic and Statistical Manual of Mental Disorders (DSM-5), including the succeeding elements [70] given hereunder.

- Cataloguing primarily in the United States, also employed by other countries.
- Most commonly implemented by psychiatrists.
- Primarily concerned with delivering secondary psychiatric care in high-income nations.
- It appears to have a proclivity for extra diagnoses with each successive iteration.
- The diagnostic technique includes a polythetic procedure based on operating parameters.

The "American Psychiatric Association" (APA) published the current edition of "Diagnostic and Statistical Manual of Mental Diseases" DSM-TR, which was released in March 2022. This can be used for the identification of psychological disorders employing a universal language and standard measurements. It is the predominant commodity employed in the diagnosis and treatment of psychological issues across the United States of America [71].

Similarities and Dissimilarities Between DSM and ICD

A. The following are the most significant commonalities between the DSM and ICD's psychiatric disorder subdivisions.

- Natural psychological ailments encompassing manifestations.
- Personality disorders.
- Psychological development disorders.
- Psychological pathologies coupled with physiologic issues and external elements.
- Delusional, schizophrenic, and schizotypal syndromes.
- Disorders of mood and motivation.
- Emotional and behavioural abnormalities typically manifest in adolescent and childhood.
- Somatic disorders, neurotic and stress-related illnesses.
- Unidentified mental illnesses.
- Cognitive and behavioural disorders spurred on by the consumption of psychoactive substances.
- Mental immaturity.

B. The following are the major variations between both the DSM and ICD's categorization of mental illnesses.

Diagnostic and Statistical Manual of Mental Disorders (DSM)	The International Classification of Mental and Behavioural Disorders (ICD)
• US designation for mental disorders • Preponderantly used by psychologists Primarily centred on subsequent psychiatric treatment in high-income nations. • No affects clinical efficacy. • Has a propensity to add additional diagnoses for each revised edition. • Includes primary operational parameter.	• Universally recognised Organization. • Employed by all health care practitioners. • Ensure gratitude for low- and middle-income nations. • Chiefly affects clinical efficacy. • Decreasing of multitude of diagnosis. • Augment diagnostic clarifications and assistance.

CLASSIFICATION AND CLINICAL MANIFESTATIONS

Depression, despite being a mosaic disorder, is nonetheless considered a distinct clinical entity with a surfeit of underpinning manifestations showing discrete aetiologies with comparable phenotypes. In accordance with the "Spectrum of mood disorder [72]", depression is not categorised into discrete units. Conversely, a dimensional approach differentiates the forms of depression midway along a spectrum with no discernible bounds [73]. This stratification of depression is very critical for an effective therapy plan. A plethora of categorisation has been proposed to determine the number, nature, intensity, frequency, aetiology and severity of depressive episodes. Pragmatic classifications have been now entrenched in the contemporary two chief classification systems, DSM-IV [74] and ICD [75] for segmentation of depression. The DSM-IV-TR, 4th edition of the Diagnostic and Statistical Manual of Mental Disorders constitutes the basis for contemporary subtyping, divides depression into two broad categories:

- Unipolar Depression
- Bipolar Depression

In count to the above-stated organization, DSM shows a diversity of cross-sectional and transverse phase specifiers for both UD and BD distinctly conscripted as under:

Unipolar Depression

Unipolar depression is a predominant medical ailment manifested as MDD or clinical depression. It is an explicit sort of depression, not a distinct condition. Unipolar depression augments substantially the global disease burden, having a profound influence on an individual's psychosocial, physiological, and cognitive well-being [76]. All depressive disorders are not always escorted by "blues" or melancholy, and occasionally, individuals can swiftly sniff out it, but it necessitates regular medical assistance and care.

Unipolar Depression, or MDD is a multifaceted disorder with hereditary, cognitive, societal and psychological aspects triggered by the interplay of these variables. It is one of the utmost serious illnesses, often undiagnosed, affecting unevenly 8% of people in the United States annually [77]. Patients with unipolar depression partake in erroneous thought processes and beliefs, and are substantially more inclined to dive through the remission phases preceded by relapses, which infrequently alter perception power. As per 2019 statistics, about 7% of adults in the US experience unipolar depression, and the incidence upsurges dramatically, noticeably in females, surpassing 4% by the end of adolescence [78]. Studies show that by 2030, unipolar depression is anticipated to rank as the second-largest root of disease worldwide.

Manifestations

Unipolar depression is a significantly more severe form of MDD typified by one or more bouts of moderate to severe depression, a persistently gloomy mood, with the cessation of depressive cycles [73]. Individuals experiencing unipolar depression are not essentially depressed. Instead, they perceive aberrations fostering a perverted outlook on life, eliciting unpleasant sensations and emotions. They may appear to be happy or show phases when signs of depression ameliorate mildly. As a response, individuals may experience emotional anguish, bad self-image, emotional aversion, and other complications. Although researchers may not precisely comprehend the underpinning root of melancholy, implications in neurotransmitter signalling are majorly allied with mood disorders [79]. Antipsychotics stimulate the dopamine, serotonin and adrenaline signalling pathways signifying a perilous role in emotional processing [80]. Evidence-based therapies counting psychoanalysis, medications, and lifestyle variations can address both the behavioural and physical indicators of unipolar depression, which are enlisted below [81, 82].

- Common emotional shifts include a melancholy mood with feelings of sadness, pessimism, remorse, and suffering.
- Irritability allied with behavioural matters epitomizes the utmost predominant psychological concern coupled with incapacity to attain satisfaction.
- Sleeping issues like Insomnia or Hypersomnia are the prominent predictor of the incidence, nature and resurgence of unipolar depression.
- Appetite fluctuations marked by bodyweight swings, an individual may shed or gain 5% of the entire mass.
- Fatigue prompted by emotional and physical exhaustion wanes the capacity to stay energised.
- Concentration hitches instigated by cognitive fog, difficulty focusing, giving attention or making lucid conclusions.
- Recurrent suicidal predispositions by instincts of self-harm are typically spurred on by secondary stressors, such as unemployment or middling academic outcomes.
- Psychological signs of anxiousness or being bogged down on a consistent basis, in addition to substantial psychomotor regression.

Individuals experiencing UD have deteriorated emotional and physical well-being and ought to immediately seek psychological treatment and monitoring. Despite the intricacies of treating MDD, remission is still conceivable, particularly with antidepressants. As an upshot, diagnosing and treating UD is the need of an hour [83].

Types of Unipolar Depression

Unipolar depression can be prominent because of its distinctive circumstances irrespective of the condition, severity and duration of the illness. UD manifests in a plethora of forms, significantly altered by a range of variables and the manifestations are typically correlated. The primary forms of UD are detailed here, along with some of the major indications.

Anxious Depression

MDD coupled with "psychological anxiety" is referred to as anxious depression, characterised by substantial perceived stress departing from other psychiatric illnesses. In terms of pathophysiology, asymmetry in neural activity across the right and left hemispheres, specifically in the right frontal lobe, has been implicated in poor stress management in individuals suffering from AD [84].

Seasonal Affective Disorder

SAD, colloquially known as "Seasonal affective disorder", manifests itself during specified epochs of the year. The vast majority of individuals endure this predicament during the colder months when the hours extend and the temperature falls [85]. The severity and pattern of SAD signs are testified by the patient's contrasting behaviour. This may be exacerbated by undiagnosed psychological conditions or hormonal variations [86], usually in adolescence and early adulthood, accentuated further during certain seasons of the calendar [87].

The suprachiasmatic nuclei in the brain are considered to be the imaginary keeper of the biological circadian clock, to receive stimulus *via* the ganglion cells upon daylight perception. Later, successive impulses generated are passed to the pineal gland, which suppresses the melatonin release to culminate the wake cycle [88]. In addition, the serotonin signalling pathway is implicated in SAD, besides polymorphism associated with the 5-HTTLPR gene [89]. Thus, the main underlying driver force of SAD is a synergistic process coupled with melatonin misalignment and serotonin depletion in response to light cycles [90].

Postpartum Depression

Postpartum depression (PPD) or Maternal Depression is a predominant, moderate to severe psychological condition. This is underexplored and frequently overlooked in nearly 13% to 19% of childbearing women. This makes it one of the most widespread morbidities associated with pregnancy [91]. Maternal depression begins during the first three months of pregnancy due to hormonal variations, which can potentially stifle maternal-child communication and exacerbate bonding issues [92].

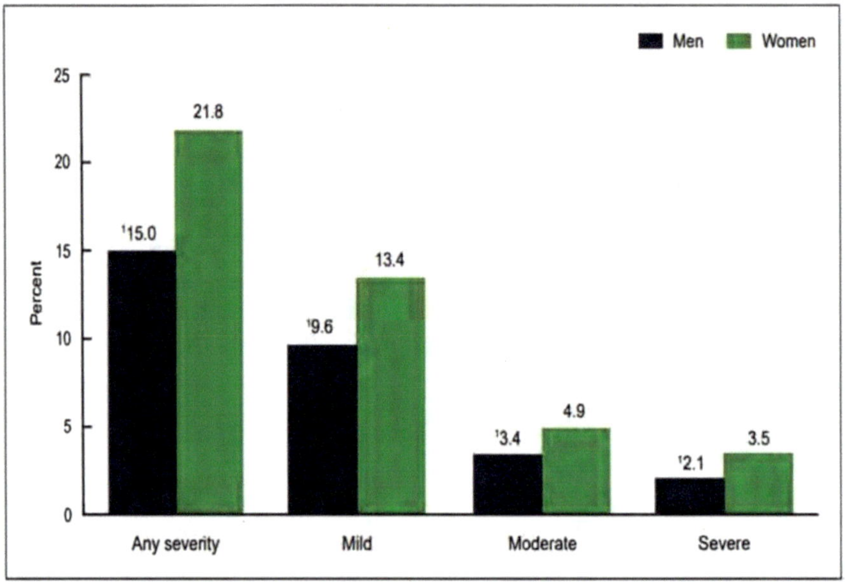

Fig. (2). Adapted from: National center for health statistics, national health interview survey, 2019.

Hormonal oscillations may play a significant role in the pathophysiology of postpartum mood disorders, characterised by hasty and profound hormonal variations, dysregulated peptides, and neurotrophic steroid production [93]. Prolonged PPD can also have severe repercussions both on the mother and child's well-being, resulting in a long-term impact on the child's cognitive, behavioural, and emotional growth. As a response, discovering the appropriate interventions for superlative maternal and neonate care is imperative. Novel revelations into the pathophysiology of PPD, along with cutting edge therapeutics, propose the outlook to proactively design the treatment options along with the augmentation of a medication regime [94].

Melancholic Depression

Melancholic depression is a "circuit sickness" epitomized by neurocircuit breakdown. MD has variably been alluded to as "intrinsic," "endogenous," "Type A," "autonomous," and "melancholic" depression [95]. It is categorized either as a much more chronic form of clinical depression or a distinct disease that seems to be more quintessentially physiological. In terms of clinical manifestations and probable aetiology, melancholy sometimes is also referred to as "neurotic" or "receptive" depression [96].

Melancholy has remained a distinct entity owing to its neuropsychiatric, physiological, and unpredictable treatment response. Antidepressant medications, including the Tricyclic antidepressants (TCA), electroconvulsive therapy (ECT), and other pharmacological interventions, are more effective on melancholic patients than selective serotonin reuptake inhibitors (SSRIs) [97]. In contrast to non-melancholic depression, melancholic depression occasionally responds to the placebo effect, interpersonal psychotherapy, or social interventions [98].

Abulia and psychomotor agitation are diagnostic biomarkers for MD that possibly will be distinctive in some individuals yet mild or non-existent in others. Melancholia has been clinically implicated with hypercortisolaemia, chronic insomnia, neuroimaging abnormalities, and alterations in circadian architecture [99]. This form of depression might emerge from a magnified perception of physical loss, which mainly impairs mood and cognitive integrity. Patients experiencing MD have a worse prognosis and a reduced risk of relapse compared to non-melancholic forms [98].

Catatonic Depression

Catatonia is a multifaceted neuropsychological cognitive condition epitomized by deteriorating schizophrenia, mania, or melancholy, headed by dissociative episodes [100]. In spite of owning the physiological capacity to move ordinarily, individuals with catatonia demonstrate a momentous loss of mobility, psychomotor agitation, or a blend of the two symptoms inextricably impeding critical functions [101].

Catatonia can foray abruptly or progressively, and manifestations typically fluctuate in intensity or switch over during bouts of atypical motions, stiffness, aberrant behaviour and seclusion [102]. A relapse of catatonia might emerge after consuming benzodiazepines or receiving ECT. These effects are reversed by NMDA antagonists such as amantadine and memantine [103]. Antipsychotics are infrequently prescribed, but they also come with risky adverse effects and, therefore might exacerbate symptoms and need medical assistance or motivational acquaintance.

Dysthymic Depression

Dysthymic disorder or Persistent Depressive Disorder (PDD) is a smouldering persistent state that persists for a minimum of two years and is preceded by transitory instants of normality in between. Robert Spitzer substituted this notion for "depressive personality" in 1970 and suggested PDD as a prevalent syndrome that can strike any individual, regardless of age. Although the aetiology of PDD is obscure, there are numerous indications that the disorder may be genetically programmed in response to a varied assortment of stressful events, implying a complicated pathophysiology [104].

PDD is indicated by pathological changes with clinical variability blighting the cognitive and physiological systems, compounding sad sensations with darkness [105]. In dysthymia patients, the amygdala, cingulate gyrus, and insula were found to be more engaged, culminating in dullness and impaired emotions coupled with HPA axis abnormalities and adrenal impairment [106]. Women suffering from PDD have distinct frontal lobe and corpus callosum architecture in comparison to normal women representing early neurological manifestations of PDD [107]. Although psychotherapy and pharmaceuticals can be employed to alleviate persistent depressive illness, the effectiveness and intensity of therapeutic response are marginally lower than in non-chronic depressive episodes, and a blend of medications and psychotherapy deliver the best outcomes [106]. Dysthymia exists in partial form with other psychiatric illnesses, especially co-occurrence of MDD with dysthymia is eluded as "double depression". It is a hallmark of cyclothymia, a mild form of bipolar illness when an individual fluctuates between episodes of dysthymic and hypomanic moods [108].

Bipolar Depression

Manic depression, often identified as bipolar illness, is a long-lasting psychological condition that causes considerable morbidity and imposes a substantial economic impact [109]. BD is the leading cause of chronic depression, which encompasses short spurts of abnormally elevated or irritable mood associated with episodes of anxiety, which typically lasts from a few days to a few weeks [110]. Mania and hypomania are two primary debilitating emotional elevations that typify bipolar disorder. Mania alludes to an intense altered state of mind accompanied by psychosis, whereas hypomanic episodes refer to a less severe illness [114]. In bipolar depression, anti-depressant responses are often suboptimal and frequently mistreated. Emerging therapies such as a multitude of anticonvulsants and modern psychotropic medications, besides employing lithium, alone or in unique combinations, are only partially effective in treating BD patients. Thus, studies towards more efficacious, targeted, and guarded treatments are required.

The prevalence of BD is pre-disposed by both inherited and environmental factors, which is estimated to be around 1.06% of the population. The determinants of BD include an enhanced risk of morbidity, persistence, and suicidal conduct. BD has a predictive correlation with recurring depression, and the therapeutic approach is typically ineffective in ensuring symptomatic alleviation [111]. Owing to the intricacy of BD's clinical presentation and the significant risk of misdiagnosis [113], it is imperative to diagnose BD precisely and manage it promptly. Furthermore, accurate assessment is essential to avoid misdiagnosis-related complications and delayed therapeutic intervention.

Manifestations

Bipolar disorder is a persistent clinical condition epitomized by severe alterations in mood, activity levels, and behaviour. This disorder is majorly prompted during adolescent and early adulthood [115] and is typified by episodes of no manifestation amid recurring bouts of mania, hypomania and depression [116]. In accordance with the DSM-5 criteria, the variation among manic and hypomanic events is determined by the extent of episodes. Hypomanic is prevalent if the sensation of elevated or irritability lasts for 4 days in a row, whereas manic is apparent if the symptoms last for more than one week. Mania is more severe than hypomania and leads to more significant issues like psychosis. Hypomania, in comparison to mania, is not necessarily preceded by reduced efficiency [118]. The signalling pathways underpinning this transition from a manic phase or a hypomanic phase to a depressive state, likewise, are currently unclear [117].

BD patients exhibit widely divergent indications reliant on the prevalence, intensity, and frequency of the symptoms [114]. Although some individuals switch equally across the two forms of episodes, other individuals are more susceptible either to depressive or manic episodes, enduring bouts of depression periodically or sporadically during their lifespan. The four specific forms of mood episodes that can emerge with BD are mania, hypomania, depression, and mixed episodes, and the indications for these episodes vary considerably [117].

Manic Episodes

Manic episodes denoted as mania, are a crucial component of bipolar disorder 1, defined as discrete periods with a minimum of one week of persistently elevated or agitated mood, composed of rapid fluctuations in emotions, thought processes and energetic intensity. Manic people may initially feel ecstatic, typically spiral out and engage in behaviours that affect them both psychologically and economically. Some manic patients also encounter delusions and become unrealistic, impatient and angry. Manic episode onset is usually preceded by sleep disturbances [119] and emerges as a consequence of long-term consumption of drugs as "self-medication." The Young Mania Rating Scale (YMR) is most commonly employed to gauge the degree of the disease and determines the severity of manic symptoms enlisted as under [120].

- The state of very high or extremely low emotions; this state can range from exhilaration to.
- Frequent and extreme emotional variations, such as transitioning from a pleasant to an enraged or aggressive condition.
- An upbeat attitude coupled by elation, brisk speech, restlessness, and intrusive thoughts.
- Impulsive behavioural tendencies as a consequence of increased vigour and decreased desire to sleep.
- An escalation in hyperactivity, poor decision making, and suicidal ideation with unrealistic ambitions.
- Enhanced grandiosity, obsessive thoughts, irresponsible and risk-taking conduct including substance misuse.
- An escalation in the frequency of psychomotor engagement associated with delusional thoughts and Hallucinations and, occasionally require psychiatric inpatient treatment.

Hypomanic Episodes

Hypomania is a milder variant of mania marked by the less intense episodes that typically continue for four days. Hypomanic episodes do not frequently cause the substantial difficulty in everyday activities. However, the stress experienced is excruciating. There have been sporadic reports of hypomanic depressed episodes, where hypomania progresses progressively to full-fledged manic states or is preceded by a severe depressive phase that might impair cognitive performance with multiple diagnostic traits enlisted as under [121].

- Absence of psychiatric indicators like delusions or hallucinations.
- Optimistic enhancement of cognitive behaviour during hypomanic episodes.
- Improved creativity escorted with agitated mood and impaired decision making.
- Lack of conception of the way others are impacted by their activities.
- Hypomanic states are not distressing, exclusive of changes that are uncontrollable or violent.

Depressive Episodes

The earliest couple of manic or hypomanic bouts that persist noticeably are bipolar depressive episodes that are erroneously diagnosed as MDD and deteriorate with time. The manifestations of bipolar illness during bouts of depression are comparable to those of severe depression. They entail [122] the following attributes.

- Acute melancholy, irritability, and nervousness.
- Loss of excitement coupled with thoughts of remorse and hopelessness.

- Variations in physical attributes, weight loss or gain, and appetite shifts.
- Low vitality and fatigue.
- Lack of determination and concentric challenges.
- Sentiments of worthlessness or self-loathing.
- Suicidal ideation.

Mixed Effective Episodes

Mixed effective episodes or a hybrid state is a condition when both maniacal and melancholic symptoms coexist. Individuals exhibiting suicidal ideology and behaviour, laterally with depressive episodes, are alleged to be at a higher risk. Panic attacks are substantially more prevalent as comorbidity in mixed episodes than in non-bipolar mania. A similar trend can be observed in substance abuse, suggesting that bipolar symptoms are predominantly the product of substance abuse [123]. The primary indications and features of mixed episodes encompass:

- Extravagant ideas coupled with manic and depressive traits like overwhelming guilt or suicidal opinions.
- Despondency-related emotions followed by panic disorder or impulsive actions.

Types of Bipolar Depression

Bipolar disorder is a mental and neurological health issue, can be diagnosed at any age, typically observed in adolescence or during early adulthood. Adolescents and young adults may endure unique substantial manic, hypomanic or depressive episodes, although the rhythm may differ from individual to individual. BD is diagnosed and categorised by the severity of the episodes, in addition to the highs and lows associated with disorder. Bipolar disorder is identified by the DSM-5 [125] and ICD-11 [124] as a range of diseases which oscillate over time and comprise five distinct subtypes, defined as follows:

Bipolar I Disorder

This is the most prominent and debilitating type of BD, epitomized by minimum of one manic event with an extent of 7 days, coupled either with or without depressed mood enduring noticeably for more than two weeks. Hypomanic or profound bouts of depression may occasionally occur before or during a manic episode. Mania may potentially result in psychosis with some depressive traits, or severe depression with the manic symptoms [126].

Bipolar II Disorder

Bipolar II is a distinct diagnosis, not a milder form of bipolar disorder. A unique aspect of bipolar II disorder is the switching between depressive episodes and less severe hypomanic episodes. However, a few individuals with bipolar II progress to develop bipolar I. Bipolar II disorder encompasses hypomanic and depressing phases, with at least one significant depressive episode and one hypomanic episode occurring over their lifespan. Bipolar II hypomanic episodes are less prevalent than depressive episodes and are sometimes misdiagnosed as MDD, manifested as periods of high efficiency [127].

Cyclothymic Disorder

Cyclothymia is a mild, unique form of bipolar illness that manifests as recurring mood alterations between hypomanic and depressive states during adolescence. It can persist a maximum of two years in adults and one year in children. The extremes and lows of cyclothymic disorder are not as intense as those of bipolar I and II to be designated as bipolar disorder episodes. Individuals with cyclothymic disorder display periods of normalcy interspersed with mania and depression, and it may escalate to bipolar 1 or bipolar 2 if untreated [128].

Unspecified Bipolar Disorder

Individuals diagnosed with some other recognized or unrecognized bipolar illness display threshold indications that elicit clinically substantial anxiety or dysfunction, need not to satisfy the DSM-5 or ICD-11 criteria, and are categorized into three subtypes:

Bipolar Disorder with Mixed Features

Bipolar disorder with "mixed episodes" manifests manic and depressed episodes simultaneously at the same time. Individuals with this condition might have high levels of energy and also have trouble sleeping, yet they could also be depressed or have suicidal ideation at the same time [129].

Bipolar with Seasonal Features

Depressive episodes can also progress in the autumnal or winter seasons, referred to as seasonal bipolar disorder. Individuals with bipolar I experience manic episodes in the late spring or early summer, whereas those who have bipolar II exhibit hypomanic episodes [131].

Bipolar with Rapid Cycling

It is a variant of bipolar illness marked by four or even more events of mood disruption, such as manic episodes, hypomania, or bouts of depression, over the span of a year. Rapid cycling is typically transient, with phases interrupted by periods of remission or reversal in mood polarity. There are relatively few pharmaceuticals for managing rapid cycling, and sufferers are typically more challenging to treat and significantly less responsive to medications than other BD sufferers [130].

NEUROBIOLOGY OF DEPRESSION, PATHOGENESIS AND IMPLICATED PATHWAYS

Depression is a terminal, nonhomogeneous progressive condition with societal and therapeutic repercussions that may be traced directly to its manifold aetiologies [131]. Because of the challenging availability of human brain tissues, neurochemical analysis and clinical variability evaluating the psychopathological condition of depression is difficult to explicate arguing for a coherent elucidation of the neurobiology of depression [132].

Pathophysiology of Depression

Neurotransmitters are at the vanguard of the brain, released and intercepted by bridges spanning across the neurons to mediate physiological interconnectivity in the central nervous system by eliciting impulses which modulate the serotonin, norepinephrine and Dopamine signalling pathways [133].

Serotonin (Happy Hormone)

The Raphe-Serotonin Mechanism modulates emotional expressions, anxiety, nervousness, circadian cycles and excitement. It maintains the process of homeostasis, emotional regulation and resilience to adverse experiences. The "Serotonin Theory" hypothesizes the decreased functioning of serotonergic circuits correlated with the pathophysiology of depression [134].

Dopamine (Motivation Messenger)

Dopamine mediates motivation and impulses in the hippocampus of the normal brain. Impaired dopaminergic signalling is correlated with decreased DA production from presynaptic nerve terminals or reduced cell signalling [135]. In contrast to healthy subjects, PET imaging trials on depressed patients exhibiting anhedonia revealed substantially reduced DA transporter (DAT) affinity. DAT dysfunction has similarly been correlated to incentive prediction, psychological excitation, and sensitivity to learned incentive stimuli implicated in severe depression [136].

Adrenaline (Promising Fix)

Norepinephrine augments concentration, attitude, and efficiency. Many studies specify the role of NE in modulating the locus coeruleus, which has been allied to emotional disorders, found to be implicated in Post-mortem brains from depressed patients and healthy controls, revealing substantial alterations in NE mechanisms stipulating the role of NE in the aetiology and treatment of depression [137].

Studies have reported inadequate levels of neurotransmitters and hormones implicated in depressive states with alterations in neural circuit crosstalk associated with the CNS [138]. Depression is correlated with dysfunctional neurotransmitters such as glutamate, dopamine, and gamma-aminobutyric acid (GABA), and alterations in neurocircuit, neurotrophic factors, and circadian rhythms [132]. The maladaptive behaviours discussed here thereby focus on the elements considered to be the heart of clinical depression [133].

Pathways Implicated

Mechanisms that disrupt the normal functioning of the human central nervous system are implicated in depression pathophysiology that, includes the following:

- Neurochemical Dysregulation
- Dysfunctional Cytokines
- Neuroendocrine Deregulation
- Neuroanatomic Dysfunction
- Predisposition to other Factors

Neurochemical Dysregulation

Monoamine Hypothesis (Biogenic Amine Hypothesis)

Monoaminergic circuits foster depression-related behavioural symptoms, such as melancholy, anxiety, reduced motivation, fatigue, and psychomotor agitation [139]. According to the monoamine-deficiency hypothesis, proposed three decades ago, the brain monoaminergic transmitters norepinephrine (NE), Serotonin and dopamine preponderate the midbrain and brainstem nuclei [140], displaying substantial extensions throughout the brain and are speculated to be biologically impaired in depression [141]. Dysregulation in neurotransmitter modulation at pre- and post-synaptic cleft contributes to impaired cognitive function, predisposing to the symptomatic aspects of depression [142, 143].

Antidepressant medications enhance serotonergic, dopaminergic, and noradrenaline synaptic concentrations [144]. Serotonin (5-hydroxytryptamine: 5HT) actuates the cortical regions and constitutes the brain's most prevalent integrated neurotransmitter network implicated in depression. Reduced tryptophan is correlated with deprived serotonin levels, which seems to be related to the pathophysiology of psychological distress [134]. Norepinephrine (NE) endorses behaviour and concentration primarily by modulating the efficacy of pre frontal cortex. This encodes cognitive function and is involved in the propagation of noradrenergic neurons outspreading from the brain stem to other areas of the brain [145]. Impairment in the noradrenergic system is speculated to be correlated with enhanced tyrosine hydroxylase activity, reduced norepinephrine metabolism and lowered density of NE transporter in the locus coeruleus [146]. Dopamine (DA) promotes incentive and emotion regulation, in addition to cognitive memory and focus. Dopamine re-uptake inhibitors (Nomifensine) and dopaminergic agonists (pramipexole) have shown significant antidepressant activity in placebo-controlled trials in MDD, implying implications in depressive patients [147].

Deficiency of Monoamine Oxidase (MAO)

Neurotransmitter biological impairments ascend as a consequence of degradation interceded by the enzyme monoamine oxidases in the synaptic space, reducing the bioavailability of biogenic amines [142]. Antidepressant medications augment monoamine reuptake, upsurge monoamine concentration in the synaptic cleft, and suppress the enzyme monoamine oxidase [148]. These results are consistent with the most pertinent monoamine-deficiency proposition for melancholy [149]. The application of MAO inhibitors as antidepressants is based on the notion that increasing the significantly reduced amounts of monoamines will reduce MDD [150]. Elevated neurotransmitter concentrations are also allied with a reduction in psychological distress [151], adding credence to the notion that monoamine deficiency might contribute to the progression of depression. Various neurotransmitters, such as glutamate, histamine and NE, interact to reduce substrate release triggered by depression's stress response.

Reduced Protein Functioning

Transport proteins play an indispensable role in cell-to-cell crosstalk, nerve-nerve connections, and monoaminergic propagation, facilitating presynaptic reuptake of neurotransmitters in normal brain activity [152]. Transport mechanisms regulate the multitude of neurotransmitters accessible in the synaptic cleft, minimizing the amount of neurotransmitter breakdown prompted by monoamine oxidase enzymes [145]. Studies have depicted serotonin dysregulation triggered by an upsurge in the predominance of monoamine oxidase, associated with decreased protein transporter functioning, indicating potential implications in the aetiology of depression [153].

Receptor Aberrations

Disparities in receptor activity culminate in aberrant neurotransmitter functioning, ultimately inducing depressive states [152]. Such aberrations may be prompted by altered downstream signalling cascades, inefficient or erroneous transmission, and impaired neurotransmitter-receptor coupling, typically driven by reduced receptor binding affinity or diminished receptor numbers. Countless bio-molecular studies have revealed the role of receptor imperfections, sensitivity of presynaptic 2-adrenoceptors, modulation in cerebral production of NE and alterations in the quantity and affinity of serotonin receptors especially (5-HT1 and 5-HT2) in depressed individuals [154], showing new targets for therapy [155]. The serotonin-1A receptor thatpredominantly coordinates serotonergic activity, is the clearest indication for serotonin receptor anomalies in depression, with substantially reduced levels in MDD patients [156].

A distinctive possible consequence of depression appears to be the loss of function in the gene encoding the specific enzyme tryptophan hydroxylase-2 [157]. Post-mortem studies from the brains of depressive individuals who committed suicide revealed lower locus coeruleus neuronal densities, reduced alpha-1 adrenergic receptor mass and increased alpha-2 adrenergic receptor richness [158]. Disparities in the G-protein receptors and kinases have also been implicated in the aetiology of depressive states [159]. The monoamine systems constitute the principal targets of all approved antidepressants [160]. Yet, the complete or partial resilience to these medications and the sluggish onset of effectiveness indicate that malfunctioning monoaminergic schemes are only indirect upshots of MDD. Despite this limitation, the paradigm has emerged as the most therapeutically relevant neurological explanation for depression.

Neuroendocrine Deregulation

A multitude of hormonal anomalies show substantial drivers concerning neuroendocrine circuit imbalance and depressive aetiology under two main principal assumptions:

Neurotrophic Hypothesis of Depression

This theory is an offshoot of the “Monoamine Hypothesis of Depression,” emphasizing on hippocampal degeneration, decreased neuroplasticity with reduced BDNF expression in the brain as a consequence of imperfect Pro BDNF-receptor complex setting off apoptotic proteins inducing Long Term Depression (LTD). On the contrary, the formation of the intricate mBDNF-receptor complex excites synapses to mediate Long Term Potentiation (LTP), enhancing the survival mechanisms essential for maintaining neuronal plasticity and proliferation.

Brain-derived neurotrophic factor (BDNF) is severely implicated in depressed responses associated with low hippocampal BDNF levels. However, BDNF upregulation is perceived following pharmaceutical intervention [161]. Severe depression has been allied to hippocampus atrophy, augmented stress sensitivity, and an increased risk of relapse [162]. Reduced neurotrophic components, decreased neurogenesis, glutamatergic excitotoxicity, and glucocorticoid impairment are putative causes of brain volume reduction in depressive episodes, resulting in decreased BDNF production in the hippocampus inducing atrophy.

Endocrine Implications

A plethora of anomalies allied with the endocrine system potentially influence the aetiology of depression. These comprise aberrant thyroid function and elevated concentrations of growth hormone (GH) [163], as specified below.

Growth Hormones (GH)

GH has been studied for their putative role in the onset of depressive symptoms [145]. Catecholaminergic pathways are compromised in depression [164], inducing flat GH expression in depressive subjects, arbitrated by an inherent defect in the GH system. Animal studies have shown the implication of GH hormone that correlates with morbidly depressive behaviour. However, the exact pathophysiology is obscure [165].

Thyroid Hormones

The bioactive isoforms of thyroid hormones, T3(tri-iodothyronine) and T4(tetra-iodothyronine) are synthesised following the stimulation by Thyroid Stimulating Hormone (TSH). The hypothalamic hormone, Thyrotropin Releasing Hormone (TRH), oversees THS secretion and modulates the overall metabolism of the human body by regulating the levels of T3 and T4 [166]. Reports have depicted that variations in hormonal levels may have an impact on the onset of depressive symptoms [167]. Aberrant thyroid function may be the origin of certain psychological issues, specifically weight loss, agitation, and anxiety [168]. T3 serves as an affective ancillary treatment [169], augmenting cortical 5HT exudation, assuming the intervention of the serotoninergic and adrenergic frameworks. However, the specific mechanism of hormonal anomalies allied with the genesis of depression remains uncertain [170].

Hypothalamus Pituitary Adrenal Dysfunction (HPA)

The hypothalamic-pituitary dysfunction is an altered mechanism implicated in 20-30% of cases of profound depression. Depression has been allied to Corticotrophin Releasing factor (CRF) and cortisol hypersecretion, ineffective glucocorticoid feedback systems, deficient HPA axis modulation and altered corticosteroid receptor signalling (CRF) [171]. CRF modulates the functioning of the HPA axis [172]. Pituitary corticotropic (ACTH) is secreted in response to stressful events and stimulates the discharge of Corticotropin-releasing hormone (CRH) from the hypothalamus, which prompts the adrenal gland to produce cortisol into the plasma [173]. CRF is a neurotransmitter that chiefly integrates stress-related cognitive, autonomic, hormonal, and inflammatory responses. It is also expressed in non-hypothalamic regions of the brain, alluding to the involvement of CRF in the emergence of depression [174].

Depressed people display pre-eminent CRH levels in the cerebrospinal fluid [175]. Post-mortem studies revealed an augmented proportion of CRH-releasing neurons in limbic regions of depressed patients and diminished CRF receptors in PFC, inferring a compensatory reflex to elevated CRH concentrations [176]. In depressive subjects, CRH induces a plethora of behavioural and physiological aberrations, including weakened appetite, poor sleep, libido loss, and psychomotor shifts [177]. The CRH stimulation assay (also referred to as the dex/CRH test) has little specificity for MDD despite being a sensitive indicator of HPA axis impairment in depressive episodes [178].

Dysfunctional Cytokines

Lymphoid cells are the chief producers of biochemical inflammatory signals referred to as cytokines in response to pathogenic antigens [179]. Cytokines encompass interferons (INF), inflammatory mediators, interleukins (IL), the colony-stimulating factor, the tumour necrosis factor (TNF), serum amyloid proteins and C- reactive elements correlated with the emergence of depression. Diverse theories have been postulated concerning the straight and secondary implications of interleukins (IL-1, IL-2, IL-4, IL-6, IL-8, IL-10), interferon-gamma and chemokine monocyte protein 1in the aetiology of depression [180].

Depressive inflammatory responses predispose to certain manifestations, including fatigue, melancholy, perceptual allowing and cognitive deficits, referred to as "sickness behaviour. "Pro-inflammatory cytokines like TNF, IL-1and IL-6 are supposed to be mediators of central serotonin impairment [152]. Antidepressant-like effects have been observed in mice after the suppression of pro-inflammatory cytokines, suggesting their implication in a subset of depressive populations suffering from comorbid illness [155].

Neuroanatomic Dysfunction

MDD patients display impaired cognitive activity in the cerebellar, lateral frontal and temporal cortices of the brain [181]. Intervention with a serotonin reuptake inhibitor augmented activity in brain regions that had previously indicated signs of progressive decline [182]. Parallel alterations could occur in the striatum, ventromedial frontal areas, and presumably other subcortical regions [183]. In MDD-related anomalies, the ventromedial PFC, specifically the orbitofrontal region and the left anterior cingulate, exhibited significant volumetric losses [184]. Moderate volume reduction was also observed in the Hippocampal, striatal and lateral PFC regions of the brain [181]. Post-mortem studies have shown a decrease in the number of glia cells in the dorsal, orbital, and subgenual prefrontal cortices and amygdala [183, 184]. This was particularly apparent with a volume loss in this area [185].

Individuals with cortical brain injuries displayed aberrant physiological responses to external stimuli [186]. Therapies such as deep neural stimulation potentially target specific sections of the brain, showing positive developments and depicting the potential of neuropsychological data, which could be exploited to envisage the probability of responses to explicit treatments [188].

Neuroinflammation

Manifold epidemiological provisions that induce neuroinflammation in the brain comprise, autoimmune systemic lupus erythematosus, brain injury, and multiple sclerosis, which are typically linked to significant rates of major depression, indicating the relationship between neuroinflammation and major depression [189]. Peripheral pro-inflammatory cytokines traversing the BBB aggravate neuroinflammation and induce psychological distress [190]. Thus, recognising specific biomarkers exclusively neurological in genesis implies a more prominent influence on exploring the role of neuroinflammation in depressive aetiologies.

Neuroinflammation in specific areas of the brain culminates in cognitive behaviours mimicking MDD pathophysiology depicting a correlation between chronic depression and inflammation [191]. Translocator Protein Density (TSPO VT) levels upsurge during microglial stimulation in the PFC, insula and anterior cingulate cortex, depicting the presence of neuroinflammatory changes or reflexes during depressive episodes [192].

Neurogenesis

Neurogenesis, or neuronal growth, is the genesis of radically new-fangled neurons and synaptic acquaintances amid the hippocampus's dentate gyrus and the lateral ventricle's sub ventricular regions [193]. Impaired neuroplasticity as a consequence of several diseases predisposes to anxiety characteristics, culminating in volumetric deterioration of hippocampal structure and functioning [194]. Numerous antidepressant therapies comprising MAO reuptake inhibitors, SSRIs, ECT, Mood stabilisers and TCAs specifically enhance the process of neurogenesis by significantly decreasing ceramide concentrations, a lipid moiety that suppresses cell growth in the brain, subsequently enhancing neuronal cell proliferation [195]. Even though multiple antidepressants function independently of neurogenesis, still neurogenic process remains a crucial component in comprehending the pathophysiology and management of depression [196].

Predisposition to other Factors

Genetic Factors

Studies have found that the inheritance of psychological disorders does not imitate a reliable circadian rhythm; therefore, upholding just one inheritable trait does not substantially decrease the likelihood of mental illnesses ascending within the close circle [197]. MDD impressions include both the hereditary element and severity, directly influenced by underlying biological factors. A specific genetic variation in the gene promoter of the serotonin transporter encompasses stressful situations leading to anxiety [198]. There is less evidence of the serotonin transporter gene, either alone or in conjunction with other genes, which induces disease manifestations, despite the strong scientific and neurobiological plausibility of this association. However, it has been particularly challenging to recognize pertinent modifications in mental diseases employing robust gene mapping [199].

Environment Influences

The heterogeneity in the propensity to MDD is interceded by specific environmental parameters such as gene environmental implications and erroneous impacts [200]. Environmental variables are mediated by immunological reactions, and chromosomal variances induce severe metabolic fluctuations across neural circuits, culminating in disrupted neurogenesis and neurotoxicity, ultimately manifested as the assortment of symptoms referred to as depression [201]. MDD manifestations are predisposed by adverse developmental experiences and continuous or former anxiety from psychosocial adversity, such as sexual assault, severe long-term trauma, minimal social interaction, marriage strife, and separation.

Gender Specificity

Psychological responsiveness in melancholy is predominantly gender-specific. Both genders are relatively susceptible to the depressogenic consequences of traumatic incidents. Individual sensitivities vary conditionally based on the level of distress. Menfolk are far more inclined to experience depressive bouts after divorce, separation, and work-related issues. However, women are more susceptible to catastrophes in their immediate social circle, chronic sickness or mortality and mostly postpartum depression [202]. This highlights the significance of gender-responsive psychosocial strategies in the diagnosis and conduct of MDD.

Several heritable traits, such as environmental elements, immune-mediated factors, cellular proliferation, a deficiency of monoamine oxidase, and hormonal fluctuations, influence the pathophysiology of depression. Moreover, comparatively low efficacy and long remission time of anti-depressive medications indicate the emergence of a unified elucidation of depression. This suggests that depression is a diagnostic and aetiologically pluralistic condition. Therefore, integrating genomics and biomarkers studies for cross-functional and cross-variability in stress susceptibility and psychopharmacological action will certainly assist in enhancing the responsiveness of individual therapeutic elements.

Therapeutic Interventions

Depression is among the most curable psychiatric conditions, yet, it is stigmatised, and treatment is predicated on the intensity and complexity of the manifestations. Untreated depression can persist for months or even years and result in a diverse range of negative repercussions in a given situation. The intensity of depressive bouts determines the pattern of depression treatment. To effectively alleviate depression, it is imperative to seek medical treatment [203]. When opposed to mild depression, moderate depression has a significant impact on life, whereas severe depression appears to be more intricate and makes the experience challenging [204].

Understanding the disease, implementing lifestyle modifications, and undergoing psychotherapy can all assist in alleviating moderate symptoms. For mild to profound depression, pharmaceutical interventions may be necessitated in addition to these other therapies [205]. Neurostimulation could be an alternative therapeutic option if such approaches are ineffectual at improving symptoms. In milder cases of depression, psychotherapy alone may be employed as the initial line of treatment, supplemented with pharmaceuticals if required. Many mental health professionals employ multiple-line combinational therapies enlisted for managing depressive patients [203].

Therapies

Therapy is the ideal course of action for treating anxiety and depression. Pharmaceuticals should only be used in conjunction with the former if an individual suffers from severe depression or is unresponsive to therapy independently. The following are the various counselling modalities to treat mental illness.

Psychotherapy

The phrase "psychotherapy," "talk therapy," or "psychological treatments" applies primarily to conferring depression and associated complications with a psychologist. Psychological therapies have proven to be an effective approach to relieve the symptoms by recognizing and altering negative beliefs and practices. These approaches encourage individuals to examine the patterns that lead to melancholy and encourage innovative ideas in analysing the trends that predispose them to depression [206]. Psychotherapy assists in the management of behaviour, the enhancement of delight, and the resolution of social and psychological challenges. Multiple psychotherapeutic models, encompassing evidence-based and pseudoscience-based approaches, have been designed to address established mental health issues and depressive behaviour [207].

Cognitive Behaviour Therapy (CBT)

Behaviour therapy, usually referred to as cognitive behavioural therapy (CBT) or behavioural activation, is a collective term for psychiatric therapeutic interventions that integrate behavioural psychology or cognitivism. Behaviour therapy employs a combination of strategies instead of just one approach to address depressed and anxious moods, enabling patients to comprehend, challenge, evaluate, and alter detrimental cognitive habits and attitudes [208]. Current revelations in CBT include the merging of contemplation ideas and the design of specific programs that explicitly target illnesses such as sleeplessness and other associated depressive manifestations [209].

Interpersonal Therapy (IPT)

IPT is a rapid, emotional treatment that emphasizes symptomatic treatment and the reconciliation of interpersonal conflicts. IPT is intended to assist people in confronting emergencies that may be exacerbating or deteriorating mental mood by enhancing communication [210].

Emotionally Focussed Therapy

An assortment of closely interrelated psychotherapeutic modalities, stated as emotion-focused treatment (EFT) or emotionally focused therapy (EFT), decreases anxiety by diagnosing and alleviating sensitive states. This is the core principle of EFT therapies, which are predicated on the premise that emotions and feelings are inextricably associated with human needs [211].

Acceptance and Commitment Therapy

ACT is an awareness-based CBT with cognitive diagnostic underpinnings, and may be more productive than the conventional CBT, explicitly when anxiousness is predominant and refractory to classical CBT. It is an empirically corroborated therapeutic intervention that endorses psychological resilience by integrating approaches to motivational and behavioural patterns [212].

Psychodynamic psychotherapy

This therapy is a combination of multifaceted thoughts and therapeutic approaches with a unique societal and interpersonal orientation that highlights the reconciliation of unconscious mental confrontations and is employed to manage patients experiencing mild to severe depression [213].

Medical Procedures

Brain stimulators, also denoted as neuromodulators, are one of the therapeutic approaches currently explored for the treatment of depressive disorders in individuals, unresponsive to medication or psychotherapy. Electrical or magnetic waves are employed in neurostimulation therapy to directly stimulate or repress the brain. Individuals suffering from severe depression or melancholy combined with psychosis potentially benefit from below mentioned brain stimulation intervention:

Electroconvulsive Therapy

Electroconvulsive therapy or ECT, is a prevalent psychological treatment that chiefly entails shooting electrical impulses across the brain to modify neurotransmitter interaction and function by eliciting immediate anticonvulsant effects primarily in the anterior and medial temporal lobes of the brain. ECT is used as a last resort therapy for severely depressed patients, those with unipolar or bipolar depression who have refractory phases and individuals who are at high risk of committing suicide [214].

ECT characteristically comprises manifold sessions, often administered twice or thrice weekly under anaesthetic effect in blend with relaxant to alleviate depressive symptoms. Three conceivable executions of ECT have emerged. This involves sensor positioning, treatment intensity, and electrotherapy, with notable variations in both negative side effects and symptom remission. Given the possibility of complications like dizziness, nauseous, disorientation, and impaired memory, pharmaceutical therapy is frequently maintained after ECT [215].

Transcranial Magnetic Stimulation (TMS)

The unobtrusive approach to TMS (Transcranial magnetic stimulation) or (DTMS) Deep Transcranial Magnetic Stimulation employs electromagnetism to stimulate specific sections of the brain [216]. Periodic magnetic waves stimulate brain cells, retaining magnetic fields to alleviate psychological anguish. TMS is characteristically cast off when other antipsychotic therapies prove to be ineffective [217].

TMS, also referred to as rTMS or repetitive TMS was approved by the FDA in 2008 for the control of depressive bouts. TMS's negative effects incorporate dizziness and convulsions, in addition to distress, pain, manic episodes, behavioural impairment, sensory impairment, and inadvertent circuit activation in implantable devices like defibrillators or pacemakers [218].

Vagus Nerve Stimulation (VNS)

VNS, broadly identified as the brain's pacemaker, is a form of neuromodulation that modifies nerve function. This process directly stimulates the nervous system in the neck to deliver periodic, moderate electrical impulses to the brainstem. The interplay of the brain cells is altered when charged particles pass through the brainstem and are distributed to particular areas of the brain to induce transmission [219].

The treatments of depressive disorders in patients who have experienced either partial improvement or relapse with conventional therapeutic approaches are subjected to VNS. Vagus nerve stimulation serves as a feasible therapy for a variety of pathologies, such as inflammatory arthritis, intestinal disease, bipolar disorder, obesity, and Alzheimer's disease. This is also employed in treatment-resistant epilepsy, treatment-resistant depression (TR-MDD) and super refractory epilepticus [220].

Pharmaceutical Interventions

The pharmaceutical drug intervention, cast-off in appropriate proportions and diverse combinations, is the mainstay of treating depression. There is no specific effective antidepressant; instead, the optimal one varies on medical history and symptomology, drug type and the individualized needs. Antidepressants primarily contribute to ensuring the proper equilibrium of the brain's neurotransmitters, such as norepinephrine, dopamine, and serotonin. Typically, decreased levels of psychological distress are correlated with higher levels of these neurotransmitters. Antidepressant medication can combat depression by enhancing neurotransmitter levels. However, their effectiveness varies depending on a person's response to drugs, the drug's half-life, and the mode of action. Presently, there are six distinct pharmacotherapy types that can be employed to treat psychological disorders, which are given hereunder.

Selective Serotonin Reuptake Inhibitors (SSRIs)

SSRIs are frequently directed antidepressants to manage severe depression, nervousness, and other associated psychological disorders. SSRIs augment the neurotransmitter serotonin's cytoplasmic level and have substantial selectivity for the serotonin transporter by suppressing its re-uptake into the presynaptic terminal [221]. SSRIs are the utmost extensively implemented drugs because of fewer detrimental consequences, comprehensive impressions, and an abridged probability of accidental overdose. Sertraline, Fluoxetine, paroxetine and citalopram are the most broadly used SSRIs, either separately or in combinational therapy for MDD subjects. However (SSRIs) may be upshot in the following undesirable consequences [222].

- Agitation coupled with fatigue, anxiousness, and sleeplessness.
- Persistent diarrhoea, dry mouth, and vomiting.
- Frequent headaches, tremors while feeling lightheaded.

Serotonin and Noradrenaline Reuptake Inhibitors (SNRIs)

SNRIs are basically the monoamine reuptake antagonists, an arrangement of antidepressant medication cast-off to treat a wide array of disorders encompassing Major depressive disorder, panic disorder, anxiety symptoms, attention deficit hyperactivity disorder (ADHD), obsessive-compulsive disorder (OCD) and fibromyalgia syndrome (FMS) symptoms as well as persistent neuropathic pain [223]. The absorption of neurotransmitters implicated in mood regulation is suppressed by SNRIs. The reuptake of norepinephrine and serotonin from the synaptic gap into the postsynaptic nerve ending is accomplished by the mammalian integral membrane transporters encompassing the serotonin transporter (SERT) and noradrenaline transporters (NAT) alleviating by concurrently decreasing serotonin and noradrenaline reuptake. Commonly employed SNRIs include Desvenlafaxine, Venlafaxine and Duloxetine, with the following possible negative effects [224].

- Pervasive Headaches with disorientation.
- Profuse sweating, nausea. and dry mouth.
- Constipation and bloating.
- Insomnia

Tricyclic Antidepressants (TCAs)

TCAs are the first antipsychotics endorsed for the treatment of MDD, alluded to as the second line of prescription drugs after SSRIs. Unfortunately, TCAs have been substantially replaced by relatively new antidepressants such as SSRIs, SNRIs, and norepinephrine in diagnosis and therapy, yet they are still effective in managing treatment-resistant depression as compared to contemporary antipsychotics [225]. Majorly employed TCAs include amitriptyline, imipramine and nortriptyline, having few negative consequences enlisted as under [226].

- Difficulties in urination, incontinence, and dry mouth.
- Ocular fogginess, excessive fatigue, and sleepiness.
- Dizzy spells, shivering, and an elevated heart rate.
- Increasing weight with a dysfunctional metabolism.

Monoamine Oxidase Inhibitors (MAOIs)

MAOIs are a group of medications that suppress the functioning of the monoamine oxidase A (MAO-A) and monoamine oxidase B (MAO-B) enzymes. These are universally acknowledged to be effective antipsychotics, notably for the management of panic disorder, interpersonal anxiety symptoms, Parkinson's disease, and a variety of other maladies. Newer pharmaceuticals in this class (RIMA) have been designed with a milder profile of side effects and enhanced potency in the wake of the fact that monoamine oxidase inhibitors have a history of doubtful performance and potentially fatal adverse events [227].

A subclass of MAOIs classified as rescindable inhibitors of monoamine oxidase A (RIMAs) suppress the MAO-A enzyme preferentially. RIMAs are widely used for the treatment of dysthymia and emotions of hopelessness. Since their irrevocability, these are much less severe in single-drug misuse and more efficacious at boosting monoamine levels that are significant in psychiatric illnesses [228]. Phenelzine, tranylcypromine, and isocarboxazid are some instances of MAOIs with few possible side effects:

- Fatigue, vertigo, and headaches.
- Increasing weight and urinary issues.
- High levels of perspiration and reduced blood pressure.
- Constipation or diarrhoea coupled with persistent nausea.

Norepinephrine and Dopamine Reuptake Inhibitors (NDRIs)

NDRIs are prescribed to alleviate a multitude of “off-prescription” psychiatric conditions comprising nervousness, bipolar disorder, and hyperactivity disorder as well as severe depression and seasonal affective disorders (ADHD). The only pharmaceutical in this subcategory is bupropion, which is marketed under the trademark Wellbutrin, with a few of its recognised detrimental consequences [229].

- Chronic headache and sleeplessness.
- Parched mouth and sweaty.
- Convulsions while vomiting, tiredness, and loose stools.

Non-competitive N-methyl-D-aspartate Receptor Antagonists

NMDA receptor blockers are a subclass of medications that function as an anaesthetic to diminish NMDA receptor functionality (NMDAR) by inducing dissociative anaesthesia typified by Extrapyramidal symptoms, amnesia, and analgesia. Impaired NMDA receptor activity has been associated with a number of negative consequences. These include memory deficits induced by ageing that may be predominantly induced by NMDA receptor hypofunction, which develops disproportionately as the brain grows [230].

NMDA antagonists have exhibited substantial promise in the treatment of neurotoxic conditions such as concussion, cerebrovascular illness, and neurodegenerative disarrays comprising Parkinson's, Alzheimer's, and Huntington disease and are currently being explored for anti-depressive potential [231]. Furthermore, ketamine displays abiding antidepressant properties following clinical administration. In 2019, the NMDA blocker enantiomer of ketamine was accepted to be used as an antipsychotic in the United States for individuals suffering from depression who had botched to respond to standard therapies. Spravato (esketamine), a non-competitive NMDA blocker, is accessible as a nasal spray given with an antidepressant drug. Esketamine has the budding for exploitation and misuse and has been correlated to a higher probability of suicidal attitudes and behaviours with the below mentioned side effects [232].

- Dizzy spells, sedation, and nauseous.
- Elevated blood pressure, agitation, and tiredness.
- Dissociative symptoms (temporal, spatial, and perception deformation).

Challenges and Future Prospects

The therapeutic management of depressive episodes presently has significant flaws, minimal efficiency, poor safety profile, pharmacokinetic interrelations, low recovery and remission, evidenced by the astonishingly high rate of non-responsiveness and resistance to medications even after successive antipsychotic trials [233]. New approaches and pathophysiological paradigms are therefore obligated to exploit the multifaceted neurotransmitter pathways implicated in depressive disorders. Furthermore, a new generation of speculative pharmaceuticals, spanning from triple reuptake inhibitors to antipsychotic drugs, is being explored in severely depressed patient populations [2234], depicting optimism for novel therapeutics to enhance the response rate of these patients by uncovering alternative pathogenetic pathways.

The aforementioned new speculative pharmaceuticals currently undergoing trials for antidepressant potential are given hereunder [236].

A. Molecules in the pipeline targeting the MAO pathway.

S. no	Name of drug	Targeted pathway
1	Ansofaxine	Triple reuptake inhibitor of SE, NE,DA
2	Edivoxetine	NE reuptake inhibitor
3	SEP-4199	Non racemic amisulpride
4	Psilocybin	5HT2A receptor antagonist
5	Min-117	Orexin receptor modulators
6	Pimavanserin	5HT2A receptor antagonist
7	Cariprazine	Atypical antipsychotic

B. Molecules in the pipeline for inhibiting the C0X2 pathway and anticytokine therapies.

S. no	Name of drug	Targeted pathway
1	Ustekinumab	Human IgG1 monoclonal antibody
2	Infliximab	Chimeric Mouse/Human IgG1 monoclonal antibody
3	Ixekizumab	Humanized IgG monoclonal antibody
4	Losmapimod	Selective p38 MAPK inhibitor
6	Adalimumab	Human IgG1 monoclonal antibody
7	Etanercept	TNF inhibitor

C. Molecules in the pipeline acting as orexin receptor antagonists

S. no	Name of drug	Targeted pathway
1	Seltorexant (Min-202)	OX2 receptor antagonist

D. Neurosteroid analogues and GABA-A modulators in the pipeline.

S. no	Name of drug	Targeted pathway
1	Brexanolone	Positive allosteric modulator of intra and inter-synaptic GABA-A receptors
2	PRAX-114	Positive allosteric modulator of extrasynaptic GABA-A receptors
3	Zuranolone	Neuroactive steroid modulating GABA-A receptor

cont.....

S. no	Name of drug	Targeted pathway
4	Ganaxolone	Allopregnanolone analogue serves as an allosteric positive modulator of GABA-A

CONCLUSION

Depression represents the most significant, persistent and treatable psychiatric condition encompassing several complicated processes with moderate and transitory consequences. The prognosis of depression is quite difficult, therefore, comprehending depressive facets is critical for the proper diagnosis and management. There are legitimate and effective treatment options, like targeted approaches, that have a substantial influence on enhancing diagnosis and increasing treatment frequencies.

As the stigma around psychological health is now being confronted on a global basis, it is vital for us to put a spotlight on the negative consequences associated with depression. The preceding section provides an overview of the various processes implicated in underpinning the neurobiology of depression and the effect of population heterogeneity, chronology of symptom onset, a predilection for negative life events, and required therapeutic approaches. This is important as we move on from the COVID-19 fallout since many more people went through depression and other psychological illnesses. With these details, it becomes clear that the development of precision medicine useful for depression has to address all the issues discussed in this chapter. However, when once we succeed, like other diseases, depression too may be treated in a precise manner. Clearly, a search for more specific drug molecules and an exploration of herbal formulations will go a long way to ameliorate neurological disorders. In the meantime, a healthy lifestyle, positive attitude, regular exercise and plant-based food coupled with nuts and fruits may be considered to keep the body and mind fit and fine.

REFERENCES

[1] Prince M, Patel V, Saxena S, *et al.* No health without mental health. Lancet 2007; 370(9590): 859-77. [http://dx.doi.org/10.1016/S0140-6736(07)61238-0] [PMID: 17804063]

[2] Charles J. Lynch, Faith M. Gunning, Conor Liston, Causes and Consequences of Diagnostic Heterogeneity in Depression: Paths to Discovering Novel Biological Depression Subtypes. Biological Psychiatry 2020; 83-94. [http://dx.doi.org/10.1016/j.biopsych.2020.01.012]

[3] Akil Huda, Gordon Joshua, Hen Rene, *et al.* Nestler, Treatment resistant depression: A multi-scale, systems biology approach. Neuroscience & Biobehavioural Reviews 2018; 84: 27288. [http://dx.doi.org/10.1016/j.neubiorev.2017.08.019]

[4] Global, regional, and national incidence, prevalence, and years lived with disability for 310 diseases and injuries, 1990–2015: a systematic analysis for the Global Burden of Disease Study 2015 Vos, Theo *et al.* The Lancet, Volume 388, Issue 10053, 1545 – 1602.

[5] The Lancet Commission on global mental health and sustainable development Patel, Vikram *et al.* The

Lancet, :392(10157) pp.1553–1598.

[6] Global, regional, and national burden of 12 mental disorders in 204 countries and territories, 1990–2019: a systematic analysis for the Global Burden of Disease Study 2019 The Lancet Psychiatry, Volume 9, Issue 2, 137 - 150.

[7] Available from: https://worldpopulationreview.com/country-rankings/depression-rates-by-country

[8] Global prevalence and burden of depressive and anxiety disorders in 204 countries and territories in 2020 due to the COVID-19 pandemic. 2020.

[9] Available from: https://www.nimh.nih.gov/health/statistics/major-depression

[10] Symptoms of Depression Among Adults: United States, 2019 Maria A. Villarroel, Ph.D., and Emily P. Terlizzi, M.P.H. NCHS Data Brief , No. 379 , September 2020.

[11] Available from: https://www.cdc.gov/nchs/nhis.htm

[12] Perou R, Bitsko RH, Blumberg SJ, *et al.* Mental health surveillance among children – United States. 2013; 62: 1-35.

[13] Bitsko RH, Claussen AH, Lichtstein J, *et al.* Surveillance of Children's Mental Health : United States, 2013 : 2019. MMWR 2022; 71 (2): 1-42.

[14] Ghandour RM, Sherman LJ, Vladutiu CJ, *et al.* Prevalence and treatment of depression, anxiety, and conduct problems in U.S. children. The Journal of Pediatrics, 2018. Published online before print. 2018.

[15] Dunn V, Goodyer IM. Longitudinal investigation into childhood-and adolescence-onset depression: Psychiatric outcome in early adulthood. Br J Psychiatry 2006; 188(3): 216-22. [http://dx.doi.org/10.1192/bjp.188.3.216] [PMID: 16507961]

[16] Thapar A, Collishaw S, Pine DS, Thapar AK. Depression in adolescence. Lancet 2012; 379(9820): 1056-67. [http://dx.doi.org/10.1016/S0140-6736(11)60871-4] [PMID: 22305766]

[17] Racine N, McArthur BA, Cooke JE, Eirich R, Zhu J, Madigan S. Global Prevalence of Depressive and Anxiety Symptoms in Children and Adolescents During COVID-19. JAMA Pediatr 2021; 175(11): 1142-50. [http://dx.doi.org/10.1001/jamapediatrics.2021.2482] [PMID: 34369987]

[18] Geir Scott B, Jasmina Burdzovic A. Increase in time spent on social media is associated with modest increase in depression, conduct problems, and episodic heavy drinking. J Adolesce 2019; 74.

[19] Comsa M, Anderson KN, Sharma A, Yadav VC, Watson S. The relationship between sleep and depression and bipolar disorder in children and young people. BJPsych Open 2022; 8(1): e27. [http://dx.doi.org/10.1192/bjo.2021.1076] [PMID: 35027099]

[20] Kroenke K, Strine TW, Spitzer RL, Williams JBW, Berry JT, Mokdad AH. The PHQ-8 as a measure of current depression in the general population. J Affect Disord 2009; 114(1-3): 163-73. [http://dx.doi.org/10.1016/j.jad.2008.06.026] [PMID: 18752852]

[21] Alexopoulos GS, Buckwalter K, Olin J, Martinez R, Wainscott C, Krishnan KRR. Comorbidity of late life depression: An opportunity for research on mechanisms and treatment. Biol Psychiatry 2002; 52(6): 543-58. [http://dx.doi.org/10.1016/S0006-3223(02)01468-3] [PMID: 12361668]

[22] Blazer DG. Depression in late life: review and commentary. J Gerontol A Biol Sci Med Sci 2003; 58(3): M249-65. [http://dx.doi.org/10.1093/gerona/58.3.M249] [PMID: 12634292]

[23] Butters MA, Becker JT, Nebes RD, *et al.* Changes in cognitive functioning following treatment of late-life depression. Am J Psychiatry 2000; 157(12): 1949-54. [http://dx.doi.org/10.1176/appi.ajp.157.12.1949] [PMID: 11097959]

[24] Wu Q, Feng J, Pan C-W. Risk factors for depression in the elderly: An umbrella review of published meta-analyses and systematic reviews. Journal of Affective Disorders, 2022; 307: 37-45. [http://dx.doi.org/10.1016/j.jad.2022.03.062]

[25] United Nation. Ageing UN 2019. Available from: https://www.un.org/en/global-issues/ageing (Accessed October 15 2019).

[26] World Health Organization (WHO). World report on ageing and health. 2015.

[27] World Health Organization. Aging and health. Available online: Available from: https://www.who.int/news-room/factsheets/detail/ageing-and-health (Accessed 4 Oct 2021).

[28] Botoseneanu A, Allore HG, Mendes de Leon CF, Gahbauer EA, Gill TM. Sex differences in concomitant trajectories of self-reported disability and measured physical capacity in older adults. J Gerontol A Biol Sci Med Sci 2016; 71(8): 1056-62. [http://dx.doi.org/10.1093/gerona/glw038] [PMID: 27071781]

[29] Joan S. Kaite Yang, Gender and depression. Current Opinion in Psychology 2015; 4: 53-60. [http://dx.doi.org/10.1016/j.copsyc.2015.01.019]

[30] Girgus J, Yang K, Ferri C. The Gender Difference in Depression: Are Elderly Women at Greater Risk for Depression Than Elderly Men? Geriatrics 2017; 2(4): 35. [http://dx.doi.org/10.3390/geriatrics2040035] [PMID: 31011045]

[31] Hyde Janet S, Mezulis Amy H. Gender differences in depression: Biological, affective, cognitive, and sociocultural factors. Harvard Rev Psych 2020; 28(1): 4-13. [http://dx.doi.org/10.1097/HRP.0000000000000230]

[32] Mojtabai R, Olfson M, Han B. National trends in the prevalence and treatment of depression in adolescents and young adults. Pediatrics 2016; 138(6): e20161878. [http://dx.doi.org/10.1542/peds.2016-1878] [PMID: 27940701]

[33] Wiens K, Williams JVA, Lavorato DH, *et al.* Is the prevalence of major depression increasing in the Canadian adolescent population? Assessing trends from 2000 to 2014. J Affect Disord 2017; 210: 22-6. [http://dx.doi.org/10.1016/j.jad.2016.11.018] [PMID: 28012349]

[34] Haroz EE, Ritchey M, Bass JK, *et al.* How is depression experienced around the world? A systematic review of qualitative literature. Social Science & Medicine 2017; 183: 151-62. [http://dx.doi.org/10.1016/j.socscimed.2016.12.030]

[35] Zimmerman M, Ellison W, Young D, Chelminski I, Dalrymple K. How many different ways do patients meet the diagnostic criteria for major depressive disorder? Comprehensive Psychiatry 2015; 56: 29-34.

[36] Santor DA, Gregus M, Welch A. FOCUS ARTICLE: Eight Decades of Measurement in Depression. Measurement 2006; 4(3): 135-55. [http://dx.doi.org/10.1207/s15366359mea0403_1]

[37] Hedlund JL, Viewig BW. The Hamilton rating scale for depression: a comprehensive review. J Oper Psychiatr 1979; 10: 149-65.

[38] Hamilton M. Assessment of change in psychiatric state by means of rating scales. Proc R Soc Med 1966; 59(Suppl 1) (Suppl.): 10-3. [PMID: 5922401]

[39] Hamilton M. Development of a rating scale for primary depressive illness. British Journal of Social and Clinical Psychology 1967; 6(4): 278-96. [http://dx.doi.org/10.1111/j.2044-8260.1967.tb00530.x]

[40] Hamilton M. Standardised assessment and recording of depressive symptoms. Psychiatria, Neurologia, Neurochirurgia 1969; 72(2): 201-5.

[41] Hamilton M. Rating depressive patients. J Clin Psychiatry 1980; 41(12 Pt 2): 21-4. [PMID: 7440521]

[42] Firestone RW, Firestone LA. Firestone Assessment of Self-Destructive Thoughts Manual. San Antonio, TX: Psychological Corporation 1996.

[43] Firestone RW, Firestone LA. Firestone Assessment of Self-Destructive Thoughts Manual. San Antonio, TX: Psychological Corporation 1996.

[44] Wechsler H, Grosser GH, Busfield BL Jr. Jr (1963) The depression rating scale: a quantitative approach to the assessment of depressive symptomatology. Arch Gen Psychiatry 1963; 9(4): 334-43. [http://dx.doi.org/10.1001/archpsyc.1963.01720160024003] [PMID: 14045262]

[45] Raskin A, Schulterbrandt J, Reatig N, McKeon JJ (1969). "Replication of factors of psychopathology in interview, ward behavior and self-report ratings of hospitalized depressives". Journal of Nervous and Mental Disease. 148 (1): 87–98. 1969. [http://dx.doi.org/10.1097/00005053-196901000-00010]

[46] Inventory of Depressive Symptomatology (IDS) & Quick Inventory of Depressive Symptomatology (QIDS) Archived 2007-06-26 at the Wayback Machine in IDS/QIDS: Instruments in English and Multiple Translations by the University of Pittsburgh Epidemiology Data Center, 2008. Retrieved June 27, 2008. 2008.

[47] Psychiatric Rating Scales for Depression in www.neurotransmitter.net website by Shawn M. Thomas. Retrieved June 30, 2008.

[48] Boyle GJ. Self report measures of depression: Some psychometric considerations. British Journal of Clinical Psychology 1985; 24: 45-9. [http://dx.doi.org/10.1111/j.2044-8260.1985.tb01312.x]

[49] Hamilton M. A rating scale for depression. J Neurol Neurosurg Psychiatry 1960; 23: 56-62.

[50] Bagby RM, Ryder AG, Schuller DR, Marshall MB. The Hamilton Depression Rating Scale: Has the gold standard become a lead weight? Am J Psychiatry 2004; 161(12): 2163-77. [http://dx.doi.org/10.1176/appi.ajp.161.12.2163] [PMID: 15569884]

[51] Zimmerman M, Martinez JH, Young D, Chelminski I, Dalrymple K. Severity classification on the Hamilton depression rating scale. J Affect Disord 2013; 150(2): 384-8. [http://dx.doi.org/10.1016/j.jad.2013.04.028] [PMID: 23759278]

[52] Tabuse H, Kalali A, Azuma H, *et al.* The new GRID Hamilton Rating Scale for Depression demonstrates excellent inter-rater reliability for inexperienced and experienced raters before and after training, Psychiatry Research, 2007; 153(1): 61-7. [http://dx.doi.org/10.1016/j.psychres.2006.07.004]

[53] Lin CH, Park C, McIntyre RS. Early improvement in HAMD-17 and HAMD-7 scores predict response and remission in depressed patients treated with fluoxetine or electroconvulsive therapy. J Affect Disord 2019; 253: 154-61. [http://dx.doi.org/10.1016/j.jad.2019.04.082] [PMID: 31035216]

[54] Williams JBW, Kobak KA. Development and reliability of a structured interview guide for the Montgomery-Åsberg Depression Rating Scale (SIGMA). Br J Psychiatry 2008; 192(1): 52-8. [http://dx.doi.org/10.1192/bjp.bp.106.032532] [PMID: 18174510]

[55] Relationship Between the Hamilton Depression Rating Scale and the Montgomery–Åsberg Depression Rating Scale in Depressed Elderly: A Meta-analysis from the American Journal of Geriatric Psychiatry

[56] Test: Montgomery-Åsberg Depression Rating Scale (MADRS) in BioPsychoSocial Assessment Tools for the Elderly - Assessment Summary Sheet. The University of Western Ontario, London, Ontario, Canada. In turn citing: 2015.

[57] Fish J. Raskin Rating Scale. In: Kreutzer JS, DeLuca J, Caplan B, Eds. Encyclopedia of Clinical Neuropsychology. New York, NY: Springer 2011.

[http://dx.doi.org/10.1007/978-0-387-79948-3_1960]

[58] Beck AT. Depression: Causes and treatment. Philadelphia: University of Pennsylvania Press 1972; p. 333.

[59] "Beck Depression Inventory — 2nd Edition". Nova Southeastern University Center for Center for Psychological Studies. Archived from the original on 2008.

[60] Yesavage JA. Geriatric Depression Scale. Psychopharmacol Bull 1988; 24(4): 709-11. [PMID: 3249773]

[61] Katz IR (1998). "Diagnosis and treatment of depression in patients with Alzheimer's disease and other dementias. The Journal of Clinical Psychiatry 1998; 59(9): 38-44.

[62] Zung WWK. A self-rating depression scale. Arch Gen Psychiatry 1965; 12(1): 63-70. [http://dx.doi.org/10.1001/archpsyc.1965.01720310065008] [PMID: 14221692]

[63] Spitzer RL, Kroenke K, Williams JB. Validation and utility of a self-report version of PRIME-MD: the PHQ primary care study. Primary Care Evaluation of Mental Disorders. Patient Health Questionnaire. JAMA 1999; 282(18): 1737-44. [http://dx.doi.org/10.1001/jama.282.18.1737] [PMID: 10568646]

[64] World Health Organization. Archived from the original on 2014.

[65] The ICD-10 Classification of Mental and Behavioural Disorders. Clinical descriptions and diagnostic guidelines 1992.

[66] World Health Organization. Archived from the original on 2013.

[67] classification-of-diseases Available from: www.who.int

[68] Editorial. The Lancet 2019; 393: 2275. [http://dx.doi.org/10.1016/S0140-6736(19)31205-X]

[69] Reed GM, First MB, Kogan CS, Hyman SE, Gureje O, Gaebel W, *et al.* Innovations and changes in the ICD-11 classification of mental, behavioural and neurodevelopmental disorders. World Psychiatry 2019; 18(1): 3-19. [http://dx.doi.org/10.1002/wps.20611]

[70] Joyce-Beaulieu D, Sulkowski ML. The Diagnostic and Statistical Manual of Mental Disorders 2016. [http://dx.doi.org/10.1007/978-1-4899-7996-4_8]

[71] Wakefield JC. DSM-5: An Overview of Changes and Controversies. Clinical Social Work Journal 2013; 41(2): 139-54. [http://dx.doi.org/10.1007/s10615-013-0445-2]

[72] American Psychiatric Association. Diagnostic and Statistical Manual of Mental Disorders. 4th ed, Text Revision., Washington, DC: American Psychiatric Association 2000.

[73] Angst J, Sellar R, Merikangas KR. Depressive spectrum diagnoses. Compr Psychiatry 2000; 41(2) (Suppl. 1): 39-47. [http://dx.doi.org/10.1016/S0010-440X(00)80007-3] [PMID: 10746903]

[74] Diagnostic APA. and Statistical Manual of Mental Disorders 2000.

[75] Sullivan PF, Kessler RC, Kendler KS. Latent class analysis of lifetime depressive symptoms in the national comorbidity survey. Am J Psychiatry 1998; 155(10): 1398-406. [http://dx.doi.org/10.1176/ajp.155.10.1398] [PMID: 9766772]

[76] Tucci V, Moukaddam N. We are the hollow men: The worldwide epidemic of mental illness, psychiatric and behavioral emergencies, and its impact on patients and providers. J Emerg Trauma Shock 2017; 10(1): 4-6. [http://dx.doi.org/10.4103/0974-2700.199517] [PMID: 28243005]

[77] Kumar K, Gupta M. Clinical and socio-demographic determinants of psychological health and burden

in family caregivers of patients with unipolar depression. Asian Journal of Psychiatry, 2014; 9: 51-6. [http://dx.doi.org/10.1016/j.ajp.2014.01.002]

[78] Siegel-Ramsay JE, Bertocci MA, Wu B, Phillips ML, Strakowski SM, Almeida JRC. Distinguishing between depression in bipolar disorder and unipolar depression using magnetic resonance imaging: A systematic review. Bipolar Disord 2022; 24(5): 474-98. [http://dx.doi.org/10.1111/bdi.13176] [PMID: 35060259]

[79] MitchellPB.MalhiGS.Bipolar depression. phenomenological overview and clinical characteristics Bipolar Disord

[80] Benazzi F. Family history validation of a definition of mixed depression. Compr Psychiatry 2005; 46(3): 159-66. [http://dx.doi.org/10.1016/j.comppsych.2004.07.034] [PMID: 16021584]

[81] National Collaborating Centre for Mental Health (UK). 2010.

[82] The ICD-10 Classification of Mental and Behavioural Disorders – Clinical Descriptions and Diagnostic Guidelines. Geneva: WHO 1992.

[83] Pariante CM, Nemeroff CB. Unipolar depression. Handb Clin Neurol 2012; 106: 239-49. [http://dx.doi.org/10.1016/B978-0-444-52002-9.00014-0] [PMID: 22608625]

[84] Hamilton M. A rating scale for depression. J Neurol Neurosurg Psychiatry 1960; 23(1): 56-62. [http://dx.doi.org/10.1136/jnnp.23.1.56] [PMID: 14399272]

[85] National Institute of Mental Health. U.S. Department of Health and Human Services. Seasonal affective disorder Available from: https://www.nimh.nih.gov/health/publications/seasonal-affectiv--disorder (Accessed: October 22, 2022).

[86] Roecklein KA, Wong PM. Seasonal affective disorder. Encyclopedia of Behavioral Medicine. 2013; pp. 1722-4. [http://dx.doi.org/10.1007/978-1-4419-1005-9_836]

[87] Mayo Clinic. Mayo Foundation for Medical Education and Research 2021.https://www.mayoclinic.org/diseases-conditions/seasonal-affecti-e-disorder/symptoms-causes/syc-20364651

[88] Pfizer. The science behind the winter blues. Available from: https://www.pfizer.com/news/articles/the_science_behind_the_winter_blues (Accessed: October 22, 2022).

[89] Rosenthal NE, Sack DA, Jacobsen FM, *et al.* Melatonin in seasonal affective disorder and phototherapy. J Neural Transm Suppl 1986; 21: 257-67. [PMID: 3462335]

[90] Terman M, Amira L, Terman JS, Ross DC. Predictors of response and nonresponse to light treatment for winter depression. Am J Psychiatry 1996; 153(11): 1423-9. [http://dx.doi.org/10.1176/ajp.153.11.1423] [PMID: 8890675]

[91] American College of Obstetricians and Gynecologists Committee on Obstetric Practice. Committee Opinion No. 630. Obstet Gynecol 2015; 125(5): 1268-71. [http://dx.doi.org/10.1097/01.AOG.0000465192.34779.dc] [PMID: 25932866]

[92] Martins C, Gaffan EA. Effects of early maternal depression on patterns of infant-mother attachment: A meta-analytic investigation. J Child Psychol Psychiatry 2000; 41(6): 737-46. [http://dx.doi.org/10.1111/1469-7610.00661] [PMID: 11039686]

[93] Postpartum depression. MedlinePlus. 2016. Available from: https://medlineplus.gov/ency/article/007215.htm (Accessed January 11, 2017).

[94] Brummelte S, Galea LAM. Postpartum depression: Etiology, treatment and consequences for maternal care, Hormones and Behavior 2016; 77: 153-66. [http://dx.doi.org/10.1016/j.yhbeh.2015.08.008]

[95] McGrath PJ, Khan AY, Trivedi MH, *et al.* Response to a selective serotonin reuptake inhibitor (citalopram) in major depressive disorder with melancholic features: a STAR*D report. J Clin Psychiatry 2008; 69(12): 1847-55.
[http://dx.doi.org/10.4088/JCP.v69n1201] [PMID: 19026268]

[96] Monzón S, Gili M, Vives M, *et al.* Melancholic versus non-melancholic depression: differences on cognitive function. A longitudinal study protocol. BMC Psychiatry 2010; 10(1): 48.
[http://dx.doi.org/10.1186/1471-244X-10-48] [PMID: 20565743]

[97] Perry P. Pharmacotherapy for major depression with melancholic features: relative efficacy of tricyclic versus selective serotonin reuptake inhibitor antidepressants. J Affect Disord 1996; 39(1): 1-6.
[http://dx.doi.org/10.1016/0165-0327(96)00014-6] [PMID: 8835647]

[98] McGrath PJ, Khan AY, Trivedi MH, *et al.* Response to a selective serotonin reuptake inhibitor (citalopram) in major depressive disorder with melancholic features: A STAR*D report. J Clin Psychiatry 2008; 69(12): 1847-55.
[http://dx.doi.org/10.4088/JCP.v69n1201] [PMID: 19026268]

[99] Leventhal A, Rehm L. The empirical status of melancholia: Implications for psychology. Clin Psychol Rev 2005; 25(1): 25-44.
[http://dx.doi.org/10.1016/j.cpr.2004.09.001] [PMID: 15596079]

[100] Burrow Jeffrey P, Spurling Benjamin C, Marwaha Raman. Catatonia. StatPearls 2022.

[101] Zisselman MH, Jaffe RL. ECT in the treatment of a patient with catatonia: consent and complications. Am J Psychiatry 2010; 167(2): 127-32.
[http://dx.doi.org/10.1176/appi.ajp.2009.09050703] [PMID: 20123920]

[102] Fink M, Taylor MA. The catatonia syndrome: forgotten but not gone. Arch Gen Psychiatry 2009; 66(11): 1173-7.
[http://dx.doi.org/10.1001/archgenpsychiatry.2009.141] [PMID: 19884605]

[103] Fink M, Taylor MA. Catatonia: A Clinician's Guide to Diagnosis and Treatment. Cambridge University Press 2003.
[http://dx.doi.org/10.1017/CBO9780511543777]

[104] Dysthymia. Harvard Health Publications. Harvard University. February 2005. Archived from the original (February 2005 issue of the Harvard Mental Health. 2005.

[105] American Psychiatric Association. Diagnostic and Statistical Manual of Mental Disorder. 5th ed. Washington, DC: American Psychiatric Publishing 2013; pp. 168-71.

[106] Ravindran AV, Smith A, Cameron C, *et al.* Toward a functional neuroanatomy of dysthymia: A functional magnetic resonance imaging study. Journal of Affective Disorders 2009; 119(1-9): 9-15.
[http://dx.doi.org/10.1016/j.jad.2009.03.009]

[107] Lyoo In Kyoon, Kwon Jun Soo, Lee Soo Jin, Han Moon Hee, Chang Chang-Gok, Seo Cheon Seok. Decrease in genu of the corpus callosum in medication-naïve, early-onset dysthymia and depressive personality disorder. Biological Psychiatry 2002; 52(12): 1134-43.
[http://dx.doi.org/10.1016/S0006-3223(02)01436-1]

[108] Double Depression: Hopelessness key component of mood disorder. Science Daily 2007.

[109] Anderson IM, Haddad PM, Scott J. Bipolar disorder. BMJ. 2012.
[http://dx.doi.org/10.1136/bmj.e8508]

[110] American Psychiatry Association. Diagnostic and Statistical Manual of Mental Disorders. 5th ed. Arlington: American Psychiatric Publishing 2013; pp. 123-54.

[111] Xue C, Zhang X, Cao P, Yuan Q, Liang X. Chaoyong Xiao,Evidence of functional abnormalities in the default mode network in bipolar depression: A coordinate-based activation likelihood estimation meta-analysis. Journal of Affective Disorders 2023; 0165-327.
[http://dx.doi.org/10.1016/j.jad.2023.01.088]

[112] Clemente AS, Diniz BS, Nicolato R, *et al.* Bipolar disorder prevalence: A systematic review and meta-analysis of the literature. Rev Bras Psiquiatr 2015; 37(2): 155-61. [http://dx.doi.org/10.1590/1516-4446-2012-1693] [PMID: 25946396]

[113] Woo YS, Shim IH, Wang HR, Song HR, Jun TY, Bahk WM. A diagnosis of bipolar spectrum disorder predicts diagnostic conversion from unipolar depression to bipolar disorder: A 5-year retrospective study. J Affect Disord 2015; 174: 83-8. [http://dx.doi.org/10.1016/j.jad.2014.11.034] [PMID: 25486276]

[114] Anderson IM, Haddad PM, Scott J. Bipolar disorder 2012. [http://dx.doi.org/10.1136/bmj.e8508]

[115] Goodwin FK, Jamison KR. Manic–depressive illness: bipolar disorders and recurrent depression. 2nd ed., Oxford University Press 2007.

[116] Chen CH, Suckling J, Lennox BR, Ooi C, Bullmore ET. A quantitative meta-analysis of fMRI studies in bipolar disorder. Bipolar Disord 2011; 13(1): 1-15. [http://dx.doi.org/10.1111/j.1399-5618.2011.00893.x] [PMID: 21320248]

[117] Salvadore G, Quiroz JA, Machado-Vieira R, Henter ID, Manji HK, Zarate CA. The neurobiology of the switch process in bipolar disorder: A review. The Journal of Clinical Psychiatry 2010; 71(11): 1488-501. [http://dx.doi.org/10.4088/JCP.09r05259gre]

[118] Grande I, Berk M, Birmaher B, Vieta E. Bipolar disorder. Lancet 2016; 387(10027): 1561-72. [http://dx.doi.org/10.1016/S0140-6736(15)00241-X]

[119] McKenna BS, Eyler LT. Overlapping prefrontal systems involved in cognitive and emotional processing in euthymic bipolar disorder and following sleep deprivation: A review of functional neuroimaging studies. Clin Psychol Rev 2012; 32(7): 650-63. [http://dx.doi.org/10.1016/j.cpr.2012.07.003] [PMID: 22926687]

[120] Titmarsh S. Characteristics and duration of mania: implications for continuation treatment. Progress in Neurology and Psychiatry 2013; 17(3): 26-7. [http://dx.doi.org/10.1002/pnp.283]

[121] Beentjes TAA, Goossens PJJ, Poslawsky IE. Caregiver burden in bipolar hypomania and mania: a systematic review. Perspect Psychiatr Care 2012; 48(4): 187-97. [http://dx.doi.org/10.1111/j.1744-6163.2012.00328.x] [PMID: 23005586]

[122] Carvalho AF, Firth J, Vieta E. 2020; Bipolar Disorder. N Engl J Med 383(1): 58-66. [http://dx.doi.org/10.1056/NEJMra1906193]

[123] Swann AC, Lafer B, Perugi G, *et al.* Bipolar mixed states: An international society for bipolar disorders task force report of symptom structure, course of illness, and diagnosis. Am J Psychiatry 2013; 170(1): 31-42. [http://dx.doi.org/10.1176/appi.ajp.2012.12030301] [PMID: 23223893]

[124] ICD-11 for Mortality and Morbidity Statistics. World Health Organization 2019; 60-2.

[125] American Psychiatry Association. Diagnostic and Statistical Manual of Mental Disorders. 5th ed. Arlington: American Psychiatric Publishing 2013; pp. 123-54.

[126] Barnett JH, Smoller JW. The genetics of bipolar disorder. Neuroscience 2009; 164(1): 331-43. [http://dx.doi.org/10.1016/j.neuroscience.2009.03.080] [PMID: 19358880]

[127] Renk K, White R, Lauer BA, McSwiggan M, Puff J, Lowell A. Bipolar disorder in children. Psychiatry J 2014; 2014(928685): 1-19. [http://dx.doi.org/10.1155/2014/928685] [PMID: 24800202]

[128] Van Meter AR, Youngstrom EA, Findling RL. Cyclothymic disorder: A critical review. Clin Psychol Rev 2012; 32(4): 229-43. [http://dx.doi.org/10.1016/j.cpr.2012.02.001] [PMID: 22459786]

[129] American Psychiatry Association. Diagnostic and Statistical Manual of Mental Disorders. 5th ed. Arlington: American Psychiatric Publishing 2013; pp. 123-54.

[130] Angst J, Sellaro R. Historical perspectives and natural history of bipolar disorder. Biological Psychiatry Review 2000; 48(6): 445-57.
[http://dx.doi.org/10.1016/S0006-3223(00)00909-4]

[131] Brigitta B. Pathophysiology of depression and mechanisms of treatment. Dialogues Clin Neurosci 2002; 4(1): 7-20.
[http://dx.doi.org/10.31887/DCNS.2002.4.1/bbondy] [PMID: 22033824]

[132] Angst J. How recurrent and predictible is depressive illness?Long-Term Treatment in Depression. New York, NY: John Wiley 1992; pp. 29-39. [Google Scholar]

[133] Hasler G. Pathophysiology of depression: Do we have any solid evidence of interest to clinicians? World Psychiatry 2010; 9(3): 155-61.
[http://dx.doi.org/10.1002/j.2051-5545.2010.tb00298.x] [PMID: 20975857]

[134] Cowen PJ, Browning M. What has serotonin to do with depression? World Psychiatry 2015; 14(2): 158-60.
[http://dx.doi.org/10.1002/wps.20229] [PMID: 26043325]

[135] Dunlop BW, Nemeroff CB. The role of dopamine in the pathophysiology of depression. Arch Gen Psychiatry 2007; 64(3): 327-37.
[http://dx.doi.org/10.1001/archpsyc.64.3.327] [PMID: 17339521]

[136] Tamura T, Sugihara G, Okita K, *et al.* Dopamine dysfunction in depression: Application of texture analysis to dopamine transporter single-photon emission computed tomography imaging. Transl Psychiatry 2022; 12(1): 309.
[http://dx.doi.org/10.1038/s41398-022-02080-z] [PMID: 35922402]

[137] Briley M, Chantal M. The importance of norepinephrine in depression. Neuropsychiatr Dis Treat 2011; 7 (Suppl. 1): 9-13.
[http://dx.doi.org/10.2147/NDT.S19619] [PMID: 21750623]

[138] McCance KL, Huether SE. Pathophysiology: The Biological Basis for Disease in Adults and Children. 7th ed., St. Louis, MO: Elsevier 2014.

[139] Atzori M, Cuevas-Olguin R, Esquivel-Rendon E, *et al.* Locus ceruleus norepinephrine release: A central regulator of cns spatio-temporal activation? Front Synaptic Neurosci 2016; 8(25): 25.
[http://dx.doi.org/10.3389/fnsyn.2016.00025] [PMID: 27616990]

[140] Coppen A. The biochemistry of affective disorders. Br J Psychiatry 1967; 113(504): 1237-64.
[http://dx.doi.org/10.1192/bjp.113.504.1237] [PMID: 4169954]

[141] Delgardo P, Morena F. Neurochemistry of mood disorders. In: Stein DK, Kupfer DJ, Schatzberg AF, Eds. The textbook of mood disorders. Washington, DC: American Psychiatric Publishing Inc 2006; pp. 101-16.

[142] Brigitta B. Pathophysiology of depression and mechanisms of treatment. Dialogues Clin Neurosci 2002; 4(1): 7-20.
[http://dx.doi.org/10.31887/DCNS.2002.4.1/bbondy] [PMID: 22033824]

[143] Belmaker RH, Agam G. Major depressive disorder. N Engl J Med 2008; 358(1): 55-68.
[http://dx.doi.org/10.1056/NEJMra073096] [PMID: 18172175]

[144] Maletic V, Eramo A, Gwin K, Offord SJ, Duffy RA. The role of norepinephrine and its α-adrenergic receptors in the pathophysiology and treatment of major depressive disorder and schizophrenia: A systematic review. Front Psychiatry 2017; 8: 42.
[http://dx.doi.org/10.3389/fpsyt.2017.00042] [PMID: 28367128]

[145] Maletic V, Eramo A, Gwin K, Offord SJ, Duffy RA. The role of norepinephrine and its α-adrenergic receptors in the pathophysiology and treatment of major depressive disorder and schizophrenia: A

systematic review. Front Psychiatry 2017; 8: 42.
[http://dx.doi.org/10.3389/fpsyt.2017.00042] [PMID: 28367128]

[146] Charney DS, Manji HK. Life stress, genes, and depression: multiple pathways lead to increased risk and new opportunities for intervention. Sci STKE 2004.
[http://dx.doi.org/10.1126/stke.2252004re5]

[147] Goldberg JF, Burdick KE, Endick CJ. Preliminary randomized, double-blind, placebo-controlled trial of pramipexole added to mood stabilizers for treatment-resistant bipolar depression. Am J Psychiatry 2004; 161(3): 564-6.
[http://dx.doi.org/10.1176/appi.ajp.161.3.564] [PMID: 14992985]

[148] Stahl SM. Basic psychopharmacology of antidepressants, part 1: Antidepressants have seven distinct mechanisms of action. J Clin Psychiatry 1998; 59(4) (Suppl. 4): 5-14.
[PMID: 9554316]

[149] Neumeister A, Konstantinidis A, Stastny J, *et al.* Association between serotonin transporter gene promoter polymorphism (5HTTLPR) and behavioral responses to tryptophan depletion in healthy women with and without family history of depression. Arch Gen Psychiatry 2002; 59(7): 613-20.
[http://dx.doi.org/10.1001/archpsyc.59.7.613] [PMID: 12090814]

[150] Ramesh M, Dokurugu YM, Thompson MD, Soliman ME. Therapeutic, molecular and computational aspects of novel monoamine oxidase (mao) inhibitors. Comb Chem High Throughput Screen 2017; 20(6): 492-509.
[PMID: 28294055]

[151] Yamana M, Atake K, Katsuki A, *et al.* Blood biological markers for prediction of escitalopram response in patients with major depressive disorder: Preliminary study. J Depress Anxiety 2016; 5(2): 1-3.
[http://dx.doi.org/10.4172/2167-1044.1000222]

[152] Owens MJ, Nemeroff CB. Role of serotonin in the pathophysiology of depression: Focus on the serotonin transporter. Clin Chem 1994; 40(2): 288-95.
[http://dx.doi.org/10.1093/clinchem/40.2.288] [PMID: 7508830]

[153] Lesch KP, Wolozin BL, Murphy DL, Riederer P. Primary structure of the human platelet serotonin uptake site: Identity with the brain serotonin transporter. J Neurochem 1993; 60(6): 2319-22.
[http://dx.doi.org/10.1111/j.1471-4159.1993.tb03522.x] [PMID: 7684072]

[154] Jacobsen JPR, Krystal AD, Krishnan KRR, Caron MG. Adjunctive 5-Hydroxytryptophan slow-release for treatment-resistant depression: Clinical and preclinical rationale. Trends Pharmacol Sci 2016; 37(11): 933-44.
[http://dx.doi.org/10.1016/j.tips.2016.09.001] [PMID: 27692695]

[155] Hrdina PD, Bakish D, Ravindran A, Chudzik J, Cavazzoni P, Lapierre YD. Platelet serotonergic indices in major depression: up-regulation of 5-HT2A receptors unchanged by antidepressant treatment. Psychiatry Res 1997; 66(2-3): 73-85.
[http://dx.doi.org/10.1016/S0165-1781(96)03046-6] [PMID: 9075272]

[156] Drevets WC, Frank E, Price JC, *et al.* Pet imaging of serotonin 1A receptor binding in depression. Biol Psychiatry 1999; 46(10): 1375-87.
[http://dx.doi.org/10.1016/S0006-3223(99)00189-4] [PMID: 10578452]

[157] Zhang X, Gainetdinov RR, Beaulieu JM, *et al.* Loss-of-function mutation in tryptophan hydroxylase-2 identified in unipolar major depression. Neuron 2005; 45(1): 11-6.
[http://dx.doi.org/10.1016/j.neuron.2004.12.014] [PMID: 15629698]

[158] Pandey GN, Dwivedi Y. Noradrenergic function in suicide. Arch Suicide Res 2007; 11(3): 235-46.
[http://dx.doi.org/10.1080/13811110701402587] [PMID: 17558608]

[159] Duman RS, Malberg J, Thome J. Neural plasticity to stress and antidepressant treatment. Biol Psychiatry 1999; 46: 1181-91.

[160] Stahl SM. Mechanism of action of serotonin selective reuptake inhibitors. J Affect Disord 1998; 51(3): 215-35.
[http://dx.doi.org/10.1016/S0165-0327(98)00221-3] [PMID: 10333979]

[161] Martinowich K, Manji H, Lu B. New insights into BDNF function in depression and anxiety. Nat Neurosci 2007; 10(9): 1089-93.
[http://dx.doi.org/10.1038/nn1971] [PMID: 17726474]

[162] Frodl TS, Koutsouleris N, Bottlender R, *et al.* Depression-related variation in brain morphology over 3 years: effects of stress? Arch Gen Psychiatry 2008; 65(10): 1156-65.
[http://dx.doi.org/10.1001/archpsyc.65.10.1156] [PMID: 18838632]

[163] Hoehe M, Valido G, Matussek N. Growth hormone response to clonidine in endogenous depressive patients: Evidence for a trait marker in depression. In: Shagass C, Josiassen RC, Bridger WH, Weiss KJ, Stoff D, Simpson GM, Eds. Proceedings of the IVth World Congress of Biological Psychiatry. 862-5.

[164] Matussek N. Catecholamines and mood: Neuroendocrine aspects. Current Topics in Neuroendocrinology 1988; 8: 141-82.
[http://dx.doi.org/10.1007/978-3-642-72738-2_6]

[165] Mullur R, Liu YY, Brent GA. Thyroid hormone regulation of metabolism. Physiol Rev 2014; 94(2): 355-82.
[http://dx.doi.org/10.1152/physrev.00030.2013] [PMID: 24692351]

[166] Chiamolera MI, Wondisford FE. Minireview: Thyrotropin-releasing hormone and the thyroid hormone feedback mechanism. Endocrinology 2009; 150(3): 1091-6.
[http://dx.doi.org/10.1210/en.2008-1795] [PMID: 19179434]

[167] Hage MP, Azar ST. The link between thyroid function and depression. J Thyroid Res 2012; 8.

[168] Peng R, Li Y. Low serum thyroid-stimulating hormone levels are associated with lipid profile in depressive patients with long symptom duration. J Affect Disord 2017; 217: 99-104.
[http://dx.doi.org/10.1016/j.jad.2017.03.055] [PMID: 28395210]

[169] Cooper R, Lerer B. [The use of thyroid hormones in the treatment of depression]. Harefuah 2010; 149(8): 529-534, 550, 549. [Hebrew].
[PMID: 21341434]

[170] Gordon JT, Kaminski DM, Rozanov CB, Dratman MB. Evidence that 3,3′,5-triiodothyronine is concentrated in and delivered from the locus coeruleus to its noradrenergic targets *via* anterograde axonal transport. Neuroscience 1999; 93(3): 943-54.
[http://dx.doi.org/10.1016/S0306-4522(99)00146-3] [PMID: 10473259]

[171] Holsboer F. The corticosteroid receptor hypothesis of depression. Neuropsychopharmacology 2000; 23(5): 477-501.
[http://dx.doi.org/10.1016/S0893-133X(00)00159-7] [PMID: 11027914]

[172] Young EA. Sex differences and the HPA axis: Implications for psychiatric disease. J Gend Specif Med 1998; 1(1): 21-7.
[PMID: 11279849]

[173] Vreeburg SA, Hoogendijk WJG, van Pelt J, *et al.* Major depressive disorder and hypothalamic-pituitary-adrenal axis activity: Results from a large cohort study. Arch Gen Psychiatry 2009; 66(6): 617-26.
[http://dx.doi.org/10.1001/archgenpsychiatry.2009.50] [PMID: 19487626]

[174] Bonfiglio JJ, Inda C, Refojo D, Holsboer F, Arzt E, Silberstein S. The corticotropin-releasing hormone network and the hypothalamic-pituitary-adrenal axis: Molecular and cellular mechanisms involved. Neuroendocrinology 2011; 94(1): 12-20.
[http://dx.doi.org/10.1159/000328226] [PMID: 21576930]

[175] Nemeroff CB, Widerlöv E, Bissette G, *et al.* Elevated concentrations of CSF corticotropin-releasing factor-like immunoreactivity in depressed patients. Science 1984; 226(4680): 1342-4. [http://dx.doi.org/10.1126/science.6334362] [PMID: 6334362]

[176] Nemeroff CB, Owens MJ, Bissette G, Andorn AC, Stanley M. Reduced corticotropin releasing factor binding sites in the frontal cortex of suicide victims. Arch Gen Psychiatry 1988; 45(6): 577-9. [http://dx.doi.org/10.1001/archpsyc.1988.01800300075009] [PMID: 2837159]

[177] Nemeroff CB. The corticotropin-releasing factor (CRF) hypothesis of depression: new findings and new directions. Mol Psychiatry 1996; 1(4): 336-42. [PMID: 9118360]

[178] Heuser I, Yassouridis A, Holsboer F. The combined dexamethasone/CRH test: A refined laboratory test for psychiatric disorders. J Psychiatr Res 1994; 28(4): 341-56. [http://dx.doi.org/10.1016/0022-3956(94)90017-5] [PMID: 7877114]

[179] Song C, Halbreich U, Han C, Leonard BE, Luo H. Imbalance between pro- and anti-inflammatory cytokines, and between Th1 and Th2 cytokines in depressed patients: the effect of electroacupuncture or fluoxetine treatment. Pharmacopsychiatry 2009; 42(5): 182-8. [http://dx.doi.org/10.1055/s-0029-1202263] [PMID: 19724980]

[180] Miller AH, Maletic V, Raison CL. Inflammation and its discontents: The role of cytokines in the pathophysiology of major depression. Biol Psychiatry 2009; 65(9): 732-41. [http://dx.doi.org/10.1016/j.biopsych.2008.11.029] [PMID: 19150053]

[181] Fitzgerald PB, Laird AR, Maller J, Daskalakis ZJ. A meta-analytic study of changes in brain activation in depression. Hum Brain Mapp 2008; 29(6): 683-95. [http://dx.doi.org/10.1002/hbm.20426] [PMID: 17598168]

[182] Hercher C, Turecki G, Mechawar N. Through the looking glass: Examining neuroanatomical evidence for cellular alterations in major depression. J Psychiatr Res 2009; 43(11): 947-61. [http://dx.doi.org/10.1016/j.jpsychires.2009.01.006] [PMID: 19233384]

[183] Simpson D. Phrenology and the neurosciences: contributions of F. J. Gall and J. G. Spurzheim. ANZ J Surg 2005; 75(6): 475-82. [http://dx.doi.org/10.1111/j.1445-2197.2005.03426.x] [PMID: 15943741]

[184] Sullivan RM, Gratton A. Lateralized effects of medial prefrontal cortex lesions on neuroendocrine and autonomic stress responses in rats. J Neurosci 1999; 19(7): 2834-40. [http://dx.doi.org/10.1523/JNEUROSCI.19-07-02834.1999] [PMID: 10087094]

[185] Koolschijn PCMP, van Haren NEM, Lensvelt-Mulders GJLM, Hulshoff Pol HE, Kahn RS. Brain volume abnormalities in major depressive disorder: A meta-analysis of magnetic resonance imaging studies. Hum Brain Mapp 2009; 30(11): 3719-35. [http://dx.doi.org/10.1002/hbm.20801] [PMID: 19441021]

[186] Mayberg HS, Lozano AM, Voon V, *et al.* Deep brain stimulation for treatment-resistant depression. Neuron 2005; 45(5): 651-60. [http://dx.doi.org/10.1016/j.neuron.2005.02.014] [PMID: 15748841]

[187] MacQueen GM. Magnetic resonance imaging and prediction of outcome in patients with major depressive disorder. J Psychiatry Neurosci 2009; 34(5): 343-9. [PMID: 19721844]

[188] Rajkowska G, Miguel-Hidalgo JJ, Wei J, *et al.* Morphometric evidence for neuronal and glial prefrontal cell pathology in major depression See accompanying Editorial, in this issue. Biol Psychiatry 1999; 45(9): 1085-98. [http://dx.doi.org/10.1016/S0006-3223(99)00041-4] [PMID: 10331101]

[189] Maes M, Kubera M, Obuchowiczwa E, Goehler L, Brzeszcz J. Depression's multiple comorbidities explained by (neuro)inflammatory and oxidative & nitrosative stress pathways. Neuroendocrinol Lett 2011; 32(1): 7-24.

[PMID: 21407167]

[190] McCusker RH, Kelley KW. Immune–neural connections: how the immune system's response to infectious agents influences behavior. J Exp Biol 2013; 216(1): 84-98. [http://dx.doi.org/10.1242/jeb.073411] [PMID: 23225871]

[191] Turkheimer FE, Rizzo G, Bloomfield PS, *et al.* The methodology of TSPO imaging with positron emission tomography. Biochem Soc Trans 2015; 43(4): 586-92. [http://dx.doi.org/10.1042/BST20150058] [PMID: 26551697]

[192] McCusker RH, Kelley KW. Immune–neural connections: how the immune system's response to infectious agents influences behavior. J Exp Biol 2013; 216(1): 84-98. [http://dx.doi.org/10.1242/jeb.073411] [PMID: 23225871]

[193] Gandy K, Kim S, Sharp C, Dindo L, Maletic-Savatic M, Calarge C. Pattern Separation: A potential marker of impaired hippocampal adult neurogenesis in major depressive disorder. Front Neurosci 2017; 11: 571. [http://dx.doi.org/10.3389/fnins.2017.00571] [PMID: 29123464]

[194] Malberg JE, Duman RS. Cell proliferation in adult hippocampus is decreased by inescapable stress: Reversal by fluoxetine treatment. Neuropsychopharmacology 2003; 28(9): 1562-71. [http://dx.doi.org/10.1038/sj.npp.1300234] [PMID: 12838272]

[195] Mnie-Filali O, Faure C, Mansari ME, *et al.* R-citalopram prevents the neuronal adaptive changes induced by escitalopram. Neuroreport 2007; 18(15): 1553-6. [http://dx.doi.org/10.1097/WNR.0b013e3282f04047] [PMID: 17885600]

[196] Vollmayr B, Mahlstedt MM, Henn FA. Neurogenesis and depression: what animal models tell us about the link. Eur Arch Psychiatry Clin Neurosci 2007; 257(5): 300-3. [http://dx.doi.org/10.1007/s00406-007-0734-2] [PMID: 17401725]

[197] Burton PR, Clayton DG, Cardon LR, *et al.* Wellcome Trust Case Control Consortium. Genome-wide association study of 14,000 cases of seven common diseases and 3,000 shared controls. Nature 2007; 447(7145): 661-78. [http://dx.doi.org/10.1038/nature05911] [PMID: 17554300]

[198] Caspi A, Sugden K, Moffitt TE, *et al.* Influence of life stress on depression: Moderation by a polymorphism in the 5-HTT gene. Science 2003; 301(5631): 386-9. [http://dx.doi.org/10.1126/science.1083968] [PMID: 12869766]

[199] Risch N, Herrell R, Lehner T, *et al.* Interaction between the serotonin transporter gene (5-HTTLPR), stressful life events, and risk of depression: a meta-analysis. JAMA 2009; 301(23): 2462-71. [http://dx.doi.org/10.1001/jama.2009.878] [PMID: 19531786]

[200] Bear MF, Connors BW, Paradiso MA. Neuroscience: Exploring the brain. 3rd ed., Baltimore, MD: Lippincott, Williams & Wilkins 2007.

[201] Charney DS. Psychobiological mechanisms of resilience and vulnerability: implications for successful adaptation to extreme stress. Am J Psychiatry 2004; 161(2): 195-216. [http://dx.doi.org/10.1176/appi.ajp.161.2.195] [PMID: 14754765]

[202] Kendler KS, Gardner CO, Prescott CA. Toward a comprehensive developmental model for major depression in women. Am J Psychiatry 2002; 159(7): 1133-45. [http://dx.doi.org/10.1176/appi.ajp.159.7.1133] [PMID: 12091191]

[203] Kendler KS, Thornton LM, Prescott CA. Gender differences in the rates of exposure to stressful life events and sensitivity to their depressogenic effects. Am J Psychiatry 2001; 158(4): 587-93. [http://dx.doi.org/10.1176/appi.ajp.158.4.587] [PMID: 11282693]

[204] Khan A, Faucett J, Lichtenberg P, Kirsch I, Brown WA. A systematic review of comparative efficacy of treatments and controls for depression. plos one 2012; 7(7): 41778. [http://dx.doi.org/10.1371/journal.pone.0041778]

[205] Dale J, Sorour E, Milner G. Do psychiatrists perform appropriate physical investigations for their patients? A review of current practices in a general psychiatric inpatient and outpatient setting. Journal of Mental Health 2008; 17(3): 293-8.
[http://dx.doi.org/10.1080/09638230701498325]

[206] NICE. NICE Guidelines:depression in children and adolescents. London: NICE 2005; p. 5.

[207] McAleavey, Andrew A.; Castonguay, Louis G. (2015). "The process of change in psychotherapy: common and unique factors". In Gelo, Omar C. G.; Pritz, Alfred; Rieken, Bernd (eds.). Psychotherapy research: foundations, process, and outcome. Vienna. New York: Springer-Verlag 2015; 293: pp. 293-310.
[http://dx.doi.org/10.1007/978-3-7091-1382-0_15]

[208] Thase ME. When are psychotherapy and pharmacotherapy combinations the treatment of choice for major depressive disorder? The Psychiatric Quarterly 1999; 70(4): 333-46.
[http://dx.doi.org/10.1023/A:1022042316895]

[209] Roth A, Fonagy P. “Cognitive-Behavioral Therapy Alone and in Combination with medication: University of Minnesota and University of Pennsylvania–Vanderbilt University Studies” What Works for Whom?: A Critical Review of Psychotherapy Research. 2nd ed. Guilford Press 2006; pp. 76-8.

[210] Antony MM, Roemer E. Behaviour therapy.Essential psychotherapies. 2nd ed. New York: Guilford 2003; pp. 182-223.

[211] Klerman GL, Weissman MM, Rounsaville BJ, Chevron ES. Interpersonal psychotherapy of depression. New York: Basic Books 1984.

[212] Greenberg LS, Rice LN, Elliott R. Facilitating emotional change: the moment-by-moment process. New York: Guilford Press 1993.

[213] Hayes Steven C. Acceptance & Commitment Therapy (ACT). ContextualPsychologyorg

[214] de Maat S, Dekker J, Schoevers R, van Aalst G, Gijsbers-van Wijk C, Hendriksen M, *et al.* Short psychodynamic supportive psychotherapy, antidepressants, and their combination in the treatment of major depression: A mega-analysis based on three randomized clinical trials. Depression and Anxiety 2007; 25(7): 565-74.
[http://dx.doi.org/10.1002/da.20305]

[215] Rudorfer MV, Henry ME, Sackeim HA. Electroconvulsive therapy (PDF). In: Tasman A, Kay J, Lieberman JA, Eds. Psychiatry. 2nd ed. Chichester: John Wiley & Sons Ltd. 2003; pp. 1865-901.

[216] Abbott CC, Gallegos P, Rediske N, Lemke NT, Quinn DK. A review of longitudinal electroconvulsive therapy: Neuroimaging investigations. J Geriatr Psychiatry Neurol 2014; 27(1): 33-46.
[http://dx.doi.org/10.1177/0891988713516542] [PMID: 24381234]

[217] Transcranial magnetic stimulation for treating and preventing migraine. NiCE January 2014 Archived from the original 2015.

[218] Melkerson MN. Special premarket 510(k) notification for neurostar® tms therapy system for major depressive disorder. Food and Drug Administration Retrieved 2008.

[219] Groppa S, Oliviero A, Eisen A, *et al.* A practical guide to diagnostic transcranial magnetic stimulation: Report of an IFCN committee. Clin Neurophysiol 2012; 123(5): 858-82.
[http://dx.doi.org/10.1016/j.clinph.2012.01.010] [PMID: 22349304]

[220] Englot DJ, Chang EF, Auguste KI. Vagus nerve stimulation for epilepsy: a meta-analysis of efficacy and predictors of response. Journal of Neurosurgery 2011; 115(6): 1248-55.
[http://dx.doi.org/10.3171/2011.7.JNS11977]

[221] Kron Thomas. Vagus Nerve Stimulation: A little-known option for depression. Medscape 2022.

[222] Mechanism of Action of Antidepressants Psychopharmacology Bulletin. 36. Summer 2002. S2CID 4937890 Archived from the original 2019.

[223] Hetrick SE, McKenzie JE, Bailey AP, Sharma V, Moller CI, Badcock PB, *et al.* Cochrane Common Mental Disorders Group (ed.). "New generation antidepressants for depression in children and adolescents: a network meta-analysis". The Cochrane Database of Systematic Reviews. 2021; p. (5): CD013674.
[http://dx.doi.org/10.1002/14651858.CD013674.pub2]

[224] Cashman JR, Ghirmai S. Inhibition of serotonin and norepinephrine reuptake and inhibition of phosphodiesterase by multi-target inhibitors as potential agents for depression. Bioorg Med Chem 2009; 17(19): 6890-7.
[http://dx.doi.org/10.1016/j.bmc.2009.08.025] [PMID: 19740668]

[225] Spina E, Santoro V, D'Arrigo C. Clinically relevant pharmacokinetic drug interactions with second-generation antidepressants: An update. Clin Ther 2008; 30(7): 1206-27.
[http://dx.doi.org/10.1016/S0149-2918(08)80047-1] [PMID: 18691982]

[226] Paumier K L, Siderowf A D, Auinger P, *et al.* Parkinson Study Group Genetics Epidemiology Working Group. Tricyclic antidepressants delay the need for dopaminergic therapy in early Parkinson's disease. Movement Disorders 2012; 27(7): 880-7.
[http://dx.doi.org/10.1002/mds.24978]

[227] Trindade E, Menon D, Topfer LA, Coloma C. Adverse effects associated with selective serotonin reuptake inhibitors and tricyclic antidepressants: a meta-analysis. CMAJ 1998; 159(10): 1245-52.
[PMID: 9861221]

[228] Krishnan KR. Revisiting monoamine oxidase inhibitors. J Clin Psychiatry 2007; 68 (Suppl. 8): 35-41.
[PMID: 17640156]

[229] Mottram PG, Wilson K, Strobl JJ. Antidepressants for depressed elderly. Cochrane Libr 2006; 2009(1): CD003491.
[http://dx.doi.org/10.1002/14651858.CD003491.pub2] [PMID: 16437456]

[230] Ceber M, Salihoglu T. Ketamine may be the first choice for anesthesia in burn patients. J Burn Care Res 2006; 27(5): 760-2.
[http://dx.doi.org/10.1097/01.BCR.0000238091.41737.7C] [PMID: 16998413]

[231] Newcomer JW, Krystal JH. NMDA receptor regulation of memory and behavior in humans. Hippocampus 2001; 11(5): 542.
[http://dx.doi.org/10.1002/hipo.1069]

[232] FDA approves new nasal spray medication for treatment-resistant depression; available only at a certified doctor's office or clinic 2020.

[233] Sun L, Li Q, Li Q, *et al.* Chronic ketamine exposure induces permanent impairment of brain functions in adolescent cynomolgus monkeys. Addiction Biology 2014; 19(2): 185-94.
[http://dx.doi.org/10.1111/adb.12004]

[234] Vasiliu O. Effect of the selective serotonin reuptake inhibitors over coagulation in patients with depressive disorders – a systematic review and retrospective analysis. Romanian Journal of Military Medicine 2019; 122(2): 7-11.
[http://dx.doi.org/10.55453/rjmm.2019.122.2.1]

[235] Mi W, Yang F, Li H, *et al.* Efficacy, safety, and tolerability of ansofaxine (ly03005) extended-release tablet for major depressive disorder: A randomized, double-blind, placebo-controlled, dose-finding, phase 2 clinical trial. Int J Neuropsychopharmacol 2022; 25(3): 252-60.
[http://dx.doi.org/10.1093/ijnp/pyab074] [PMID: 34747448]

[236] SYSTEMATIC review article Front. Pharmacol 2022; 13
[http://dx.doi.org/10.3389/fphar.2022.884143]

CHAPTER 9

Artificial Intelligence, Deep Learning and Precision Medicine

Khalid Umar Fakhri[1], Sugandh Kumar[2], Md Zubbair Malik[3], Chirag N. Patel[4,5], Yogesh Kumar[6], Khalid Imtiyaz[1], Farhan Jalees Ahmad[7] and **Moshahid Alam Rizvi[1,*]**

[1] *Genome Biology Lab, Department of Biosciences, Jamia Millia Islamia, New Delhi-110025, India*

[2] *School of Medicine, University of California San Francisco (UCSF), San Francisco-94115, CA, USA*

[3] *Department of Genetics and Bioinformatics, Dasman Diabetes Institute, Dasman, P.O. Box 1180, Kuwait City-15462, Kuwait*

[4] *Chemical Biology Laboratory, Center for Cancer Research, National Cancer Institute, National Institute of Health, Frederick, MD-21702, USA*

[5] *Department of Botany, Bioinformatics and Climate Change Impacts Management, School of Science, Gujarat University, Ahmedabad-380 009, India*

[6] *Department of General, Visceral and thoracic surgery, University Medical Centre Hamburg-Eppendorf, Martiniatrasse 52/ building N27, Hamburg-20246, Germany*

[7] *Department of Pharmaceutics, School of Pharmaceutical Education and Research, Jamia Hamdard, New Delhi-110062, India*

Abstract: Cancer is often described as a complex and diverse collection of cells, encompassing many distinct subtypes. To address the challenges presented by this heterogeneity, artificial intelligence (AI) has emerged as a pivotal technology for advanced cancer research and clinical management. AI leverages computer systems to perform tasks that traditionally rely on human cognitive abilities. One integral component of AI is Deep Learning (DL), which empowers algorithms to autonomously acquire knowledge from vast datasets, enabling them to make accurate predictions. The application of AI in cancer research has witnessed continuous growth, particularly in the realm of disease prognosis. This advancement has empowered pathologists to precisely diagnose various cancer types, and classify them into different grades and subtypes while considering factors such as invasion patterns, genetic mutations, and metastasis. Such precise characterization of cancers facilitates the implementation of tailored treatment strategies, ultimately leading to more favorable clinical outcomes. Moreover, AI plays a pivotal role in the field of precision medicine, aiding in overcoming challenges like drug resistance and cancer relapse.

* **Corresponding author Moshahid Alam Rizvi:** Genome Biology Lab, Department of Biosciences, Jamia Millia Islamia, New Delhi-110025, India; E-mail: mrizvi@jmi.ac.in

Farzana Mahdi & Abbas Ali Mahdi (Eds.)

In comparison to traditional methods, AI offers superior predictive accuracy and enhances the overall clinical perspective. This chapter aims to showcase the evolving roles of AI in diagnosing and prognosticating various cancer types and their subtypes. The applications of AI in cancer prediction warrant further assessment and validation, supporting not only routine tasks for pathologists but also complex diagnostic scenarios. Within these pages, we will highlight various instances where AI, particularly DL, has effectively addressed challenges that were previously deemed insurmountable. Additionally, we will focus on the resources and datasets available to foster a deeper understanding of the intricacies of AI in cancer research. The continued expansion of advanced computational methodologies and AI is expected to facilitate the study of interactomes, significantly enriching our insights into oncology and advancing the concept of personalized medicine.

Keywords: Artificial Intelligence, Cancer, Diagnosis, Deep Learning, Machine Learning.

INTRODUCTION

An interdisciplinary approach involves the fusion of two or more fields of research, enabling a more comprehensive, expansive, and innovative perspective, and developing a coherent understanding of a subject. Recent advancements in both biological and computer sciences have spurred scientists to explore the role of computational methods in cancer research. According to the Center for Disease Control and Prevention (CDC), cancer ranks as the second leading cause of death on a global scale [1]. In 2022, the National Cancer Institute (NCI) reported an estimated mortality rate of 609,360 in the United States alone, with 194,451 individuals succumbing to lung cancer, 42,260 to breast cancer, 31,620 to prostate cancer, and 17,760 to brain malignancies (as per the American Cancer Society's 2020 new cancer release report) [2].

Timely cancer detection emerges as an imperative goal that has the potential to save countless lives worldwide. Early detection not only significantly enhances survival rates but also reduces mortality and minimizes the chances of its future recurrence. Initial and accurate diagnosis of cancer is one of the major challenges for the treatment as misdiagnosis is caused because of the lack of molecular markers [3]. Recent studies have shown that nearly 46% of cancer cases have missed diagnosis at the primary health care centre [4] due to the use of traditional pathology techniques. Historically, the diagnosis of malignant disorders has relied heavily on the visual examination of clinical images and the judgment of pathologists. However, this traditional approach is plagued by both time-consuming processes and susceptibility to errors.

Since malignant growth can occur due to a variety of reasons, the genesis is often not clearly known. Ever since, the first malignant cells were detected from sputum in 1851, several devices and systems have been developed to recognize malignant growth at an early stage. A brief history of diagnosis of malignant growth is shown in Fig. **(1)**. It depicts the significant leaps that changed the course of cancer diagnosis and treatment over the century. Early prediction of any chronic ailment is useful in limiting complications of the disease. It also helps in determining treatment options available to the patients leading to better management. Multiple analyses and treatment conventions have established that AI is a beneficial approach having great implications in the healthcare sector. The fundamental premise of this area of research is to make computers progressively helpful in elucidating complex healthcare challenges and decipher the correct inference using data from different pathological conditions. In the mid-1980s, computer-aided diagnosis (CAD) was developed to aid specialists in improving the interpretation of medical images with precision and within the limit of time [5].

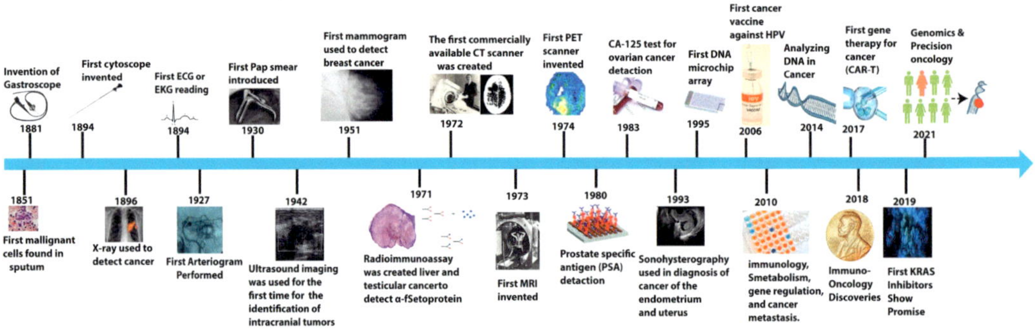

Fig. (1). History of cancer diagnostics [10].

Machine learning (ML) is an interdisciplinary field that complements AI and use computer resources focusing on different disciplines such as neurology, psychology, and statistics to create mathematical algorithms. This in turn facilitates the diagnosis and provides possible treatment options that may vary for different patients [6]. Feature extraction is the key principle that underlines ML reducing the resources and data dimensions while dealing with large datasets. Feature extraction also plays crucial role in over and under fitting of desired models [7]. Several techniques for feature extraction in different types of cancers have been reported in the literature [8, 9], and they have demonstrated their utility. Here we discuss interdisciplinary approaches of cancer detection/prognosis in the context of AI and ML.

However, these extraction-based approaches have their flaws. To address these flaws and enhance quality, a new paradigm known as (DL) has been developed [11]. DL is therefore, a sub-area of ML aimed at permitting abstract portrayal of data through multilayer neural network systems or deep neural systems. From video/board games to the world of health, it has increasingly proved its potential in replicating human vision and assessing human intellectual capacity. DL offers the benefit of directly creating a significantly high-level feature depiction from raw photos. Similar to DL, Graphics Processing Units (GPU) are employed in combination with data augmentation and picture recognition. Convolution neural networks, in particular, have the potential to detect cancerous development with high precision [12]. AI and ML-based approaches have imperative advantages over current techniques for diagnosing and treating oncological disorders. It may be noted that a health expert may miss minor details from an image but machines backed by powerful algorithms do not show such vulnerability. Over the past decade, there has been a significant advancement in cancer diagnostics, showcasing high precision and fidelity through the utilization of AI and ML [13, 14]. AI has been utilized for clinical data examination and classification. The success of AI lies in the identification and classification of skin sores [15], malignant lung growths [16], metastases in women with breast cancer [17], and forecast oncogenesis and tumor silencing [18]. AI protocols are mostly based on various mathematical algorithms [19] implemented through computer resources.

AI is a vibrant field of science that investigates and develops technology systems capable of coping with difficult issues in ways that mimic human intelligence [20]. With the combination of technology, information science, and other related fields, this invention is supplementing core domains of applied research strengthening robotics, machine learning, computer vision, and large scale data handling. Digital marketing may cause huge conventional and socio-economic changes in the economic framework [21], which is also relevant to human healthcare systems. ML has grown enormously encompassing the domain of AI for the past few decades. This is true for biological sciences, especially in classifying cancers and predicting the prognosis. DL in the context of ML is a collection of mathematical techniques, which a program trains itself *via* learning from a massive database of examples that demonstrate the ideal behavior, without the need to explicitly establish the rules [22]. AI harnesses algorithms and statistical models, enabling computer systems to proficiently execute specific tasks without the need for explicit rules, relying instead on patterns and inferences. AI systems create mathematical models using labeled "training data" samples to make predictions and determinations without requiring explicit training for each task. DL is one of the various AI approaches based on artificial cognitive domains [23]. Deep neural network (DNN) systems, deep belief networks, convolutional neural processes, and CNN (CNN) are all illustrative examples of DL models. ML, voice and audio recognition, web screening, computational linguistics, bioinformatics, drug design process, medical picture research, histopathological analysis, and material inspection are just a few of the disciplines where these models were frequently utilized. These models have delivered remarkable results, perhaps even better than human specialists [24]. This significant advancement, particularly in deep learning classifiers, holds the promise of precisely enhancing the optimization of cancer diagnosis and prognosis assessment. The adaptive intelligence system is a sort of cognitive computing that is dependent on classifiers that simulate human cognitive abilities. Brain systems play a vital role throughout the processing of large-scale data, which becomes common in scientific experiments. The development of DL algorithms is employed to assess tumor growth more effectively than traditional approaches since they eliminate the requirement for invasive procedures. Furthermore, neural systems have been designed in such a way that they can accurately examine individual prognoses and treatment plans similar to those of experienced clinicians. Hence, these systems can guide both clinical experts and patients in a settling on ideal medicinal choices. A large number of computing projects attempting to "treat" oncological disorders using bioinformatics have been developed. This will impact the transformation of clinical studies involving advances such as neural networking and other kinds of AI.

ARTIFICIAL INTELLIGENCE (AI) VS DEEP LEARNING (DL)

The utilization of AI-based technology in the healthcare sector, aimed at enhancing the diagnosis, management, therapy, prognosis, and development of effective medicines, has witnessed tremendous growth. Given the substantial number of cancer patients and their pressing needs for accurate diagnosis and effective treatment, artificial intelligence is poised to significantly improve both healthcare and therapy outcomes. AI, initially conceived in the 1950s, defines a computer's ability to perform tasks typically associated with intelligent behavior [25]. It brings together various disciplines within computational mathematics and science and can be thought of as a series of heuristic, self-learning systems. This concept bears a resemblance to Mandelbrot patterns, which identify hidden connections within datasets that can be unraveled and optimized. Moreover, AI can be seamlessly integrated with an array of emerging mobile health interfaces, including mobile applications and handheld devices, to create "digital biomarkers" capable of predicting clinical outcomes.

Significant applications of AI within the medical and healthcare domains involve the utilization of machine learning (ML) algorithms, which constitute a crucial component of AI applications in pharmaceutical and healthcare services. More as training information is collected to ML algorithms, they may recognize hidden patterns within the data and hence complete a task without explicit programming [26]. Many ML algorithms have been presented across latest generations, and the more common forms of ML, such as multiple regressions, were validated as effective elements during clinical oncology [27]. ML applications have been thoroughly categorised as both supervised and unsupervised learning. To construct the ML algorithms, supervised learning employs a specified collection containing upstream and downstream sources. The algorithm attempts to become familiar with a generic paradigm which outlines insight into yields. Supervised learning algorithms may learn data designs and patterns for categorization as compared to regression. Unsupervised learning techniques, on the other hand, leverage unlabeled data to unveil patterns within the input information. Unsupervised ML approaches are normally employed to rearrange reduction in dimensionality and organize (categorizing or convergence) statistics. The pre-requisite for periodically restructuring statistical features into internal processing has been one disadvantage of classical ML methods. This inability associated with specific classification methods to use large datasets at the start has hampered their value in medical care. DL is one of the most suited ML algorithms for investigating unstructured data. In the field of AI within computer science, the aim is to emulate human intelligence in machines through the use of algorithms and programming, enabling them to perform predefined tasks without requiring direct human input [28]. There was a time in the 1980s known as the "AI winter" that saw big economic concerns and challenges pertaining to this sector. The resurgence of interest in AI, however, started in 2000. One of the most recent disciplines of DL was created as a result of increased processing capacity and fewer budgetary barriers. The approximate overlaps and links between the areas of AI, ML, and DL have been illustrated in Fig. (**2**) [29]. In most cases, they serve as a branch of computer science that coordinates the formation and growth of intelligent machines [30]. AI effectively employs algorithms to perform tasks that depend on them, such as learning from experience, adapting to new sources of information, and executing jobs akin to those carried out by humans [31]. In the past, an AI application was used in the medical profession. A type of AI known as an expert system has already been used to make medical judgments with respect to the principles that computers might implement [32]. The diversity of pharmaceuticals and the variety of illnesses make it difficult to encode a set of principles for every clinical situation. As a result, throughout the 1990s, ML replaced classifiers since "rules would be learnt by algorithms directly from a large number of cases instead of being encoded by hand" [32].

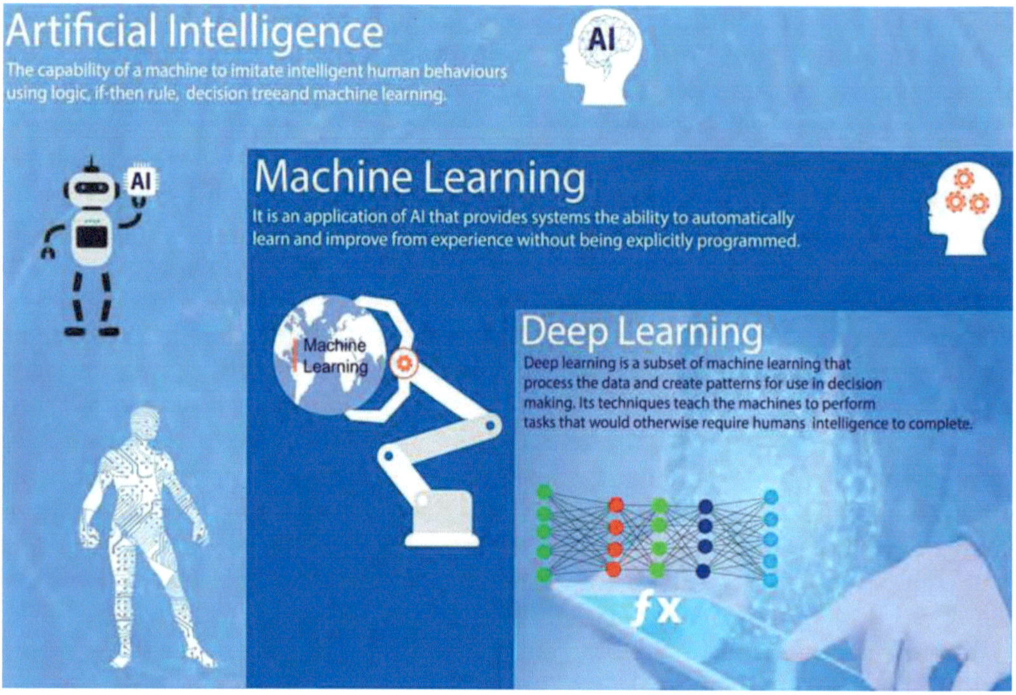

Fig. (2). Artificial Intelligence, Machine Learning and Deep Learning: Their Relationship [29].

Machine learning (ML) is a subset of AI, and it would be accurate to say that in today's context, when one mentions AI, ML and its related disciplines take precedence. When provided with databases of raw data, ML employs computer algorithms, simulations, and techniques to unveil patterns and correlations through the learning process. Both oncology and radiation treatment have reaped the benefits of machine learning methods. Support Vector Machine (SVM), Artificial Neural Network (ANN), and the latest (DL) approaches are among the ML techniques applied to radiotherapy target delineation [33]. ML research draws inspiration from the working models of the human brain and strives to mimic the neural structure of the nervous system by creating artificial neural networks (ANNs), which are composed of units called artificial neurons organized into layers [34]. The framework identifies patterns from information given to the system in an instructional session. ANNs were built on the understanding of human physiology and the brain's ability to grasp complicated patterns by layering, descending, and shifting variations in nerve cells (Fig. **3**). The fundamental structure of the first ANNs was created by simulating the operation of biological receptors using computational approaches [35]. Every "neuron" in a progressive network receives input, produces an output, and may determine the importance of a given link using the artificial neural network (ANN) method of machine learning. ANN is made up of multi-layered connected neural systems. Since ANN is constructed from several interconnected layers of neural networks, the algorithm is able to reassign the level of relevance to each operation until it discovers a relationship or correlation. Radical radiation for the growth of prostate cancer was already predicted using ANN [36] and successfully chemo-radiotherapy was used for the treatment of head and neck cancer [37]. ANNs have also been applied to different parts of malignancy medication for a significant time. More recent endeavors in this area of research were augmented by new information about the biological aspects of malignant growth [38]. However, computational strategies are getting fundamentally more powerful and effective than ever before.

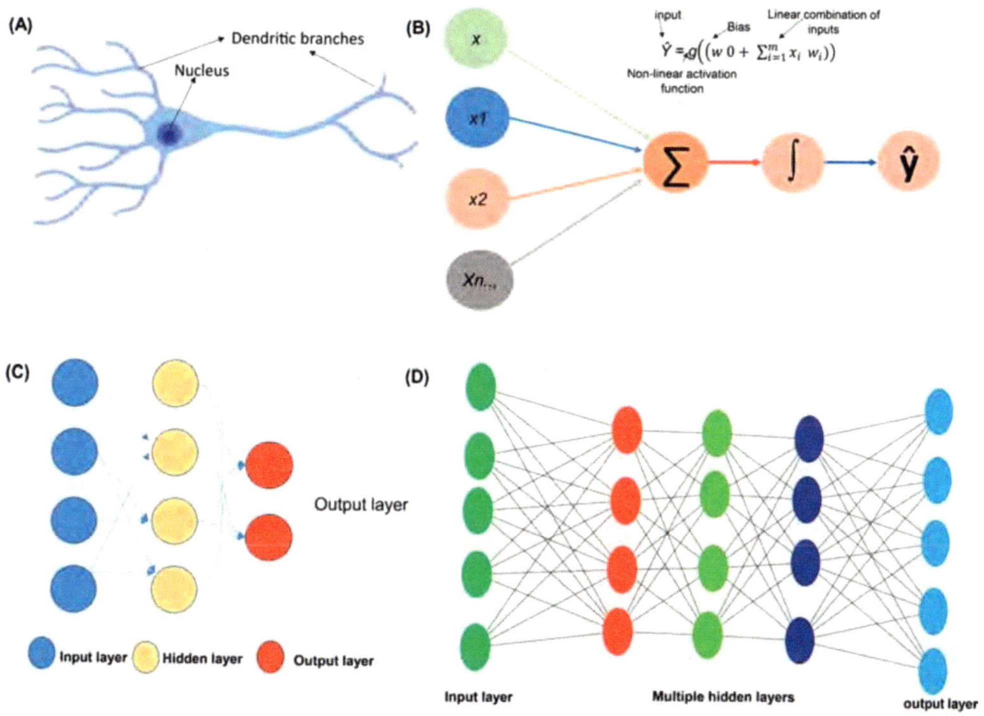

Fig. (3). Neurological Basis of the Neural Network System [39].

Recently, an intriguing and incredible branch in ML called DL exhibited significant accomplishment in terms of solving pattern recognition and computer vision as compared to traditional ML systems. These learning algorithms were based on NN structures with an excess of two hidden layers and hence called "deep". An ANN with several layers-typically over five than a regular neural network (ANN) and better prediction accuracy is called Deep Neural Network

(DNN). Imperative preference is given nowadays to DNNs as their performances persistently improve the sizes of the training datasets expansion [32]. Consequently, as ML's DL subsection, which makes use of techniques like DNN, CNN systems are born. It is a kind of ANN that incorporates multi-layered neural network systems with a greater prominence of concealed layers [29]. These supervised and unsupervised learnings may be accomplished with DL. The DL technique has been applied to radiotherapy targeting OAR (organ-at-risk) delineation in head and neck cancers [40]. It has been shown that DL is capable of helping students learn well from difficult assignments [41], mostly due to a built-in quality termed the model-based control features [42]. This characteristic of CNNs may be understood as training data representation in a supervised manner simultaneously improving performance prediction for the specific task with little risk of imbalanced datasets [43]. Instead of just serving as a classifier, as demonstrated by the example with ML, this neural system may also serve as a feature extractor [41, 44]. This favors end-to-end training since DNN figures out the output category from the input signal directly [32]. CNNs are for the most part applied to image segmentation and classification. In general, AI and DL algorithms are interchangeable. A subset of machine learning known as DL employs layers of "ANN" to make predictions that can understand data at different levels of complexity [45]. While ML algorithms relied on pre-designed features to advance forecasting, DL algorithms may learn about the appropriate features that match the data the best through the preparation process, avoiding the requirement of using constructive complex data. Due to this ability, DL algorithms have outperformed classic ML algorithms in a number of fundamental AI problems, including object recognition, natural language processing and sequence prediction [45, 46].

The ML, AI and DL are used for classification and forecasting, by analyzing the properties of the complex cancer network to understand the drug-disease relationship [47]. These methods are widely used for structure-activity relationship analysis of the drugs [48]. It can also be used to study the response of cancer cell lines to drug treatment from which one can study the impact of drugs on these cancer diseases [49].

As a result, during the past several years, there have been an increasing number of study publications publicly released in the medical sector that include DL (Fig. **4**). This has evolved into a crucial helper in oncology's pursuit of therapeutic approach [50, 51], heterogeneous datasets to better diagnose disease burden, foresee patient results and tailor the management.

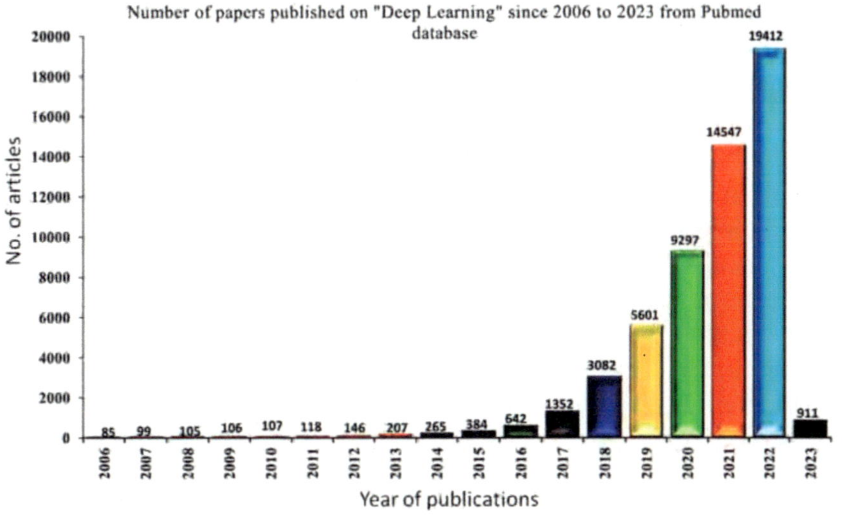

Fig. (4). Rise in year-wise publications in DL [52].

Most DL strategies utilize neural system designs, which is the reason DL models are frequently alluded to as DNN systems. The term "deep" often refers to the amount of buried computation nodes system (Fig. **5**). DNNs can include as many as 150 convolution layers, compared to conventional neural networks which contain 2-3 hidden layers. DL models are constructed using massive amounts of correctly classified data and neural network architectures that properly extract descriptors without the need for human feature extraction.

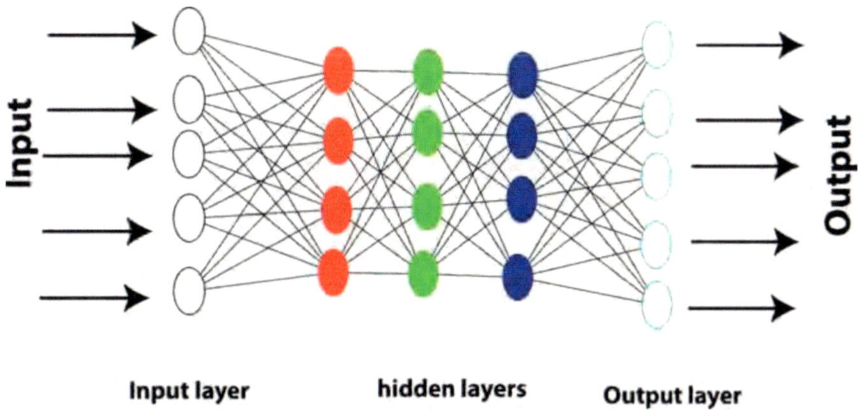

Fig. (5). Classical example of Neural network model for input and output structure with demonstrating different layers.

One of the popular ANNs is the most common deep neural system (CNN or ConvNet) (Fig. **6**). A CNN is a DL approach that excels at learning and extracting highlights from datasets, particularly when dealing with 2D data such as images. CNNs eliminate the need for manual feature extraction, which involves identifying specific characteristics required to categorize pictures. Instead, CNNs work by autonomously identifying relevant features within images during the network's training process using a dataset. This automated feature extraction makes DL models highly accurate for various computer vision tasks, including object recognition. In CNNs, a multitude of convolutional nodes is used to detect distinctive features within an image. As the model progresses through its layers, these nodes become more adept at learning complex features. For example, the initial convolutional layers may learn to distinguish edges and basic shapes, while the latter layers can recognize intricate patterns and more advanced characteristics within the objects being identified. This ability to automatically learn and extract features from images is what makes CNNs a powerful tool in the field of computer vision.

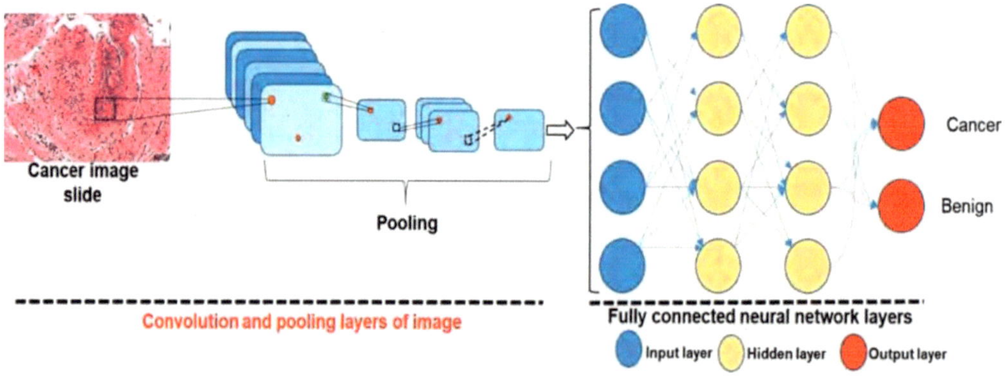

Fig. (6). A convolutional neural network has three layers: convolution, pooling and a fully connected layers. These layers may be repeated depending on the parameters, before reaching the final fully connected layers. The output of a convolutional layer is a feature map. CNNs are the most commonly used DL models for processing two-dimensional data representations, particularly color images.

These CNNs typically consist of convolutional and pooling layers, followed by fully connected layers that enable the network to classify images based on the features it has learned. Researchers have proposed a two-stage technique that involves the use of two separate CNNs. The first CNN identifies nuclei within a specific tissue image, while the second CNN utilizes features extracted from the detected nuclei to assess the likelihood of cancer presence on the map. DL algorithms, including CNNs, have been applied to analyze a wide range of malignancies, achieving accuracy levels equivalent to or surpassing those of human experts. For instance, by training a dataset of 12,940 clinical images, CNNs were able to distinguish one of the most common and deadly types of skin disorders [53]. In the field of pathology, the top-performing algorithm for detecting lymph node cancers in carcinoma from pathology images relied on supervised learning CNNs [54]. This algorithm outperformed a group of 11 pathologists in a simulated clinical workflow, demonstrating not only excellent predictive accuracy but also cost-effective efficiency provided by machine learning algorithms.

Among AI methods, DL has demonstrated great success in a variety of automated real - time applications [55]. In addition to various applications in pathology, several DL-based algorithms have emerged in recent years for identifying the site of breast cancer metastases in lymph nodes [56, 57]. Initial findings suggest that a few algorithms can outperform a pathologist's ability to identify specific cancer hotspots within the automated pictures. However, as we strive for precision, this approach is also susceptible to errors [58] which necessitates human supervision. Additionally, DL algorithms are innately restricted to the task for which they have been explicitly trained. In view of the strength of these algorithms, exhaustive searches are comprehended. The shortcomings of these algorithms, including their sensitivity to poor optical focus, tumor mimics, and their potential clinical utility, need to be further established. Despite our understanding of the capabilities and limitations of algorithms like exhaustive search, a comprehensive assessment of the potential clinical usefulness of these algorithms is still lacking. It is worth noting that a precise algorithm alone would not aid pathologists or assist in the clinical interpretation of an object. These benefits can be realized through the appropriate integration of algorithmic predictions into the clinical workflow [59].

ARTIFICIAL INTELLIGENCE TECHNOLOGY IN CANCER PREDICTION

Cancer research is crucial in leveraging modern computational biology, statistics, and learning methodologies in order to provide increasingly precise and rapid diagnosis. As the significance of predictive and personalized medicine continues to grow, there is an increasing interest in employing AI-driven models to facilitate predictions and diagnoses in cancer research and clinical trials [60]. The application of AI strategies for classification in cancer growth and malignancy studies lays the knowledge-based groundwork for precise and rapid testing of cancer prediction and prognosis, often in shorter timeframes [61]. Predictions and prognoses regarding malignant growth progression revolve around three pivotal areas: hazard assessment or prognosis in tumorigenesis, recurrence diagnosis, and mortality risk estimation. This major area involves anticipating the potential formation of specific malignant growths before clinical investigations [62]. For approximately three decades, ANNs and decision trees (DTs) have been instrumental in cancer screening and diagnosis [60, 62, 63]. Support Vector Machine-based models have also played a significant role in cancer prediction tasks for nearly two decades [64]. Moreover, the utilization of deep networks in cancer research has exhibited substantial promise for widespread adoption, although this presents certain implementation challenges for specific issues. A study by Liang, M. *et al.* [65] generated and evaluated several instances of the efficient use of DL or DL-related models for integrative data analysis. The researchers looked at the possibility of DL-based techniques for classifying and recognizing major disease subgroups in non-linear and non structure large scale datasets. Another study [66] introduces a DL-based multi-omics model that predicts optimal differential grouping for patient survival rates. This prediction is based on the expression of malignant immune cells across histopathology due to the dysregulation of several oncogenic signature genes. Both of these examinations were grounded in integrative data analysis methodologies, which can effectively untangle a unified representation of input vectors while maintaining a certain degree of stability. The standard protocol used for machine learning and DL is outlined in Fig. (7).

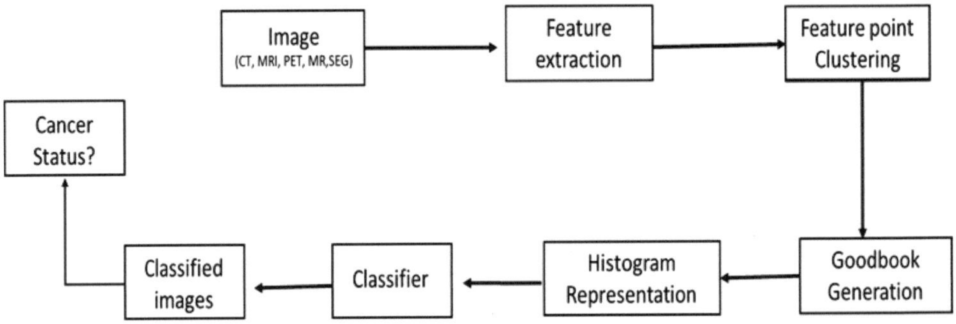

Fig. (7). Machine learning workflow showing extraction of the features from whole slide or patch images cluster to generate "goodbook" clusters, then determine slide status based on the goodbook clusters.

An AI framework consists of an artificial neural network comprising multiple layers of mathematical operations [67]. Each numerical layer receives data input, resulting in another data output. The data output then becomes an input source for the following layer. Each layer transmits only the necessary data to the next layer while filtering out unwanted information. The AI framework analyzes the data throughout the process, identifying patterns. This is how it learns from the provided data and can apply that knowledge to solve problems. For instance, in the case of brain metastasis diagnosis [68], the AI framework can utilize information from individuals with similar data, such as symptoms, radiological images, or genetic markers used in diagnosing cancer under similar circumstances. Another application of an AI framework is its ability to assess data to determine whether a patient has cancer, based on the analysis of nearly 100,000 cancer cases [69]. This large-scale data evaluation allows the identification of an unusual type of cancer. In any case, if it was a single candidate with comparative records that might not include cancers during the learning process, in that case, the patient may be given the wrong diagnosis. Consider the situation that someone has cancer, but the AI framework does not recognize it because it learned that individuals with similar symptoms did not have cancer. As a result, AI-based innovation and a few studies revealed a new field, DL, being widely employed for the categorization of chest, urinary, and respiratory cancers [70]. Thus, AI does take into consideration the possibility of false positives or negatives to ensure the reliability of the outcome. Data output refinement from across the spectrum of diseases using AI is a continuous process. The development of novel, cheap, relevant, and effective AI protocols has made training bigger and increasingly complex. This has resulted in the plan of designing new deep CNNs that are robust enough to achieve complex visual recognition assignments. Coudray *et al.* [71], reported that DL technology, specifically CNNs, can significantly improve medical care by outperforming other techniques and achieving accuracy in cancer classification that is similar to that of a pathologist, enabling the selection of appropriate treatment regimens. In addition to performing well on independent datasets of frozen tissues and biopsy images, these models have also shown success when CNNs are used for the classification of lung patterns on CT scans. This discovery was made possible by Google Corporation, which achieved the Image-Net Large-Scale Visual Recognition Challenge in 2014. The Image-Net program is a massive graphical repository designed for the purpose of graphical visual recognition software development. About 14 million images have been manually curated by the project to show what objects are envisioned and in at least one million of the images, bounding boxes are likewise provided. Image-Net, building up the Google-Net architecture expanded the strength to translation and nonlinear learning capacities by utilizing microarchitecture units called "inception units". Every inception unit incorporates several non-linear convolution modules at different resolutions [72].

The inception architecture is particularly effective in processing information at various resolutions, which makes it a potentially useful tool for medical applications, particularly in the field of pathology. This complicated CNF has been successfully modified to targeted treatment categories, such as skin cancer and diabetic retinopathy detection [73]. In certain cases, such as glaucoma, which is the most common cause of irreversible blindness whose diagnosis mainly rests on the subjective judgment of the clinicians. New AI techniques based on DL models can help pathologists recognize cancer subtypes or gene mutations in any form of cancer, while reducing time and expenses. Additionally, these AI advancements enable locations with limited transportation to access healthcare services by sending digital images to labs in other countries, closing the gap in healthcare technology access between nations. CNNs have emerged as the most recent trend in the DL field for diagnosing and analyzing carcinogenic tissues and tumors to facilitate data-driven learning [74].

There are essentially three ways to implement a CNN model: building the model from scratch, using supervised training (where the CNN model learns from available data), and using unsupervised training. Crowd-sourcing might be a more effective approach to developing DL models. It is a collaborative process by which a person, a collective assembly, and an organization execute a job on purpose. The information gathered from the action or survey assists in developing an AI model. In clinical research, it is now common to acquire ground information which can form the basis of artificial intelligence. The quality of the crowd is fundamental to limit "noisy" observations. The information is gathered mainly from two credible (knowledge) and unreliable (community) repositories, making the performance of the produced learning algorithm unclear. Learning via crowd annotations differs from average supervised approaches. In that case, many labels are taken for a similar sample, whereas average supervised techniques are taken together in a framework with bottom cognition material [75]. DL from crowd-sourcing has been used for mitosis detection in breast cancer. Her2Net, another DL framework, has been employed in breast cancer evaluation enabling feature extraction as well as the classification of cytoplasmic membrane and nucleus. Her2Net becomes a machine learning algorithm that recognizes and fragments distinct transmembrane domains including the nucleus from labelled carcinoma cell pictures. After lung cancer, breast cancer occupies the second most common kind of carcinoma. Breast cancer was diagnosed in the United States and Europe's women around 10% at some point of time in their lives. The microscopic observation of the biopsy tissue slides were examined by professionals with an error-prone method (Fig. **7**). Even before an individual develops malignant growth, AI technological models have been reported to provide insight into one's susceptibility to developing the disease. In this context, Naushad *et al.* [76] created an ANN-based framework that analyzes the potential collaboration of genetics, micronutrients, and epidemiological factors that could predict the probability of breast cancer. There is a precise, 94.2% accuracy and a marked number of factors that added to the risk of occurrence of breast cancer, including folate inadequacy and estrogen exposure illustrated by this method [76]. There has long been a recognition that ANNs can be used for diagnostic purposes, and a survey in the early 90s concluded that AI methods are more powerful than conventional statistical techniques, especially for large datasets [77]. There have been several examples such as the ANN created by He *et al.* [78], to analyze breast cancer at an appropriate level. Another study reported a method for developing ANNs utilizing hereditary algorithms. This was done with the goal that the networks adapt similar to how natural evolution occurs so that the system can be utilized in computer-supported mammographic mass detection [79].

AI methods, for example, those for which we have indicated accuracy exactness rates practically identical to humans or even better, provides a specific ANN foundation for diseased melanoma scan that shows a categorization veracity of 93% [81]. Mobadersany *et al.* [84], used survival CNN (SCNNs) to integrate data from both histopathology images and genomic information as a biomarker into a single unified structure to predict time-to-event outcomes and showed higher prediction accuracy that exceeds the current clinical paradigm for predicting the overall survival of patients diagnosed with glioma (Fig. **8**). Table 1 depicts various DL techniques employed so far in the detection and segmentation of cancer cells.

Table 1. An overview of the potential research studies which implemented DL techniques for cancer cell detection and segmentation.

Serial No.	Problem Areas	Technology used	Reference
1.	Brain Tumor	Brain Tumor Image Segmentation	[82]
2.	Cancer cell and tumor detection	CNN Architectures, Dataset Characteristics and Transfer Learning	[74]
3.	Prostate cancer detection	Targeted Contrast-Enhanced Ultrasound based detection	[83]
4.	Breast cancer	DL from crowdsourcing	[75]
5.	To detect morphologic changes in chromatin arrangement	A decision support system	[85]
6.	Breast cancer evaluation	Her2Net: A deep framework for semantic segmentation and classification	[85]
7.	Prostate cancer recurrence	CNN (CNN)	[86]
8.	Colon cancer histology images	Locality Sensitive DL	[87]

ARTIFICIAL INTELLIGENCE TECHNOLOGY AND CANCER TREATMENT

Multiple studies have suggested AI technology may be relied on to provide accurate cancer therapy to patients [88, 89]. For instance, research has provided proof to make cancer treatment less toxic [90]. Recently, the utilization of AI in proliferative disease modeling has emerged as a useful pattern in research because of the capacity of AIs to decode complex datasets for both disease recurrence and patient survival [27, 97]. With access to public information; these methods can be very helpful. The publicly available resources data such as genomics, proteomics, epigenetics, and image data along with the tools used to predict the cancer status and survival are given in Table **2**. The CAMELYON16 research challenge competition focused on developing automated DL algorithms for detecting lymph node metastases of breast cancer using whole slide images (WSI) stained with hematoxylin and eosin [91].

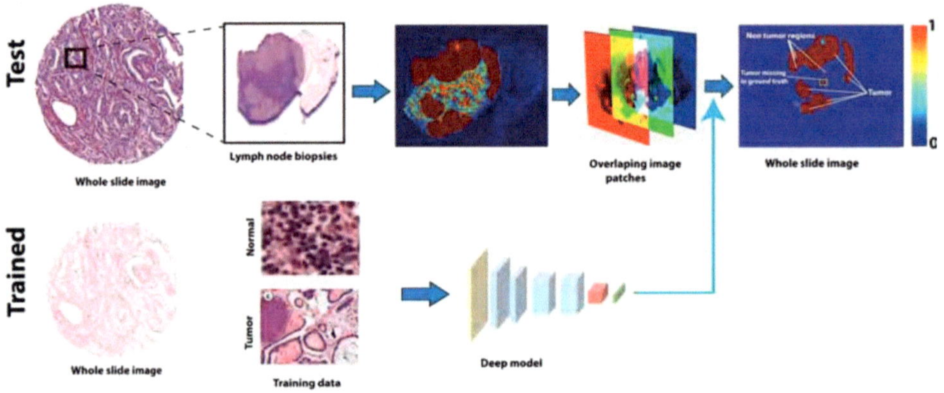

Fig. (8). The Left images showed two lymph node biopsies. The middle image depicts earlier results via DL methods in tumor detection. The last image shows the current results. Notice the visibly reduced noise (potential false positives) between the two versions [80].

Table 2. List of various cancer image repositories available for machine learning study.

Serial No.	Dataset	Slide	Stain	Disease	Additional Sata	Reference
1.	TCGA (Image) https://www.cancerimagingarchive.net/	18,462	H&E	Cancer	Genome/transcriptome/ epigenome/ mutations/ clinical info	[98]
2.	GTEx https://biospecimens.cancer.gov/resources/tissue_image_library.asp	25,380	H&E	Normal	Transcriptome	[99]
3.	TMAD https://www.hsls.pitt.edu/obrc/index.php?page=URL1208277760	3726	H&E	Breast Cancer	Proliferation score for 500 WSIs, position for mitosis for 73 WSI, ROI for 148 cases	[100]
4.	Camelyon17 https://camelyon17.grand-challenge.org	1000	H&E	Breast Cancer (lymph node metastasis)	Mask for cancer region (in 500 WSIs) with 5 WSIs per patients	[101]
5.	KIMIA960 http://kimia.uwaterloo.ca/kimia_lab_data_Path960.html	960	H&E/IH	Various tissue	None	[102]
6.	BreakHis https://web.inf.ufpr.br/vri/databases/breast-cancer-histopathological-database-breakhis/	7909	H&E	Breast Cancer	None	[103]
7.	Linder *et al.* http://fimm.webmicroscope.net/supplements/epistroma	1377	IHC	Colorectal Cancer	Mask for epithelium and stroma	[104]

Table **2** is based on TCGA (The Cancer Genome Atlas); GTEx (Genotype-Tissue Expression); TMAD (The Stanford Tissue Microarray Database) and BreakHis (Breast Cancer Histopathological Database).

This was a goldmine study of the whole slide image analysis in cancer biology by applying DL and AI. In this study, several researchers across the world participated to predict the correct stratification of metastasis vs. non-metastasis using several DL models such as GoogLeNet, ResNet, VGG-16, SegNet, CNN, AlexNet, SVM, Adaboost, Radmon Forests, etc. There are several reports available in connection with different cancer vs normal classifications by utilizing DL and AI in the prediction of the overall survival rate in the context of several cancers. Recently, Cheerla *et al.* [92], demonstrated a study on pan-cancer by applying a multimodal DL approach for the prediction of prognosis using genomics, whole slide image, and clinical information (Fig. **9**). Pan-Cancer research aimed at exploring the similarities and discrepancies between genomic and cellular alterations observed in different tumors. Another research used ANN to categorize women having ovarian disorders. Women were classified in three diagnostic groups based on clinical data, each of which represented a distinct level of severity, in order to develop a decision-support score system [93]. Studies similar to this represent a present flow pattern since many studies have focused on personalized clinical guidelines, and as a result, many of the processes used to determine ANN models may support those programs. Another capacity of ANNs that can often aid in the development of personalized treatment strategies is their ability to predict treatment outcomes. Specialists from MIT created ML methods to decide the doses required for patients experiencing chemotherapy or radiotherapy for cases like glioblastoma [90]. Such a cancer is very malignant and individuals suffering from this disease have an optimum mortality time of approximately 5 years. To combat this, physicians try with several drug types including combinations using chemotherapy and radiation. For maintaining a strategic distance from adverse reactions, machine learning algorithms could really determine the most effective and most feasible drug proportion to provide to the individuals. In actuality, this AI program becomes sustainable from previous patient's treatments and trained to adjust dose quantities and recurrence [90].

It is relevant to offer the minimum effective measure of medications to a cancer patient. It does, provide a fair knowledge to determine a sufficient drug quantity to diminish the growth of the cancer. A few authors like Walczak and Velanovich [94], have claimed that AI frameworks potentially help patients and clinicians to identify the best possible treatment options. For instance, analysts made an ANN framework in decision-making for surgical resection to treat pancreatic malignant growth [94]. The pancreatic cancer is reported to have only about a 7-month survival. At this juncture, if AI or ANN can predict the survival rate accurately, that would either save the money or protect the patient. Regardless of the fascinating outcomes concerning the use of AI to treat cancerous growth, various inquiries need to be addressed. Studies in this area are newer and began only towards the end of 2017. The fundamental unresolved challenge seems to be whether experts could construct an ANN that determines the outcome of selecting a specific therapy? This response could be influenced by the latest reported outcomes for pancreatic cancer. Additionally, it should be beneficial for individuals beyond those with a seven-month survival rate. Francis *et al.* [95] conducted a study employing a neural network system to analyze post-operative data from patients who underwent colorectal cancer surgery. The results of this investigation were consistent with standard regression strategies and identified two factors that contributed to readmission within the first 30 days after the surgery. ANNs were also simple to operate with a little technological understanding. Thus, making it more beneficial for the clinicians to capitalize on advances of such technologies [96]. As research progressed in the interface of health and technology, the therapy will be more inclusive for AI techniques. It will extend enormous practical usefulness for people with cancer.

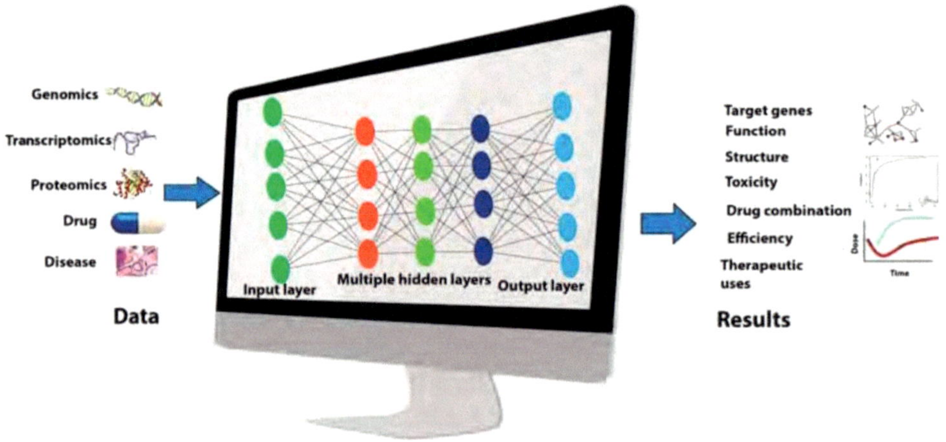

Fig. (9). DL approach for cancer diagnostic and treatment.

MAJOR DRAWBACKS OF AI

The application of AI in oncology presents significant challenges that must be addressed. The key challenge among these is the imperative need for rigorous validation to demonstrate the AI models' capacity to generalize their findings reliably. Moreover, concerns loom over the interpretation of AI-generated results, potentially exacerbating the information gap between clinical practitioners and data science specialists. Nevertheless, if these formidable challenges can be effectively tackled and surmounted, AI stands poised to usher in a transformative era in the field of oncology. By harnessing the immense potential of big data, AI holds the promise of revolutionizing the way we diagnose and treat cancer, offering unprecedented insights and advancements in this critical field.

CONCLUSION

In recent years, there has been a remarkable upsurge in the application of machine learning (ML) techniques across various facets of oncology. This encompasses the creation of predictive models for cancer diagnosis, early detection, streamlining of workflows, predictive analytics, and interventions aimed at treatment. As ML technology and its methodologies continue to advance, it is foreseeable that ML will keep reshaping the landscape of cancer and disease management. AI holds immense potential to revolutionize the delivery of medications and treatments to patients while enhancing the decision-making process for healthcare professionals. It offers the promise of quicker, cost-effective, and highly precise diagnoses. Nonetheless, it is imperative to develop a comprehensive understanding of both the advantages and limitations of this technology to ensure its seamless integration into healthcare practices. The incorporation of AI in healthcare hinges on the availability of extensive datasets for training and evaluation, which brings forth pertinent concerns surrounding data sharing and privacy. Thus, addressing these concerns stands as a paramount step in the successful implementation of AI strategies within the healthcare sector. With the proliferation of computational resources, technological advancements, and substantial progress in deep learning neural network models, AI is poised to reshape clinical practices and oncological treatments. AI has demonstrated its potential in various areas, including medical imaging, therapy diagnostics, assessment of therapeutic responses, forecasting survival rates, and even catalyzing innovations in personalized chemotherapy approaches.

To conclude, DL and AI in general may assist health professionals and clinicians by improving their clinical competence, institutionalizing quality, and providing improved prognosis. Despite the fact that AI innovation models are likely to modify pathologists' and other doctors' work processes. The pathologists' and other doctors' commitments to patient consideration will remain vital in disease management. Most studies evaluating AI in cancer and other fields of therapeutic sciences have received mixed reviews in terms of repeatability and universal applicability of outcomes.

FUTURE POSSIBILITES

AI could make healthcare more effective, personalized, and cheaper through the creation of intelligent processes and workflows. Changing clinical workflows is AI's most immense promise in healthcare as it can both facilitate or enhance the quality of work of clinicians and staff. Healthcare professionals can also use AI to improve performance and patient outcomes by automating many repetitive tasks. Although the use of different classifiers for clinical treatment seems intriguing, several challenges still persist that can impede our progress in ordinary clinical cancer practice. Thus, additional research on AI is warranted to make it play much broader roles in the human health care systems.

LIST OF ABBREVIATIONS

AI	Artificial Intelligence
ML	Machine Learning
DL	Deep Learning
DNN	Deep Neural Network
ANN	Artificial Neural Network
SVM	Support Vector Machine
CNN	Convolutional Neural Network
CAD	Computer-aided diagnosis
GPU	Graphics Processing Units
OAR	Organ-at-risk
2D	Two dimensional
DT	Decision tree
CT	Computed tomography
SCNN	Survival CNN
H & E	Haemotoxylin and Eosin
IHC	Immunohistochemistry
IH	Image histology
WSI	Whole Slide image
TCGA	The Cancer Genome Atlas
GTEx -	Genotype-Tissue expression
TMAD	The Stanford Tissue Microarray Database
AlexNet	Deep Convolutional Neural Network
SegNet	Semantic Segmentation Model
ResNet	Residual Neural Network
VGG	Visual Geometry Group

ACKNOWLEDGEMENTS

KUF thanks the Indian Council of Medical Research-SRF, Govt. of India for providing financial assistance (File No.: 45/75/2020-Nan-BMS).

AUTHOR CONTRIBUTIONS

Khalid Umar Fakhri - Conceptualization and design, Critical review, Intellectual input and Writing-Original draft. Email id: fakhri.khalid@rediffmail.com

Sugandh Kumar – Intellectual input, Critical Review & Writing-review & editing.

Email id: skjobs0123@gmail.com

Md Zubbair Malik - Critical review and Intellectual input. Email id: zubbairmalik@jnu.ac.in

Chirag N. Patel - Writing–review & editing. Email id: chiragpatel269@gmail.com

Yogesh Kumar - Writing–review & editing. Email id: kumar.yogesh601@gmail.com

Khalid Imtiyaz – Writing-review & editing. Email id: khaliddar123@gmail.com

Farhan Jalees Ahmad - Writing-review & editing. Email id: fjahmad@jamiahamdard.ac.in

M. Moshahid Alam Rizvi – Supervision, Writing- review & editing and final editing.

REFERENCES

[1] Torre LA, Bray F, Siegel RL, Ferlay J, Lortet-Tieulent J, Jemal A. Global cancer statistics, 2012. CA Cancer J Clin 2015; 65(2): 87-108. [http://dx.doi.org/10.3322/caac.21262] [PMID: 25651787]

[2] Siegel RL, Miller KD, Fuchs HE, Jemal A. Cancer statistics, 2022. CA Cancer J Clin 2022; 72(1): 7-33. [http://dx.doi.org/10.3322/caac.21708] [PMID: 35020204]

[3] Holtedahl K. Challenges in early diagnosis of cancer: the fast track. Scand J Prim Health Care 2020; 38(3): 251-2. [http://dx.doi.org/10.1080/02813432.2020.1794415] [PMID: 32791936]

[4] Aaronson EL, Quinn GR, Wong CI, *et al.* Missed diagnosis of cancer in primary care: Insights from malpractice claims data. J Healthc Risk Manag 2019; 39(2): 19-29. [http://dx.doi.org/10.1002/jhrm.21385] [PMID: 31338938]

[5] Doi K. Computer-aided diagnosis in medical imaging: Historical review, current status and future potential. Comput Med Imaging Graph 2007; 31(4-5): 198-211. [http://dx.doi.org/10.1016/j.compmedimag.2007.02.002] [PMID: 17349778]

[6] Mitchell TM, *et al.* Machine learning. Wcb/McGraw-Hill Science 1997.

[7] Spiewak C, Islam MR, Zaman MAU. A Comprehensive Study on EMG Feature Extraction and Classifiers. Open Access J Biomed Eng Biosci 2018; 1(1) . [http://dx.doi.org/10.32474/OAJBEB.2018.01.000104]

[8] Han F, Wang H, Zhang G, *et al.* Texture feature analysis for computer-aided diagnosis on pulmonary

nodules. J Digit Imaging 2015; 28(1): 99-115.
[http://dx.doi.org/10.1007/s10278-014-9718-8] [PMID: 25117512]

[9] Barata C, Ruela M, Mendonca T, Marquees JS. A bag-of-features approach for the classification of melanomas in dermoscopy images: The role of color and texture descriptors.Computer Vision Techniques for the Diagnosis of Skin Cancer. Berlin/Heidelberg, Germany: Springer 2014; pp. 49-69.
[http://dx.doi.org/10.1007/978-3-642-39608-3_3]

[10] DeVita VT Jr, Chu E. A history of cancer chemotherapy. Cancer Res 2008; 68(21): 8643-53.
[http://dx.doi.org/10.1158/0008-5472.CAN-07-6611]

[11] Sarker IH. Deep Learning: A Comprehensive Overview on Techniques, Taxonomy, Applications and Research Directions. SN Computer Science 2021; 2(6): 420.
[http://dx.doi.org/10.1007/s42979-021-00815-1] [PMID: 34426802]

[12] Xu B, Wang N, Chen T, Li M. Empirical evaluation of rectified activations in convolutional network. Machine Learning. Computer Vision and Pattern Recognition. 2015.

[13] Lynch CJ, Liston C. New machine-learning technologies for computer-aided diagnosis. Nat Med 2018; 24(9): 1304-5.
[http://dx.doi.org/10.1038/s41591-018-0178-4] [PMID: 30177823]

[14] Azuaje F. Artificial intelligence for precision oncology: beyond patient stratification. NPJ Precis Oncol 2019; 25: 3-6.
[http://dx.doi.org/10.1038/s41698-019-0078-1]

[15] National Institute for Health and Care Excellence. Melanoma: assessment and management. 2015. https://www.nice.org.uk/guidance/ng142015.

[16] Ardila D, Kiraly AP, Bharadwaj S, *et al.* End-to-end lung cancer screening with three-dimensional deep learning on low-dose chest computed tomography. Nat Med 2019; 25(6): 954-61.
[http://dx.doi.org/10.1038/s41591-019-0447-x] [PMID: 31110349]

[17] Apple SK. Sentinel lymph node in breast cancer: review article from a pathologist ?(tm)s point of view. J Pathol Transl Med 2016; 50(2): 83-95.
[http://dx.doi.org/10.4132/jptm.2015.11.23] [PMID: 26757203]

[18] Bailey MH, Tokheim C, Porta-Pardo E, *et al.* Comprehensive characterization of cancer driver genes and mutations. Cell 2018; 173(2): 371-385.e18.
[http://dx.doi.org/10.1016/j.cell.2018.02.060] [PMID: 29625053]

[19] Li Y, Wu FX, Ngom A. A review on machine learning principles for multi-view biological data integration. Brief Bioinform 2018; 19(2): 325-40.
[PMID: 28011753]

[20] Iafrate F. Artificial intelligence and big data the birth of a new intelligence. ISTE Ltd and John Wiley & Sons 2018.
[http://dx.doi.org/10.1002/9781119426653]

[21] Geuna A, Guerzoni M, Nuccio M, Pammolli F, Rungi A. Digital Disruption and the Transformation of Italian Manufacturing Piemonte Region and Northern Italy in the Global Competition. Robotics. Aspen Institute Italia 2017.

[22] Goodfellow I, Yoshua B, Courville A. MIT Press 2018.

[23] Madabhushi A, Lee G. Image analysis and machine learning in digital pathology: Challenges and opportunities. Med Image Anal 2016; 33: 170-5.
[http://dx.doi.org/10.1016/j.media.2016.06.037] [PMID: 27423409]

[24] Esteva A, Kuprel B, Novoa RA, *et al.* Dermatologist-level classification of skin cancer Litjens G, S nchez CI, Timofeeva N, et al. DL as a tool for increased accuracy and efficiency of histopathological diagnosis. (2016), Sci Rep, 6:26286. 2016.

[25] Russell SJ, Norvig P. Artificial intelligence: a modern approach. 3rd ed., Upper Saddle River, New

Jersey: Prentice-Hall 2003.

[26] Samuel AL. Some studies in machine learning using the game of checkers. IBM J Res Develop 1959; 3(3): 210-29.
[http://dx.doi.org/10.1147/rd.33.0210]

[27] Kourou K, Exarchos TP, Exarchos KP, Karamouzis MV, Fotiadis DI. Machine learning applications in cancer prognosis and prediction. Comput Struct Biotechnol J 2015; 13: 8-17.
[http://dx.doi.org/10.1016/j.csbj.2014.11.005] [PMID: 25750696]

[28] Meyer P, Noblet V, Mazzara C, Lallement A. Survey on deep learning for radiotherapy. Comput Biol Med 2018; 98: 126-46.
[http://dx.doi.org/10.1016/j.compbiomed.2018.05.018] [PMID: 29787940]

[29] Hunter B, Hindocha S, Lee RW. The role of artificial intelligence in early cancer diagnosis. Cancers 2022; 14(6): 1524.
[http://dx.doi.org/10.3390/cancers14061524] [PMID: 35326674]

[30] Xu Y, Liu X, Cao X, *et al.* Artificial intelligence: A powerful paradigm for scientific research. Innovation 2021; 2(4): 100179.
[http://dx.doi.org/10.1016/j.xinn.2021.100179] [PMID: 34877560]

[31] Venkatesan M. Artificial intelligence vs machine learning vs DL https://www.datasciencecentral.com/profiles/blogs/artificial-intelligence-vs-machine-learning-vs-deep-learning2018.Data Science Central.

[32] Schmidt-Erfurth U, Sadeghipour A, Gerendas BS, Waldstein SM, Bogunovi H. Artificial intelligence in retina. Prog Retin Eye Res 2018; 67: 1-29.
[http://dx.doi.org/10.1016/j.preteyeres.2018.07.004] [PMID: 30076935]

[33] Bibault JE, Giraud P, Burgun A. Big Data and machine learning in radiation oncology: State of the art and future prospects. Cancer Lett 2016; 382(1): 110-7.
[http://dx.doi.org/10.1016/j.canlet.2016.05.033] [PMID: 27241666]

[34] Pearson D. Artificial intelligence in radiology: the game-changer on Everyone ?(tm)s Mind https://www.radiologybusiness.com/topics/technology-management/artificial-intelligen-e-radiology-game-changer-everyones-mind2017.

[35] Hopfield JJ. Artificial neural networks. IEEE Circuits Devices 1988; 4(5): 3-10.
[http://dx.doi.org/10.1109/101.8118]

[36] Gulliford SL, Webb S, Rowbottom CG, Corne DW, Dearnaley DP. Use of artificial neural networks to predict biological outcomes for patients receiving radical radiotherapy of the prostate. Radiother Oncol 2004; 71(1): 3-12.
[http://dx.doi.org/10.1016/j.radonc.2003.03.001] [PMID: 15066290]

[37] Cho DD, Wernicke AG, Nori D, Chao KC, Chang J, Parashar B. Predicting radiation therapy outcome for head and neck cancer patients using artificial neural network (ANN). Int J Radiat Oncol Biol Phys 2014; 90(1): S852.
[http://dx.doi.org/10.1016/j.ijrobp.2014.05.2442]

[38] Russakovsky O, Deng J, Su H, *et al.* ImageNet large scale visual recognition challenge. Int J Comput Vis 2015; 115(3): 211-52.
[http://dx.doi.org/10.1007/s11263-015-0816-y]

[39] Nelsen M. Neural Networks and DL Press 2015.

[40] Nikolov S, Blackwell S, Mendes R, *et al.* DL to achieve clinically applicable segmentation of head and neck anatomy for radiotherapy. arXiv:180904430 2018.

[41] Turing AM. Computing machinery and intelligence. Mind 1950; LIX(236): 433-60.
[http://dx.doi.org/10.1093/mind/LIX.236.433]

[42] Hornik K. Approximation capabilities of multilayer feedforward networks. Neural Netw 1991; 4(2):

251-7.
[http://dx.doi.org/10.1016/0893-6080(91)90009-T]

[43] Zeiler MD, Fergus R. Visualizing and understanding convolutional networks. In: Fleet D, Pajdla T, Schiele B, Tuytelaars T, Eds. Computer Vision ?" ECCV. Cham: Springer International Publishing 2014; pp. 818-33.

[44] Ahuja AS, Halperin LS. Understanding the advent of artificial intelligence in ophthalmology. J Curr Ophthalmol 2019; 31(2): 115-7.
[http://dx.doi.org/10.1016/j.joco.2019.05.001] [PMID: 31317087]

[45] Lighthill J. Lighthill report: artificial intelligence: a paper symposium 2017.

[46] Wang S, Summers RM. Machine learning and radiology. Med Image Anal 2012; 16(5): 933-51.
[http://dx.doi.org/10.1016/j.media.2012.02.005] [PMID: 22465077]

[47] Freeman TC, Goldovsky L, Brosch M, *et al.* Construction, visualisation, and clustering of transcription networks from microarray expression data. PLOS Comput Biol 2007; 3(10): e206.
[http://dx.doi.org/10.1371/journal.pcbi.0030206] [PMID: 17967053]

[48] Lee HK, Hsu AK, Sajdak J, Qin J, Pavlidis P. Coexpression analysis of human genes across many microarray data sets. Genome Res 2004; 14(6): 1085-94.
[http://dx.doi.org/10.1101/gr.1910904] [PMID: 15173114]

[49] Menden Michael P, *et al.* Machine learning prediction of cancer cell sensitivity to drugs based on genomic and chemical properties. PLoS one 2013; 61318.
[http://dx.doi.org/10.1371/journal.pone.0061318]

[50] FrAhlich H, Balling R, Beerenwinkel N, *et al.* From hype to reality: Data science enabling personalized medicine. BMC Med 2018; 16(1): 150.
[http://dx.doi.org/10.1186/s12916-018-1122-7] [PMID: 30145981]

[51] Ding MQ, Chen L, Cooper GF, Young JD, Lu X. Precision oncology beyond targeted therapy: Combining omics data with machine learning matches the majority of cancer cells to effective therapeutics. Mol Cancer Res 2018; 16(2): 269-78.
[http://dx.doi.org/10.1158/1541-7786.MCR-17-0378] [PMID: 29133589]

[52] Mousavi SM, Beroza GC. Deep-learning seismology. Science 2022; 377(6607): eabm4470.
[http://dx.doi.org/10.1126/science.abm4470] [PMID: 35951699]

[53] Esteva A, Kuprel B, Novoa RA, *et al.* Dermatologist-level classification of skin cancer with deep neural networks. Nature 2017; 542(7639): 115-8.
[http://dx.doi.org/10.1038/nature21056] [PMID: 28117445]

[54] Spanhol A, Oliveira LS, Petitjean C, Heutte L. Breast cancer histopathological image classification using CNN. 2016 international joint conference on neural networks, IJCNN 2016, Vancouver, BC, Canada, July 24-29, (2016) (pp. 2560-2567.

[55] Han Z, Wei B, Zheng Y, Yin Y, Li K. LiBreast cancer multi-classification from histopathological images with structured DL modelSci Rep. 2017; 7(1): 4172.

[56] Liu Y, Gadepalli K, Norouzi M, *et al.* Detecting cancer metastases on gigapixel pathology images. 2017; 2017.

[57] Ehteshami Bejnordi B, Veta M, Johannes van Diest P, *et al.* Diagnostic assessment of DL algorithms for detection of lymph node metastases in women with breast cancer. JAMA 2017; 318(22): 2199-210.
[http://dx.doi.org/10.1001/jama.2017.14585] [PMID: 29234806]

[58] Litjens G, SA nchez CI, Timofeeva N, *et al.* Deep learning as a tool for increased accuracy and efficiency of histopathological diagnosis. Sci Rep 2016; 6(1): 26286.
[http://dx.doi.org/10.1038/srep26286] [PMID: 27212078]

[59] Hinton GEPereira F, Burges CJC, Bottou L, Weinberger KQ ImageNet classification with deep CNN. Krizhevsky A, Sutskever I. Advances in Neural Information Processing SystemsSan Francisco, CA:

Curran Associates Inc 2012; 25: pp. 1097-105.

[60] Cruz JA, Wishart DS. Applications of machine learning in cancer prediction and prognosis. Cancer Inform 2007; 2(2): 59-77.
[PMID: 19458758]

[61] Weston AD, Hood L. Systems biology, proteomics, and the future of health care: toward predictive, preventative, and personalized medicine. J Proteome Res 2004; 3(2): 179-96.
[http://dx.doi.org/10.1021/pr0499693] [PMID: 15113093]

[62] Hagerty RG, Butow PN, Ellis PM, Dimitry S, Tattersall MHN. Communicating prognosis in cancer care: a systematic review of the literature. Ann Oncol 2005; 16(7): 1005-53.
[http://dx.doi.org/10.1093/annonc/mdi211] [PMID: 15939716]

[63] Liu Y, Wang C, Zhang L. Decision Tree Based Predictive Models for Breast Cancer Survivability on Imbalanced Data. 3rd International Conference on Bioinformatics and Biomedical Engineering 2009; 1-4.
[http://dx.doi.org/10.1109/ICBBE.2009.5162571]

[64] Delen D, Walker G, Kadam A. Predicting breast cancer survivability: A comparison of three data mining methods. Artif Intell Med 2005; 34(2): 113-27.
[http://dx.doi.org/10.1016/j.artmed.2004.07.002] [PMID: 15894176]

[65] Liang M, Li Z, Chen T, Zeng J. Integrative Data Analysis of Multi-Platform Cancer Data with a Multimodal DL Approach. IEEE/ACM Trans. Comput Biol Bioinform 2015; 12: 928-37.
[PMID: 26357333]

[66] Chaudhary K, Poirion OB, Lu L, Garmire LX. Deep Learning ?"Based Multi-Omics Integration Robustly Predicts Survival in Liver Cancer. Clin Cancer Res 2018; 24(6): 1248-59.
[http://dx.doi.org/10.1158/1078-0432.CCR-17-0853] [PMID: 28982688]

[67] Abbass HA. An evolutionary artificial neural networks approach for breast cancer diagnosis. Artif Intell Med 2002; 25(3): 265-81.
[http://dx.doi.org/10.1016/S0933-3657(02)00028-3]

[68] Portnoi T, Yala A, Schuster T, *et al.* DL Model to Assess Cancer Risk on the Basis of a Breast MR Image Alone. AJR Am J Roentgenol 2019; 213(1): 227-33.

[69] Vobugari N, Raja V, Sethi U, Gandhi K, Raja K, Surani SR. Advancements in Oncology with Artificial Intelligence ?"A Review Article. Cancers (Basel) 2022; 14(5): 1349.
[http://dx.doi.org/10.3390/cancers14051349] [PMID: 35267657]

[70] Khosravi P, Kazemi E, Imielinski M, Elemento O, Hajirasouliha I. Deep CNN Enable Discrimination of Heterogeneous Digital Pathology Images. EBioMedicine 2018; 27: 317-28.
[http://dx.doi.org/10.1016/j.ebiom.2017.12.026] [PMID: 29292031]

[71] Coudray N, Ocampo PS, Sakellaropoulos T, *et al.* Classification and mutation prediction from non ?"small cell lung cancer histopathology images using deep learning. Nat Med 2018; 24(10): 1559-67.
[http://dx.doi.org/10.1038/s41591-018-0177-5] [PMID: 30224757]

[72] Russakovsky O, Deng J, Su H, *et al.* ImageNet Large Scale Visual Recognition Challenge, Journal of International Journal of Computer Vision 2015.
https://arxiv.org/abs/1409.0575

[73] Gulshan V, Peng L, Coram M, *et al.* Development and validation of a DL algorithm for the detection of diabetic retinopathy in retinal fundus photographs. JAMA 2016; 316(22): 2402-10.
[http://dx.doi.org/10.1001/jama.2016.17216] [PMID: 27898976]

[74] Hoo-Chang S, Roth H R, Gao M, Lu L, Xu Z, Nogues I, *et al.* IEEE Trans Med Imaging 2016; 35(5): 1285.
[http://dx.doi.org/10.1109/TMI.2016.2528162] [PMID: 26886976]

[75] Albarqouni S, Baur C, Achilles F, Belagiannis V, Demirci S, Navab N. Aggnet: DL from crowds for

mitosis detection in breast cancer histology images. IEEE Trans Med Imaging 2016; 35(5): 1313-21. [http://dx.doi.org/10.1109/TMI.2016.2528120] [PMID: 26891484]

[76] Naushad SM, Janaki Ramaiah M, Pavithrakumari M, *et al.* Artificial neural network-based exploration of gene-nutrient interactions in folate and xenobiotic metabolic pathways that modulate susceptibility to breast cancer. Gene 2016; 580(2): 159-68. [http://dx.doi.org/10.1016/j.gene.2016.01.023] [PMID: 26784656]

[77] Abbod MF, Catto JWF, Linkens DA, Hamdy FC. Application of artificial intelligence to the management of urological cancer. J Urol 2007; 178(4): 1150-6. [http://dx.doi.org/10.1016/j.juro.2007.05.122] [PMID: 17698099]

[78] He S, Wu QH, Saunders JR. Breast cancer diagnosis using an artificial neural network trained by group search optimizer. Trans Inst Meas Contr 2009; 31(6): 517-31. [http://dx.doi.org/10.1177/0142331208094239]

[79] Tan M, Pu J, Zheng B. Optimization of network topology in computer-aided detection schemes using phased searcing with NEAT in a time-scaled framework. Cancer Inform 2014; 13(1) (Suppl. 1): 17-27. [PMID: 25392680]

[80] Martin Stumpe, Lily Peng. Assisting pathologist in detecting cancer with DL 2017.

[81] Premaladha J, Ravichandran KS. Novel Approaches for Diagnosing Melanoma Skin Lesions Through Supervised and DL Algorithms. J Med Syst. (2016) Apr;40(4):96. 2016.

[82] Menze B H, Jakab A, Bauer S, Kalpathy-Cramer J, Farahani K, Kirby J, *et al.* The multimodal brain tumor image segmentation benchmark (BRATS). IEEE transactions on medical imaging, 34(10), 2015.

[83] Feng Y, Yang F, Zhou X, *et al.* A DL Approach for Targeted Contrast-Enhanced Ultrasound Based Prostate Cancer Detection IEEE/ACM Trans Comput Biol Bioinform. (2019) Nov-Dec;16(6):179--1801. 2019.

[84] Mobadersany P, Yousefi S, Amgad M, *et al.* Predicting cancer outcomes from histology and genomics using convolutional networks. Proc Natl Acad Sci U S A (2018) Mar 27;115(13):E2970-E2979 2018. [http://dx.doi.org/10.1073/pnas.1717139115]

[85] Saha M, Chakraborty C. Her2net: A deep framework for semantic segmentation and classification of cell membranes and nuclei in breast cancer evaluation. IEEE Trans Image Process 2018; 27(5): 2189-200. [http://dx.doi.org/10.1109/TIP.2018.2795742] [PMID: 29432100]

[86] Kumar N, Verma R, Arora A, *et al.* CNN for prostate cancer recurrence prediction. In Medical Imaging 2017: Digital Pathology. International Society of Optics and Photonics 2017; 10140: 101400H.

[87] Sirinukunwattana K, Raza SEA, Tsang Y-W, Snead DRJ, Cree IA, Rajpoot NM. Locality sensitive DL for detection and classification of nuclei in routine colon cancer histology images. IEEE Trans Med Imaging 2016; 35(5): 1196-206. [http://dx.doi.org/10.1109/TMI.2016.2525803] [PMID: 26863654]

[88] Kickingereder P, Isensee F, Tursunova I, *et al.* Automated quantitative tumour response assessment of MRI in neuro-oncology with artificial neural networks: a multicentre, retrospective study. Lancet Oncol (2019) May;20(5):728-740 2019. [http://dx.doi.org/10.1016/S1470-2045(19)30098-1]

[89] Davenport T, Kalakota R. The potential for artificial intelligence in healthcare. Future Healthc J 2019; 6(2): 94-8. [http://dx.doi.org/10.7861/futurehosp.6-2-94]

[90] Matheson R. MIT News Office. Artificial intelligence model "learns" from patient data to make cancer treatment less toxic 2018.

[91] Ehteshami Bejnordi B, Veta M, Johannes van Diest P, *et al.* Diagnostic Assessment of DL Algorithms for Detection of Lymph Node Metastases in Women With Breast Cancer. JAMA. (2017) Dec 12;318(22):2199-2210. 2017.

[92] Cheerla A, Gevaert O. Deep learning with multimodal representation for pancancer prognosis prediction. Bioinformatics 2019; 35(14): i446-54. [http://dx.doi.org/10.1093/bioinformatics/btz342] [PMID: 31510656]

[93] Kyrgiou M, Pouliakis A, Panayiotides JG, *et al.* Personalised management of women with cervical abnormalities using a clinical decision support scoring system. Gynecol Oncol 2016; 141(1): 29-35. [http://dx.doi.org/10.1016/j.ygyno.2015.12.032] [PMID: 27016226]

[94] Walczak S, Velanovich V. An Evaluation of Artificial Neural Networks in Predicting Pancreatic Cancer Survival. J Gastrointest Surg. (2017) Oct;21(10):1606-1612. 2017.

[95] Francis NK, Luther A, Salib E, *et al.* The use of artificial neural networks to predict delayed discharge and readmission in enhanced recovery following laparoscopic colorectal cancer surgery. Tech Coloproctol 2015; 19(7): 419-28. [http://dx.doi.org/10.1007/s10151-015-1319-0] [PMID: 26084884]

[96] Li Q, Chan MF. Predictive time-series modeling using artificial neural networks for Linac beam symmetry: An empirical study J Ambient Intell Humaniz Comput 2017; 1387(1): 84-94. [http://dx.doi.org/10.1111/nyas.13215]

[97] Kumar Y, Koul A, Singla R, Ijaz MF. Artificial intelligence in disease diagnosis: a systematic literature review, synthesizing framework and future research agenda. J Ambient Intell Humaniz Comput 2022; 13: 1-28.

[98] Tomczak K, Czerwi ska P, Wiznerowicz M. Review The Cancer Genome Atlas (TCGA): An immeasurable source of knowledge. Contemp Oncol 2015; 1A(1A): 68-77. [http://dx.doi.org/10.5114/wo.2014.47136] [PMID: 25691825]

[99] GTEx Consortium. The Genotype-Tissue Expression (GTEx) project. Nat Genet 2013; 45(6): 580-5.

[100] Marinelli RJ, Montgomery K, Liu CL, *et al.* The stanford tissue microarray database. Nucleic Acids Res 2008.

[101] Bandi P, Geessink O, Manson Q, *et al.* From Detection of Individual Metastases to Classification of Lymph Node Status at the Patient Level: The CAMELYON17 Challenge. IEEE Trans Med Imaging 2019; 38(2): 550-60.

[102] Kumar MD, Babaie M, Zhu S, Kalra S, Tizhoosh HR. A comparative study of CNN, BoVW and LBP for classification of histopathological images. 2017 IEEE Symposium Series on Computational Intelligence (SSCI). 1-7.

[103] Spanhol FA, Oliveira LS, Petitjean C, Heutte L. A dataset for breast cancer histopathological image classification. IEEE Trans Biomed Eng 2016; 63(7): 1455-62. [http://dx.doi.org/10.1109/TBME.2015.2496264] [PMID: 26540668]

[104] Linder E, Lundin M, Thors C, *et al.* Web-based virtual microscopy for parasitology: A novel tool for education and quality assurance. PLoS Negl Trop Dis 2008; 2(10): e315. [http://dx.doi.org/10.1371/journal.pntd.0000315] [PMID: 18941514]

CHAPTER 10

Precision Medicine in Fibromyalgia Syndrome

Ghizal Fatima[1,*]

[1] *Department of Biotechnology, Era University, Lucknow-226003, India*

Abstract: Individualized remedy for patients is a middle objective of today's clinical approach and the need of our society. Many elements, starting from genes to proteins, all stay unknown for their unique roles in human physiology. The accurate prognosis, monitoring, and remedy of various problems require dependable biomarkers, for the development of correct healing interventions. Precision medicine within the treatment of Fibromyalgia Syndrome (FMS) has attracted a whole lot of attention, particularly with the gene discovery pushing toward more modern know-how of the biology of disorders. Genome-huge association research has proven that in fibromyalgia pathogenesis, genetic factors are accountable for as much as 50% of the sickness susceptibility. Candidate genes determined to be associated with fibromyalgia are SLC64A4, TRPV2, MYT1L, and NRXN3. Fibromyalgia is an extensive musculoskeletal pain disorder followed by fatigue, sleep, memory, and mood troubles.

Fibromyalgia syndrome (FMS) exacerbates painful sensations by altering the way the brain and spinal cord process both painful and non-painful signals. While some targeted treatments have shown promise in improving the condition of FMS patients in the short term, there is an opportunity to delve deeper into the mechanisms at play. With the aid of animal models, we can further explore the intricate interplay between the brain and the spinal cord, identifying specific genes, loci, and potential failures within the spinal cord that contribute to FMS.

Additionally, FMS has been linked to biogenic amine depletion and mitochondrial dysfunction. These factors represent crucial avenues for investigation. This chapter aims to spotlight the significant advancements in technology that facilitate personalized or precision medicine approaches for FMS. Since FMS is closely tied to the functioning of the brain and spinal cord, research using animal models offers a promising avenue, as conducting experiments on patients presents logistical challenges.

Keywords: Animal model, Anxiety disorders, Amine depletion, Fibromyalgia prognosis, Precipitated fibromyalgia, Sleep aetiology.

* **Corresponding author Ghizal Fatima:** Department of Biotechnology, Era University, Lucknow-226003, India; Tel: 9616283669; E-mail: ghizalfatima8@gmail.com

Farzana Mahdi & Abbas Ali Mahdi (Eds.)

INTRODUCTION

Precision medicine (PM) is defined as an approach to an individual's genetics, environment, and lifestyle to help determine the exceptional preventable method to treat a disorder [1]. PM was well-documented [2] and has now and again proven an excellent impact on some diseases inclusive of FMS [2]. Dramatic progress in the area has enabled achievements in FMS genetics [4]. PM in the narrower aspect assumes that a drug concentrated on a molecular stage might be the satisfactory possible method to attain accuracy, justifying the term "precision remedy. The primary issue is that the definition of what is particular and what is not can most effectively consult with the present-day (molecular and pathogenetic) information. The feasibility of diagnostic tests and their ability to provide additional precision directly influences the accuracy of treatment. The application of genetics has recognized the cause of many severe, regularly treatment-resistant diseases producing a paradigm for PM extending from genetic discovery to *in vitro* and *in vivo* models. Further, this enabled rational drug selection, repurposing, or the discovery of the more recent drug molecules for human beings with mutations within the gene that can be used for clinical trials. Fibromyalgia syndrome (FMS) is a commonplace sickness, characterised by way of persistent generalized aches with an anticipated prevalence of one–5% of the population [5]. FMS is likewise related to a variety of somatic and mental issues, which include fatigue, sleep disturbances, stiffness, anxiety, and cognitive disorder [6].

Over the last couple of decades, research has been devoted drastically closer to the development of newer pharmacological solutions for the fibromyalgia spectrum. This fact is properly predicted in view of the overpowering financial burden posed by using persistent pain in popular and FMS. These efforts have led to 3 medications gaining FDA acclaim for the FMS treatment. nevertheless, at the same time as reviewing the progress made on this location of untreated FMS disease, it should be acknowledged that pharmacological remedy has been met, in widespread, with rather modest prices of success. Actual-lifestyles data published over recent years [7], showed that only a minority of FMS patients took drug treatments for a quick time period both due to lack of efficacy or aspect results, or each. Current suggestions published regarding the remedy of this disorder, unanimously propose, a multidisciplinary approach, with the aid of combining pharmacological remedy with complementary modalities, inclusive of cognitive behavioral therapy (CBT), aerobic and strengthening bodily training, and meditative movement cures [8, 9].

However, studies have proven the reason for a few treatments to be extra powerful than others and proven to be a possible remedy earlier than the identification of the cause of the disorder. The capacity of PM seems big and huge and the enthusiasm is comprehensible: The PM provides rational powerful care for each person affected by FMS [10]. Throughout human diseases, PM has attracted tons of attention in the direction of the discovery and progress of genetics as this line of work is envisaged to assist in picking out and broadening the makers by using know-how the disorder biology. The rise and the autumn of the preceding revolutions inside the field of FMS bear witness to the idea that a particular exhilaration can also be the simplest quick-lived dream [11].

PM perhaps gets towards disease biology more than any other previous efforts made for sickness diagnosis. However, PM for FMS requires clarity of experimental strategies to increase markers reliable enough to be useful across the spectrum of FMS patients. The modern status of PM in FMS for diagnosis, diagnosis, choice of remedy, and choice to lessen remedy could be discussed here. Development of markers for analysis of FMS involves several additives encompassing genomics, genetics, environmental publicity, assessment of epigenetic amendment, imaging, and radiological surveillance, and getting admission to to health care device (Fig. **1**). Prognostic precision (P.P) is properly set up for FMS, such as markers of sickness activity or its shape, as well as autoantibodies and genetics. Eventually, the latest, and most reliable markers for a secure remedy continue to be inside the lower ranges of disease activity and longer presence of remission of the sickness.

PURPOSE OF PRECISION MEDICINE IN FMS

Character and behavioral environmental exposure get the right of entry to Healthcare Genetics and Genomics customized medicinal drug modifications in Epigenetic Biomarkers Imaging and Radiology (Fig. **1**). An outline of personalized medicine for understanding the underlying factors of Fibromyalgia Syndrome (FMS) should encompass multiple aspects. Purpose of Precision Medication in FMS-vital unmet want of remedy in FMS is the identity of biomarkers that predict which of the medications can be only for a man or woman suffering from FMS, which will decrease sickness activity. Here we strive to outline goal measures for remedy and response therein for the development of personalised medicine for FMS [12].

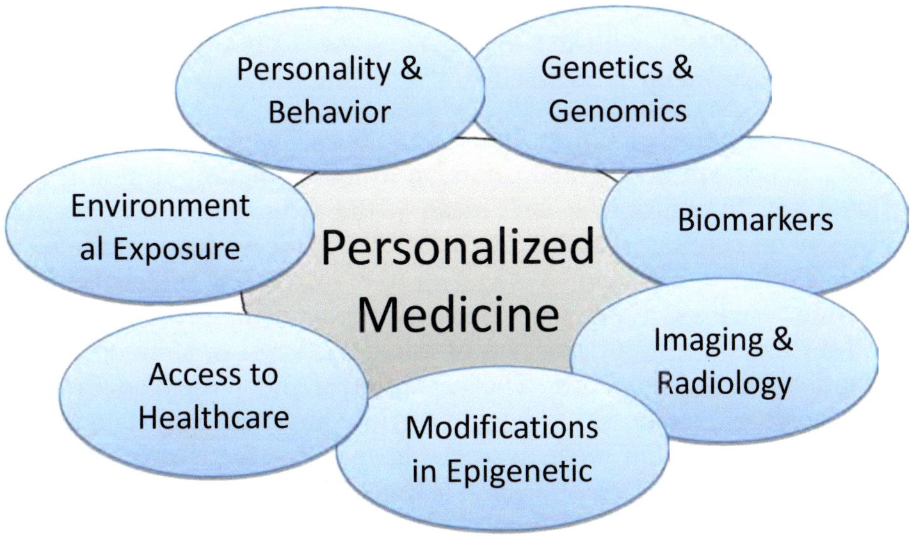

Fig. (1). Elements in personalized medicine.

PRECISION MEDICINAL DRUG AND ITS FRAMEWORK

Several targeted remedy options are emerging, a few with substantial sophistication geared toward individual-level tailor-made remedies. There have been achievements in enhancing a few patients. In conjunction with a good deal-needed success, problems are also springing up. Precision remedies do not always paint, and every so often those are inaccessible or do not not exist. Failures of PM might not locate their way to broader scrutiny. However, PM isn't always a new idea; It has already been boosted by means of genetics and is regularly much centered on genetically decided disorders, usually considered to be driven in a man or woman by means of a single genetic variation. Often the mechanisms generating the total medical phenotype from this sort of perceived single motive are incompletely understood. The effect of additional genetic variants and different factors that could have an effect on the medical presentation represents complexities that are not typically taken into possible consideration.

Precision fulfillment and precision failure are also need to be explained. There is a need for a more comprehensive evaluation and rigorous framework, bringing together records that are both essential and sufficient to explain clinical presentation and its responses to precision remedies for FMS. All this provides a brand new or an awful lot narrower definition of PM, which suggests the use of the unique molecular traits of a patient for management. However, for FMS-affected persons, the search for a unique feature for diagnosis is not feasible because of several bodily, physiological, genetic, genomically, and hormonal variants. Due to the fact brain and spinal cord both are involved, each has to be studied independently or interdependently to determine out root cause of the trouble correlating that with the disorder's signs. Consequently, a huge set of information has ended up as an essential part before PM may be attempted.

The modern reputation of PM in FMS inside the management areas of analysis, prognosis, choice of remedy, and selection to lessen therapy has no longer been formulated yet. In addition, it isn't clean if the drug molecules prescribed are based totally on cautious titration for his or her choicest dose or related to one-time trial. Similarly, it isn't always known how many drug molecules have been re-purposing used as a precision remedy. Prognostic precision is properly mounted for FMS, including markers of ailment interest or structure, in addition to autoantibodies and genetics. The selection of the proper compound in an affected person is recognized to have a terrible analysis, but, stays extensively arbitrary. In the end, the most dependable markers for a safe withdrawal of remedy stay decreased stages of disease activity and longer presence of remission. As we can be on the point of a remedy revolution, progress ought to be considered and reasoned: One viable framework is proposed for the evaluation of precision treatment is highlighted in Fig. (**2**).

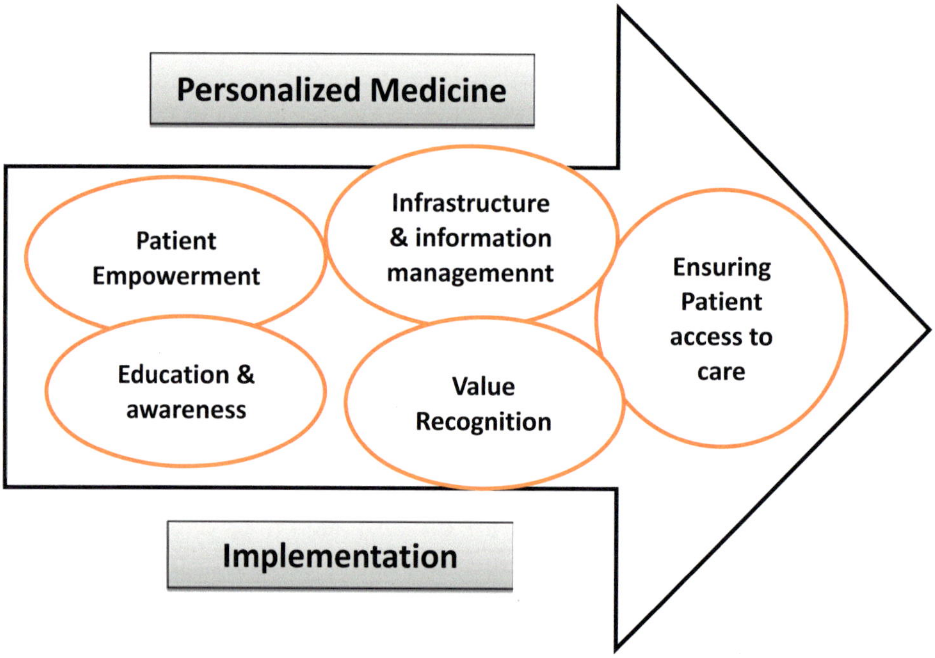

Fig. (2). Strategies for integrating personalized medicine into healthcare practice.

Personalized remedy patient empowerment infrastructure and statistics control training and focus value recognition implementation ensuring patient get right of entry to care (Fig. **2**). Techniques for integrating personalized medication into healthcare practices.

PRECISION MEDICINE AND GENETICS

Genetic variations and inheritance mechanisms in FMS genes were proven to contribute about 50% of inside the development of chronic ache problems, as shown *via* linkage studies, showing the correlation between the genetic variations and pain reaction [13]. Currently, loads of pains-regulated genes potentially relevant to ache sensitivity or analgesia have been diagnosed, out of which genes encoding for sodium channels, GTP cyclohydrolase 1 (GTPCH-1), mu-opioid receptors, catechol-O-methyltransferase, and GABAergic pathway proteins are commonplace [14]. The diagnostic phenotype of FMS isn't discernible. In FMS, as for most other rheumatic situations, category criteria are to be had, but those fluctuate conceptually from the diagnostic standards. The principle distinction is the identification of category criteria. Therefore, trying to pick out homogeneous companies of patients for enrolment in scientific trials studies could be distinctively compared to diagnostic standards that will have a practical effect on getting the analysis right within the given ailment. The putative genetic causes of increasing illnesses were identified; aiming that additional rational healing procedures will emerge quickly [15]

The new genetic discovery sets the direction for decided-on or engineered answers. Accordingly, if a particular disease is shown to be because of pathogenic variations in a gene encoding an ion channel, as an example, the well-trodden pathway is to decide whether or not a specific phenotype is because of loss- or gain-of function of the encoded mutant protein and then to pick out a treatment which can reverse this proximal practical consequence. This sort of remedy may be already known to have the desired impact at the channel in query, or a repurposed drug on the way to be used to lower the severity of the sickness symptoms by means of correcting the genetic mutations in that gene, or it is able to be that a brand new remedy desires invention.

Correction of the genes *in vivo* is possible conceptually but not practically. Therefore, the most effective choice left is to either provide the correct protein from outside or inject an expression vector, safe and powerful enough that in the human body, it continues to code for the lively protein. However, there comes the law of the expression of protein. If the body's homeostasis is capable sufficient to just accept outside protein expression vector and redirect its function with no side impact, which could be ideal state of affairs. This will be resource intensive but would still vary throughout the FMS sufferers. Consequently, not most effective reliable markers for FMS are to be advanced, however, the ones have to comply with consensus as well.

These strategies can take widespread time and effort to accomplish, with excellent complexity viable even for a single mutation in one gene [16-17]. Furthermore, locating a mutation does not not always imply it's far the reason for the affected person's disease, in spite of *in vitro* proof that there may be a trade in channel body structure. Additional evidence can be required, together with segregation of the variant within a family. If the pathogenic version is in a gene encoding a part of a metabolic or nutrition-related pathway, as an example, then there may be reputedly simple treatments that could replace what is lacking or bypass the relevant step(s) in the pathway (for instance, in FMS because of mutations within the gene COMT). In other instances, there may not but be an apparent instantaneous remedy alternative (as an instance, FMS because of mutations in numerous genes SLC64A4, TRPV2, MYT1L, and NRXN3).

To clarify the ability amalgamation between gene polymorphisms in five-HTT, COMT, and five- HT2A genes and FMS susceptibility, a meta-analysis on FMS genetic predisposition, highlighting the capability vital position of 102T/C polymorphism in 5-HT2A receptor; the great associations of five-HTTLPR S/L allele and COMT Val158Met with FMS were now not shown [18]. Greater investigations want to understand the position of these genes in pain biology and continual pain diseases such as FMS. Genome-wide affiliation research has contributed to maintain the feasible involvement of relevant fearful gadget (CNS) disorder in FMS. Recently, genome-extensive association studies and duplicate range version analyses in 952 FM instances and 644 controls have been carried out. The consequences showed FMS-associated variations, rs11127292 SNP and an intronic reproduction wide variety version, belonging to MYT1L (myelin transcription element 1-like gene), which performs a key role in neuronal differentiation and involved in cognitive incapacity, and to NRXN3 (neurexin 3 gene), which acts in the nervous system as receptor and cell adhesion molecule. Further, its genetic variants have been found to be involved in autism spectrum disorder [19].

These studies improved the knowledge about FMS and supported the genetic speculation underlying its pathogenesis, suggesting capacity genetic markers for susceptibility of FMS, even though universally confirmed SNPs have not yet been discovered. Ability motives are the populace specificity of genetic variations and being FMS a multifactorial condition, haplotypes, combinations of various editions, may have an effect on the advanced chance of FMS development more than an unmarried version. A correlation between the disease and the "high ache sensitivity" haplotype (ACCG) belonged to the COMT gene in a Spanish population [20] and the B2- AR AC haplotype in Mexican and Spanish populations which have already been recognized [21]. Achievement of precision medicinal drugs and their evaluation could consist of measures of their real mechanistic effects. Whilst PM is "a fulfillment", there needs to be direct mechanistic proof that it has achieved, and what it was supposed to achieve. The severity of signs in FMS may also enhance, however, remedy X reversed the disorder as a result of putatively pathogenic variant Y in gene Z, or due to the fact something else might come about. But, in such a situation, proof is not often received, or expected, in the people treated with the precision medicinal drug. We then need to offer a "precision failure" rationalization. Failed PM attempts are posted.

Frequently taken into consideration hypothesis about the motives for failure; however, it is not clear how many failed tries are not posted, and the hypothesis will not rework into the real explanation. Within the absence of a mechanistic cause of these eventualities, can we easily claim the remedy is a precision remedy? Precision therapy is based totally on prevention, analysis, and remedy of sickness in its early section (Fig. **3**), or, are we again into the scenario in which a present drug brings about the symptoms under control in an unexplained way in an affected person, for example;the patient feels higher after certain medications but as he stops medications, symptoms reverse returned again. We will keep in mind PM without the round argument only if it works exactly in the majority of the patients if not in all the sufferers. What is important and enough?

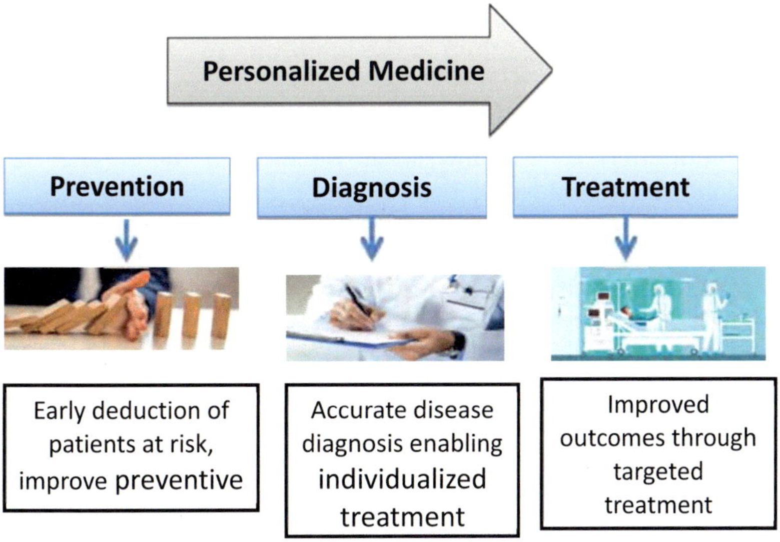

Fig. (3). Therapeutic strategies in Personalized Medicine.

Personalized medication, prevention and early diagnosis of patients at the risk enhance preventive measure for improved prognosis permitting results *via* individualized focused treatment. An overview of the therapeutic strategies in customized medication is shown in Fig. (**3**).

CONCLUSION

Despite the high prevalence of FM, many studies included small-size samples and, due to FM comorbidities, and enrolled patients were less and not using specific exclusion standards and attention and ongoing cures were followed. In addition, to make clear, the temporal onset among FM and its additional signs and symptoms, the usage of longitudinal follow-ups might be considered. Info on patients' history may want to enhance everyday clinical practice: nutritional and way of life that may lead to alteration in the gastrointestinal microbiome, observed in this complex disease must be taken into consideration.

Further future research could focus on the identification of more selective analgesics or new pharmacological approaches, as currently being used against the pain of diverse etiologies. This includes Postherpetic Neuralgia, Inherited Erythromelalgia, and Lumbosacral Radiculopathy, with three phase II clinical trials on selective blocker drugs for sodium channels. Since epigenetics play a major role in regulating the expression of pro- or anti-nociceptive genes, epigenetic drug might potentially reverse aberrant gene expression associated with FMS states. First, preclinical data suggest chromatin-modifying drugs' relevance for treating pain in the context of inflammation 5- azacytidine administration in rats following tissue damage resulted in the inhibition of global DNA methylation increment and MeCP2 expression with subsequent decrease of painful behavior. Drugs targeting epigenetic mediators such as histone deacetylase and acetylase or involving DNA methylation maintenance have been developed for different pathological conditions, following the PM approach.

Similarly, by improving FMS biomarkers research, a new treatment scenario based on personalized medicine may be revealed, with major benefits and less side effects for FMS patients and reduced costs for the national healthcare systems.

ABBREVIATIONS

FMS	Fibromyalgia Syndrome
PM	Precision Medicinal Drug
FDA	Food and Drug Administration
CBT	Cognitive Behavioral Remedy
RA	Rheumatoid Arthritis

COMT	Catechol-O-methyltransferase
PP	Prognostic precision
GTPCH-1	Guanosine triphosphate cyclohydrolase I
TRPV-2	Brief Receptor Capability Vanilloid Type 2
NRXN3	Neurexin-3-alpha
MYT1L	Myelin transcription issue 1 like five
HTT	Five-Hydroxy Tryptamine Transporter
HT2A	Serotonin HT2A
ACCG	Anterior cingulate cortex gyrus
MeCP-2	Methyl-CpG-binding protein 2

REFERENCES

[1] Toward precision medicine: Building a knowledge network for biomedical research and a new taxonomy of disease/Committee on A Framework for Developing a New Taxonomy of Disease, Board on Life Sciences, Division on Earth and Life Sciences, National Research Council of the National Academies. Washington, DC: National Academies Press 2011.

[2] Møller RS, Hammer TB, Rubboli G, Lemke JR, Johannesen KM. From next-generation sequencing to targeted treatment of non-acquired epilepsies. Expert Rev Mol Diagn 2019; 19(3): 217-28. [http://dx.doi.org/10.1080/14737159.2019.1573144] [PMID: 30661434]

[3] Kim J, Hu C, Moufawad El Achkar C, *et al.* Patient-customized oligonucleotide therapy for a rare genetic disease. N Engl J Med 2019; 381(17): 1644-52. [http://dx.doi.org/10.1056/NEJMoa1813279] [PMID: 31597037]

[4] Parvez S, Fatima G, Mahdi F, Fedacko J, Hadi NR. Unraveling the clinico-genetic association of catechol-o-methyltransferase-rs4680 g>a gene polymorphism in women with fibromyalgia syndrome. Wiad Lek 2022; 75(10): 2439-44. [http://dx.doi.org/10.36740/WLek202210123] [PMID: 36472276]

[5] Jones GT, Atzeni F, Beasley M, Flüß E, Sarzi-Puttini P, Macfarlane GJ. The prevalence of fibromyalgia in the general population: A comparison of the American College of Rheumatology 1990, 2010, and modified 2010 classification criteria. Arthritis Rheumatol 2015; 67(2): 568-75. [http://dx.doi.org/10.1002/art.38905] [PMID: 25323744]

[6] Mahdi AA, Fatima G. A quest for better understanding of biochemical changes in fibromyalgia syndrome. Indian J Clin Biochem 2014; 29(1): 1-2. [http://dx.doi.org/10.1007/s12291-013-0395-z] [PMID: 24478541]

[7] Kim J, Hu C, Moufawad El Achkar C, *et al.* Patient-customized oligonucleotide therapy for a rare genetic disease. N Engl J Med 2019; 381(17): 1644-52. [http://dx.doi.org/10.1056/NEJMoa1813279] [PMID: 31597037]

[8] Macfarlane GJ, Kronisch C, Dean LE, *et al.* EULAR revised recommendations for the management of fibromyalgia. Ann Rheum Dis 2017; 76(2): 318-28. [http://dx.doi.org/10.1136/annrheumdis-2016-209724] [PMID: 27377815]

[9] Sosa-Reina MD, Nunez-Nagy S, Gallego-Izquierdo T, Pecos-Martín D, Monserrat J, Álvarez-Mon M. Effectiveness of therapeutic exercise in fibromyalgia syndrome: A systematic review and meta-analysis of randomized clinical trials. BioMed Res Int 2017; 2017: 1-14. [http://dx.doi.org/10.1155/2017/2356346] [PMID: 29291206]

[10] Wolff M, Brunklaus A, Zuberi SM. Phenotypic spectrum and genetics of *SCN 2A* -related disorders,

treatment options, and outcomes in epilepsy and beyond. Epilepsia 2019; 60(S3): S59-67. [http://dx.doi.org/10.1111/epi.14935] [PMID: 31904126]

[11] Fitzcharles MA, Ste-Marie PA, Goldenberg DL, *et al.* 2012 Canadian Guidelines for the diagnosis and management of fibromyalgia syndrome: Executive summary. Pain Res Manag 2013; 18(3): 119-26. [http://dx.doi.org/10.1155/2013/918216] [PMID: 23748251]

[12] Amit L, Melanie HS, Laura TD. Rheumatology in the era of precision medicine: Synovial tissue molecular patterns and treatment response in rheumatoid arthritis. Curr Opin Rheumatol 2021; 33(1): 58-63. [http://dx.doi.org/10.1097/BOR.0000000000000767]

[13] Epi PM. A roadmap for precision medicine in the epilepsies. Lancet Neurol 2015; 14(12): 1219-28. [http://dx.doi.org/10.1016/S1474-4422(15)00199-4] [PMID: 26416172]

[14] Mogil JS. Pain genetics: Past, present and future. Trends Genet 2012; 28(6): 258-66. [http://dx.doi.org/10.1016/j.tig.2012.02.004] [PMID: 22464640]

[15] Oertel B, Lötsch J. Genetic mutations that prevent pain: implications for future pain medication. Pharmacogenomics 2008; 9(2): 179-94. [http://dx.doi.org/10.2217/14622416.9.2.179] [PMID: 18370847]

[16] Atkin TA, Maher CM, Gerlach AC, *et al.* A comprehensive approach to identifying repurposed drugs to treat *SCN 8A* epilepsy. Epilepsia 2018; 59(4): 802-13. [http://dx.doi.org/10.1111/epi.14037] [PMID: 29574705]

[17] Bechi G, Rusconi R, Cestèle S, Striano P, Franceschetti S, Mantegazza M. Rescuable folding defective NaV1.1 (SCN1A) mutants in epilepsy: Properties, occurrence, and novel rescuing strategy with peptides targeted to the endoplasmic reticulum. Neurobiol Dis 2015; 75: 100-14. [http://dx.doi.org/10.1016/j.nbd.2014.12.028] [PMID: 25576396]

[18] Lee YH, Choi SJ, Ji JD, Song GG. Candidate gene studies of fibromyalgia: A systematic review and meta-analysis. Rheumatol Int 2012; 32(2): 417-26. [http://dx.doi.org/10.1007/s00296-010-1678-9] [PMID: 21120487]

[19] Docampo E, Escaramís G, Gratacòs M, *et al.* Genome-wide analysis of single nucleotide polymorphisms and copy number variants in fibromyalgia suggest a role for the central nervous system. Pain 2014; 155(6): 1102-9. [http://dx.doi.org/10.1016/j.pain.2014.02.016] [PMID: 24582949]

[20] Vargas-Alarcón G, Fragoso JM, Cruz-Robles D, *et al.* Catechol-O-methyltransferase gene haplotypes in Mexican and Spanish patients with fibromyalgia. Arthritis Res Ther 2007; 9(5): R110. [http://dx.doi.org/10.1186/ar2316] [PMID: 17961261]

[21] Vargas-Alarcón G, Fragoso JM, Cruz-Robles D, *et al.* Association of adrenergic receptor gene polymorphisms with different fibromyalgia syndrome domains. Arthritis Rheum 2009; 60(7): 2169-73. [http://dx.doi.org/10.1002/art.24655] [PMID: 19565482]

CHAPTER 11

Circadian Clock Modulation: A Novel Therapeutic Approach to Cancer Treatment and Management

Armiya Sultan[1,*], **Khalid Umar Fakhri**[2], **Tahira Sultan**[3], **Mohd Yasir Khan**[1] and **Sher Ali**[4]

[1] *Department of Biotechnology, Jamia Millia Islamia, New Delhi, India.*

[2] *Department of Biosciences, Jamia Millia Islamia, New Delhi, India.*

[3] *Department of Clinical Biochemistry, University of Kashmir, Srinagar, India.*

[4] *Department of Personalized and Molecular Medicine, Era University, Lucknow, India.*

Abstract: There is a time code to the genome instructing temporal regulation of cellular activities. The time code is expressed in the form of circadian clocks composed of many transcription, co-activator, and co-repressor factors. The transcription-translation feedback loops generated collectively by these factors regulate daily ~24-hour rhythms in physiology, metabolism, and behavior across divergent phyla. Genome-wide studies reflect that chronic disruption of circadian rhythms provides a plinth for the occurrence and progression of multiple diseases across our lifespan. Increasing epidemiological and experimental evidence are confirming that circadian clocks are compromised in cancer. Altered expression of circadian clock components is likely to be associated with the onset and progression of cancer. The concept of targeting circadian clocks at the molecular level is rapidly evolving and opening a new therapeutic window in cancer. Here we discuss the approaches and recent advancements that have been made for the identification and development of clock-modulating small molecules bearing drug-like properties for the therapeutics and therapeutic management of cancer. It is envisaged that this chapter will augment the concepts of precision medicine in general and circadian-related system anomalies.

Keywords: Cancer, Circadian clock, Clock-modulating small molecules, Drug-like properties, Precision medicine, System anomalies, Time code.

INTRODUCTION

Circadian clocks refer to the internal biological timing systems that regulate various physiological and behavioral processes in organisms. These clocks operate on a roughly 24-hour cycle and are found in a wide range of organisms, including humans, animals, plants, and even some microorganisms [1].

* **Corresponding author Armiya Sultan:** Department of Biotechnology, Jamia Millia Islamia, New Delhi, India. E-mail: armia86bms@gmail.com.

Farzana Mahdi & Abbas Ali Mahdi (Eds.)

The circadian clock enables organisms to synchronize their biological activities with the Earth's daily cycle of light and dark. Circadian clocks are molecular systems consisting of various transcription factors, co-activators, and co-repressors [2, 3]. These components work together to create transcription-translation feedback loops, which play a crucial role in regulating daily rhythms lasting approximately 24 hours. These rhythms affect diverse aspects such as physiology, metabolism, and behavior across different phyla. The circadian timing system plays a crucial role in regulating sleep-wake cycles, hormone production, body temperature, metabolism, immune function, and many other physiological processes. Disruptions to the circadian timing system, such as shift work, jet lag, or certain sleep disorders, can have significant impacts on overall health and well-being [2].

In mammals, the circadian timing system encompasses the interconnected network of biological processes and mechanisms that regulate the body's circadian rhythms. It includes the central clock (pacemaker), known as the suprachiasmatic nucleus (SCN), located in the hypothalamus of the brain [1]. The SCN, consisting of around 20,000 neurons, is synchronized by the natural light-dark cycle, acting as the dominant zeitgeber (time giver). The SCN receives light input from the eyes and coordinates the timing of various physiological and behavioral functions. In addition to the SCN, the circadian timing system involves peripheral clocks found in various tissues and organs throughout the body. These peripheral clocks are influenced by signals from the SCN and help synchronize the timing of local processes with the central rhythm. Fig. (**1**) represents the general organization of the circadian timing system in mammals. In mammals, light signals are detected by special cells in the retina called intrinsically photosensitive retinal ganglion cells (ipRGCs). These cells transmit chemical messages, like glutamate and pituitary adenylate cyclase-activating polypeptide, to the suprachiasmatic nucleus (SCN) through a pathway known as the retinohypothalamic tract [2]. These chemical messages trigger the influx of calcium ions into the SCN, leading to the activation of specific protein kinases. Consequently, the Ca2+/cAMP-response element binding protein (CREB) becomes phosphorylated [3]. The phosphorylated CREBs then bind to specific regions called Ca2+/cAMP-response elements (CREs) within gene promoters. This binding initiates the expression of certain genes called early immediate genes (EIGs), which include Per1 and Per2 [4]. The expression of these EIGs drives neuroendocrine signals that communicate with cell-autonomous peripheral clocks instructing temporal regulation of cellular activities [3, 4]. In addition, peripheral clocks are likely to be influenced by feeding [5, 6], activity [7], and strong social interactions [8].

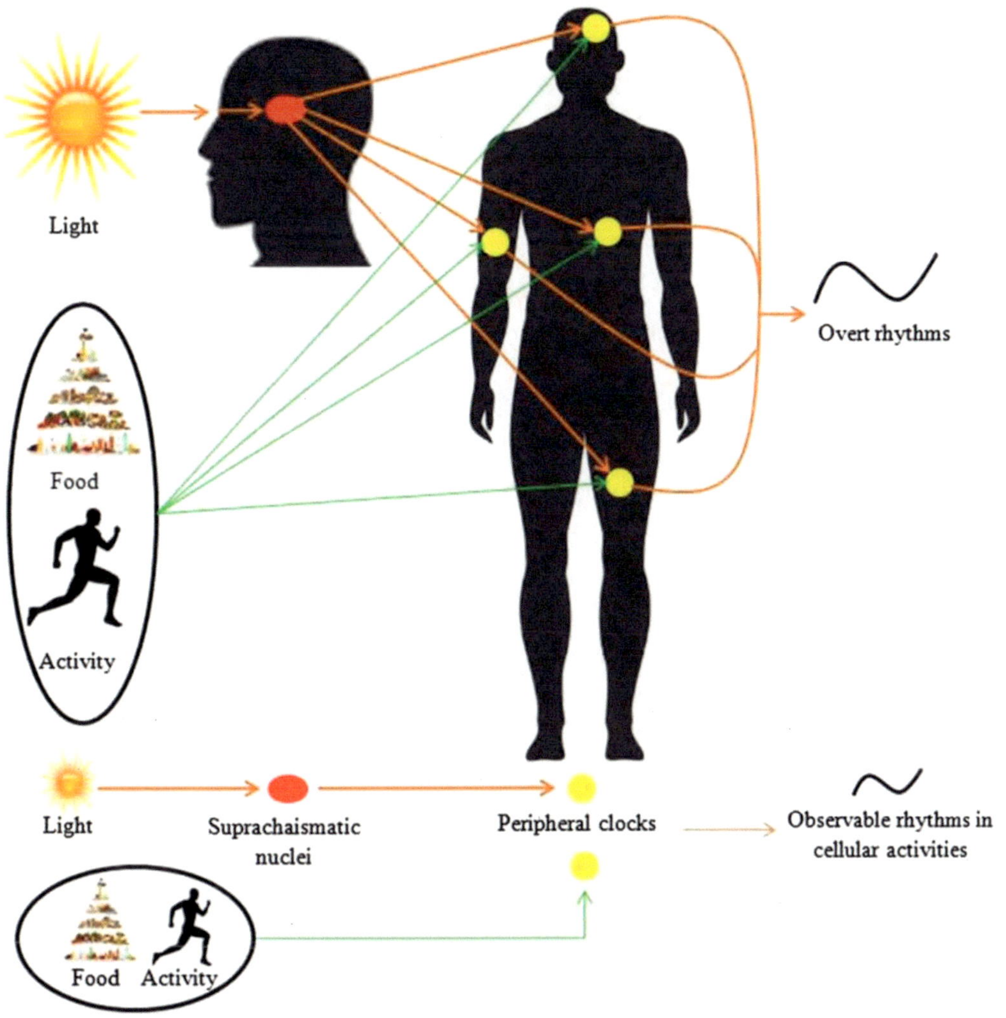

Fig. (1). Circadian clocks system in mammals. Circadian clocks in mammals are organized in a hierarchical system. The master clock "suprachaismatic nuclei (SCN)" is present in hypothalamic region of brain. Light signals are received in eyes by the photosensitive cells. These cells generate chemical messages that travel through retinohypothalamic tract to reach SCN. SCN communicate with peripheral clocks to transducer them the "internal day" and generates overt rhythms in cellular activities. High degree of intercellular coupling of SCN neuronal cellular clocks is a key feature to orchestrate circadian programme. Clocks in peripheral organs also respond to signals generated by feeding, activity, and strong social interactions.

Genome-wide transcriptome, proteome, and metabolome studies reflect that optimized daily rhythms sustain health; their disruption increases the risk of humans to multiple diseases including cancer [9 - 18]. Increasing epidemiological and experimental evidence supports the idea that circadian rhythms are disrupted in various types of cancer, including breast cancer [19 - 21], oral cancer [22], colorectal cancer [23], ovarian cancer [24], prostate cancer [25 - 28], non-small cell lung cancer [29], gastric cancer [30, 31], thyroid cancer [32], head and neck cancer [33, 34], metastatic melanoma [35], chronic lymphocytic leukemia [36], and chronic myeloid leukemia [37 - 39]. The involvement of the circadian clock directly or indirectly in different diseases provide a notion that these clocks can be used as plinths in therapeutics [40]. Recent studies indicate three primary approaches to target circadian clocks in disease conditions:

- "training the clocks" for optimizing the circadian lifestyle [41],
- "clocking the drugs" for optimization of 3 the timing of therapy [42] and,
- "drugging the clock" by targeting specific circadian clock components [43].

All three ways are intended to pave for the optimization of the circadian rhythms to prevent or treat chronic diseases [44 - 46]. Here in the current review, our focus is on the concept of "drugging the clock" in cancer.

MOLECULAR COMPONENTS AND FEEDBACK LOOPS IN CIRCADIAN CLOCK REGULATION

Circadian clocks consist of numerous transcription factors, co-activators, and co-repressors, working together to form a core loop as well as additional accessory transcription/translation feedback loops (TTFLs) (Fig. **2a**). These intricate mechanisms guide cells in regulating daily approximately 24-hour rhythms, governing various cellular activities that control physiology, metabolism, and behavior. By orchestrating these processes, circadian clocks play a vital role in maintaining the temporal order and coordination of biological systems.

In mammals, the core transcription/translation feedback loop (TTFL) of the circadian clock is initiated by the activation of two essential transcription factors, CLOCK and BMAL1, during the daytime. These factors form a complex that binds to specific promoter sites on Per and Cry genes, promoting their transcription process in the afternoon [47, 48]. The Per and Cry genes encode crucial repressor proteins, namely period (Per1, Per2, and Per3) and cryptochrome (Cry1 and Cry2), which gradually accumulate in the cytoplasm during the late afternoon and evening [49, 50]. Due to their relatively short half-lives, the stability of these repressor proteins is regulated through ubiquitination and proteasomal degradation processes [48, 51]. Once a sufficient accumulation of the repressor proteins occurs in the cytoplasm, they interact with each other and with casein kinases (CK1ε and CK1δ), forming a complex that translocates into the nucleus at night. In the nucleus, this complex interacts with the transcription factors CLOCK and BMAL1, leading to the repression of their own transcription process. Consequently, the levels of PER and CRY proteins in the cytoplasm decline during the night [48 - 50, 52]. When the repression complex is relieved, the activity of CLOCK-BMAL1 is restored, initiating a new cycle [14, 53]. The stability of PER and CRY proteins in the nucleus is regulated through the ubiquitination and proteasomal degradation of CRY proteins, with FBXL21, a homolog of FBXL3, playing an antagonistic role in the nucleus [48, 54 - 56]. This intricate mechanism constitutes the core loop that is essential for the proper functioning of the circadian clock [48].

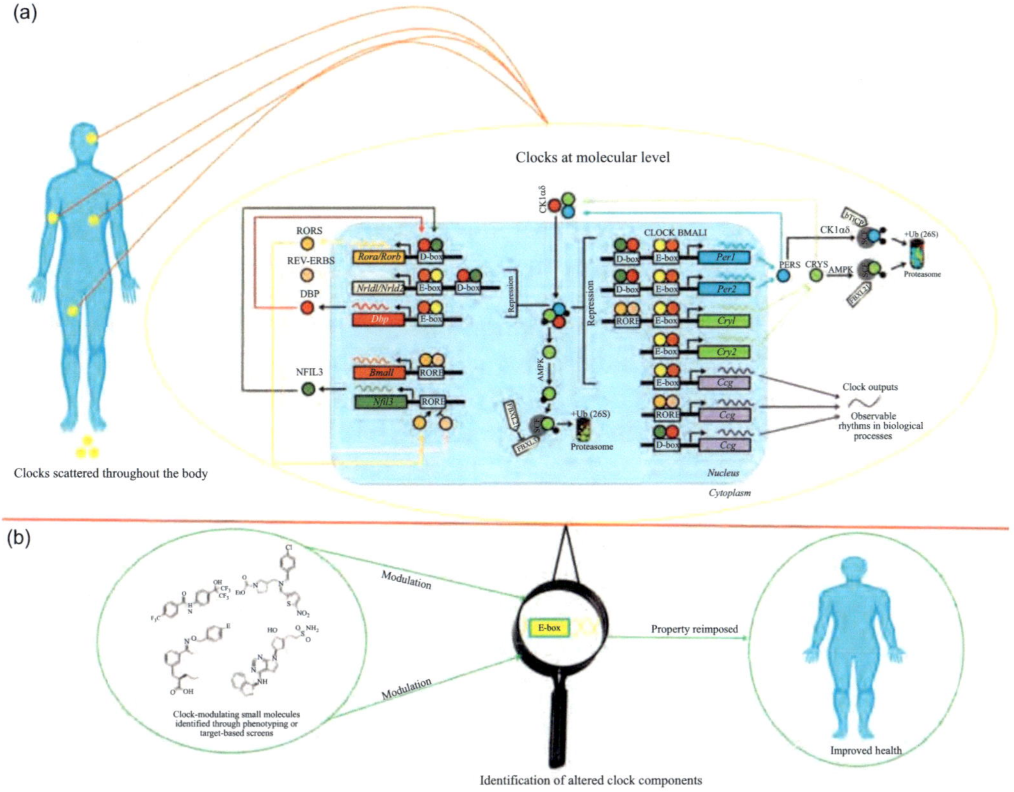

Fig. (2). Circadian clock at molecular level in mammals. (a) In the beginning of the cycle, two transcription factors, CLOCK and BMAL1, form a complex that binds to E-box cis-regulatory sequences of *Per1, Per2, Per3, Cry1, and Cry2* and other clock-controlled target genes. The encoded proteins PER and CRY interact with each other as well as with casein kinases to form a complex. This complex translocates into the nucleus and interacts with CLOCK-BMAL1 transcription factor complex to suppress their activity leading to inhibition of their own expression as well as the expression of other clock-controlled genes. A time delay between the activation and repression of genes generates oscillations in their expression, thereby stretching the period length to ~ 24 h.

Nuclear receptors, specifically RORs (retinoic acid-related orphan receptor α/β/γ) and REV-ERBs (reverse orientation c-erbA α/β), play a crucial role in generating oscillations in the BMAL1 gene [14, 56 - 58]. The transcription factor complex CLOCK-BMAL1 binds to promoter sites on the Nr1d1/Nr1d2 genes, which encode REV-ERBα and REV-ERBβ nuclear receptors [48, 58, 59]. The robust circadian expression of these genes mediates a negative feedback loop [60]. In the promoter region of Bmal1, there are cis-regulatory elements known as Rev-DR2 and ROR-binding elements. REV-ERBs and RORs (encoded by RorA, RorB, and RorC) engage in competition to bind to these regulatory elements [58 - 60]. The Rev-DR2/RORE motifs exhibit a consensus sequence characterized by RGGTCA half-sites, which are preceded by a region rich in (A/T) nucleotides [48]. When RORs bind to these motifs, it leads to the activation of Bmal1 transcription. Conversely, when REV-ERBs bind to these motifs, it results in the repression of Bmal1 expression [59, 61]. Dual degradation of BMAL1 is mediated by proteasome- and autophagosome-dependent mechanisms [62]. This entire procedure creates the first accessory loop, which interacts with the core loop to create a stable and reliable clock mechanism [48, 60, 61]. Additionally, the ROR-REV-ERB loop controls the expression of the nuclear factor interleukin-3 regulated (NFIL3), which represses the target genes *via* the D-box [63, 64].

A different group of Timeless Transcription Factor-Like proteins (TTFL) consist of the PARbZip transcription factors, namely the D-box binding protein (DBP), thyrotroph embryonic factor (TEF), hepatic leukemia factor (HLF), and repressor protein nuclear factor interleukin-3 regulated (NFIL3) [64 - 66]. The activation of the PAR-bZip transcription factors is facilitated by the CLOCK-BMAL1 transcription factor complex, while NFIL3 is regulated through the ROR-RE--ERB loop [67]. These transcription factors exert their influence on target genes by binding to the D-box element, thus forming an additional accessory loop that enhances the stability and resilience of the circadian clock mechanism [48, 60, 61].

The intrinsic timing of the molecular clock is determined by the occurrence of subsequent circadian oscillations in the expression of clock genes and their encoded proteins. This regulation is dependent on the combination of regulatory sequences, such as D-boxes, E-boxes, and ROREs, present on the promoter and enhancer regions of target genes [48, 68]. These regulatory elements govern the rhythmic expression patterns, ensuring the proper functioning of the circadian system.

RATIONALE OF THE CONCEPT "DRUGGING THE CLOCK"

The concept of "drugging the clock" by targeting and modulating circadian clock components in cancer is rapidly evolving. The concept is mainly based on the rationale that circadian clocks are resilient to wide fluctuation in the cellular biochemical environment, pleiotropic effects of clock-modulating drugs, and their roles in the reduction of secondary health burden [69]. One of the most important expectations of the use of circadian clock modulators is to reimpose the temporal restraint of cancer cells on necessary pathways to control tumour growth [70]. One recent important study [43] has reported the anticancer activity of two clock-modulating pyrrole derivative small molecules (SR9009 and SR9011 - agonists of REV-ERBs), originally developed 5 by Solt and his colleagues in 2012 [71]. This study reported that the activation of the circadian clock component “REV-ERB” by these two agonists is lethal to cancer cells and oncogene-induced senescent cells. Both molecules affected the activity of multiple oncogenic drivers (such as HRAS, BRAF, PIK3CA, and others). The anticancer activity of both molecules persisted even under hypoxic conditions and in the absence of P53. The regulation of autophagy and de novo lipogenesis by these agonist molecules is critical to evoke apoptotic responses in cancer cells. Moreover, this study showed that the treatment with these agonist molecules altered the glioblastoma growth and improved survival in mice. Pharmacological modulation of circadian clocks by such small drug-like molecules represents an effective strategy to discover and develop anticancer agents that can be implemented for the treatment and clinical management of cancer.

METHODS EMPLOYED FOR THE DISCOVERY OF CIRCADIAN CLOCK- MODULATING SMALL MOLECULES

There are two primary strategies extensively utilized for the exploration of clock-modulating small molecules (Fig. **2b**). The first strategy encompasses the detection of molecules *via* phenotypic screening, utilizing kinetic assays for identification, as well as endpoint assays for activity screening. The second approach is centered on target-based screening, utilizing biochemical assays [60, 72]. The Phenotypic screening approach first involves the multiple-day recording of bioluminescence signals generated by the expression of luciferase from an exogenous clock gene promoter or fused PER2: luciferase from the endogenous Per2 locus of a stable cell line [60, 73 - 79]. The collected data, representing circadian bioluminescence signals, is then subjected to analysis using relevant tools to calculate parameters such as the period, phase, and amplitude of the circadian rhythm [47]. The activity screening approach serves the purpose of tracing and identifying explicit transcription activities. To achieve this, the method employs the creation of reporter cell lines that are engineered to express luciferase [60]. In this approach, the rhythmic expression of the reporter is regulated and governed by the promoter of the clock genes [80, 81]. By utilizing this technique, researchers can observe and analyze the periodic changes in luciferase expression, providing valuable insights into the transcriptional dynamics and behavior of the clock genes. These two screening approaches have resulted in the identification of several clock-modulating small molecules [73, 75 - 78, 82]. One of the small molecules is "KL001" reported by Hirota and his colleagues in 2012 [77]. This molecule is first-in-class CRY stabilizer. It specifically interacts with CRY proteins (CRY1 and CRY2) and prevents them from ubiquitin-dependent degradation, leading to lengthening of the circadian period.

The target-based screening approach, utilizing biochemical assays, encompasses the comprehensive evaluation of various aspects such as protein modification, ligand binding, and protein-protein interactions [60, 72]. This methodology holds an advantage over cell-based assays due to its ability to directly assess these specific biochemical interactions. By employing the target-based screening approach, researchers have successfully identified a range of small molecules that have the capacity to modulate the circadian properties of clock factors. Notably, these molecules have been found to influence the behavior and function of key clock factors, including protein casein kinases and the nuclear receptor REV-ERBs [71, 83]. Two clock-modulating pyrrole derivative small molecules (SR9009 and SR9011) were reported by Solt and his colleagues in 2012 [71]. These two small molecules are agonists of REV-ERBs. One recent important study has reported the anticancer activity of these two molecules [43]. Authors reported that the activation of the circadian clock component "REV-ERB" by these two agonists is lethal to cancer cells and oncogene-induced senescent cells. Through the application of this approach, valuable insights have been gained regarding the molecular mechanisms underlying the regulation of circadian rhythms.

SOME IMPORTANT CIRCADIAN CLOCK-MODULATING SMALL MOLECULES HAVE SHOWN PROMISING DRUG-LIKE PROPERTIES IN CANCER

SR1078

In 2010, Wang and his colleagues reported SR1078 as the first synthetic and highly selective RORα/γ agonist [84]. It has been observed that treatment with SR1078 induces apoptosis in HepG2 cells through RORα and p53-dependent processes [84, 85]. The authors of the study further demonstrated that SR1078 stabilizes p53 in cancer cells and enhances the expression of p21 and PUMA, both of which are important regulators of cell cycle arrest and apoptosis [85]. Additionally, SR1078 has also been found to increase the expression of Sox4 and REV-ERBα in HepG2 cells. These findings highlight the multifaceted effects of SR1078 on cellular processes and gene expression, indicating its potential as a therapeutic agent with diverse regulatory properties.

SR9009

SR9009 is a small molecule derived from pyrrole that functions as a specific agonist of the nuclear receptor REV-ERB-α/β [71]. This molecule demonstrates direct and reversible binding to REV-ERB-α, with a dissociation constant (Kd) of 800 nM. Importantly, it exhibits remarkable selectivity over a panel of 46 other nuclear receptors. Upon binding, SR9009 effectively enhances REV-ERB dependent repressor activity, as evidenced by an IC_{50} of 670 nM and 800 nM in Gal4-REV-ERB-α and β transfected HEK 293 cells, respectively. Additionally, this ligand exerts its effects by reducing the expression of BMAL1 mRNA in HepG2 cells, with an IC_{50} value of 710 nM. These findings demonstrate the potent and specific regulatory properties of SR9009 on REV-ERB-dependent processes, highlighting its potential as a valuable tool compound for studying and modulating circadian rhythms.

Recent studies have shed light on the promising anticancer potential of SR9009 [43, 86, 87]. Notably, Sulli, Rommel, *et al.* [43] conducted a study revealing that the activation of the circadian clock component REV-ERB by SR9009 resulted in a lethal effect on cancer cells as well as oncogene-induced senescent cells. Importantly, this effect was not observed in normal cells, indicating a selective cytotoxicity towards cancerous cells. Furthermore, the study demonstrated that SR9009 treatment had a profound impact on the activity of multiple oncogenic drivers, including HRAS, BRAF, PIK3CA, and others. This alteration in oncogenic driver activity was associated with the inhibition of glioblastoma growth and improved survival in mice. Remarkably, SR9009's anticancer activity was shown to persist even under hypoxic conditions and in the absence of the tumor suppressor protein P53. These findings highlight the potential of SR9009 as a therapeutic candidate for cancer treatment, particularly in targeting oncogenic drivers and overcoming challenging tumor microenvironments.

In a study conducted by Wagner *et al.* [87], the effects of SR9009 on cell viability, chemotherapy time responses, and underlying metabolic processes were investigated in T98G and HepG2 cells. These effects were compared with the proteasome inhibitor Bortezomib treatment. The authors found that SR9009 treatment led to alterations in tumor metabolism, resulting in a significant impact on cell viability and a decrease in ROS levels in T98G and HepG2 cancer cells.

Similarly, Shen *et al.* [86] conducted a study using chemosensitive cells (H69 and H446) as well as the corresponding chemoresistant cells (H69AR and H446DDP) from small-cell lung cancer. They aimed to evaluate the efficacy of SR9009 treatment in these cells. The authors reported that SR9009 treatment specifically induced cell death in both chemosensitive and chemoresistant small-cell lung cancer cells. Furthermore, they found that SR9009 treatment suppressed the core autophagy gene "Atg5," leading to alterations in autophagy activity. This, in turn, contributed to SR9009-induced cytotoxicity in small-cell lung cancer cells.

MLN4924

MLN4924 is a small molecule inhibitor of NEDD8 activating enzyme with potential antineoplastic activity, triggering cell-cycle arrest, apoptosis, and senescence in cancer cells [88 - 91]. Zhang and his colleagues [91] discovered that MLN4924 exerts an anti-proliferative effect on osteosarcoma cells through the mediation of RORα and Bmal1. Authors reported that this molecule suppressed the proliferation of osteosarcoma cells by inducing their apoptosis and cell cycle arrest in the G2/M phase. MLN4924 stabilized the RORα and RNA interference of RORα attenuated its anti-proliferative effect. MLN4924 increased the expression of two ROR transcriptional targets, p21 and Bmal1. Bmal1 suppression by siRNA attenuated the anti-proliferative effect of MLN4924 in U2OS osteosarcoma cells, indicating that the MLN4924-mediated cell growth inhibition is mediated by Bmal1.

KS15

KS15 is a remarkable small molecule that possesses a unique chemical structure, comprising a 2-ethoxypropanoic scaffold and two aryl rings linked together by an oxime ether linker. This intriguing compound was first described by Chun and his colleagues in 2014 [80]. Research on this small molecule unveiled that KS15 directly interacts with the C-terminal region of cryptochromes (CRY1 and CRY2), resulting in the inhibition of their repressive function and the facilitation of the E-box-mediated transcription process [92]. Further investigations conducted by Chun *et al.* [93] aimed to assess the potential therapeutic properties of KS15. The authors specifically explored its anti-proliferative and pro-apoptotic effects. Their findings demonstrated that KS15 exhibits anti-proliferative properties and enhances chemosensitivity in human breast cancer cells. Treatment with KS15 was shown to significantly impede the rate of cell growth and augment the sensitivity of MCF-7 cells to two widely used chemotherapeutic drugs, namely doxorubicin, and tamoxifen.

CONCLUSION

In conclusion, the accumulating evidence highlighting the dysregulation of circadian clocks in cancer underscores the significance of targeting these molecular timekeepers as a novel therapeutic avenue. Extensive research efforts are necessary to identify and optimize clock-modulating small molecules with drug-like properties. Implementing these compounds in cancer treatment holds great potential for improving patient outcomes and revolutionizing the clinical management of cancer.

LIST OF ABBREVIATIONS

CREB	Ca2+/cAMP-response element binding protein
CREs	Ca2+/cAMP-response elements
DBP	D-box binding protein
EIGs	Early immediate genes
HLF	Hepatic leukemia factor
ipRGCs	Intrinsically photosensitive retinal ganglion cells
NFIL3	Nuclear factor interleukin-3
SCN	Suprachiasmatic nuclei
TEF	Thyrotroph embryonic factor
TTFLs	Transcription/translation feedback loops

REFERENCES

[1] Dibner C, Schibler U, Albrecht U. The mammalian circadian timing system: Organization and coordination of central and peripheral clocks. Annu Rev Physiol 2010; 72(1): 517-49. [http://dx.doi.org/10.1146/annurev-physiol-021909-135821] [PMID: 20148687]

[2] Panda S, Nayak SK, Campo B, Walker JR, Hogenesch JB, Jegla T. Illumination of the melanopsin signaling pathway. Science 2005; 307(5709): 600-4. [http://dx.doi.org/10.1126/science.1105121] [PMID: 15681390]

[3] Zhang X, Odom DT, Koo SH, *et al.* Genome-wide analysis of cAMP-response element binding protein occupancy, phosphorylation, and target gene activation in human tissues. Proc Natl Acad Sci 2005; 102(12): 4459-64. [http://dx.doi.org/10.1073/pnas.0501076102] [PMID: 15753290]

[4] Golombek DA, Rosenstein RE. Physiology of circadian entrainment. Physiol Rev 2010; 90(3): 1063-102. [http://dx.doi.org/10.1152/physrev.00009.2009] [PMID: 20664079]

[5] Damiola F, Le Minh N, Preitner N, Kornmann B, Fleury-Olela F, Schibler U. Restricted feeding uncouples circadian oscillators in peripheral tissues from the central pacemaker in the suprachiasmatic nucleus. Genes Dev 2000; 14(23): 2950-61. [http://dx.doi.org/10.1101/gad.183500] [PMID: 11114885]

[6] Xie X, Kukino A, Calcagno HE, Berman AM, Garner JP, Butler MP. Natural food intake patterns have little synchronizing effect on peripheral circadian clocks. BMC Biol 2020; 18(1): 160. [http://dx.doi.org/10.1186/s12915-020-00872-7] [PMID: 33158435]

[7] Sasaki H, Hattori Y, Ikeda Y, *et al.* Phase shifts in circadian peripheral clocks caused by exercise are dependent on the feeding schedule in PER2:LUC mice. Chronobiol Int 2016; 33(7): 849-62. [http://dx.doi.org/10.3109/07420528.2016.1171775] [PMID: 27123825]

[8] Krupp JJ, Kent C, Billeter JC, *et al.* Social experience modifies pheromone expression and mating behavior in male Drosophila melanogaster. Curr Biol 2008; 18(18): 1373-83. [http://dx.doi.org/10.1016/j.cub.2008.07.089] [PMID: 18789691]

[9] Depner CM, Melanson EL, McHill AW, Wright KP Jr. Mistimed food intake and sleep alters 24-hour time-of-day patterns of the human plasma proteome. Proc Natl Acad Sci 2018; 115(23): E5390-9. [http://dx.doi.org/10.1073/pnas.1714813115] [PMID: 29784788]

[10] Dyar KA, Lutter D, Artati A, *et al.* Atlas of circadian metabolism reveals system-wide coordination and communication between clocks. Cell 2018; 174(6): 1571-1585.11. [http://dx.doi.org/10.1016/j.cell.2018.08.042] [PMID: 30193114]

[11] Hatori M, Vollmers C, Zarrinpar A, *et al.* Time-restricted feeding without reducing caloric intake prevents metabolic diseases in mice fed a high-fat diet. Cell Metab 2012; 15(6): 848-60. [http://dx.doi.org/10.1016/j.cmet.2012.04.019] [PMID: 22608008]

[12] Kettner NM, Voicu H, Finegold MJ, *et al.* Circadian homeostasis of liver metabolism suppresses hepatocarcinogenesis. Cancer Cell 2016; 30(6): 909-24. [http://dx.doi.org/10.1016/j.ccell.2016.10.007] [PMID: 27889186]

[13] Ruben MD, Wu G, Smith DF, *et al.* A database of tissue-specific rhythmically expressed human genes has potential applications in circadian medicine. Sci Transl Med 2018; 10(458): eaat8806. [http://dx.doi.org/10.1126/scitranslmed.aat8806] [PMID: 30209245]

[14] Sultan A, Parganiha A, Sultan T, Choudhary V, Pati AK. Circadian clock, cell cycle, and breast cancer: An updated review. Biol Rhythm Res 2017; 48(3): 353-69. [http://dx.doi.org/10.1080/09291016.2016.1263011]

[15] Sutton EF, Beyl R, Early KS, Cefalu WT, Ravussin E, Peterson CM. Early time-restricted feeding improves insulin sensitivity, blood pressure, and oxidative stress even without weight loss in men with prediabetes. Cell Metab 2018; 27(6): 1212-1221.e3. [http://dx.doi.org/10.1016/j.cmet.2018.04.010] [PMID: 29754952]

[16] Wefers J, van Moorsel D, Hansen J, *et al.* Circadian misalignment induces fatty acid metabolism gene profiles and compromises insulin sensitivity in human skeletal muscle. Proc Natl Acad Sci 2018; 115(30): 7789-94. [http://dx.doi.org/10.1073/pnas.1722295115] [PMID: 29987027]

[17] Zhang J, Lv H, Ji M, Wang Z, Wu W. Low circadian clock genes expression in cancers: A meta-analysis of its association with clinicopathological features and prognosis. PLoS One 2020; 15(5): e0233508. [http://dx.doi.org/10.1371/journal.pone.0233508] [PMID: 32437452]

[18] Zhou L, Zhang Z, Nice E, Huang C, Zhang W, Tang Y. Circadian rhythms and cancers: the intrinsic links and therapeutic potentials. J Hematol Oncol 2022; 15(1): 21. [http://dx.doi.org/10.1186/s13045-022-01238-y] [PMID: 35246220]

[19] Grundy A, Schuetz JM, Lai AS, *et al.* Shift work, circadian gene variants and risk of breast cancer. Cancer Epidemiol 2013; 37(5): 606-12. [http://dx.doi.org/10.1016/j.canep.2013.04.006] [PMID: 23725643]

[20] Hadadi E, Taylor W, Li XM, *et al.* Chronic circadian disruption modulates breast cancer stemness and immune microenvironment to drive metastasis in mice. Nat Commun 2020; 11(1): 3193. [http://dx.doi.org/10.1038/s41467-020-16890-6] [PMID: 32581213]

[21] Lesicka M, Jabłońska E, Wieczorek E, *et al.* Altered circadian genes expression in breast cancer tissue according to the clinical characteristics. PLoS One 2018; 13(6): e0199622. [http://dx.doi.org/10.1371/journal.pone.0199622] [PMID: 29958276]

[22] Yang K, Fu X-J, Li H-X, Chen D, Tang H. The important tumor suppressor role of PER1 in regulating the cyclin–CDK–CKI network in SCC15 human oral squamous cell carcinoma cells. OncoTargets Ther 2016; 9: 2237-45. [http://dx.doi.org/10.2147/OTT.S100952] [PMID: 27143919]

[23] Zeng Z, Luo H, Yang J, *et al.* Overexpression of the circadian clock gene Bmal1 increases sensitivity to oxaliplatin in colorectal cancer. Clin Cancer Res 2014; 20(4): 1042-52.

[http://dx.doi.org/10.1158/1078-0432.CCR-13-0171] [PMID: 24277452]

[24] Yeh CM, Shay J, Zeng TC, *et al.* Epigenetic silencing of ARNTL, a circadian gene and potential tumor suppressor in ovarian cancer. Int J Oncol 2014; 45(5): 2101-7. [http://dx.doi.org/10.3892/ijo.2014.2627] [PMID: 25175925]

[25] Cao Q, Gery S, Dashti A, *et al.* A role for the clock gene per1 in prostate cancer. Cancer Res 2009; 69(19): 7619-25. [http://dx.doi.org/10.1158/0008-5472.CAN-08-4199] [PMID: 19752089]

[26] Markt SC, Valdimarsdottir UA, Shui IM, *et al.* Circadian clock genes and risk of fatal prostate cancer. Cancer Causes Control 2015; 26(1): 25-33. [http://dx.doi.org/10.1007/s10552-014-0478-z] [PMID: 25388799]

[27] Yu CC, Chen LC, Chiou CY, *et al.* Genetic variants in the circadian rhythm pathway as indicators of prostate cancer progression. Cancer Cell Int 2019; 19(1): 87. [http://dx.doi.org/10.1186/s12935-019-0811-4] [PMID: 30996687]

[28] Zhu Y, Stevens RG, Hoffman AE, *et al.* Testing the circadian gene hypothesis in prostate cancer: A population-based case-control study. Cancer Res 2009; 69(24): 9315-22. [http://dx.doi.org/10.1158/0008-5472.CAN-09-0648] [PMID: 19934327]

[29] Gapstur SM, Diver WR, Stevens VL, Carter BD, Teras LR, Jacobs EJ. Work schedule, sleep duration, insomnia, and risk of fatal prostate cancer. Am J Prev Med 2014; 46(3) (Suppl. 1): S26-33. [http://dx.doi.org/10.1016/j.amepre.2013.10.033] [PMID: 24512928]

[30] Gery S, Komatsu N, Kawamata N, *et al.* Epigenetic silencing of the candidate tumor suppressor gene Per1 in non-small cell lung cancer. Clin Cancer Res 2007; 13(5): 1399-404. [http://dx.doi.org/10.1158/1078-0432.CCR-06-1730] [PMID: 17332281]

[31] Hu ML, Yeh KT, Lin PM, *et al.* Deregulated expression of circadian clock genes in gastric cancer. BMC Gastroenterol 2014; 14(1): 67. [http://dx.doi.org/10.1186/1471-230X-14-67] [PMID: 24708606]

[32] Mannic T, Meyer P, Triponez F, *et al.* Circadian clock characteristics are altered in human thyroid malignant nodules. J Clin Endocrinol Metab 2013; 98(11): 4446-56. [http://dx.doi.org/10.1210/jc.2013-2568] [PMID: 23979949]

[33] Hsu CM, Lin SF, Lu CT, Lin PM, Yang MY. Altered expression of circadian clock genes in head and neck squamous cell carcinoma. Tumour Biol 2012; 33(1): 149-55. [http://dx.doi.org/10.1007/s13277-011-0258-2] [PMID: 22081375]

[34] Li Y, Jin F, Zhou JJ, *et al.* Downregulation of the circadian period family genes is positively correlated with poor head and neck squamous cell carcinoma prognosis. Chronobiol Int 2019; 36(12): 1723-32. [http://dx.doi.org/10.1080/07420528.2019.1648486] [PMID: 31609143]

[35] de Assis LVM, Kinker GS, Moraes MN, Markus RP, Fernandes PA, Castrucci AML. Expression of the circadian clock gene *bmal1* positively correlates with antitumor immunity and patient survival in metastatic melanoma. Front Oncol 2018; 8: 185. [http://dx.doi.org/10.3389/fonc.2018.00185] [PMID: 29946530]

[36] Rana S, Munawar M, Shahid A, *et al.* Deregulated expression of circadian clock and clock-controlled cell cycle genes in chronic lymphocytic leukemia. Mol Biol Rep 2014; 41(1): 95-103. [http://dx.doi.org/10.1007/s11033-013-2841-7] [PMID: 24190490]

[37] Wang N, Mi M, Wei X, Sun C. Circadian clock gene Period2 suppresses human chronic myeloid leukemia cell proliferation. Exp Ther Med 2020; 20(6): 147. [http://dx.doi.org/10.3892/etm.2020.9276] [PMID: 33093885]

[38] Yang MY, Chang JG, Lin PM, *et al.* Downregulation of circadian clock genes in chronic myeloid leukemia: Alternative methylation pattern of *hPER3*. Cancer Sci 2006; 97(12): 1298-307. [http://dx.doi.org/10.1111/j.1349-7006.2006.00331.x] [PMID: 16999817]

[39] Yang MY, Yang WC, Lin PM, *et al.* Altered expression of circadian clock genes in human chronic myeloid leukemia. J Biol Rhythms 2011; 26(2): 136-48.
[http://dx.doi.org/10.1177/0748730410395527] [PMID: 21454294]

[40] Lee Y. Roles of circadian clocks in cancer pathogenesis and treatment. Exp Mol Med 2021; 53(10): 1529-38.
[http://dx.doi.org/10.1038/s12276-021-00681-0] [PMID: 34615982]

[41] Roenneberg T, Merrow M. The Circadian Clock and Human Health. Curr Biol 2016; 26(10): R432-43.
[http://dx.doi.org/10.1016/j.cub.2016.04.011] [PMID: 27218855]

[42] Lévi F, Okyar A, Dulong S, Innominato PF, Clairambault J. Circadian timing in cancer treatments. Annu Rev Pharmacol Toxicol 2010; 50(1): 377-421.
[http://dx.doi.org/10.1146/annurev.pharmtox.48.113006.094626] [PMID: 20055686]

[43] Sulli G, Rommel A, Wang X, *et al.* Pharmacological activation of REV-ERBs is lethal in cancer and oncogene-induced senescence. Nature 2018; 553(7688): 351-5.
[http://dx.doi.org/10.1038/nature25170] [PMID: 29320480]

[44] Kelly KP, Borsetti H, Wenzler ME, *et al.* Screen for Small-Molecule Modulators of Circadian Rhythms Reveals Phenazine as a Redox-State Modifying Clockwork Tuner. ACS Chem Biol 2022; 17(7): 1658-64.
[http://dx.doi.org/10.1021/acschembio.2c00240] [PMID: 35679588]

[45] Sulli G, Manoogian ENC, Taub PR, Panda S. Training the circadian clock, clocking the drugs, and drugging the clock to prevent, manage, and treat chronic diseases. Trends Pharmacol Sci 2018; 39(9): 812-27.
[http://dx.doi.org/10.1016/j.tips.2018.07.003] [PMID: 30060890]

[46] Sultan A, Ali R, Sultan T, Ali S, Khan NJ, Parganiha A. Circadian clock modulating small molecules repurposing as inhibitors of SARS-CoV-2 M ^{pro} for pharmacological interventions in COVID-19 pandemic. Chronobiol Int 2021; 38(7): 971-85.
[http://dx.doi.org/10.1080/07420528.2021.1903027] [PMID: 33820462]

[47] Sultan A. Identification and development of clock-modulating small molecules – an emerging approach to fine-tune the disrupted circadian clocks. Biol Rhythm Res 2019; 50(5): 769-86.
[http://dx.doi.org/10.1080/09291016.2018.1498197]

[48] Takahashi JS. Transcriptional architecture of the mammalian circadian clock. Nat Rev Genet 2017; 18(3): 164-79.
[http://dx.doi.org/10.1038/nrg.2016.150] [PMID: 27990019]

[49] Gallego M, Virshup DM. Post-translational modifications regulate the ticking of the circadian clock. Nat Rev Mol Cell Biol 2007; 8(2): 139-48.
[http://dx.doi.org/10.1038/nrm2106] [PMID: 17245414]

[50] Lee C, Etchegaray JP, Cagampang FRA, Loudon ASI, Reppert SM. Posttranslational mechanisms regulate the mammalian circadian clock. Cell 2001; 107(7): 855-67.
[http://dx.doi.org/10.1016/S0092-8674(01)00610-9] [PMID: 11779462]

[51] Preußner M, Heyd F. Post-transcriptional control of the mammalian circadian clock: Implications for health and disease. Pflugers Arch 2016; 468(6): 983-91.
[http://dx.doi.org/10.1007/s00424-016-1820-y] [PMID: 27108448]

[52] Chaix A, Zarrinpar A, Panda S. The circadian coordination of cell biology. J Cell Biol 2016; 215(1): 15-25.
[http://dx.doi.org/10.1083/jcb.201603076] [PMID: 27738003]

[53] Ko CH, Takahashi JS. Molecular components of the mammalian circadian clock. Hum Mol Genet 2006; 15(Spec No 2) (2): R271-7.
[http://dx.doi.org/10.1093/hmg/ddl207] [PMID: 16987893]

[54] Siepka SM, Yoo SH, Park J, *et al.* Circadian mutant Overtime reveals F-box protein FBXL3 regulation of cryptochrome and period gene expression. Cell 2007; 129(5): 1011-23. [http://dx.doi.org/10.1016/j.cell.2007.04.030] [PMID: 17462724]

[55] Hirano A, Yumimoto K, Tsunematsu R, *et al.* FBXL21 regulates oscillation of the circadian clock through ubiquitination and stabilization of cryptochromes. Cell 2013; 152(5): 1106-18. [http://dx.doi.org/10.1016/j.cell.2013.01.054] [PMID: 23452856]

[56] Yoo SH, Mohawk JA, Siepka SM, *et al.* Competing E3 ubiquitin ligases govern circadian periodicity by degradation of CRY in nucleus and cytoplasm. Cell 2013; 152(5): 1091-105. [http://dx.doi.org/10.1016/j.cell.2013.01.055] [PMID: 23452855]

[57] Preitner N, Damiola F, Luis-Lopez-Molina , *et al.* The orphan nuclear receptor REV-ERBalpha controls circadian transcription within the positive limb of the mammalian circadian oscillator. Cell 2002; 110(2): 251-60. [http://dx.doi.org/10.1016/S0092-8674(02)00825-5] [PMID: 12150932]

[58] Sato TK, Panda S, Miraglia LJ, *et al.* A functional genomics strategy reveals Rora as a component of the mammalian circadian clock. Neuron 2004; 43(4): 527-37. [http://dx.doi.org/10.1016/j.neuron.2004.07.018] [PMID: 15312651]

[59] Lowrey PL, Takahashi JS. Genetics of circadian rhythms in mammalian model organisms. Adv Genet 2011; 74: 175-230. [http://dx.doi.org/10.1016/B978-0-12-387690-4.00006-4] [PMID: 21924978]

[60] Chen Z, Yoo SH, Takahashi JS. Development and therapeutic potential of small-molecule modulators of circadian systems. Annu Rev Pharmacol Toxicol 2018; 58(1): 231-52. [http://dx.doi.org/10.1146/annurev-pharmtox-010617-052645] [PMID: 28968186]

[61] Zhang Y, Fang B, Emmett MJ, *et al.* Discrete functions of nuclear receptor Rev-erbα couple metabolism to the clock. Science 2015; 348(6242): 1488-92. [http://dx.doi.org/10.1126/science.aab3021] [PMID: 26044300]

[62] Jeong K, He B, Nohara K, *et al.* Dual attenuation of proteasomal and autophagic BMAL1 degradation in ClockΔ19/+ mice contributes to improved glucose homeostasis. Sci Rep 2015; 5(1): 12801. [http://dx.doi.org/10.1038/srep12801] [PMID: 26228022]

[63] Gachon F, Fonjallaz P, Damiola F, *et al.* The loss of circadian PAR bZip transcription factors results in epilepsy. Genes Dev 2004; 18(12): 1397-412. [http://dx.doi.org/10.1101/gad.301404] [PMID: 15175240]

[64] Mitsui S, Yamaguchi S, Matsuo T, Ishida Y, Okamura H. Antagonistic role of E4BP4 and PAR proteins in the circadian oscillatory mechanism. Genes Dev 2001; 15(8): 995-1006. [http://dx.doi.org/10.1101/gad.873501] [PMID: 11316793]

[65] Ohno T, Onishi Y, Ishida N. A novel E4BP4 element drives circadian expression of mPeriod2. Nucleic Acids Res 2006; 35(2): 648-55. [http://dx.doi.org/10.1093/nar/gkl868] [PMID: 17182630]

[66] Ueda HR, Hayashi S, Chen W, *et al.* System-level identification of transcriptional circuits underlying mammalian circadian clocks. Nat Genet 2005; 37(2): 187-92. [http://dx.doi.org/10.1038/ng1504] [PMID: 15665827]

[67] He B, Chen Z. Molecular targets for small-molecule modulators of circadian clocks. Curr Drug Metab 2016; 17(5): 503-12. [http://dx.doi.org/10.2174/1389200217666160111124439] [PMID: 26750111]

[68] Gustafson CL, Partch CL. Emerging models for the molecular basis of mammalian circadian timing. Biochemistry 2015; 54(2): 134-49. [http://dx.doi.org/10.1021/bi500731f] [PMID: 25303119]

[69] Sulli G, Lam MTY, Panda S. Interplay between circadian clock and cancer: New frontiers for cancer

treatment. Trends Cancer 2019; 5(8): 475-94.
[http://dx.doi.org/10.1016/j.trecan.2019.07.002] [PMID: 31421905]

[70] Panda S. The arrival of circadian medicine. Nat Rev Endocrinol 2019; 15(2): 67-9.
[http://dx.doi.org/10.1038/s41574-018-0142-x] [PMID: 30602736]

[71] Solt LA, Wang Y, Banerjee S, *et al.* Regulation of circadian behaviour and metabolism by synthetic REV-ERB agonists. Nature 2012; 485(7396): 62-8.
[http://dx.doi.org/10.1038/nature11030] [PMID: 22460951]

[72] Wallach T, Kramer A. Chemical chronobiology: Toward drugs manipulating time. FEBS Lett 2015; 589(14): 1530-8.
[http://dx.doi.org/10.1016/j.febslet.2015.04.059] [PMID: 25957770]

[73] Chen Z, Yoo SH, Park YS, *et al.* Identification of diverse modulators of central and peripheral circadian clocks by high-throughput chemical screening. Proc Natl Acad Sci 2012; 109(1): 101-6.
[http://dx.doi.org/10.1073/pnas.1118034108] [PMID: 22184224]

[74] He B, Nohara K, Park N, *et al.* The small molecule nobiletin targets the molecular oscillator to enhance circadian rhythms and protect against metabolic syndrome. Cell Metab 2016; 23(4): 610-21.
[http://dx.doi.org/10.1016/j.cmet.2016.03.007] [PMID: 27076076]

[75] Hirota T, Lewis WG, Liu AC, Lee JW, Schultz PG, Kay SA. A chemical biology approach reveals period shortening of the mammalian circadian clock by specific inhibition of GSK-3β. Proc Natl Acad Sci 2008; 105(52): 20746-51.
[http://dx.doi.org/10.1073/pnas.0811410106] [PMID: 19104043]

[76] Hirota T, Lee JW, Lewis WG, *et al.* High-throughput chemical screen identifies a novel potent modulator of cellular circadian rhythms and reveals CKIα as a clock regulatory kinase. PLoS Biol 2010; 8(12): e1000559.
[http://dx.doi.org/10.1371/journal.pbio.1000559] [PMID: 21179498]

[77] Hirota T, Lee JW, St John PC, *et al.* Identification of small molecule activators of cryptochrome. Science 2012; 337(6098): 1094-7.
[http://dx.doi.org/10.1126/science.1223710] [PMID: 22798407]

[78] Isojima Y, Nakajima M, Ukai H, *et al.* CKIε/δ-dependent phosphorylation is a temperature-insensitive, period-determining process in the mammalian circadian clock. Proc Natl Acad Sci 2009; 106(37): 15744-9.
[http://dx.doi.org/10.1073/pnas.0908733106] [PMID: 19805222]

[79] Yagita K, Yamanaka I, Koinuma S, Shigeyoshi Y, Uchiyama Y. Mini screening of kinase inhibitors affecting period-length of mammalian cellular circadian clock. Acta Histochem Cytochem 2009; 42(3): 89-93.
[http://dx.doi.org/10.1267/ahc.09015] [PMID: 19617956]

[80] Chun SK, Jang J, Chung S, *et al.* Identification and validation of cryptochrome inhibitors that modulate the molecular circadian clock. ACS Chem Biol 2014; 9(3): 703-10.
[http://dx.doi.org/10.1021/cb400752k] [PMID: 24387302]

[81] Hu Y, Spengler ML, Kuropatwinski KK, *et al.* Selenium is a modulator of circadian clock that protects mice from the toxicity of a chemotherapeutic drug *via* upregulation of the core clock protein, BMAL1. Oncotarget 2011; 2(12): 1279-90.
[http://dx.doi.org/10.18632/oncotarget.411] [PMID: 22249125]

[82] Lee JW, Hirota T, Peters EC, *et al.* A small molecule modulates circadian rhythms through phosphorylation of the period protein. Angew Chem Int Ed 2011; 50(45): 10608-11.
[http://dx.doi.org/10.1002/anie.201103915] [PMID: 21954091]

[83] Meng QJ, Maywood ES, Bechtold DA, *et al.* Entrainment of disrupted circadian behavior through inhibition of casein kinase 1 (CK1) enzymes. Proc Natl Acad Sci USA 2010; 107(34): 15240-5.
[http://dx.doi.org/10.1073/pnas.1005101107] [PMID: 20696890]

[84] Wang Y, Kumar N, Nuhant P, *et al.* Identification of SR1078, a synthetic agonist for the orphan nuclear receptors RORα and RORγ. ACS Chem Biol 2010; 5(11): 1029-34. [http://dx.doi.org/10.1021/cb100223d] [PMID: 20735016]

[85] Wang Y, Solt LA, Kojetin DJ, Burris TP. Regulation of p53 stability and apoptosis by a ROR agonist. PLoS One 2012; 7(4): e34921. [http://dx.doi.org/10.1371/journal.pone.0034921] [PMID: 22509368]

[86] Shen W, Zhang W, Ye W, *et al.* SR9009 induces a REV-ERB dependent anti-small-cell lung cancer effect through inhibition of autophagy. Theranostics 2020; 10(10): 4466-80. [http://dx.doi.org/10.7150/thno.42478] [PMID: 32292508]

[87] Wagner PM, Monjes NM, Guido ME. Chemotherapeutic Effect of SR9009, a REV-ERB Agonist, on the Human Glioblastoma T98G Cells. ASN Neuro 2019; 11. [http://dx.doi.org/10.1177/1759091419892713] [PMID: 31825658]

[88] Brownell JE, Sintchak MD, Gavin JM, *et al.* Substrate-assisted inhibition of ubiquitin-like protein-activating enzymes: The NEDD8 E1 inhibitor MLN4924 forms a NEDD8-AMP mimetic *in situ*. Mol Cell 2010; 37(1): 102-11. [http://dx.doi.org/10.1016/j.molcel.2009.12.024] [PMID: 20129059]

[89] Milhollen MA, Traore T, Adams-Duffy J, *et al.* MLN4924, a NEDD8-activating enzyme inhibitor, is active in diffuse large B-cell lymphoma models: rationale for treatment of NF-κB–dependent lymphoma. Blood 2010; 116(9): 1515-23. [http://dx.doi.org/10.1182/blood-2010-03-272567] [PMID: 20525923]

[90] Soucy TA, Smith PG, Milhollen MA, *et al.* An inhibitor of NEDD8-activating enzyme as a new approach to treat cancer. Nature 2009; 458(7239): 732-6. [http://dx.doi.org/10.1038/nature07884] [PMID: 19360080]

[91] Zhang S, Zhang J, Deng Z, *et al.* Circadian clock components RORα and Bmal1 mediate the anti-proliferative effect of MLN4924 in osteosarcoma cells. Oncotarget 2016; 7(40): 66087-99. [http://dx.doi.org/10.18632/oncotarget.11807] [PMID: 27602774]

[92] Jang J, Chung S, Choi Y, *et al.* The cryptochrome inhibitor KS15 enhances E-box-mediated transcription by disrupting the feedback action of a circadian transcription-repressor complex. Life Sci 2018; 200: 49-55. [http://dx.doi.org/10.1016/j.lfs.2018.03.022] [PMID: 29534992]

[93] Chun SK, Chung S, Kim HD, *et al.* A synthetic cryptochrome inhibitor induces anti-proliferative effects and increases chemosensitivity in human breast cancer cells. Biochem Biophys Res Commun 2015; 467(2): 441-6. [http://dx.doi.org/10.1016/j.bbrc.2015.09.103] [PMID: 26407844]

CHAPTER 12

A Roadmap towards Precision Medicine for Multiple Sclerosis

Nimisha Gupta[1] and **Saima Wajid**[1,*]

[1] *Department of Biotechnology, School of Chemical and Life Sciences, Jamia Hamdard, Jamia Nagar, New Delhi – 110062, India*

Abstract: Multiple Sclerosis (MS) is an autoimmune inflammatory disease and this affects roughly 2.8 million people worldwide. This is a highly heterogeneous disease in terms of course, clinical symptoms and response treatment. The exact pathogenesis and aetiology of this disease remain unknown. The lack of successful treatment can be explained by the heterogeneous nature of MS with patients exhibiting widely disparate clinical features and progression patterns resulting in phenotypic heterogeneity. Therefore, there is a need for the development of biomarkers for MS. The "Omics" approaches have been exploited for the development of biomarkers although the system biology was taken into consideration. With the introduction of Omics approaches, personalized medicine has gained potential revealing hitherto unseen elements of illness causation, initiation and progression. This chapter will focus on the potential role of genomics, transcriptomics, proteomics and metabolomics in MS for the possible identification of biomarkers facilitating and augmenting the concept of precision medicine.

Keywords: Biomarkers, Early diagnosis and precision medicine, Multiple sclerosis, Omics approaches.

INTRODUCTION

The term "Personalized medicine" (PM) refers to the medical treatment that takes into account factors such as the disease status of the patient and their background to select the most appropriate treatment. This strategy gives patients and medical staff the chance to gain from more focused and efficient treatments, potentially increasing healthcare gains and boosting the effectiveness of the healthcare system. Finding the right drug for the right patient at the right time is the main aim of personalised medicine [1, 2].

* **Corresponding author Saima Wajid:** Department of Biotechnology, School of Chemical and Life Sciences, Jamia Hamdard, Hamdard Nagar, New Delhi – 110062, India; Tal: 9899823898; E-mails: swajid@jamiahamdard.ac.in; wajid.saima@gmail.com

Farzana Mahdi & Abbas Ali Mahdi (Eds.)

OMICS covers genomics, transcriptomics, proteomics, metabolomics, epigenomics and lipidomics, among other high-throughput technologies that have rapidly grown in recent years, allowing us to elucidate the complex pathophysiology behind complicated biological events (Fig. **1**). Additionally, it is concentrated on the customization and timing of therapeutic and preventive actions based on biological data, omics biomarkers and molecular disease pathways. The non-invasive, high-throughput and cost-effective methods of metabolomics and proteomics study of biomarkers show promise for diagnosing early-stage prognosis, monitoring therapy effectiveness, and contributing to the creation of innovative targeted medicines. Therefore, "omics" has seen a sharp increase in studies on biomarkers' discovery in recent times and it is very important to understand system biology. With the introduction to Omics approaches, personalised medicine has gained momentum and now has potential to uncover hitherto 'unseen' elements of illness causation, initiation, and disease progression [3].

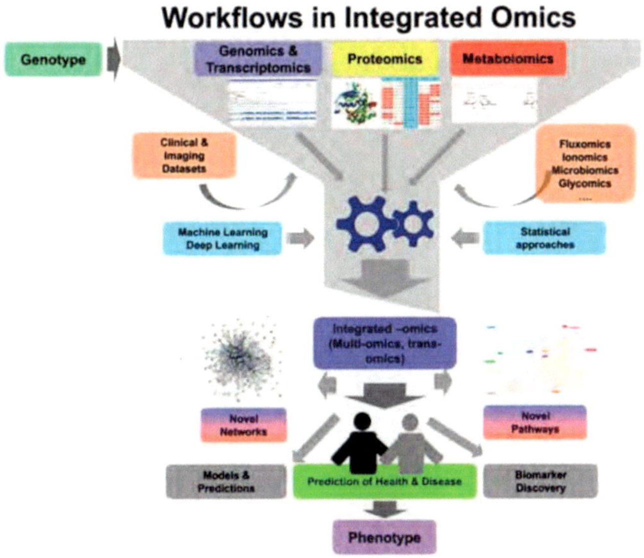

Fig. (1). Integrated Omics workflow adapted from B.B. Mishra *et al.*, 2019 [3].

Multiple Sclerosis (MS) is an inflammatory, chronic, autoimmune disease of the central nervous system (CNS) resulting in neuronal demyelination and axonal damage in the brain and spinal cord. MS affects roughly 2.8 million people worldwide. The MS is a leading cause of non-traumatic medical disability in young people of 20-45 years. This disease commonly affects women (Female to male ratio 3:1) though the cause is still unknown.

The scientific community generally agrees that various environmental conditions in genetically susceptible persons produce an aberrant activation of the immune system against CNS myelin. MS is a highly heterogeneous disease in terms of course, clinical symptoms and response to treatment. It is characterized by inflammatory demyelinating relapsing-remitting multiple sclerosis (RRMS) which progresses over time to a progressively degenerative stage characterized by scar formation and axonal loss, resulting in cognitive disability [4, 5].

MS complexity has been characterised more thoroughly using epigenetic, transcriptomic, proteomic, and metabolomic techniques. A combination of techniques provides unique insights into the molecular underpinnings of disease pathogenesis. This enables its integration and translation into clinical neurology. Given the scarcity of prognostic markers for MS, the importance of "omics" techniques that can build a fingerprint for each patient appears to be a suitable approach for accomplishing "ad hoc" therapeutic therapy [4]. However, according to available data, personalized therapies for MS are still at the preliminary stage. This chapter will concentrate on the potential role of genomics, transcriptomics, proteomics and metabolomics in MS, for the possible identification of biomarkers useful in the context of personalized medicine.

DIAGNOSTIC CRITERIA FOR MULTIPLE SCLEROSIS

MS is classified into four subtypes based on empirical evidence which includes relapsing-remitting multiple sclerosis (RRMS), primary progressive multiple sclerosis (PPMS), secondary progressive multiple sclerosis (SPMS), and progressive relapsing multiple sclerosis (PRMS). Thus far, there is no specific laboratory marker for the diagnosis of MS. McDonald criteria for diagnosis were first developed in 2001. The International Panel on Diagnosis of MS developed the McDonald criteria in 2001, giving magnetic resonance imaging (MRI) increasingly more weight in the diagnosis of MS as a result of the technology's increased availability. These criteria were subsequently revised in 2005 and 2010, with the most recent revision occurring in 2017. The 2017 revisions to the McDonald criteria allow for early diagnosis of MS, and an increasing number of approved disease-modifying therapies (DMTs) provide the best treatment for MS patients by altering the disease course [6]. Presently, there are 13 MS disease-modifying therapies for MS that have received FDA approval [7]. MS is diagnosed through clinical evaluation and supported by laboratory findings such as MRI, and CSF analysis. Another important examination is lumbar puncture for CSF examination, cytopathological evaluation, microbiological test, test for IgG index and qualitatively oligoclonal band analysis. The risks of misdiagnosis MSt be weighed against the advantages of early diagnosis [8].

Imaging techniques such as MRI, spinal fluid analysis and evoked potentials are used for MS. White matter lesions on an MRI typically show a patient's progression from clinically isolated syndrome (CIS) to a clinically identified MS subtype. In case of MS with low-grade disease activity, CSF biomarkers are more sensitive than clinical / MRI assessments. CSF immunoglobulin (IgG)-Index and neurofilament light chain (cNfL) levels have been found to be significantly higher in some patients whose disease was determined by clinical scales and/or MRI. The assessment of neural conduction in different pathways can be done using evoked potentials, which include visual evoked potentials, somatosensory evoked potentials, and brainstem auditory evoked responses. It is carried out by stimulating the corresponding system and measuring the latency and amplitude with a scalp electrode placed over the corresponding cortex. Indicators of demyelination damage, such as prolonged latency can be used to diagnose MS and evaluate particular pathways [9]. Molecular biomarkers can complement MRI and clinical characteristics and are easily quantifiable. Now, there are a number of potential molecular biomarkers available for the diagnosis of MS, prognosis, disease activity, and treatment response.

PERSONALIZED MEDICINE IN MULTIPLE SCLEROSIS

MS is a very heterogeneous disease, so individualised care is highly desired. In this context, it becomes important to use right drug for the patient at the right time using the right dose. If drug titration is required, that too MSt be done to ensure the optimum dose [1, 2]. An approach that prioritises the patient is necessary for personalised medicine, and disease taxonomy MSt be based on the characterization of pathophysiological processes. Profiling and patient characterization are essential for ensuring that MS patients receive the proper care, taking into account the many clinical and immunopathological aspects of the disease. Three essential elements are necessary for the use of personalised medicine in MS. First, prognosis evaluation soon after diagnosis; second, early therapeutic planning based on risk-benefit analysis and patient preferences; third, early evaluation of therapy response and use of alternative therapies in the event of failure. Moreover, there is no effective treatment for MS despite significant research in this area. At this juncture, drug repurposing options may also be explored. It has been found that some drugs are effective not only for the disease they were developed but also for other diseases. Drug repurposing is an area that needs our serious attention. This will broaden the spectrum of the use of drug enabling far more patients to be covered and even cutting the cost of the new drug development. There are a number of disease-modifying drugs available for RR subtype patients, classified as first- and second-line therapies with varying efficacy and safety profiles. Furthermore, due to the dearth of reliable biomarkers and the complexity of the pathogenesis of MS, personalised medicine, as opposed to precision medicine would be the preferred management strategy today. Therefore, it is necessary to achieve more accurate assessments of important MS predictors. Such MS patients will have more opportunities for early preventive interventions, more accurate diagnoses and treatment. Beyond the notion of precision medicine, personalised medicine has recently been taken into consideration in the therapeutic strategy for MS. Biomarkers are crucial for understanding the disease diagnosis, prognosis and forecasting of the disease course in MS patients. Additionally, they play a crucial role in determining the advantages and disadvantages of novel treatments for patients [10]. It would be a rewarding proposition if drug bank is systematically searched for the potent drug molecules to be used for MS in a more individualized manner. It would be equally important to work out the involvement of all the genes, their mutational load and involvement in signal transduction. Thus, detailed genetic background information would enable better diagnosis allowing more accurate treatment. Such genetic information for every single disease may be generated by highly focused independent research and development. This would be the part of actual translational research.

TREATMENT RESPONSE BIOMARKERS IN MULTIPLE SCLEROSIS

Several Cerebrospinal Fluids (CSF) and blood biomarkers have been developed so far to monitor the treatment response. Neutralizing antibodies, Oligoclonal bands (OCBs), interferon-beta (IFN-β) and natalizumab (NTZ) are currently used clinically.

OCBs are clinically validated biomarkers having diagnostic and prognostic values. OCBs improve the sensitivity of RRMS diagnosis in patients with a first clinical event, implying MS and criteria for 'dissemination in space' (DIS) [11].

The injectable recombinant IFN-β was the first approved disease-modifying treatment (DMT) drug used most commonly to treat MS. IFN - β helped patients experience fewer relapses and delayed the onset of disability. IFN-treated patients most frequently experience injection site reactions and flu-like symptoms [12]. However, because of their excellent long-term cost-effectiveness and safety, they are still widely used. Glatiramer acetate (GA) is another injectable medication that is useful to block the immune system's attack on myelin. GA is also the first-line disease-modifying treatment (DMT) prescribed for relapsing types of MS as compared to IFN-β, but for this, fewer pharmacogenomic trials have been conducted [13]. Moreover, Ocrelizumab, a monoclonal antibody, and siponimod, a sphingosine-1-phosphate receptor modulator, have recently received approval for the treatment of MS progression [14].

Additionally, natalizumab (Monoclonal antibody) is directed against the VLA-4 integrin's alpha chain (CD49d) and it is a powerful inhibitor of cell migration toward tissues, including the CNS. When the disease is in the relapsing remitting stage, it significantly lowers relapses and active brain lesions. It may be considered as a first line of treatment for people suffering from severe MS. The severe infectious complication progressive multifocal leukoencephalopathy (PML) has been linked to long-term treatment. This susceptibility, is seen in other immunosuppression states, that has not been linked to any particular biological risk related to NAT properties [15].

Moreover, protein-based medications can cause the production of neutralising antibodies (NAbs), which can disrupt the drug's mechanism of action. Following DMT exposure in MS, the emergence of NAbs has been noted. NAbs serve as a clinically relevant biomarker for therapeutic decision-making purposes at the moment. Neutralizing antibodies can be found in patients treated with IFN-β, a protein with potential immunogenicity (NAbs). The radiological activity, clinical course, and disability progression are all adversely affected by neutralising antibodies, which also decrease IFN's therapeutic efficacy. Comparing the rate of relapse, radiological activity, and disability progression between patients with NAbs and those without them reveals that neutralising antibodies to natalizumab are associated with lower serum levels of the medication and, consequently, a lower therapeutic efficacy of natalizumab [16].

GENOMICS OF MULTIPLE SCLEROSIS

During the past few years, genome-wide association studies with growing sample sizes have resulted in the discovery of substantially related genetic variations at an exponential rate. Genetic research contributes significantly to our understanding of the disease's genesis. More than 200 susceptibility loci have been found, accounting for around half of the hereditary diseases [17]. Currently, 233 genome-wide loci linked to MS susceptibility have been discovered. Further, the largest genetic study of 47,351 cases of MS was conducted together with 68,284 healthy controls. Approximately, 200 of these loci are found in the autosomal non-MHC genome and account for 20% of the genetics of MS. As predicted by the CVCD hypothesis, the sizes of these loci are modest, ranging from ORs of 1.05 to 1.2 [18]. Recent studies in a variety of MS cohorts have demonstrated that the HLA-DRB1*1501 allele is primarily responsible for genetic risk in the MS population. Furthermore, observations in a Japanese cohort established a positive correlation of HLA-DRB1*1501 allele with oligoclonal bands in the CSF of MS patients, which was supported by subsequent studies [19 - 22]. The functional characterization of the MS risk variant on chromosome 12p13.31 containing the gene TNFRSF1A, which encodes for the tumour necrosis factor (TNF) receptor superfamily member 1A with apoptotic activity, is a significant step forward. TNFRSF1A is linked to MS risk and provides insight into the pathophysiology, which may lead to novel therapeutic strategies. TNFRSF1A shows that systematic follow-up of specific variants display strong link with MS risk of the underlying effect. This is envisaged to help assess the cause and condition providing cutting-edge treatment options [23]. In addition to this, the association of non-HLA genes with MS risk has been examined. The results of this study suggest that interleukin IL2RA and IL7R, two cytokine genes, may contribute to MS development [24]. Whether these two genes also show sequence heterogeneity or specific mutations amongst the MS patients is not clear. However, a systematic search of mutations and expression of these genes would enrich our understanding of the additional causative factors associated with MS.

TRANSCRIPTOMICS FOR MULTIPLE SCLEROSIS

Gene expression profiling has been widely utilized to fish out biomarkers for MS diagnosis, disease progression, and disease activity. Nali *et al.* [25] performed global transcriptomic profiling of 9 patients with their corresponding control samples. In this study, a total of 435 and 731 differentially expressed genes were identified in RRMS and SPMS, respectively. TANC2, SIPA1L1, IRS2, RERE and PLAGL1 genes showed over-expression in both SPMS and RRMS, while PAD4 and PAD2 were downregulated in SPMS and upregulated in RRMS [25]. In another study, RNA-Seq data analysis showed that non-coding and coding transcriptomic changes of monocytes in MS patients as compared to healthy controls involved several still uncharacterized genes. These genes are PRKY, DDX3Y, XIST, RPS4Y1, KDM5D, EIF1AY, UTY and KDM6A. Furthermore, gene ontology analysis shows the top 5 upregulated pathways (JAK-STAT signalling, NOD-like receptor signalling, Toll-like receptor signalling, B-cell receptor signalling and apoptosis) that were found to be upregulated and one pathway (Ribosome) was found to be significantly downregulated. These genes and their associated pathways are envisaged to improve diagnosis and help guide therapies of MS [26].

Interestingly, single cell transcriptomics makes unbiased biological research possible and holds a promise for individualised medicine. In one such study, single cell RNA-Sequencing to CSF specimens from MS patients and controls were analysed. In the process, they validated the first transcriptional atlas of single CSF leukocytes and identified T follicular helper cells as drivers of local inflammation in MS [27]. In another study, Derakhshani *et al.* [28] assessed PD-L1 and CTLA-4 gene expression in peripheral blood mononuclear cells of MS patients using single cell RNA-Seq. This sequencing results revealed a substantial expression of PD-L1 and CTLA-4 in the native T cells and activated CD8+ T cells, which seems to plays a key role in restraining autoreactive T-cells and ceasing the development of MS autoimmunity [28].

A recent study confirmed the involvement of BACH2 and MICAL3 genes in paediatric and adult MS patients when compared to age matched control group. This study also observed upregulation of TNFSF13B gene in paediatric MS patients that were under concomitant disease modifying treatments [29]. Another study examined changes in microRNA expression in response to IFN-β and discovered downregulation of the miR-29 family of miRNAs. These miRNAs were found to be associated with IFN feedback loops and apoptotic processes [30]. However, further studies will be needed to determine the prognostic value of the above the reported genes, requiring validation in longitudinal samples from a larger cohort of MS patients.

PROTEOMICS FOR MULTIPLE SCLEROSIS

Proteomics approach allows a detailed separation of proteins in biological fluids. Biomarkers are predictors and indicators of specific pathophysiological processes. As a result, a validated set of proteoform biomarkers would support early accurate prognosis and diagnosis. Furthermore, biomarkers that can aid in disease diagnosis/ prognosis, patient stratification, and objectively tracking treatment progression and response are crucial during the development and implementation of various treatments. Clinically, the most important step in identifying biomarker candidates is the collection of biological samples using less invasive techniques. Biochemical markers for MS have been derived from various sources, such as blood, serum, CSF, saliva, brain tissues, urine and tears. Due to their many connections, these biological fluids have a diverse range of molecules and protein composition. Biomarkers for MS are important because they can aid in early diagnosis, which enables better disease management and they are non-invasive [31].

Biofluid / Tissue Proteomic Studies in MS

Blood and CSF

There have been a number of proteomic studies using blood and Cerebrospinal fluid (CSF) of MS patients focusing on individual proteins for their role as biomarkers. One such study used Orbitrap Mass Spectrometry analysis and isobaric tags for relative abundance and quantitation (iTRAQ) labelling to identify seven biomarker candidates in CSF samples from MS patients. This included chitinase-3-like protein 1 (CHI3L1), cerebellin-1, neuroserpin, cell surface glycoprotein MUC18, secretogranin-1 (Sg1), and glutamate receptor 4. Furthermore, the intracellular calcium binding protein Sg1 showed higher protein levels in early-MS patients compared to RRMS in the follow-up validation study from an independent sample set of MS patients [32]. Interestingly, Shi *et al.* [33] identified 83 CSF specific differentially expressed proteins in MS patients using tandem mass tag quantitative proteomic analysis. They found that the somatostatin (SSP) and insulin-like growth factor-binding protein 7 (IGFBP7) were significantly differentially expressed in both CSF and serum samples. They also identified the coagulation and complement cascades, PI3K-Akt signalling pathway and Ras signalling pathway as main components [33]. In another study, Probert *et al.* [34] identified a number of independent CSF biomarkers that could help distinguish MS from non-MS controls as compared to (oligoclonal IgG bands) OCGB positivity. High sensitivity (85%) and low specificity (67%) were used by OCGB to distinguish between clinically definite MS and non-MS. The determination of Connective tissue growth factor (CCN5), von Willebrand factor (vWF) and glial fibrillary acidic protein (GFAP) levels enhances the diagnostic accuracy, sensitivity and specificity as compared to OCGB alone [34]. Recently, SERPINA3 and S100A4 were found to be more prevalent in the CSF of MS patients compared to controls [35]. Regardless of the disease subtype, a Danish study conducted in 2021 discovered that trypsin-1, augurin, receptor-type tyrosine-protein phosphatase, apolipoprotein C-I, and apolipoprotein A-II were all upregulated in the CSF of MS patients when compared to healthy controls [36]. Jankovska *et al.* [37] found 69 proteins to be differentially expressed between CSF of women with newly diagnosed RRMS and control samples. Among them, eosinophil-derived neurotoxin, ceruloplasmin and lysozyme-C were found to be upregulated in MS patients while the Nogo receptor was downregulated [37].

Some potential prognostic biomarkers, including C-X-C motif chemokine 13 (CXCL13), chitinase-3-like protein 1 (CHI3L1) and osteopontin were discovered through MS analysis of CSF and blood samples from MS patients. Several studies demonstrated increased level of CXCL13 protein in CSF of MS patients as well as in other neuroinflammatory diseases. Furthermore, CXCL13 may represent an important prognostic biomarker for the development of individualized medicine, since increased level of CXCL13 has been identified in CIS patients. This protein may have a role in monitoring therapy [38 - 40]. Proteomic profiling of CSF before and after NTZ treatment for a year revealed, in an interesting finding, that CSF CHI3L1 levels were significantly lower, indicating the possibility of CHI3L1 to be a biomarker of therapeutic response. The response to IFN was associated with peripheral blood CHI3L1 levels. Increased expression of CHI3L1 was found in the progressive forms of MS. CHI3L1 serum levels have been found to be elevated in groups of patients who are unresponsive to IFN- treatment [41 - 44]. Several studies reported higher level of osteopontin in MS patients' plasma and CSF compared to controls and strengthens the evidence regarding clinical utility of osteopontin as a promising biomarker for MS [45 - 47].

Moreover, Tremlett *et al.* [48] identified a panel of 11 serum proteins using isobaric tagging and iTRAQ methodology. These proteins were associated with inflammatory, opsonization (associated with phagocytosis), and complement activation processes [48]. Nevertheless, some investigation has uncovered the immunopathologic activity of Matrix metalloproteinases (MMPs) in MS. MMP 9 is a crucial metalloproteinase in MS pathogenesis that enhances leukocyte migration, blood-brain barrier disruption and myelin lysis. Elevated levels of MMP-9 were observed in the serum and CSF of MS patients during relapses [49, 50]. In another proteomic study on serum samples, MMP 9 was found to be decreased in MS patients treated with natalizumab. This study suggests that the proangiogenic factor MMP9 may play a role as a biomarker associated with the development of progressive multifocal leukoencephalopathy (PML) in MS patients treated with natalizumab [51].

Interestingly, Berge *et al.* [52], looking at the difference in the proteomic profiles of T cells from peripheral blood mononuclear cells, found higher protein abundance in CD4+ and CD8+ T cells from relapsing-remitting MS (RRMS) patients as compared to controls [52]. Furthermore, Amin *et al.* [53] detected 241 serum proteins using 2D-DIGE. Among these, three highly expressed proteins, namely, transthyretin, zinc alpha-2-glycoprotein and immunoglobulin kappa light chain, were validated in the serum of RRMS patients as compared to healthy controls [53].

Saliva

Saliva is easy to collect, more diluted and less complex biofluid compared to plasma. Manconi *et al.* [54] used a mass spectrometry-based top-down proteomic approach to perform the quantitative analysis on saliva samples. They found 23 proteins that were differentially expressed. Out of which eight proteins (Mono- and di-oxidized cystatin SN, mono- and di-oxidized cystatin S1, mono-oxidized cystatin SA, and mono-phosphorylated statherin) were found to be downregulated, whereas fifteen proteins (Antileukoproteinase, two proteoforms of Prolactin-inducible protein, P-C peptide, SV1 fragment of statherin, cystatin SN Des1-4, cystatin SN P11 → L variant, and cystatin A T96 → M variant) were upregulated in multiple sclerosis patients compared to control samples. Further evidence that saliva samples may be suitable for MS biomarker studies comes from the fact that these proteins are connected to pathways of neurodegeneration and inflammation [54]. Thus, the refinement of this approach on a larger sample size may prove to be more economical and less resource intensive facilitating the concept of personalized medicine.

Urine

Urine is easy to collect and may contain valuable proteins associated with MS diagnosis and prognosis. In a single proteomic study, Singh *et al.* [55] identified 1699 tryptic peptides (related to 402 proteins) in urine from 31 MS and 8 healthy controls throughout the third trimester of pregnancy and postpartum period using mass spectrometry (LTQ orbitrap). Among these proteins, the most discriminating peptides identified were lysosomal-associated membrane protein 2 and trefoil factor 3. These proteins have a crucial role in the innate immune system. The other 3 proteins with a noticeably decreased ratio in MS were osteoclast-associated immune-like receptor, plasma glutamate carboxypeptidase, and Ig mu chain C region. It appears that the improvement of disease relapse during pregnancy results from an increase in immunosuppressive proteins and a decrease in proteins related to the immunopathology of MS. Even so, additional proteomics research is required to understand the role of proteins derived from urine as biomarkers for the diagnosis and prognosis of MS [55]. However, if this approach too is refined carefully, that may prove to be yet another powerful option for MS diagnosis.

Tear

Tear biofluid is challenging due to the small sample volumes and wide dynamic range of proteins. Interestingly, an increased level of soluble interleukin -2 was found in tears of MS patients as compared to controls. In another proteomic investigation by Salvisberg *et al.* [56] 185 tear proteins were identified, of which 42 proteins were differentially expressed. Among 42 dysregulated proteins, they found alpha-1antichymotrypsin was significantly elevated in MS patients in all three experiments with a ratio ranging from 1.6 to 2.5. Traditional lumbar punctures are being replaced by the increased level of alpha-1 antichymotrypsin in tears as a potential biomarker for MS [56].

Brain tissue

Byström *et al.* [57] used affinity protein profiling and identified IRF8, IL7, SLC30A7, METTL14, and GAP43 proteins that were differentially expressed in the brain tissue of MS patients. These proteins were most indicative of disease activity and progression [57]. In another proteomics study, the pattern of protein expression in the brain tissues of EAE models was assessed using a 2-DE-based proteomics approach. Seventy out of the roughly 1000 proteins analysed showed a significant change in the EAE model compared to controls. These proteins take part in a variety of biological functions, such as the release of ions and neurotransmitters, apoptosis, and signal transduction. Additionally, these proteins are involved in the formation and operation of mitochondria and blood brain barriers [10].

METABOLOMICS FOR MULTIPLE SCLEROSIS

In recent years, metabolomics has emerged as a powerful tool to identify altered metabolites, and pathways influenced by the environment and this provides a significant insight into the pathogenesis related to MS and offers wide clinical application.

The term "metabolome" describes the entire collection of low molecular weight metabolites (900 Da or less) produced by an individual, forming a vast network of connected reactions. It is quicker and more efficient than other Omics methods. As a result, it offers a more comprehensive picture of the physiological status and cellular functions. The complexity of the analysis of metabolites is caused by the diversity of the metabolic pathway. As a result, metabolomics makes use of analytical methods like LTQ Orbitrap, nuclear magnetic resonance, gas chromatography-mass spectrometry, and liquid chromatography-mass spectrometry (GC-MS). Recently, metabolomics has been used to identify specific and sensitive metabolic biomarkers that may help in the early diagnosis/prognosis of MS at different stages and provide better insight into drug response [58].

Reinke *et al.* [59] performed NMR spectroscopic analysis of CSF specimens, identified 15 metabolites in MS and non-MS patients. In MS-derived CSF, mean levels of myo-inositol, and threonate were upregulated while 3-hydroxybutyrate, citrate, phenylalanine, 2-hydroxyisovalerate, and mannose decreased (p value less than 0.05), indicating changes in energy and phospholipid metabolism [59]. Kim *et al.* [60] performed a comparative metabolomic analysis and reported elevated amount of acetone, formate, 2-hydroxybutyrate and pyroglutamate. The levels of glucose and acetate were decreased in both MS and *Neuromyelitis optica* spectrum syndrome (NMOSD) patients [60]. Moreover, a lower level of citrate was found in MS patients [60]. Additionally, Ferreira and colleagues [61] demonstrated that serum phospholipidomics shows alterations in lipid profile that have been associated with MS. Results of this study revealed that the phospholipidomic signature of MS is significantly different from healthy controls. Particularly, the phosphatidylethanolamine and phosphotidylcholine showed lower levels in MS and RRMS patients [61]. Plasma profiling in 73 MS patients and 88 healthy controls was performed by Cocco *et al.* [62] using ^{1}H-NMR spectroscopy. They demonstrated increased levels of acetone, alanine, choline and acetoacetate while decreased levels of tryptophan and glucose in MS patients. These altered metabolites were associated with energy metabolism and tryptophan metabolism [62]. Moreover, Vingara *et al.* [63] used proton magnetic resonance spectroscopy on 27 patients with RRMS and 14 healthy controls. They found key altered metabolites N-acetyl aspartate, glutamic acid, creatinine and choline, which were found to be decreased in RRMS [63]. In another study, Tisell *et al.* [64] reported increased levels of glutamine, myo-inositol and creatinine in MS patients. Researchers considered that these metabolites are glial-specific markers and also concluded that the increased concentrations result from increased glial cell density in MS patients [64]. Interestingly, Gebregiworgis *et al.* [65] found 27 differentially expressed metabolites in urine samples of MS patients, and neuromyelitis optica-spectrum disorder (NMO-SD) using NMR-based metabolomics approach. These changes in metabolites of MS patients were associated with alterations in energy and fatty acid metabolism, mitochondrial activity, and the gut microbiota [65]. These metabolic biomarkers may provide novel insights into the MS pathophysiology, and may help in response to various disease modifying therapies in MS patients. While the discussion in this chapter has remained confined to MS, the "Omics" approach may also be extended to other such neurological disorders.

CONCLUDING REMARKS

Personalized medication for persons with MS is currently under development and will require several milestones to be met before it can be used in MS on a routine basis. The majority of the information gathered so far on the use of MS genomics, transcriptomics, proteomics and metabolomics is suggestive but encouraging. However, there is a long way to go before it can be used in clinical settings on a regular basis. Personalised treatments for future therapeutic targets will be possible by improved diagnostic and prognostic biomarkers. Therefore, extensive studies on large number of samples would confirm all the above mentioned findings. Further, for complex and heterogeneous diseases like MS, a single biomarker will be insufficient because of the heterogeneity of the disease. Thus, a panel of biomarkers will be necessary for effective and reliable diagnosis fulfilling the aspiration of precision medicine.

LIST OF ABBREVIATIONS

MS	Multiple Sclerosis
PM	Personalized Medicine
CSF	Cerebrospinal Fluid
CNS	Central nervous system
RRMS	Relapsing -remitting Multiple Sclerosis
PPMS	Primary progressive Multiple sclerosis
SPMS	Secondary progressive Multiple sclerosis
PRMS	Progressive relapsing Multiple sclerosis

DMT	Disease-modifying therapies
OCBs	Oligoclonal bands
IFN-β	Interferon -beta
NTZ	Natalizumab
DIS	Dissemination in space
FDA	Food and drug administration
CIS	Clinically isolated syndrome
NfL	Neurofilament light chain
GA	Glatiramer acetate
NAbs	Neutralising antibodies
RR	Relapsing-remitting
MRI	Magnetic resonance imaging
PML	Progressive multifocal leukoencephalopathy
CVCD	Common variant, common disease
MHC	Major histocompatibility complex
ORs	Olfactory receptors
TNF	Tumour necrosis factor
HLA	Human leukocyte antigens
iTRAQ	Isobaric tags for relative abundance and quantitation
MMP	Matrix metalloproteinases
EAE	Experimental autoimmune encephalomyelitis
GC-MS	Gas chromatography-mass spectrometry
NMOSD	Neuromyelitis optica-spectrum disorder
CXCL13	C-X-C motif chemokine 13
CHI3L1	Chitinase-3-like protein 1
CCN5	Connective tissue growth factor
VWF	Von willebrand factor
GFAP	Glial fibrillary acidic protein
NMR	Nuclear magnetic resonance
OCGB	Oligoclonal IgG bands
RNA- Seq	RNA sequencing
2-DE	2D electrophoresis
2D-DIGE	Two-dimensional difference gel electrophoresis

ACKNOWLEDGEMENT

The authors are grateful to Jamia Hamdard for facilitating their research by providing the infrastructure support and the Central Instrumentation Facility. Nimisha Gupta is supported by a Research fellowship by the Indian Council of Medical Research (ICMR), Government of India (Ref no. 3/1/2(4)/Nephrology/2019-NCD-II). The research in our laboratory is also funded by Indian Council of Medical Research (ICMR), Government of India (Grant No: 5/4/7-8/2012/NCD-II, PI) to Dr. Saima Wajid.

REFERENCES

[1] Siwy J, Mischak H, Zürbig P. Proteomics and personalized medicine: A focus on kidney disease. Expert Rev Proteomics 2019; 16(9): 773-82. [http://dx.doi.org/10.1080/14789450.2019.1659138] [PMID: 31441341]

[2] Gluba-Brzózka A, Franczyk B, Olszewski R, Banach M, Rysz J. Personalized medicine: New perspectives for the diagnosis and the treatment of renal diseases. Int J Mol Sci 2017; 18(6): 1248. [http://dx.doi.org/10.3390/ijms18061248] [PMID: 28604601]

[3] Misra BB, Langefeld C, Olivier M, Cox LA. Integrated omics: Tools, advances and future approaches. J Mol Endocrinol 2019; 62(1): R21-45. [http://dx.doi.org/10.1530/JME-18-0055] [PMID: 30006342]

[4] Del Boccio P, Rossi C, di Ioia M, Cicalini I, Sacchetta P, Pieragostino D. Integration of metabolomics and proteomics in multiple sclerosis: From biomarkers discovery to personalized medicine. Proteomics Clin Appl 2016; 10(4): 470-84. [http://dx.doi.org/10.1002/prca.201500083] [PMID: 27061322]

[5] Sandi D, Kokas Z, Biernacki T, Bencsik K, Klivényi P, Vécsei L. Proteomics in multiple sclerosis: The perspective of the clinician. Int J Mol Sci 2022; 23(9): 5162. [http://dx.doi.org/10.3390/ijms23095162] [PMID: 35563559]

[6] Ömerhoca S, Akkaş SY, İçen NK. Multiple sclerosis: Diagnosis and differential diagnosis. Noro Psikiyatri Arsivi 2018; 55 (1): S1-9. [https://doi.org/10.29399/npa.23418]. [PMID: 30692847]

[7] Robertson D, Moreo N. Disease-modifying therapies in multiple sclerosis: Overview and treatment considerations. Fed Pract 2016; 33(6): 28-34. [PMID: 30766181]. [PMID: 30766181]

[8] Ford H. Clinical presentation and diagnosis of multiple sclerosis. Clin Med 2020; 20(4): 380-3. [http://dx.doi.org/10.7861/clinmed.2020-0292] [PMID: 32675142]

[9] Yang J, Hamade M, Wu Q, *et al.* Current and future biomarkers in multiple sclerosis. Int J Mol Sci 2022; 23(11): 5877. [http://dx.doi.org/10.3390/ijms23115877] [PMID: 35682558]

[10] Jafari A, Babajani A, Rezaei-Tavirani M. Multiple sclerosis biomarker discoveries by proteomics and metabolomics approaches. Biomark Insights 2021; 16 [http://dx.doi.org/10.1177/11772719211013352] [PMID: 34017167]

[11] Ziemssen T, Akgün K, Brück W. Molecular biomarkers in multiple sclerosis. J Neuroinflammation 2019; 16(1): 272. [http://dx.doi.org/10.1186/s12974-019-1674-2] [PMID: 31870389]

[12] Filipi M, Jack S. Interferons in the treatment of multiple sclerosis. Int J MS Care 2020; 22(4): 165-72. [http://dx.doi.org/10.7224/1537-2073.2018-063] [PMID: 32863784]

[13] Javan MR, Jalali Nezhad A, Safa A, Mohammadi MH, Jamebozorgi . Personalized medicine toward multiple sclerosis; current challenges and future prospects. International Journal of Basic Science in Medicine 2017; 2(1): 11-5. [https://doi.org/10.15171/ijbsm.2017.03]. [http://dx.doi.org/10.15171/ijbsm.2017.03]

[14] Dumitrescu L, Papathanasiou A, Coclitu C, Constantinescu CS, Popescu BO, Tanasescu R. Beta interferons as immunotherapy in multiple sclerosis: A new outlook on a classic drug during the COVID-19 pandemic. QJM 2021; 114(10): 691-7. [http://dx.doi.org/10.1093/qjmed/hcaa348] [PMID: 33486513]

[15] Khoy K, Mariotte D, Defer G, Petit G, Toutirais O, Le Mauff B. Natalizumab in multiple sclerosis treatment: From biological effects to immune monitoring. Front Immunol 2020; 11: 549842. [http://dx.doi.org/10.3389/fimmu.2020.549842] [PMID: 33072089]

[16] Nociti V, Romozzi M, Mirabella M. Update on multiple sclerosis molecular biomarkers to monitor treatment effects. J Pers Med 2022; 12(4): 549. [http://dx.doi.org/10.3390/jpm12040549] [PMID: 35455665]

[17] Patsopoulos NA. Genetics of multiple sclerosis: An overview and new directions. Cold Spring Harb Perspect Med 2018; 8(7): a028951. [http://dx.doi.org/10.1101/cshperspect.a028951] [PMID: 29440325]

[18] Patsopoulos N, Ed. 200 loci complete the genetic puzzle of multiple sclerosis. American Society of Human Genetics (ASHG Annual Meeting. 2016; 2016.

[19] Bozikas VP, Anagnostouli MC, Petrikis P, *et al.* Familial bipolar disorder and multiple sclerosis: A three-generation HLA family study. Prog Neuropsychopharmacol Biol Psychiatry 2003; 27(5): 835-9. [http://dx.doi.org/10.1016/S0278-5846(03)00116-7] [PMID: 12921917]

[20] Schmidt H, Williamson D, Ashley-Koch A. HLA-DR15 haplotype and multiple sclerosis: A HuGE review. Am J Epidemiol 2007; 165(10): 1097-109. [http://dx.doi.org/10.1093/aje/kwk118] [PMID: 17329717]

[21] Oksenberg JR, Barcellos LF, Cree BAC, *et al.* Mapping multiple sclerosis susceptibility to the HLA-DR locus in African Americans. Am J Hum Genet 2004; 74(1): 160-7. [http://dx.doi.org/10.1086/380997] [PMID: 14669136]

[22] Kikuchi S, Fukazawa T, Niino M, *et al.* HLA-related subpopulations of MS in Japanese with and without oligoclonal IgG bands. Neurology 2003; 60(4): 647-51. [http://dx.doi.org/10.1212/01.WNL.0000048202.09147.9E] [PMID: 12601107]

[23] Lill CM. Recent advances and future challenges in the genetics of multiple sclerosis. Front Neurol 2014; 5: 130. [http://dx.doi.org/10.3389/fneur.2014.00130] [PMID: 25071715]

[24] Tempest A, Veettil SK, Maharajan MK, Earl JC, Ngorsuraches S, Chaiyakunapruk N. Genetic biomarkers in multiple sclerosis: An umbrella review of meta-analyses of observational studies. Mult Scler Relat Disord 2022; 63: 103834. [http://dx.doi.org/10.1016/j.msard.2022.103834] [PMID: 35526474]

[25] Nali LH, Olival GS, Sousa FTG, *et al.* Whole transcriptome analysis of multiple Sclerosis patients reveals active inflammatory profile in relapsing patients and downregulation of neurological repair pathways in secondary progressive cases. Mult Scler Relat Disord 2020; 44: 102243. [http://dx.doi.org/10.1016/j.msard.2020.102243] [PMID: 32559700]

[26] Almsned F, Lipsky RH, Jafri MS. Transcriptomic analysis of Multiple Sclerosis patient-derived monocytes by RNA-Sequencing for candidate gene discovery. Informatics in Medicine Unlocked 2021; 23: 100563. [https://doi.org/10.1016/j.imu.2021.100563]. [http://dx.doi.org/10.1016/j.imu.2021.100563]

[27] Schafflick D, Xu CA, Hartlehnert M, *et al.* Integrated single cell analysis of blood and cerebrospinal fluid leukocytes in multiple sclerosis. Nat Commun 2020; 11(1): 247.

[http://dx.doi.org/10.1038/s41467-019-14118-w] [PMID: 31937773]

[28] Derakhshani A, Asadzadeh Z, Safarpour H, *et al.* Regulation of CTLA-4 and PD-L1 expression in relapsing-remitting multiple sclerosis patients after treatment with fingolimod, IFNβ-1α, glatiramer acetate, and dimethyl fumarate drugs. J Pers Med 2021; 11(8): 721.
[http://dx.doi.org/10.3390/jpm11080721] [PMID: 34442365]

[29] Consiglio A, Nuzziello N, Liguori M. Dysregulation of Gene Expressions in Multiple Sclerosis: *TNFSF13B* and Other Candidate Genes. J Integr Neurosci 2022; 22(1): 4.
[http://dx.doi.org/10.31083/j.jin2201004] [PMID: 36722235]

[30] Hecker M, Thamilarasan M, Koczan D, *et al.* MicroRNA expression changes during interferon-beta treatment in the peripheral blood of multiple sclerosis patients. Int J Mol Sci 2013; 14(8): 16087-110.
[http://dx.doi.org/10.3390/ijms140816087] [PMID: 23921681]

[31] Housley WJ, Pitt D, Hafler DA. Biomarkers in multiple sclerosis. Clin Immunol 2015; 161(1): 51-8.
[http://dx.doi.org/10.1016/j.clim.2015.06.015] [PMID: 26143623]

[32] Kroksveen AC, Jaffe JD, Aasebø E, *et al.* Quantitative proteomics suggests decrease in the secretogranin-1 cerebrospinal fluid levels during the disease course of multiple sclerosis. Proteomics 2015; 15(19): 3361-9.
[http://dx.doi.org/10.1002/pmic.201400142] [PMID: 26152395]

[33] Shi Y, Ding Y, Li G, *et al.* Discovery of novel biomarkers for diagnosing and predicting the progression of multiple sclerosis using TMT-based quantitative proteomics. Front Immunol 2021; 12: 700031.
[http://dx.doi.org/10.3389/fimmu.2021.700031] [PMID: 34489947]

[34] Probert F, Yeo T, Zhou Y, *et al.* Determination of CSF GFAP, CCN5, and vWF levels enhances the diagnostic accuracy of clinically defined MS from non-MS patients with CSF oligoclonal bands. Front Immunol 2021; 12.
[PMID: 35185866]

[35] Fissolo N, Matute-Blanch C, Osman M, *et al.* CSF SERPINA3 levels are elevated in patients with progressive MS. Neurol Neuroimmunol Neuroinflamm 2021; 8(2): e941.
[http://dx.doi.org/10.1212/NXI.0000000000000941] [PMID: 33436375]

[36] Elkjaer ML, Nawrocki A, Kacprowski T, *et al.* CSF proteome in multiple sclerosis subtypes related to brain lesion transcriptomes. Sci Rep 2021; 11(1): 4132.
[http://dx.doi.org/10.1038/s41598-021-83591-5] [PMID: 33603109]

[37] Jankovska E, Lipcseyova D, Svrdlikova M, *et al.* Quantitative proteomic analysis of cerebrospinal fluid of women newly diagnosed with multiple sclerosis. Int J Neurosci 2022; 132(7): 724-34.
[http://dx.doi.org/10.1080/00207454.2020.1837801] [PMID: 33059501]

[38] Harris VK, Sadiq SA. Biomarkers of therapeutic response in multiple sclerosis: Current status. Mol Diagn Ther 2014; 18(6): 605-17.
[http://dx.doi.org/10.1007/s40291-014-0117-0] [PMID: 25164543]

[39] Ragheb S, Li Y, Simon K, *et al.* Multiple sclerosis: BAFF and CXCL13 in cerebrospinal fluid. Mult Scler 2011; 17(7): 819-29.
[http://dx.doi.org/10.1177/1352458511398887] [PMID: 21372118]

[40] Sellebjerg F, Börnsen L, Khademi M, *et al.* Increased cerebrospinal fluid concentrations of the chemokine CXCL13 in active MS. Neurology 2009; 73(23): 2003-10.
[http://dx.doi.org/10.1212/WNL.0b013e3181c5b457] [PMID: 19996075]

[41] Floro S, Carandini T, Pietroboni AM, De Riz MA, Scarpini E, Galimberti D. Role of Chitinase 3–like 1 as a Biomarker in Multiple Sclerosis. Neurol Neuroimmunol Neuroinflamm 2022; 9(4): e1164.
[http://dx.doi.org/10.1212/NXI.0000000000001164] [PMID: 35534236]

[42] Matute-Blanch C, Río J, Villar LM, *et al.* Chitinase 3-like 1 is associated with the response to interferon-beta treatment in multiple sclerosis. J Neuroimmunol 2017; 303: 62-5.

[http://dx.doi.org/10.1016/j.jneuroim.2016.12.006] [PMID: 28063616]

[43] Cantó E, Reverter F, Morcillo-Suárez C, *et al.* Chitinase 3-like 1 plasma levels are increased in patients with progressive forms of multiple sclerosis. Mult Scler 2012; 18(7): 983-90. [http://dx.doi.org/10.1177/1352458511433063] [PMID: 22183936]

[44] Cantó E, Tintoré M, Villar LM, *et al.* Chitinase 3-like 1: Prognostic biomarker in clinically isolated syndromes. Brain 2015; 138(4): 918-31. [http://dx.doi.org/10.1093/brain/awv017] [PMID: 25688078]

[45] Comabella M, Pericot I, Goertsches R, *et al.* Plasma osteopontin levels in multiple sclerosis. J Neuroimmunol 2005; 158(1-2): 231-9. [http://dx.doi.org/10.1016/j.jneuroim.2004.09.004] [PMID: 15589058]

[46] Börnsen L, Khademi M, Olsson T, Sørensen PS, Sellebjerg F. Osteopontin concentrations are increased in cerebrospinal fluid during attacks of multiple sclerosis. Mult Scler 2011; 17(1): 32-42. [http://dx.doi.org/10.1177/1352458510382247] [PMID: 20921238]

[47] Agah E, Zardoui A, Saghazadeh A, Ahmadi M, Tafakhori A, Rezaei N. Osteopontin (OPN) as a CSF and blood biomarker for multiple sclerosis: A systematic review and meta-analysis. PLoS One 2018; 13(1): e0190252. [http://dx.doi.org/10.1371/journal.pone.0190252] [PMID: 29346446]

[48] Tremlett H, Dai DLY, Hollander Z, *et al.* Serum proteomics in multiple sclerosis disease progression. J Proteomics 2015; 118: 2-11. [http://dx.doi.org/10.1016/j.jprot.2015.02.018] [PMID: 25753122]

[49] Leppert D, Ford J, Stabler G, *et al.* Matrix metalloproteinase-9 (gelatinase B) is selectively elevated in CSF during relapses and stable phases of multiple sclerosis. Brain 1998; 121(12): 2327-34. [http://dx.doi.org/10.1093/brain/121.12.2327] [PMID: 9874483]

[50] Avolio C, Ruggieri M, Giuliani F, *et al.* Serum MMP-2 and MMP-9 are elevated in different multiple sclerosis subtypes. J Neuroimmunol 2003; 136(1-2): 46-53. [http://dx.doi.org/10.1016/S0165-5728(03)00006-7] [PMID: 12620642]

[51] Fissolo N, Pignolet B, Matute-Blanch C, *et al.* Matrix metalloproteinase 9 is decreased in natalizumab-treated multiple sclerosis patients at risk for progressive multifocal leukoencephalopathy. Ann Neurol 2017; 82(2): 186-95. [http://dx.doi.org/10.1002/ana.24987] [PMID: 28681388]

[52] Berge T, Eriksson A, Brorson IS, *et al.* Quantitative proteomic analyses of $CD4^+$ and $CD8^+$ T cells reveal differentially expressed proteins in multiple sclerosis patients and healthy controls. Clin Proteomics 2019; 16(1): 19. [http://dx.doi.org/10.1186/s12014-019-9241-5] [PMID: 31080378]

[53] Amin B, Maurer A, Voelter W, Melms A, Kalbacher H. New poteintial serum biomarkers in multiple sclerosis identified by proteomic strategies. Curr Med Chem 2014; 21(13): 1544-56. [http://dx.doi.org/10.2174/09298673113206660311] [PMID: 24180278]

[54] Manconi B, Liori B, Cabras T, *et al.* Top-down proteomic profiling of human saliva in multiple sclerosis patients. J Proteomics 2018; 187: 212-22. [http://dx.doi.org/10.1016/j.jprot.2018.07.019] [PMID: 30086402]

[55] Singh V, Stingl C, Stoop MP, *et al.* Proteomics urine analysis of pregnant women suffering from multiple sclerosis. J Proteome Res 2015; 14(5): 2065-73. [http://dx.doi.org/10.1021/pr501162w] [PMID: 25793971]

[56] Salvisberg C, Tajouri N, Hainard A, Burkhard PR, Lalive PH, Turck N. Exploring the human tear fluid: D iscovery of new biomarkers in multiple sclerosis. Proteomics Clin Appl 2014; 8(3-4): 185-94. [http://dx.doi.org/10.1002/prca.201300053] [PMID: 24488530]

[57] Byström S, Ayoglu B, Häggmark A, *et al.* Affinity proteomic profiling of plasma, cerebrospinal fluid, and brain tissue within multiple sclerosis. J Proteome Res 2014; 13(11): 4607-19.

[http://dx.doi.org/10.1021/pr500609e] [PMID: 25231264]

[58] Gupta N, Ramakrishnan S, Wajid S. Emerging role of metabolomics in protein conformational disorders. Expert Rev Proteomics 2021; 18(5): 395-410.
[http://dx.doi.org/10.1080/14789450.2021.1948330] [PMID: 34227444]

[59] Reinke SN, Broadhurst DI, Sykes BD, *et al.* Metabolomic profiling in multiple sclerosis: Insights into biomarkers and pathogenesis. Mult Scler 2014; 20(10): 1396-400.
[http://dx.doi.org/10.1177/1352458513516528] [PMID: 24468817]

[60] Kim HH, Jeong IH, Hyun JS, Kong BS, Kim HJ, Park SJ. Metabolomic profiling of CSF in multiple sclerosis and neuromyelitis optica spectrum disorder by nuclear magnetic resonance. PLoS One 2017; 12(7): e0181758.
[http://dx.doi.org/10.1371/journal.pone.0181758] [PMID: 28746356]

[61] Ferreira HB, Melo T, Monteiro A, Paiva A, Domingues P, Domingues MR. Serum phospholipidomics reveals altered lipid profile and promising biomarkers in multiple sclerosis. Arch Biochem Biophys 2021; 697: 108672.
[http://dx.doi.org/10.1016/j.abb.2020.108672] [PMID: 33189653]

[62] Cocco E, Murgia F, Lorefice L, *et al.* ^{1}H-NMR analysis provides a metabolomic profile of patients with multiple sclerosis. Neurol Neuroimmunol Neuroinflamm 2016; 3(1): e185.
[http://dx.doi.org/10.1212/NXI.0000000000000185] [PMID: 26740964]

[63] Vingara LK, Yu HJ, Wagshul ME, *et al.* Metabolomic approach to human brain spectroscopy identifies associations between clinical features and the frontal lobe metabolome in multiple sclerosis. Neuroimage 2013; 82: 586-94.
[http://dx.doi.org/10.1016/j.neuroimage.2013.05.125] [PMID: 23751863]

[64] Tisell A, Leinhard OD, Warntjes JBM, *et al.* Increased concentrations of glutamate and glutamine in normal-appearing white matter of patients with multiple sclerosis and normal MR imaging brain scans. PLoS One 2013; 8(4): e61817.
[http://dx.doi.org/10.1371/journal.pone.0061817] [PMID: 23613944]

[65] Gebregiworgis T, Nielsen HH, Massilamany C, *et al.* A urinary metabolic signature for multiple sclerosis and neuromyelitis optica. J Proteome Res 2016; 15(2): 659-66.
[http://dx.doi.org/10.1021/acs.jproteome.5b01111] [PMID: 26759122]

CHAPTER 13

Role of Epithelial-Mesenchymal Transition (EMT) Therapy in Personalized Cancer Treatment

Rupali Ghosh[1] and **Saima Wajid**[1,*]

[1] *Department of Biotechnology, School of Chemical and Life Sciences, Jamia Hamdard, Hamdard Nagar, New Delhi, India*

Abstract: A major clinical challenge in treating cancer patients is the metastasis of cells to distant organs forming secondary tumors. Many cancers are prone to metastasis due to epithelial-mesenchymal transition (EMT), which confers motility and invasive properties to the tumor. EMT also contributes to chemotherapy resistance and facilitates metastasis by generating cancer stem cells (CSCs). Therefore, the EMT program has therapeutic potential for personalized cancer treatment. In more severe situations, this might destroy metastatic cancer cells that are already present or stop tumour progression in high-risk patients who are at risk of developing metastatic tumours. The options for developing EMT-based personalised cancer therapeutics are covered in this chapter, along with a summary of the evidence supporting some of the suggested EMT targets and a discussion on the possible benefits and drawbacks of each strategy.

Keywords: Biomarkers, cancer stem cells, epithelial-mesenchymal transition, personalized cancer therapy, tumor metastasis.

INTRODUCTION

Epithelial cells depart from their non-invasive characteristics during the EMT process and gain a more mesenchymal and invasive nature. The EMT process is characterized by the loss of apical-basal polarity and cell-to-cell adhesion and the transition into spindle-like cells with motility [1]. This process is regulated by various EMT inducers and activators whose role is to induce an EMT program in epithelial cells. At the molecular level, EMT involves the down regulation of epithelial proteins such as E-cadherin and cytokeratin, and the up regulation of mesenchymal protein markers such as vimentin. EMT infers placentation, healing of wounds, tissue fibrosis, and cancer metastasis in adults [2].

* **Corresponding author Saima Wajid:** Department of Biotechnology, School of Chemical and Life Sciences, Jamia Hamdard, Hamdard Nagar, New Delhi – 110062, India; Tal: 9899823898; E-mails: swajid@jamiahamdard.ac.in; wajid.saima@gmail.com

Farzana Mahdi & Abbas Ali Mahdi (Eds.)

The most common reason for mortality of cancer patients is metastasis. EMT plays a crucial role in cancer metastasis, as it converts an immobile epithelial phenotype into a motile invasive phenotype, which can metastasize into distant organs as secondary tumors [3]. It is critical to create novel therapeutic approaches to stop the metastasis of organ-confined tumours in patients at high risk for them, as well as to get rid of metastatic cells already present in patients with more advanced disease states. Such a technique might be made easier by the pharmaceutical targeting of the EMT process in particular cancer types [2]. In recent years, cancer treatment has been revolutionized following the identification of several molecular alterations that are responsible for cancer development. Instead of focusing on the anatomic site of tumor development as the target for treatment, biomarkers are now appropriate candidates for therapeutic intervention [4]. This change has resulted in a single targeted drug treating large groups of patients with cancer that has a specific molecular feature. This opened the door to personalized therapy. In addition to genomics, it is clear that molecular phenotyping measurements and characterization are critical for improving personalized therapy for cancer patients [5]. Further, proteomic analysis may be useful when several molecular alterations are detected, making the identification of the most critical one. Another crucial area to advance a personalised treatment strategy is metabolomics. It is crucial for not only identifying targetable biomarkers but also for developing pharmacological phenotypes that make it easier to comprehend how differently each patient responds to treatment. Additionally, metabolomics can aid in assessing drug resistance and illness relapse, resulting in the creation of fresh treatment approaches [6].

There is mounting proof that EMT, which focuses on cancer metastasis, is a clinically useful mechanism for cancer treatment. However, important issues about the viability of preventing or reducing metastasis by targeting EMT still need to be resolved. Targeting EMT as a potential adjuvant therapy for cancer treatment is covered in this chapter.

EPITHELIAL AND MESENCHYMAL PHENOTYPES

The building blocks of life are cells, which can take on a variety of morphological phenotypes and sustain the intricate intracellular and extracellular processes required for the survival and operation of the organism. One such classification of cellular phenotype is the epithelial and mesenchymal phenotype both having unique characteristics [7].

The epithelium is composed of specialized membrane junctions, including tight junctions (TJ), adherent junctions (AJ), desmosomes, and gap junctions that hold the epithelium together. Owing to localized distribution of adhesion molecules, such as cadherins and integrins, a lateral belt of intercellular junctions is formed as a result of apical-basolateral polarization. An apical structure is defined by the polarized arrangement of the intracellular actin cytoskeleton, while a lining is formed by the basement lamina, which divides the epithelium from the mesenchyme [8].

On the other hand, mesenchymal cells have no structural organisation of cell surface molecules or actin cytoskeleton, lack apical-basolateral polarity, and lack cell layer organisation. Mesenchymal cells are scattered haphazardly across the extracellular matrix and lack junctional integrity. They are distinguished by front-rear polarity, a characteristic that makes them more mobile and invasive [9]. While epithelial cells grow as "clusters" or "islands" of cells with intact intercellular cell-cell adhesion, mesenchymal cells exhibit a spindle-like, fibroblastic shape in *in-vitro* cell culture [10].

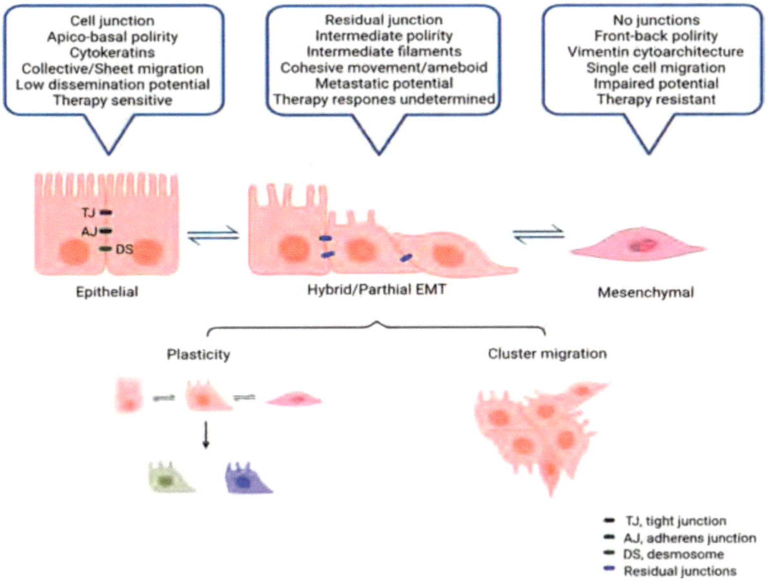

Fig. (1). Epithelial to mesenchymal transition [63].

A PERSPECTIVE ON THE TRANSITION FROM EPITHELIAL TO MESENCHYMAL CELLS

Epithelial-to-Mesenchymal Transition (EMT), a conserved evolution process, has been shown to be able to convert polarised, non-motile epithelial cells into motile mesenchymal cells. As a result of EMT, epithelial cells gradually lose many of their epithelial characteristics, including apical-basolateral polarity and dissolution of cell-cell junctions, and they consequently acquire motility-invasive qualities. As a result, the transition between the epithelial and mesenchymal stages is smooth. EMT also occurs during normal embryogenesis, wound healing, organ fibrosis, and tissue regeneration. In physiological processes like the production of somites, the development of the heart, and the kidneys, a reverse process called mesenchymal-epithelial transition (MET) is frequently observed. The junctional complexes of epithelial cells are lost during the transition to mesenchymal cells. Some of the earliest targets are proteins essential to tight junction architecture, including zonula occludens-1 (ZO-1), occludins, claudins, and E-cadherin. Chief polarity complex components, such as Crumbs protein homolog 3 (CRB3) and partitioning deficient protein-3/6 (Par-3/6), are dysregulated [11]. Actin-myosin contractility is enabled by the reorganization of the actin cytoskeleton thus enabling cytokeratin intermediate filaments to be disrupted and replaced by vimentin intermediate filaments to maintain desmosome stability.

ROLE OF EMT IN CANCER

Types 1, 2, and 3 of EMT can be distinguished by their biological processes. EMT type-1 is linked to embryogenesis, type-2 to tissue regeneration, and type-3 to the development of cancer [12]. EMT, which gives tumor cells metastatic capabilities, promotes invasion, infiltrates adjacent tissues, and colonizes distant organs, causes cancer to advance [13]. The transition from epithelial to mesenchymal cells is a dynamic and continuous process from the perspective of cancer cell energy. Cells that are intermediate in the epithelial to mesenchymal spectrum can survive, metastasize, colonize distal organs and have both epithelial and mesenchymal properties [14]. Moreover, a variety of experiments have demonstrated that EMT leads to a specific pluripotent stem cell subpopulation called cancer stem cells (CSCs), which are capable of self-renewal and tumorigenesis. Among the cellular processes affected by EMT are autophagy inhibition and cell apoptosis inhibition. This is possibly caused by epigenetic changes, reduced expression of transporters on the cell surface, and decreased chemotherapeutic drug uptake [15].

As tumor cells metastasize, they enter blood and lymphatic vessels either as individual cells or as clusters. Several studies have shown that certain cancer cells undergo transitions from tumor in situ to invasive cancer cells through development processes such as EMT. The circulating tumor cells can exist as single cells or as clusters of cells called microemboli. Various mechanisms are believed to be involved in the intravasation of single cells and microemboli. Cancer cells use the EMT program to escape from the primary tumor periphery and infiltrate into the blood vessels and lymphatic tissues as they intravasate into lymphatic vessels and blood vessels [16]. With the plasticity granted to cancer cells, they can switch between epithelial and mesenchymal states, facilitating cancer spread through EMT and MET programs. The EMT program also confers chemoresistance to certain cancer cells resulting in the failure of chemotherapy.

EMT REGULATORS AND TRANSCRIPTION FACTORS

The EMT progression is regulated by the expression of its related transcription regulators or transcription factors (TFs), such as SNAIL, ZEB, TWIST, and others. MiRNA, epigenetic modification, and post-translational modifications also control the EMT program.

Transcriptional Regulators

Transcriptional factors that regulate cell adhesion, cell polarity and motility play a crucial role in mediating the transition of epithelial cells to mesenchymal cells [17]. By inhibiting the expression of genes linked to the epithelial phenotype, transcription factors promote mesenchymal gene expression [18]. Zinc finger binding transcription factors SNAIL1 and SNAIL2, zinc finger E box binding homology frame factors ZEB1 and ZEB2, and basic helix-loop-helix (BHLH) factors TWIST1 and TWIST2 are the main transcription factors that promote EMT [19].

By attracting the polycomb repressor complex (PRC), SNAIL1 and SNAIL2 bind to the E box sequence of the CDH1 promoter region and suppress the transcription of E-cadherin genes. G9a, EZH2 (enhancer of zeste homolog 2), histone deacetylases 1, 2, and LSD1 (lys-specific demethylase 1) are among the substances found in PRC. These elements work together to suppress epithelial gene expression by coordinating histone deacetylation and hypermethylation [20]. SNAIL1 upregulates mesenchymal markers like vimentin or fibronectin while directly inhibiting the establishment of tight junctions and epithelial markers like E-cadherin and claudins. SNAIL2 confers invasion and migratory capabilities while promoting the loss of cell adhesion and polarity. Additionally, they both work in concert with additional transcription regulators to regulate gene expression [21]. For example, SNAIL1 cooperates with ETS1 (proto-oncogene) to activate the expression of proteases such as matrix metalloproteinase (MMP) that degrades ECM and provides EMT characteristic of invasive properties [22]. SNAIL1 expression level could be used as a prognostic indicator of EMT [23]. SNAIL1/2 expression is regulated by multiple signaling pathways, including TGF-β, notch, WNT, and growth factors acting on receptor tyrosine kinase (RTKs) [24].

Zinc finger E-box binding transcription factors ZEB1 and ZEB2, which belong to the human ZEB family can regulate the transcription of genes by binding at the E-box regulatory gene sequence. ZEB proteins recruited C terminal binding proteins (CTAB), thereby suppressing the transcription of epithelial genes [25]. BRG1 (Brahma-related gene 1) interacts with the switch/sucrose nonfermentable (SWI/SNF) chromatin-remodeling protein to mediate transcriptional suppression in certain cancer cells [26]. ZEB also suppresses the expression of tight junction genes and down regulates the cell polarity complex components. However, ZEB transcription regulators up-regulate the expression of mesenchymal genes like N-cadherin and vimentin, thereby driving EMT. ZEB protein expression is regulated by TGF-β, WNT, bone morphogenetic protein (BMP), and Ras-MAPK signaling pathways [19]. It should be emphasized that different cell lines respond differently to ZEB1 and ZEB2, nevertheless. This suggests that the tissue environment has an equal role in determining how well ZEB proteins work. For instance, ZEB2 inhibits tumor metastasis while ZEB1 promotes tumor development and invasion in a mouse model of melanoma. Clinical studies show that whereas ZEB1 expression is linked to worse clinical outcomes, ZEB2 deficiency reduces melanoma patient survival. The control of the bone morphogenetic protein (BMP) and transforming growth factor-β (TGF-β) signalling pathways results in distinct roles for ZEB1 and ZEB2.

TWIST1 and TWIST2 both belong to the basic helix-loop-helix (HLH) family of transcription factors and regulate the expression of genes. E12 and E47 are two helix-loop-helix transcription factors encoded by E2A genes, also known as transcription factor 3 (TCF3). Both TWIST1/2 interact with E12 and E47 as homodimers or heterodimers to regulate E-box DNA response elements in order to activate or suppress gene expression [27]. TWIST1, similar to SNAIL1, can inhibit the expression of E-catherin and induces the expression of N-catherin, thereby, decreasing cell adhesion properties and increasing cell motility [28]. TWIST transcription regulators can be activated by multiple-signaling pathways during the EMT process. Under hypoxic conditions, hypoxia-inducible transcription factor-1 α (HIF-1α) activates TWIST gene expression and promotes EMT. Additionally, TWIST1/2 is essential for the growth of benign skin tumors in mice. TWIST expression in mice skin was conditionally knocked out, which prevented tissue plasminogen activator (TPA)-induced skin cancer and markedly slowed tumor growth [29].

MicroRNA (MiRNA)

Several non-coding microRNA-mediated expressions of transcription regulator genes are related to the EMT program. By specifically attaching to mRNA, microRNA prevents translation or accelerates degradation. Different miRNA families control how genes are expressed. Five miRNAs, for instance, are part of the miR-200 family. Although they target different ZEB transcription regulator genes but enhance ZEB expression, thereby, inducing EMT [30]. On the other hand, the miR-205 family of miRNAs suppresses the expression of ZEB proteins. Additionally, miR-1 and miR-200 inhibit the expression of the SNAIL1/2 proteins in prostate adenocarcinoma cells. Furthermore, by down regulating high-mobility group A2 (HMGA2), miRNA let-7 and miR-365 control the expression of SNAIL1 and TWIST. This chromatin-binding protein stimulates the production of SNAIL1 and TWIST [31]. In addition to controlling transcription factors relevant to EMT, miRNA also has the ability to control epithelial and mesenchymal genes directly. For instance, miR-9 directly reduces the expression of genes that code for E-cadherin, which increases the invasiveness and motility of tumor cells [32]. In addition, miR-194 lowers the production of N-cadherin mRNA in advanced gastric cancer by directly interacting with its 3' untranslated region (3' UTR).

Table 1. Signals that cause EMT, transcription factors, and markers/effectors.

EMT-inducing signals	EMT-inducing transcription factors	EMT effectors/markers	
		Epithelial	Mesenchymal
TGF-β Nicotine BMP Integrins	SNAIL1/2	E-cadherin	Vimentin
EGF MMPs	TWIST1/2	Claudins	Fibronectin
FGF Bile acids	ZEB1/2	Occludins	Vitronectin
HGF	FOXC2	Desmoplakin	FSP1
PDGF	TCF3/E47	Cytokeratin	A-SMA
Notch	TCF4/E2-2	Mucin-1	N-Cadherin
Wnt	KLF-2	ZO-1	MMPs
Hypoxia			

Epigenetic Modifications

Important epigenetic alterations that are frequently linked to EMT are needed to control how EMT-TFs operate. Over time, various modifications, including DNA methylation and histone acetylation/deacetylation, as well as numerous epigenetic regulators, have been identified as important regulators of the EMT process [33]. Methylation of the CDH1 (cadherin 1) promoter area has been linked to EMT in a number of human tumours, including bladder, lung, breast, gastric, liver, and prostate cancers. This is because it prevents the production of the E-cadherin gene [34]. During embryogenesis, the transition from epithelial to mesenchymal cells in trophoblast stem cells is mediated by histone deacetylation of tight junction (TJ) promoter region by histone deacetylase HDAC6. As a result, cell-cell adhesion is reduced, and cell motility is enhanced [35]. These modifications are often reversible and provide plasticity to the EMT.

Post-Translational Modifications

At the proteome level, post-translational changes are significant for the EMT program. The most prevalent post-translational protein modification, protein phosphorylation, is necessary for the control of several pathways in transcription, metabolism, apoptosis, and differentiation [36]. Phosphorylation controls the expression of SNAIL proteins [37]. For example, glycogen synthase kinase-3β (GSK-3β) phosphorylates SNAIL protein through two consecutive motifs, thereby controlling its subcellular localization and ubiquitination. To cause the nuclear export of SNAIL, GSK-3β first attaches to and phosphorylates a serine residue in motif 1 of the SNAIL protein. Following that, GSK-3β promotes the degradation of the SNAIL proteasome by phosphorylating serine residues in SNAIL's motif 2. Many signaling pathways, including Wnt, Notch, NF-kB, and PI3K-AKT, prevent SNAIL from being phosphorylated by GSK-3β or prevent the interaction between two signaling pathways. This enhances SNAIL stability and down regulates the expression of E-cadherin, thereby activating the EMT program [38]. Other post-translation modifications can also modulate the EMT program by regulating the manifestation of significant EMT-TFs. ZEB-mediated gene regulation is stopped as a result of the polycomb complex PRC2's sumoylation of the ZEB2 protein, which encourages its export from the nucleus. Ubiquitination can also regulate the stability and activity of EMT-TFs which activate or suppress the EMT process [39]. A typical ubiquitin E3 ligase complex controls the degradation of many EMT-related transcription factors in order to regulate the EMT process. For instance, the E3 ubiquitin-ligase Hakai binds with the tyrosine-phosphorylated form of E-cadherin to cause its ubiquitination, which then causes endocytosis and degradation [40]. The p300/CBP genes, which code for the human enzyme lysine acetyltransferase, have drawn a lot of attention for post-translational modifications. Cell migration and invasion are two processes where P300/CBP acetylation is involved. The development of the repressor complex that transforms SNAIL1 into an activator protein is inhibited by the acetylation of SNAIL1 and TWIST by CBP [41].

COMPLEX MOLECULAR NETWORK CONTRIBUTING EMT

EMT is mediated by a dynamic and intricate interaction between extracellular signals, extracellular matrix (ECM) elements such as hyaluronic acid and collagen, as well as soluble growth factors [42].

The main agents of EMT are transforming growth factors (TGFs) and bone morphogenic proteins (BMPs). They trigger the TGF-β receptor, which in turn triggers the polarity-related proteins occludin and Par6 [43]. The SMAD (Suppressor of Mothers against Decapentaplegic) factors also activated EMT-TFs such as SNAIL1/2 and ZEB1/2. Other inducers of EMT include Notch, Wnt, and TGF-β signaling pathways. Hepatocyte growth factors (HGF), epidermal growth factors (EGF), insulin-like growth factors (IGF), fibroblast growth factors (FGF), and vascular endothelial growth factors (VEGF) are the ligands for receptor tyrosine kinases (RTKs), and platelet-derived growth factors (PDGF) [44]. Biochemical signaling cascades are initiated by these ligands by activating receptor-mediated signaling pathways. Due to the activation of EMT-TFs, which causes the downregulation of epithelial factors and the upregulation of mesenchymal markers, these networks support cell proliferation and survival.

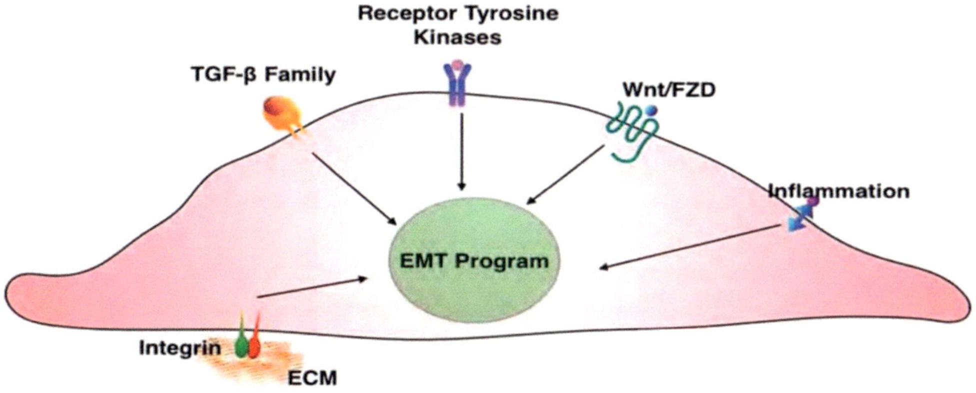

Fig. (2). EMT is influenced by complex molecular networks.

The majority of the ligands for each cell surface receptor are growth factors, and when they bind to those receptors, they dimerize the RTK, trans-phosphorylate the kinase domains, and activate their substrate by adding phosphate groups to tyrosine amino acid residues. This modulates the activation of the biochemical signaling cascade including the PI3K/Akt, Rac/Cdc4, and Ras/MAPK pathways. These signaling pathways converge by regulating EMT transcription factors, such as SNAIL1/2 and ZEB1/2 [45]. The expression of E-cadherin, which is essential for cell-cell adhesion in epithelial cells, is actively suppressed by these transcription factors. E-cadherin-dependent intercellular epithelial adherence is disrupted and β-catenin retention is decreased when junctional E-cadherin expression is down-regulated. As a result, TCF4 (TCF4) and other EMT transcription factors are activated when β-catenin is restricted to the nucleus and works in concert with the Wnt signaling pathway. A chromatin-repressed state is made by TCF4 and β-catenin complex; thereby down-regulating epithelial gene expression. IGF utilizes the RTK signal transduction pathway to induce the EMT program. Notably, the Notch, Wnt/β-catenin, TGF-β/SMAD, and RTK/Ras signal transduction cascades may interact with one another [44]. Hypoxia and inflammation can also control EMT-TFs like SNAIL1 and TWIST1 through NFkB and JAK/STAT pathways, in addition to growth factor and cytokine-induced EMT [46].

THERAPEUTIC IMPLICATION OF EMT IN PERSONALIZED TREATMENT

A patient can receive personalized treatment based on his/her physical health and environmental exposures including the past medical history. Based on these data, subjects may be categorized into different groups with clinically relevant purposes. Researchers today aim to understand the functioning of organs at multiple omics levels and characterize the effects of environmental factors on genetic predispositions [47]. Fine-tuning of every single aspect would enable scientists and doctors to predict how a particular treatment will affect patients.

Chemotherapeutic resistance to cisplatin in non-small cell lung cancer (NSCLC), gastric cancer, and docetaxel resistance in prostate cancer with significant recurrence is only in a few of the tumors that EMT modulates. Additionally, it was discovered that chemotherapy-resistant cancer stem cells (CSCs) with partial EMT states and poor clinical outcomes were present in patients with metastatic breast cancer. Chemoresistant cancer cells inhibit the microRNA that adversely controls EMT effectors, which lowers patient survival after treatment [8]. These findings point to a crucial requirement for the development of targeted therapies that prevent EMT and metastatic spread and can be combined with chemotherapy to combat drug resistance. Hence, therapies that reverse the EMT process or prevent the onset of the EMT program have clinical implications for improving chemo response and treatment outcomes.

For focused EMT therapy, there are five major methods. The first strategy is to inhibit cancer progression by blocking upstream signaling pathways. The second step is to focus on the molecular causes of EMT. The third step is to focus on how cancer cells interact with the extracellular matrix (ECM). The fourth is to inhibit the MET process, and the fifth is to target mesenchymal cell phenotype [48-51]. Additionally, numerous pro-inflammatory signals like TNF-α are also effective inducers of EMT and strategies are being developed to target these signals [52]. A permanent and reversible method of reprogramming for phenotypic switching in the EMT program is the targeted modulation of epigenetics [53].

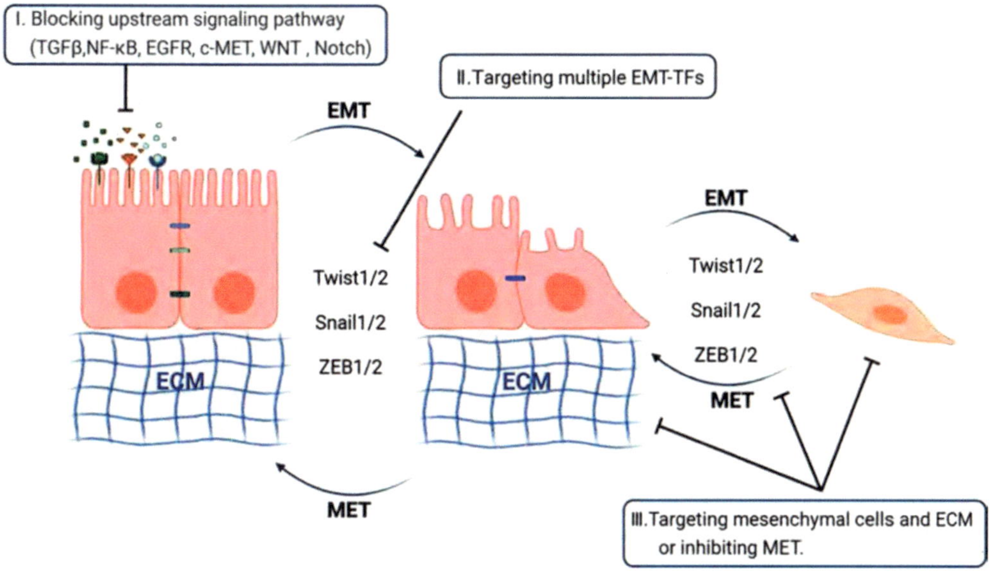

Fig. (3). Therapeutic strategies for targeting EMT.

Strategies to Block Upstream Signaling Pathways

Novel medicines that suppress the production of EMT assist patients in cancer who are at high risk of acquiring metastases. These strategies would also help prevent the EMT process in locally contained, pre-metastatic tumors. Agents that impede EMT-induced upstream signals from the tumor microenvironment and hinder crucial downstream signal transduction are examples of novel methods [54]. Additionally, strategies developed to block EMT inducers as early adjuvant therapy may increase the susceptibility of cancer cells to conventional chemotherapy given the relationship between cancers, EMT, cancer stem cells, and therapy resistance. EMT can be induced in cancer cells by many signals from tumor microenvironment. These include cytokines, growth factors, and reduced oxygen tension [55]. EMT in cancer cells could be prevented by therapeutic targeting of a particular cell surface receptor for these signals. For instance, in vitro studies demonstrate that blocking EGF-induced EMT in breast cancer cell lines by the EGF receptor kinase inhibitor AG1478. Similarly, in pancreatic cancer cells, inhibition of the TGF-β receptor by SB431542 blocks the induction of EMT by the TGF-β signal [56]. However, the diversity of signals in the tumor microenvironment capable of inducing EMT in cancer cells may limit its clinical utility [57]. For example, resistance to therapies using signal-blocking agents has been found in investigations on lung cancer.

Target the Molecular Drivers of EMT

By concentrating on shared intracellular signal transduction pathways, the aforementioned restrictions can be overcome. An alternative strategy to stop EMT induction is the therapeutic targeting of important signal transduction pathways. The transcription factor signals transducer and activator of transcription 3 (STAT3), which is essential for the development of EMT, is one instance [58]. Many cancer cells depend on the STAT3 transcription factor signaling for inducing EMT. For instance, EGF-induced EMT in MDA-MB-468 breast cancer cells and ovarian cancer cells, and interleukin-6 (IL-6)-induced EMT in head and neck squamous carcinoma cells [59]. Several molecular inhibitors have been developed for transcription factors, such as STAT3 inhibitor Stattic and S31-201 [60]. Therefore, a potential target for pharmacologically inhibiting the induction of EMT in many cancer cells is the development of novel therapeutic inhibitors for other transcription factors, such as SNAIL1/2, ZEB1/2, and TWIST1/2. Inhibition of SNAIL attenuates the development of EMT by TGF-β signal in retinal pigment epithelial cells, providing preliminary evidence for the efficacy of this tactic [61].

Upstream of transcription factors, other intracellular signal transducers that induce an EMT program by activating EMT-TFs, may also be considered a potential target. One such event is intracellular calcium signaling that regulates EMT, through calcium-dependent STAT3 activation and is turned on in MDA-MB-468 breast cancer cells by either EGF or hypoxia. Similar to this, calcium-dependent STAT3 activation and the formation of EMT are thought to be possible targets for the transient receptor potential melastatin 7 (TRPM7) channel, a plasma membrane ion channel with an integral kinase domain [2].

The existence of metastasis at the time of diagnosis is one of the drawbacks of targeting EMT-TFs and EMT regulators in cancer. Along with other forms of cancer therapy, EMT-TF inhibitors are very effective at preventing early metastasis and drug resistance in cancer patients. EMT inducer inhibitors may be more or less ineffective for patients who already have metastases or cancer cells that have already undergone transition [57].

Target the Interaction Between Cancer Cells and ECM

Targeting the interaction between cancer cells and extracellular matrix (ECM) is another EMT-related treatment. Through their attachment to the ECM, integrins, a family of cell membrane adhesion receptors, significantly influence physiological processes. Integrins are crucial in mediating interactions between cancer cells and the extracellular matrix (ECM). This further activates signals for the initiation, progression, and metastasis of cancer cells [62]. Integrins have a function in controlling oncogenic growth factor receptor (GFR) signaling pathways and regulating GFR-dependent cancer cell invasion and migration, and altered expression of integrins is commonly found in cancer metastasis [63]. Integrins also control how metastatic areas are colonized and help cancer cells in circulation survive without anchoring. Several studies have identified various integrins that have roles in EMT induction. The expression of integrins αvβ3, αvβ5, α5β1, α6β4, α4β1 and αvβ6 on cancer cells is correlated with disease progression in various tumor types. Therefore, integrins show themselves as a crucial target for cancer therapeutics. Integrins αvβ3 is up-regulated in metastatic tumors and angiogenic endothelial cells. The strategy to use anti-integrins monoclonal antibody, such as LM609, to deactivate integrins αvβ3 shows anti-angiogenic activity in model experiments [62]. Inhibiting integrins has, in fact, limited the interaction of tumor cells with the extracellular matrix and, as a result, reduced tumor metastasis in animal models.

Matrix metalloproteinase family (MMPs) is known to play a critical role in interacting ECM and tumor cells and in cancer invasion in various human cancers including hepatocellular carcinoma (HCC). MMP family proteases break down ECM proteins, allowing cancer cells to access the bloodstream and spread to other sites [63]. Studies reported that, in HCC, MMP-1 expression is associated with tumor cell invasion. Increased expression of MMP-2, MMP-7 and MM1-MMP has been associated with portal invasion, dedifferentiation, metastasis, and reoccurrence. There is transcriptional regulation of the expression of MMPs. In the promoter of MMPs family, there are promoter sites of AP-1 or EST transcription factors and these transcription factors are responsible for MMPs gene expression regulation. EMT-TFs such as SNAIL1 also regulate MMPs family proteins, but studies have shown that the E-box, which is the binding site for SNAIL was not observed in the MMPs promoter region, hence SNAIL, may not directly up-regulate the MMPs expression [64]. Therefore, MMPs and transcription factors, which regulate MMPs expression, may act as potential targets for EMT therapy.

Inhibition of the MET Process

Cancer cells eventually colonize through the MET process, and during this process, metastatic cells regain epithelial properties, resulting in distant secondary tumors that are histopathologically comparable to the main ones. Using *in vivo* microscopy, research demonstrated that mammary tumor cells in mice naturally go through the MET process after moving about, migrating, invading, and extravasating before colonizing the distal organ [65]. A more logical strategy for preventing cancer cells from colonizing secondary organs and metastasizing is to use strategies to lock cancer cells into a metastatic state by inhibiting MET. The need for ongoing counseling is one disadvantage of this strategy. By inhibiting the MET process by targeting the fibroblast growth factor receptor, one can influence the bladder cancer cells' epithelial phenotype [66].

Targeting the Mesenchymal Cells

Mesenchymal cell markers are acquired throughout the EMT process. N-cadherin, vimentin, and fibronectin are a few of these markers that are linked to the invasion and migration of cancer cells [67]. Therefore, in patients with more severe disease, targeting these mesenchymal markers may be a way to get rid of metastatic cancer cells already present. This approach can also overcome the drawback of using EMT-TF inhibitors. In addition to targeting invasive mesenchymal cells, this approach also benefits the patients with cancer of mesenchymal origin [68]. Some studies have shown that targeted inhibition of mesenchymal marker proteins eliminates metastasis which reduces chemotherapy resistance. For example, Withaferin-A is a bioactive compound extracted from the plant *Withiana somnifera* that has been shown to degrade mesenchymal cell marker vimentin. Withaferin-A is a potent inhibitor of angiogenesis.

In lung and breast cancer cell lines, Withaferin-A inhibits cancer cell invasion and migration and induces apoptosis. Studies have shown that Withaferine-A inhibits metastasis *in vivo* [69]. Targeting EMT-TFs may also affect the mesenchymal phenotype. For example, in a mouse model of breast cancer, inhibition of TWIST protein reduces lung metastasis in highly metastatic mammary carcinoma cell lines [70]. However, one limitation of targeting mesenchymal cell markers is by limiting their invasive properties that may lead to the transformation of cancer cells into a different kind of cell migration.

EMT-DERIVED MOLECULAR SUBTYPES PROVIDE PERSONALIZED THERAPEUTICS

Cancer is a disease that is generally complicated, varied, and genetically heterogeneous. It is necessary to stratify patients by analyzing the heterogeneity of genetic abnormalities and design therapeutic strategies for focusing on important drivers within each subtype in order to achieve successful treatment. In addition to concentrating on genetic changes, research is progressing towards extensive gene expression profiling [71]. One such instance is the discovery of six gene expression molecular subtypes (GEMS) in epithelial ovarian cancer (EOC) in the research. New approaches to personalized medicines can be developed based on these GEMS. These GEMS are associated with EMT molecular subtypes, each with a different expression signature and clinical prognosis [72]. Each GEMS has distinct functions and signaling pathways to regulate different drivers for the EMT process. These GEMS-specific signal transduction pathways can be used to provide personalized treatments. For instance, Vinorelbine, a microtubule destabilizer in EOC, is effective in the stem-A subtype because it exhibits the enrichment of gene sets relevant to microtubules. Targeting the TGF-β pathway might also be an option for treating Mes subtype EOC patients, as this subtype has a strong association with the gene sets involved in the route [73]. As we enter the era of personalized medicine, cancer patients can be categorized based on their individual GEMS and treated in accordance with the molecular triggers unique to each subtype.

CONCLUDING REMARKS

There are several possible treatment strategies to take advantage of the EMT in order to inhibit the spread of cancer. Strategies include targeting invasive mesenchymal cells, inhibiting the induction of EMT, and preventing MET by locking cancer cells in a metastatic state. Each of these strategies has its potential weakness and strengths in the context of developing agents for clinical utility. To target EMT in the context of personalized therapy for cancer patients, research into each of these strategies must be encouraged. It is necessary to validate such drugs for targeting EMT in conjunction with other treatments in models that accurately depict the entire metastatic process. It should be emphasized, nevertheless, that not all cancer types will metastasize unless EMT occurs. For instance, secondary metastases in cancer that were triggered by neu- and PyMT did not exhibit mesenchymal-like change [74]. This shows that even while EMT seems to play a key role in cancer spread, other mechanisms may possibly be at play. Understanding the kinds of cancer where EMT is significant and then identifying suitable biomarkers are crucial steps in the development of pharmacological medicines to target EMT in personalized cancer treatment.

ACKNOWLEDGEMENT

Rupali Ghosh is supported by a Research Fellowship from the University of Grant Commission (UGC). This chapter article comprises data gathered from several published resources, and thus we would like to extend our gratitude to all those authors whose work has been used in the present chapter.

REFERENCES

[1] Nieto MA. The ins and outs of the epithelial to mesenchymal transition in health and disease. Annu Rev Cell Dev Biol 2011; 27(1): 347-76. [http://dx.doi.org/10.1146/annurev-cellbio-092910-154036] [PMID: 21740232]

[2] Davis FM, Stewart TA, Thompson EW, Monteith GR. Targeting EMT in cancer: Opportunities for pharmacological intervention. Trends Pharmacol Sci 2014; 35(9): 479-88. [http://dx.doi.org/10.1016/j.tips.2014.06.006] [PMID: 25042456]

[3] Chaffer CL, Weinberg RA. A perspective on cancer cell metastasis. Science 2011; 331(6024): 1559-64.

[http://dx.doi.org/10.1126/science.1203543] [PMID: 21436443]

[4] Gambardella V, Tarazona N, Cejalvo JM, *et al.* Personalized medicine: Recent progress in cancer therapy. Cancers 2020; 12(4): 1009.
[http://dx.doi.org/10.3390/cancers12041009] [PMID: 32325878]

[5] Lambert AW, Pattabiraman DR, Weinberg RA. Emerging biological principles of metastasis. Cell 2017; 168(4): 670-91.
[http://dx.doi.org/10.1016/j.cell.2016.11.037] [PMID: 28187288]

[6] Harbeck N, Penault-Llorca F, Cortes J, *et al.* Breast cancer. Nat Rev Dis Primers 2019; 5(1): 66.
[http://dx.doi.org/10.1038/s41572-019-0111-2] [PMID: 31548545]

[7] Schöck F, Perrimon N. Molecular mechanisms of epithelial morphogenesis. Annu Rev Cell Dev Biol 2002; 18(1): 463-93.
[http://dx.doi.org/10.1146/annurev.cellbio.18.022602.131838] [PMID: 12142280]

[8] Antony J, Thiery JP, Huang RYJ. Epithelial-to-mesenchymal transition: Lessons from development, insights into cancer and the potential of EMT-subtype based therapeutic intervention. Phys Biol 2019; 16(4): 041004.
[http://dx.doi.org/10.1088/1478-3975/ab157a] [PMID: 30939460]

[9] Thompson E W, Newgreen D F, Tarin D. Carcinoma invasion and metastasis: a role for epithelial-mesenchymal transition? Cancer Res 2005; 65(14): 5991-5.
[http://dx.doi.org/10.1158/0008-5472.CAN-05-0616]

[10] Friedl P. Prespecification and plasticity: Shifting mechanisms of cell migration. Curr Opin Cell Biol 2004; 16(1): 14-23.
[http://dx.doi.org/10.1016/j.ceb.2003.11.001] [PMID: 15037300]

[11] Thiery JP. Epithelial-mesenchymal transitions in tumour progression. Nat Rev Cancer 2002; 2(6): 442-54.
[http://dx.doi.org/10.1038/nrc822] [PMID: 12189386]

[12] Kalluri R, Weinberg RA. The basics of epithelial-mesenchymal transition. J Clin Invest 2009; 119(6): 1420-8.
[http://dx.doi.org/10.1172/JCI39104] [PMID: 19487818]

[13] Mittal V. Epithelial mesenchymal transition in tumor metastasis. Annu Rev Pathol 2018; 13(1): 395-412.
[http://dx.doi.org/10.1146/annurev-pathol-020117-043854] [PMID: 29414248]

[14] Pal A, Barrett TF, Paolini R, Parikh A, Puram SV. Partial EMT in head and neck cancer biology: A spectrum instead of a switch. Oncogene 2021; 40(32): 5049-65.
[http://dx.doi.org/10.1038/s41388-021-01868-5] [PMID: 34239045]

[15] Chandana S, Babiker HM, Mahadevan D. Therapeutic trends in pancreatic ductal adenocarcinoma (PDAC). Expert Opin Investig Drugs 2019; 28(2): 161-77.
[http://dx.doi.org/10.1080/13543784.2019.1557145] [PMID: 30539678]

[16] Thiery JP, Acloque H, Huang RYJ, Nieto MA. Epithelial-mesenchymal transitions in development and disease. Cell 2009; 139(5): 871-90.
[http://dx.doi.org/10.1016/j.cell.2009.11.007] [PMID: 19945376]

[17] Lu W, Kang Y. Epithelial-mesenchymal plasticity in cancer progression and metastasis. Dev Cell 2019; 49(3): 361-74.
[http://dx.doi.org/10.1016/j.devcel.2019.04.010] [PMID: 31063755]

[18] Stemmler MP, Eccles RL, Brabletz S, Brabletz T. Non-redundant functions of EMT transcription factors. Nat Cell Biol 2019; 21(1): 102-12.
[http://dx.doi.org/10.1038/s41556-018-0196-y] [PMID: 30602760]

[19] Lamouille S, Xu J, Derynck R. Molecular mechanisms of epithelial-mesenchymal transition. Nat Rev

Mol Cell Biol 2014; 15(3): 178-96.
[http://dx.doi.org/10.1038/nrm3758] [PMID: 24556840]

[20] Herranz N, Pasini D, Díaz VM, *et al.* Polycomb complex 2 is required for E-cadherin repression by the Snail1 transcription factor. Mol Cell Biol 2008; 28(15): 4772-81.
[http://dx.doi.org/10.1128/MCB.00323-08] [PMID: 18519590]

[21] Zhou W, Gross KM, Kuperwasser C. Molecular regulation of Snai2 in development and disease. J Cell Sci 2019; 132(23): jcs235127.
[http://dx.doi.org/10.1242/jcs.235127] [PMID: 31792043]

[22] Jordà M, Olmeda D, Vinyals A, *et al.* Upregulation of MMP-9 in MDCK epithelial cell line in response to expression of the Snail transcription factor. J Cell Sci 2005; 118(15): 3371-85.
[http://dx.doi.org/10.1242/jcs.02465] [PMID: 16079281]

[23] Peinado H, Olmeda D, Cano A. Snail, Zeb and bHLH factors in tumour progression: An alliance against the epithelial phenotype? Nat Rev Cancer 2007; 7(6): 415-28.
[http://dx.doi.org/10.1038/nrc2131] [PMID: 17508028]

[24] Gheldof A, Hulpiau P, van Roy F, De Craene B, Berx G. Evolutionary functional analysis and molecular regulation of the ZEB transcription factors. Cell Mol Life Sci 2012; 69(15): 2527-41.
[http://dx.doi.org/10.1007/s00018-012-0935-3] [PMID: 22349261]

[25] Postigo AA, Dean DC. ZEB represses transcription through interaction with the corepressor CtBP. Proc Natl Acad Sci 1999; 96(12): 6683-8.
[http://dx.doi.org/10.1073/pnas.96.12.6683] [PMID: 10359772]

[26] Sánchez-Tilló E, Lázaro A, Torrent R, *et al.* ZEB1 represses E-cadherin and induces an EMT by recruiting the SWI/SNF chromatin-remodeling protein BRG1. Oncogene 2010; 29(24): 3490-500.
[http://dx.doi.org/10.1038/onc.2010.102] [PMID: 20418909]

[27] Franco HL, Casasnovas J, Rodríguez-Medina JR, Cadilla CL. Redundant or separate entities?--roles of Twist1 and Twist2 as molecular switches during gene transcription. Nucleic Acids Res 2011; 39(4): 1177-86.
[http://dx.doi.org/10.1093/nar/gkq890] [PMID: 20935057]

[28] Meng J, Chen S, Han JX, *et al.* Twist1 regulates Vimentin through Cul2 circular RNA to promote EMT in hepatocellular carcinoma. Cancer Res 2018; 78(15): 4150-62.
[http://dx.doi.org/10.1158/0008-5472.CAN-17-3009] [PMID: 29844124]

[29] Lee TK, Poon RTP, Yuen AP, *et al.* Twist overexpression correlates with hepatocellular carcinoma metastasis through induction of epithelial-mesenchymal transition. Clin Cancer Res 2006; 12(18): 5369-76.
[http://dx.doi.org/10.1158/1078-0432.CCR-05-2722] [PMID: 17000670]

[30] Bracken CP, Gregory PA, Kolesnikoff N, *et al.* A double-negative feedback loop between ZEB1-SIP1 and the microRNA-200 family regulates epithelial-mesenchymal transition. Cancer Res 2008; 68(19): 7846-54.
[http://dx.doi.org/10.1158/0008-5472.CAN-08-1942] [PMID: 18829540]

[31] Liu Y-N, Yin JJ, Abou-Kheir W, *et al.* MiR-1 and miR-200 inhibit EMT *via* Slug-dependent and tumorigenesis *via* Slug-independent mechanisms. Oncogene 2013; 32(3): 296-306.
[http://dx.doi.org/10.1038/onc.2012.58] [PMID: 22370643]

[32] Diepenbruck M, Tiede S, Saxena M, *et al.* miR-1199-5p and Zeb1 function in a double-negative feedback loop potentially coordinating EMT and tumour metastasis. Nat Commun 2017; 8(1): 1168.
[http://dx.doi.org/10.1038/s41467-017-01197-w] [PMID: 29079737]

[33] Hawkins RD, Hon GC, Lee LK, *et al.* Distinct epigenomic landscapes of pluripotent and lineage-committed human cells. Cell Stem Cell 2010; 6(5): 479-91.
[http://dx.doi.org/10.1016/j.stem.2010.03.018] [PMID: 20452322]

[34] Fukagawa A, Ishii H, Miyazawa K, Saitoh M. δ EF1 associates with DNMT1 and maintains DNA

methylation of the E□cadherin promoter in breast cancer cells. Cancer Med 2015; 4(1): 125-35. [http://dx.doi.org/10.1002/cam4.347] [PMID: 25315069]

[35] Mobley RJ, Raghu D, Duke LD, *et al.* MAP3K4 controls the chromatin modifier HDAC6 during trophoblast stem cell epithelial-tomesenchymal transition. Cell Rep 2017; 18(10): 2387-400. [http://dx.doi.org/10.1016/j.celrep.2017.02.030] [PMID: 28273454]

[36] Ubersax JA, Ferrell JE Jr. Mechanisms of specificity in protein phosphorylation. Nat Rev Mol Cell Biol 2007; 8(7): 530-41. [http://dx.doi.org/10.1038/nrm2203] [PMID: 17585314]

[37] Saitoh M. Epithelial-mesenchymal transition is regulated at post-transcriptional levels by transforming growth factor-β signaling during tumor progression. Cancer Sci 2015; 106(5): 481-8. [http://dx.doi.org/10.1111/cas.12630] [PMID: 25664423]

[38] Zhou BP, Deng J, Xia W, *et al.* Dual regulation of Snail by GSK-3β-mediated phosphorylation in control of epithelial-mesenchymal transition. Nat Cell Biol 2004; 6(10): 931-40. [http://dx.doi.org/10.1038/ncb1173] [PMID: 15448698]

[39] Long J, Zuo D, Park M. Pc2-mediated sumoylation of Smad-interacting protein 1 attenuates transcriptional repression of E-cadherin. J Biol Chem 2005; 280(42): 35477-89. [http://dx.doi.org/10.1074/jbc.M504477200] [PMID: 16061479]

[40] Fujita Y, Krause G, Scheffner M, *et al.* Hakai, a c-Cbl-like protein, ubiquitinates and induces endocytosis of the E-cadherin complex. Nat Cell Biol 2002; 4(3): 222-31. [http://dx.doi.org/10.1038/ncb758] [PMID: 11836526]

[41] Chang R, Zhang Y, Zhang P, Zhou Q. Snail acetylation by histone acetyltransferase p300 in lung cancer. Thorac Cancer 2017; 8(3): 131-7. [http://dx.doi.org/10.1111/1759-7714.12408] [PMID: 28296173]

[42] Zoltan-Jones A, Huang L, Ghatak S, Toole BP. Elevated hyaluronan production induces mesenchymal and transformed properties in epithelial cells. J Biol Chem 2003; 278(46): 45801-10. [http://dx.doi.org/10.1074/jbc.M308168200] [PMID: 12954618]

[43] Heldin CH, Vanlandewijck M, Moustakas A. Regulation of EMT by TGFβ in cancer. FEBS Lett 2012; 586(14): 1959-70. [http://dx.doi.org/10.1016/j.febslet.2012.02.037] [PMID: 22710176]

[44] Yang J, Weinberg RA. Epithelial-mesenchymal transition: At the crossroads of development and tumor metastasis. Dev Cell 2008; 14(6): 818-29. [http://dx.doi.org/10.1016/j.devcel.2008.05.009] [PMID: 18539112]

[45] Thiery JP, Acloque H, Huang RYJ, Nieto MA. Epithelial-mesenchymal transitions in development and disease. Cell 2009; 139(5): 871-90. [http://dx.doi.org/10.1016/j.cell.2009.11.007] [PMID: 19945376]

[46] Tsai JH, Yang J. Epithelial-mesenchymal plasticity in carcinoma metastasis. Genes Dev 2013; 27(20): 2192-206. [http://dx.doi.org/10.1101/gad.225334.113] [PMID: 24142872]

[47] Krzyszczyk P, Acevedo A, Davidoff EJ, *et al.* The growing role of precision and personalized medicine for cancer treatment. Technology 2018; 6(03n04): 79-100. [http://dx.doi.org/10.1142/S2339547818300020] [PMID: 30713991]

[48] Redfern AD, Spalding LJ, Thompson EW. The Kraken Wakes: Induced EMT as a driver of tumour aggression and poor outcome. Clin Exp Metastasis 2018; 35(4): 285-308. [http://dx.doi.org/10.1007/s10585-018-9906-x] [PMID: 29948647]

[49] Dudás J, Ladányi A, Ingruber J, Steinbichler TB, Riechelmann H. Epithelial to mesenchymal transition: A mechanism that fuels cancer radio/ chemoresistance. Cells 2020; 9(2): 428. [http://dx.doi.org/10.3390/cells9020428] [PMID: 32059478]

[50] Jonckheere S, Adams J, De Groote D, Campbell K, Berx G, Goossens S. Epithelial-mesenchymal transition (EMT) as therapeutic target. Cells Tissues Organs 2022; 211(2): 157-82. [http://dx.doi.org/10.1159/000512218] [PMID: 33401271]

[51] Xia L, Tan S, Zhou Y, *et al.* Role of the NFκB-signaling pathway in cancer. OncoTargets Ther 2018; 11: 2063-73. [http://dx.doi.org/10.2147/OTT.S161109] [PMID: 29695914]

[52] Skrypek N, Goossens S, De Smedt E, Vandamme N, Berx G. Epithelialto- mesenchymal transition: Epigenetic reprogramming driving cellular plasticity. Trends Genet 2017; 33(12): 943-59. [http://dx.doi.org/10.1016/j.tig.2017.08.004] [PMID: 28919019]

[53] Zhang L, Liao Y, Tang L. MicroRNA-34 family: A potential tumor suppressor and therapeutic candidate in cancer. J Exp Clin Cancer Res 2019; 38(1): 53. [http://dx.doi.org/10.1186/s13046-019-1059-5] [PMID: 30717802]

[54] Marino N, Woditschka S, Reed LT, *et al.* Breast cancer metastasis: Issues for the personalization of its prevention and treatment. Am J Pathol 2013; 183(4): 1084-95. [http://dx.doi.org/10.1016/j.ajpath.2013.06.012] [PMID: 23895915]

[55] Shintani Y, Okimura A, Sato K, *et al.* Epithelial to mesenchymal transition is a determinant of sensitivity to chemoradiotherapy in non-small cell lung cancer. Ann Thorac Surg 2011; 92(5): 1794-804. [http://dx.doi.org/10.1016/j.athoracsur.2011.07.032] [PMID: 22051275]

[56] Halder SK, Beauchamp RD, Datta PK. A specific inhibitor of TGF-beta receptor kinase, SB-431542, as a potent antitumor agent for human cancers. Neoplasia 2005; 7(5): 509-21. [http://dx.doi.org/10.1593/neo.04640] [PMID: 15967103]

[57] van Denderen BJW, Thompson EW. The to and fro of tumour spread. Nature 2013; 493(7433): 487-8. [http://dx.doi.org/10.1038/493487a] [PMID: 23344357]

[58] Davis FM, Azimi I, Faville RA, *et al.* Induction of epithelial-mesenchymal transition (EMT) in breast cancer cells is calcium signal dependent. Oncogene 2014; 33(18): 2307-16. [http://dx.doi.org/10.1038/onc.2013.187] [PMID: 23686305]

[59] Lo HW, Hsu SC, Xia W, *et al.* Epidermal growth factor receptor cooperates with signal transducer and activator of transcription 3 to induce epithelial-mesenchymal transition in cancer cells *via* up-regulation of TWIST gene expression. Cancer Res 2007; 67(19): 9066-76. [http://dx.doi.org/10.1158/0008-5472.CAN-07-0575] [PMID: 17909010]

[60] Schust J, Sperl B, Hollis A, Mayer TU, Berg T. Stattic: a small-molecule inhibitor of STAT3 activation and dimerization. Chem Biol 2006; 13(11): 1235-42. [http://dx.doi.org/10.1016/j.chembiol.2006.09.018] [PMID: 17114005]

[61] Li H, Wang H, Wang F, Gu Q, Xu X. Snail involves in the transforming growth factor β1-mediated epithelial-mesenchymal transition of retinal pigment epithelial cells. PLoS One 2011; 6(8): e23322. [http://dx.doi.org/10.1371/journal.pone.0023322] [PMID: 21853110]

[62] Pattabiraman DR, Bierie B, Kober KI, *et al.* Activation of PKA leads to mesenchymal-to-epithelial transition and loss of tumor-initiating ability. Science 2016; 351(6277): aad3680. [http://dx.doi.org/10.1126/science.aad3680] [PMID: 26941323]

[63] Huang Y, Hong W, Wei X. The molecular mechanisms and therapeutic strategies of EMT in tumor progression and metastasis. J Hematol Oncol 2022; 15(1): 129. [http://dx.doi.org/10.1186/s13045-022-01347-8] [PMID: 36076302]

[64] Dongre A, Rashidian M, Eaton EN, *et al.* Direct and indirect regulators of epithelial-mesenchymal transition-mediated immunosuppression in breast carcinomas. Cancer Discov 2021; 11(5): 1286-305. [http://dx.doi.org/10.1158/2159-8290.CD-20-0603] [PMID: 33328216]

[65] Gunasinghe NPAD, Wells A, Thompson EW, Hugo HJ. Mesenchymal-epithelial transition (MET) as a

mechanism for metastatic colonisation in breast cancer. Cancer Metastasis Rev 2012; 31(3-4): 469-78. [http://dx.doi.org/10.1007/s10555-012-9377-5] [PMID: 22729277]

[66] Chaffer CL, Brennan JP, Slavin JL, Blick T, Thompson EW, Williams ED. Mesenchymal-to-epithelial transition facilitates bladder cancer metastasis: role of fibroblast growth factor receptor-2. Cancer Res 2006; 66(23): 11271-8. [http://dx.doi.org/10.1158/0008-5472.CAN-06-2044] [PMID: 17145872]

[67] Yu M, Bardia A, Wittner BS, *et al.* Circulating breast tumor cells exhibit dynamic changes in epithelial and mesenchymal composition. Science 2013; 339(6119): 580-4. [http://dx.doi.org/10.1126/science.1228522] [PMID: 23372014]

[68] Yang J, Du X, Wang G, *et al.* Mesenchymal to epithelial transition in sarcomas. Eur J Cancer 2014; 50(3): 593-601. [http://dx.doi.org/10.1016/j.ejca.2013.11.006] [PMID: 24291235]

[69] Lahat G, Zhu QS, Huang KL, *et al.* Vimentin is a novel anti-cancer therapeutic target; insights from in vitro and *in vivo* mice xenograft studies. PLoS One 2010; 5(4): e10105. [http://dx.doi.org/10.1371/journal.pone.0010105] [PMID: 20419128]

[70] Yang J, Mani SA, Donaher JL, *et al.* Twist, a master regulator of morphogenesis, plays an essential role in tumor metastasis. Cell 2004; 117(7): 927-39. [http://dx.doi.org/10.1016/j.cell.2004.06.006] [PMID: 15210113]

[71] Tothill RW, Tinker AV, George J, *et al.* Novel molecular subtypes of serous and endometrioid ovarian cancer linked to clinical outcome. Clin Cancer Res 2008; 14(16): 5198-208. [http://dx.doi.org/10.1158/1078-0432.CCR-08-0196] [PMID: 18698038]

[72] Tan TZ, Miow QH, Huang RYJ, *et al.* Functional genomics identifies five distinct molecular subtypes with clinical relevance and pathways for growth control in epithelial ovarian cancer. EMBO Mol Med 2013; 5(7): 1051-66. [http://dx.doi.org/10.1002/emmm.201201823] [PMID: 23666744]

[73] Yang D, Sun Y, Hu L, *et al.* Integrated analyses identify a master microRNA regulatory network for the mesenchymal subtype in serous ovarian cancer. Cancer Cell 2013; 23(2): 186-99. [http://dx.doi.org/10.1016/j.ccr.2012.12.020] [PMID: 23410973]

[74] Trimboli AJ, Fukino K, de Bruin A, *et al.* Direct evidence for epithelial-mesenchymal transitions in breast cancer. Cancer Res 2008; 68(3): 937-45. [http://dx.doi.org/10.1158/0008-5472.CAN-07-2148] [PMID: 18245497]

CHAPTER 14

Oral Cancer and Prospects of Precision Medicine

Piyush Bhati[1], Tassaduq Hussain Wani[2], Deepti Kaushik[1], Kanu Priya[3] and Mohd. Tashfeen Ashraf[1,*]

[1] *School of Biotechnology, Gautam Buddha University, Greater Noida, India*

[2] *Department of Biological Sciences, The University of North Carolina at Charlotte, Charlotte, NC, USA*

[3] *Department of Life Sciences, School of Basic Sciences and Research, Sharda University, Greater Noida, India*

Abstract: Precision medicine is a systematic therapeutic approach that tailors the overall treatment process as per an individual's unique characteristics; taking into account the genomic makeup and lifestyle. This approach has shown promising results in treating certain types of cancers, including that of highly heterogeneous oral cancer. Oral cancer is a type of head and neck cancer mainly caused by poor oral hygiene, alcohol, and tobacco abuse, and promotes HPV infection. The conventional approaches for the treatment of oral cancer often rely on surgery, chemotherapy, and/or radiotherapy. Now, precision medicine, with the advent of newer diagnostic techniques, enables healthcare professionals to diagnose the disease early and treat the patient with appropriate medicines and optimized doses. This ensures overall safety while minimizing undesirable exposure to not-so-effective drug regimes. After a brief introduction to precision medicine, this chapter details genetic mutations as targets for precision medicine and the advantages of this approach in oral cancer treatment. It is envisaged that this approach offers improved efficacy, safety, reduced side-effects, and prepares the body's immune response against oral cancer. Targeting specific proteins, such as EGFR and HER2 to suppress tumor growth or make cancer cells more susceptible to the immune system's combat mechanism is also discussed followed by an overview of various drugs that are being used to treat patients who are positive for HER2 and EGFR. Various challenges and limitations of precision medicine and future prospects for research in this area are highlighted.

Keywords: Chemotherapy, EGFR, MAb, Oral Cancer, Precision Medicine, Small molecule inhibitors, Targeted Therapy.

[*] **Corresponding author Mohd. Tashfeen Ashraf:** School of Biotechnology, Gautam Buddha University, Greater Noida, India, E-mail: Tashfeen@gbu.ac.in

Farzana Mahdi & Abbas Ali Mahdi (Eds.)

INTRODUCTION

Though the history and origin of the term "precision medicine" remain unclear, it has a clear impact on increasing the overall survival rate in a large number of diseases. Moving forward from treatments designed for "average patients" and the "one drug fits all" hypothesis, precision medicine is developed on the basis of the genetic makeup of an individual which decides the molecular and genetic properties governing the development and progression of disease along with the responses to a particular drug [1]. This response and development are the results of the expression of different proteins at different levels. Along with genetics, an individual's lifestyle choices like diet and exercise also play a critical role in developing precision medicine. We observe phenotypic effects in patients which is a combination of both genetics and the environmental factors to which they are exposed [2].

In order to develop precision medicine, the first step requires the identification of specific biomarkers, genes, or any other factor that is unique in a way that may increase or reduce the chance of occurrence of a disease or may affect the path of progression of disease in a patient. The identification of such markers is utilized to divide patients into subpopulations. This is done in such a way that their susceptibility to disease is established and their targeted treatment response is as per the expectation [3]. This way, a person is given the best-suited treatment with limited side effects at a reduced cost of diagnosis and treatment. Thus on the basis of the lifestyle, clinical phenotype, and molecular diagnostics of a patient, precision medicine is developed in accordance with an individual's medical requirement [4]. The overall environment seems to play major roles in overpowering the genetic makeup of the patients. Thus, a healthy environment together with a healthy lifestyle, healthy foods coupled with healthy attitudes, and healthy work conditions will ensure a healthy life. Nothing can be done with the genotype one inherits. However, phenotype can be fine-tuned following the set rules of nature and nurture including regular exercise.

Oral Cancer

Cancer is one of the leading causes of death among non-communicable diseases. According to WHO, 19.3 million new cases were reported and around 10 million deaths were caused by all cancers in the year 2020. Oral cancer is among one of the leading contributors to it with around 3,77,713 new cases and 1,77,757 deaths in the year 2020 [5]. The common causes of oral cancer include poor oral hygiene, use of alcohol and tobacco, use of betel quid, an infection caused by the human papillomavirus, and Epstein Barr Virus, besides occupational hazards like exposure to radiation [6, 7]. These factors are augmented in some individuals with a genetic predisposition. Fanconi anemia is a rare genetic disorder that is characterized by a mutation in any of the 22 FANC gene families and is known to increase the possibility of oral cancer [8]. Thus, an early diagnosis of oral cancer is crucial for the survival of the patient. A large number of options are available for the purpose of diagnosis. This includes some common, non-technical but very effective approaches like a physical examination conducted by physicians and some highly advanced non-invasive methods that are not even accessible in many developing countries [9].

Genetic Mutations in Oral Cancer

A large number of genetic mutations are known to accumulate in cancerous cells. A number of studies are being conducted to identify these mutations in order to develop markers based on such mutational load and to design precision medicine targeting common mutations among subpopulations of patients. Most of these mutations are present in signaling pathways and some are present as chromosomal abnormalities [10]. Around two-thirds of oral cancer cases are known to have deletions in 9p21-22 [11]. TP53, a tumor suppressor gene involved in the regulation of the cell cycle is most commonly found to be mutated in oral cancer and plays a fundamental role in oral cancer progression. The nature of the mutation in TP53 can also be used to assess the status of exposure to tobacco, as G>T transversions are reported to show a high presence in tumors that are caused by exposure to tobacco [12]. TP53 mutations reduce the overall survival rate of patients compared to those without TP53 mutations. Mutations in tumor suppressor genes are more common among smokers while mutations in oncogenes are more frequent in non-smoker oral cancer patients [13]. Also, TP53 is found to have a lower rate of mutation in Asian patients as compared to Caucasians [14].

Thrombospondin 1 (TSP 1) and deleted in oral cancer (DOC-1) are the only known tumor suppressor genes after TP53, which are found to be mutated in oral cancer. DOC-1 gene mutation reduces the transcription and translation of the proteins. The reintroduction of wild type DOC-1 gene in tumors has shown the reversal of cancerous phenotype to normal keratinocyte cells. TSP-1 gene mutation is correlated with angiogenesis in oral cancer. TSP 1 transfection in oral cancer cells has been shown to suppress angiogenesis in the tumor [15, 16].

Epidermal growth factor receptor (EGFR) is an oncogene that is frequently found to be overexpressed in oral cancer and also in breast cancer. Aberrant expression of EGFR has been correlated to the development of oral cancer. EGFR has been shown a 5 to 50-fold increased expression in oral cancer [17]. EGFR serves as a receptor for the epidermal growth factor (EGF) and transforming growth factor alpha (TGF-alpha). The presence of TGF-Alpha along with EGFR makes oral cancer more aggressive as compared to the EGFR alone [18]. Along with the overexpression of EGFR, deletion or mutation in the N-terminal that serves as the ligand binding domain or deletion in the C-terminus is also responsible for over-activity [19].

Table 1. Commonly mutated genes and their involvement in cancer.

Gene	Function	Locus	Prevalence in cancer
TP53	Cell cycle regulator- growth arrest and apoptosis	17p13	Promoter methylation, progression of the dysplasia-Carcinoma sequence.
TSP1	Natural inhibitor of neovascularization and tumorigenesis in healthy tissue.	15q14	Suppression of tumor-induced angiogenesis.
DOC1	Negatively regulates CDK2 activity, and has a regulatory role in DNA replication.	12q24.31	Reduction of expression and protein production.
EGFR	Receptor for epidermal growth factor protein ligands.	7p11.2	Regulation of tumor cell growth and survival.
RAS family (KRAS, HRAS, NRAS)	Cell division, cell differentiation, and the self-destruction of cells (apoptosis).	12p12.1 11p14.1 1p13.2	Confer resistance to EGFR inhibitor therapy.
C-Met	Embryonic development, organogenesis and wound healing.	7q31.2	Poor prognosis *via* activation matrix metalloproteinase.
PI3K	Phosphorylation, proliferation, migration of cells, production of new proteins, and cell survival.	3q26.32	Promotes cellular proliferation through the PI3K/AKT/mTOR pathway.
PTEN	Regulates cell division, migration, adhesion, and angiogenesis.	10q23.31	

The *ras* gene mutation is another most common proto-oncogenic mutation in oral cancer. The *ras* gene family includes H-*ras*, K-*ras*, and N-*ras*, known to play a vital role in cellular differentiation and cell growth. Mutations found in codons 12, 13, and 61 are reported for converting *ras* proto-oncogene into an oncogene [20]. Though these mutations are not common in Western countries but are frequently reported in India and Taiwan. While the H-*ras* mutation is common among the Indian population, the mutation in K-*ras* is more common in the Taiwanese population. A very low mutation rate of H-*ras* and no mutation in K-*ras* was found in the western population in the same study [21, 22].

Other proto-oncogenes commonly found mutated in oral cancer are kinase receptor C-Met and phosphoinositide 3-kinase (PI3K). PI3K regulates the PI3K-AKT-mTOR pathway that regulates growth and proliferation, migration, translation, and cell survival. C-Met also known as hepatocyte growth factor receptor (HGFR) is the only receptor for the hepatocyte growth factor (HGF), expressed only on the epithelial and endothelial cell's surface. In oral cancer patients, C-Met is responsible for poor prognosis *via* activation matrix metalloproteinase MMP-1, MMP-2, and MMP-9 [23, 24]. Phosphatases and tensin homolog (PTEN) negatively regulate the PI3K pathway by acting downstream of PI3K at mitogen-activated protein kinase (MAPK), in an oral cancer patient with a reduced level of PTEN showing poor prognosis [25]. The list of commonly mutated genes discussed has been provided in Table **1**, with locus of mutation and their functions.

Host Immune Response in Oral Cancer

Tumor development is primarily controlled by cytotoxic innate and adaptive immune responses of the body. Various components of the host immune system perform different roles in oral cancer. Cytotoxic T cells, helper T cells, and tumor-infiltrating lymphocytes (TILs) target cancer cells *via* tumor-associated antigens. Tumor-associated antigen (TAG) is also found in normal body cells but is highly expressed in cancerous cells [26]. Chemokines CCL2, -3, -4, -5, Interleukin-5, -8, 10, tumor necrosis factor TNF-alpha, and interferon-gamma are hosts' defense mechanism against cancer cells that work without antigen presentation [27]. Tumor-associated neutrophils (TAN) and neutrophil type-1 (N1) are cells with anti-tumor cytotoxic activity. In oral cancer patients, an increase in the level of regulatory T cells and a decrease in CD8+ and absolute T-cell population affect the prognosis of tumors and the efficacy of treatment. In the tumor cell microenvironment, there is the presence of a large number of $CD44^{hi}/CD62^{low}$ activated/memory T-regs (T-regulatory) cells also known as amTregs that are specific to self-antigen, which provide protection against the host immune response to tumor cells [28]. Along with T-regs, other immune factors also sometimes support the growth of oral cancer such as secretory cytokines. IL-6 inhibits Nk-cells, activation of macrophages, neutrophils, dendritic cell maturation, and T-cells. STAT3 activation in oral cancer also induces IL-6, and T-regs; on the other hand, it suppresses dendritic cells and IL-12 [29]. Prostaglandins E2 (PGE2) and Vascular endothelial growth factor (VEGF) are also found to be elevated in oral cancer patients and promote angiogenesis in the tumor [30]. VEGF also results in the deactivation and dysfunction of T-cells [31]. Another key regulatory protein involved in the regulation of tumor cells is PD-1 or programmed cell death-1 present on the surface of T-cells and B-cells, which when bound to its ligand PD-L1 limits the immune response. Oral cancer cells show a higher expression of PD-L1 on its surface protecting cancer cells from T-cells and B-cells [32]. Thus in case of oral cancer, several immune system cells and other factors are found to be dysregulated and favor the progression of cancer.

Targeted Drugs and Therapies for Oral Cancer

The course of treatment is primarily based on the stage in which the tumor is presented for treatment. During the early stages, surgical removal of the tumor followed by radiotherapy, or targeted radiotherapy is the primary choice for treatment [33]. An external source of radiation is used to selectively target the tumor site in a patient and the process is known as external beam radiotherapy (EBRT). Conventional Photon beam therapy when used in intensity-modulated radiotherapy (IMRT) has a better anti-tumor effect even with a reduced dosage of radiation exposure. The exit dose in photon therapy is high and causes a toxic effect on surrounding non-cancerous cells [34]. Proton beam therapy is developed to overcome the limitation of high exit doses. Proton beam therapy not only reduces the cost of treatment but also has a very low or no exit dose. Braggs peak or the site of irradiation can be precisely controlled and targeted at any depth in proton beam therapy owing to protons' physical properties. This allows targeting of otherwise non-accessible sites in oral cancer patients. Depending upon the characteristics of the tumor, a high level of precision can be obtained with proton beam therapy for any individual patient [35].

In advanced stages of oral cancer, chemotherapy, depending upon the individual's tumor properties, is given along with radiation or radiation and surgery. Proton beam therapy along with intra-arterial infusion chemotherapy shows promising results in later or terminal stages of oral cancer. Cisplatin, an alkylating agent binds to purines resulting in DNA damage and cell cycle arrest leading to cancer cell death by apoptosis [36]. 5-fluorouracil an anti-metabolite is an antagonist of pyrimidine nucleotide. 5-FU inhibits thymidylate synthase, responsible for the conversion of deoxyuridine (dUMP) monophosphate to deoxythymidine monophosphate (dTMP). The lack of activity of thymidylate synthase results in cancer cell death due to lack of dTMP; also the accumulation of dUMP is known to exert a toxic effect on cancer cells. In cases where drug resistance is observed against 5-FU, methotrexate is given along with 5-FU [37]. Methotrexate alone is also used to treat oral cancer. Methotrexate an immunosuppressant is also a type of anti-metabolite. An anti-metabolite of folic acid, methotrexate blocks the conversion of dihydrofolate to tetrahydrofolate by binding to the enzyme dihydrofolate reductase. This blockage of conversion of dihydrofolate to tetrahydrofolate results in a deficiency of purines in the cancer cells [38]. Taxol, also known as paclitaxel is another commonly used chemotherapeutic drug in induction therapy and also for treating recurrent and metastatic oral cancer. Paclitaxel originally is a plant-based alkaloid that stabilizes microtubules thus preventing their depolymerization. This failure in the depolymerization of microtubules results in mitotic G2/M phase cell cycle arrest and ultimately cell death [39]. Table **2** summaries treatment processes mentioned and also their mode of action.

Table 2. Oral Cancer Treatment based on Radiation, Chemotherapeutic Drugs, Targeted Monoclonal Antibodies, and Small Molecules.

Treatment	Type/Effect	Mode of Action
CHEMOTHERAPY		
External beam radiotherapy (EBRT)	Radiation	External beams of radiation directed into cancerous areas with extreme precision.
Intensity-modulated radiotherapy (IMRT)	Radiation	Computer-controlled linear accelerators to deliver precise radiation doses to a malignant tumor.
Proton beam therapy	Radiation	Precisely delivers a beam of protons to disrupt and destroy tumor cells.
Cisplatin	Alkylating agent	Alkylating agent binds to purines resulting in DNA damage and cell cycle arrest leading to cancer cell. Death by apoptosis.
5-fluorouracil	Anti-metabolite	The antagonist of pyrimidine nucleotide inhibits thymidylate synthase.
Methotrexate	Immunosuppressant	The immunosuppressant blocks the enzyme required by cancer cells, affecting their growth.
Taxol	Induction	Microtubule-stabilizing drug interferes with the growth and spread of cancer cells.
TARGETED THERAPY		
Cetuximab	Monoclonal antibodies	Targets the epidermal growth factor receptor (EGFR).
Panitumumab	Monoclonal antibodies	Specific to the epidermal growth factor receptor.
Afatinib	Small molecule inhibitor	Has specific mutations in the EGFR, works by inhibiting the activity of EGFR.
Neratinib	Small molecule inhibitor	Has specific mutations in the human epidermal growth factor receptor 2 (HER2).
Trametnib	Small molecule inhibitor	Has specific mutations in the BRAF gene.

Rationale for Precision Medicine in Oral Cancer

Oral cancer is a serious and potentially life-threatening condition, but early detection and treatment can significantly improve the chances of a successful outcome. The risk of development of oral cancer, its prognosis, advancement, and response to treatment are not similar among individuals in a population. Thus, the selection of drugs, their dosage, duration of treatment, and expected response from treatment may depend upon tumor characteristics but vary among patients. A large number of causative agents are known for oral cancer. The course of development and progression of the tumor also depends on causative agents. Oral cancer developed in non-smokers is different from that of smokers. Non-smokers are known to have a higher risk of developing oral cancer. Non-smokers with oral lesions have a high probability of developing tumors from oral lesions as compared to smokers. The development of oral lesions among non-smokers indicates their high genetic susceptibility [40]. Loss-of-heterozygosity can serve as a marker for identifying high-risk lesions, selecting individuals at higher risk and developing precision medicine [41]. The rate of mortality is also higher among non-smokers as compared to smokers. The site of tumor development also varies among both. The occurrence of tumors in smokers is common at the posterior end and floor of the mouth [42]. The presence of HPV also affects the outcome of the treatment. Protein p16 known as INK4 serves as a biomarker associated with high-risk strains of HPV in oral cancer [43]. Not only the presence of HPV but also the copy number, site of integration, and virus strain also affect the progression of the tumor. HPV-positive oral cancer shows a more favorable prognosis. The outcome of chemotherapy in stage later and end stages of oral cancer, stage III and stage IV, shows outcomes affected by the presence of HPV. HPV-negative tumors show a poor prognosis as compared to HPV-positive tumors [44]. Treatment of HPV-positive tumors generally includes a combination of antiviral drugs. Also, surgical removal of HPV-positive tumors shows higher recurrence and thus demands precision medicine approach for better treatment. Along with genetic predisposition and involvement of a large number of factors depending upon the cause of the tumor, a treatment regime is required for oral cancer patients in order to remove the burden of unnecessary drugs and diagnosis. This creates a need for precision medicine in the treatment of oral cancer as some patients may experience more severe side effects from certain treatments than others. In addition, the development of precision medicine can help optimize the timing and dosing of treatment. This can be achieved by drug titration to work out the optimal dose to protect the patient from side effects. Thus, one can achieve improved efficacy, reduced side effects, and improved survival rate with better quality of life following the approaches of precision medicine.

Precision Medicine in Oral Cancer Treatment

Precision medicine is based on the identification of novel biomarkers for the purpose of diagnosis and targets with therapeutic potential in a population. Monoclonal antibodies and small molecules are used in precision medicine for the treatment of oral cancer. These small molecules and antibodies are developed against proteins that are selectively expressed or over-expressed proteins, or proteins specific to a signaling pathway activated or suppressed in certain cases of oral cancer. Mostly, these proteins include cell surface markers, surface receptors, or kinases involved in signaling pathways. These targets are found to be commonly involved in cell proliferation, survival, and evasion of apoptosis or cellular signaling.

Tipifarnib is used in precision medicine to target oncogene H-*Ras* in oral cancer patients. It is a selective inhibitor of farnesyltransferase and the activity H-*Ras* is highly dependent on Farnesylation. Thus, Tipifarnib is used for the treatment of patients with oncogene H-*Ras* mutation [45]. Abemaciclib is used to treat patients with a mutation in cyclin-dependent kinase. It targets CDK4 and CDK6 leading to the arrest of cell growth. It is known to show anticancerous effect irrespective of the EGFR or PI3K mutations [46]. Epidermal growth factor receptor (EGFR) and its family members like HER2 are common targets for developing precision medicine in squamous cell carcinomas including oral cancer. Cetuximab is a mouse/human chimeric monoclonal antibody; available under the trade name Erbitux which is an FDA-approved targeted therapy. This is approved for the treatment of oral cancer patients with wild-type K-*Ras* and a high expression of EGFR. It is a monoclonal antibody that specifically targets the EGFR. By inhibiting the activity of EGFR, Cetuximab limits the downstream pathway of EGFR responsible for cancer cell proliferation and survival [47]. Panitumumab (Vectibix) is another targeted therapy that is approved for the treatment of oral cancer. It is a human monoclonal antibody that also targets the extracellular domain of EGFR and prevents the binding of its ligand [48]. Afatinib available by the tradename Gilotrif is an FDA-approved small molecule that is also for the treatment of oral cancer where HER2 is overexpressed and is mostly given in recurrent or metastatic cancer. Neratinib or Nerlynx is another small molecule that targets surface overexpressed receptors. It works by binding to a cysteine residue in the ligand binding site of the ErbB family's HER1, HER2, and HER4 which results in the inhibition of downstream phosphorylation of ERK and AKT [49]. Trametinib is a small molecule used in precision medicine when mutations in proto-oncogene *braf* are present in a tumor. Trametinib inhibits the activity of a proto-oncogene product BRAF, which is involved in the growth and survival of tumor cells. Immunotherapy is also used in precision medicine. Pembrolizumab, Nivolumab, Atezolizumab, and Durvalumab are immune checkpoint inhibitors. Pembrolizumab and Nivolumab target cell surface receptor PD-1 protein while Atezolizumab and Durvalumab target the PD-L1 ligand. PD-1 and PD-L1 limit the ability of immune cells to target tumor cells [50]. Table **2** summaries all the monoclonal antibodies discussed here along with their specific targets.

CONCLUSION

The development of precision medicine for the treatment of oral cancer has improved the efficacy of the treatment by targeting specific genetic mutations or abnormalities that are present in an individual's tumor cells. This may lead to better treatment outcomes and an increased survival rate. It has been able to minimize the side effects as they are tailored to specific treatment regimen for each patient. Precision medicine may provide a better quality of life by maximizing the effectiveness of treatment. However, precision medicine approaches are much more expensive than standard treatments, which limits their access to many patients. The limited availability of such treatments may require patients to travel to specialized centers to access treatment. This can be challenging in underdeveloped and developing countries. With the shortage of evidence on the effectiveness of many precision, medical approaches in the treatment of oral cancer, more research is needed to fully understand their potential benefits and risks. Also, there are ethical concerns surrounding the use of precision medicine, such as the potential for discrimination based on genetic information or the allocation of limited resources to certain patients.

Overall, while precision medicine has the potential to significantly improve the treatment of oral cancer and even other diseases, there are still many challenges and limitations to its widespread adoption. It is important for healthcare providers, policymakers, and researchers to work together to address these challenges and ensure that precision medicine approaches are accessible and affordable. The future of precision medicine depends on improving the understanding of the genetic and molecular basis of oral cancer, development of new targeted therapies, optimization of the existing targeted therapies, exploring the use of immunotherapies, and evaluating the potential of gene therapies This may include the development of new gene therapies or the optimization of existing gene therapies for use in the clinical setting.

ACKNOWLEDGEMENTS

Financial assistance provided by the Council of Scientific & Industrial Research (CSIR), India to Piyush Bhati is gratefully acknowledged.

REFERENCES

[1] Phillips C J. Precision medicine and its imprecise history. Harvard Data Science Review 2020; 2(1)

[2] Jameson JL, Longo DL. Precision medicine--personalized, problematic, and promising. N Engl J Med 2015; 372(23): 2229-34. [http://dx.doi.org/10.1056/NEJMsb1503104] [PMID: 26014593]

[3] Sun W, Lee J, Zhang S, Benyshek C, Dokmeci MR, Khademhosseini A. Engineering precision medicine. Adv Sci 2019; 6(1): 1801039.

[http://dx.doi.org/10.1002/advs.201801039] [PMID: 30643715]

[4] Hockings JK, Pasternak AL, Erwin AL, Mason NT, Eng C, Hicks JK. Pharmacogenomics: An evolving clinical tool for precision medicine. Cleve Clin J Med 2020; 87(2): 91-9. [http://dx.doi.org/10.3949/ccjm.87a.19073] [PMID: 32015062]

[5] Sung H, Ferlay J, Siegel RL, *et al.* Global cancer statistics 2020: GLOBOCAN estimates of incidence and mortality worldwide for 36 cancers in 185 countries. CA Cancer J Clin 2021; 71(3): 209-49. [http://dx.doi.org/10.3322/caac.21660] [PMID: 33538338]

[6] Rivera C. Essentials of oral cancer. Int J Clin Exp Pathol 2015; 8(9): 11884-94. [PMID: 26617944]

[7] Oji C, Chukwuneke F. Poor oral hygiene may be the sole cause of oral cancer. J Maxillofac Oral Surg 2012; 11(4): 379-83. [http://dx.doi.org/10.1007/s12663-012-0359-5] [PMID: 24293926]

[8] Furquim CP, Pivovar A, Amenábar JM, Bonfim C, Torres-Pereira CC. Oral cancer in Fanconi anemia: Review of 121 cases. Crit Rev Oncol Hematol 2018; 125: 35-40. [http://dx.doi.org/10.1016/j.critrevonc.2018.02.013] [PMID: 29650274]

[9] Borse V, Konwar AN, Buragohain P. Oral cancer diagnosis and perspectives in India. Sensors International 2020; 1: 100046. [http://dx.doi.org/10.1016/j.sintl.2020.100046] [PMID: 34766046]

[10] Karunakaran K, Muniyan R. Genetic alterations and clinical dimensions of oral cancer: A review. Mol Biol Rep 2020; 47(11): 9135-48. [http://dx.doi.org/10.1007/s11033-020-05927-0] [PMID: 33085051]

[11] Nawroz H, van der Riet P, Hruban RH, Koch W, Ruppert JM, Sidransky D. Allelotype of head and neck squamous cell carcinoma. Cancer Res 1994; 54(5): 1152-5. [PMID: 8118797]

[12] Vineis P, Alavanja M, Buffler P, *et al.* Tobacco and cancer: Recent epidemiological evidence. J Natl Cancer Inst 2004; 96(2): 99-106. [http://dx.doi.org/10.1093/jnci/djh014] [PMID: 14734699]

[13] Langdon JD, Partridge M. Expression of the tumour suppressor gene p53 in oral cancer. Br J Oral Maxillofac Surg 1992; 30(4): 214-20. [http://dx.doi.org/10.1016/0266-4356(92)90263-I] [PMID: 1380822]

[14] Zanaruddin SNS, Yee PS, Hor SY, *et al.* Common oncogenic mutations are infrequent in oral squamous cell carcinoma of Asian origin. PLoS One 2013; 8(11): e80229. [http://dx.doi.org/10.1371/journal.pone.0080229] [PMID: 24224046]

[15] Polverini PJ. The pathophysiology of angiogenesis. Crit Rev Oral Biol Med 1995; 6(3): 230-47. [http://dx.doi.org/10.1177/10454411950060030501] [PMID: 8785263]

[16] Todd R, McBride J, Tsujl T, *et al.* Deleted in oral cancer-1 (*doc-l),* a novel oral tumor suppressor gene. FASEB J 1995; 9(13): 1362-70. [http://dx.doi.org/10.1096/fasebj.9.13.7557027] [PMID: 7557027]

[17] Alanazi IO, Khan Z. Understanding EGFR signaling in breast cancer and breast cancer stem cells: Overexpression and therapeutic implications. Asian Pac J Cancer Prev 2016; 17(2): 445-53. [http://dx.doi.org/10.7314/APJCP.2016.17.2.445] [PMID: 26925626]

[18] Grandis JR, Melhem MF, Gooding WE, *et al.* Levels of TGF-α and EGFR protein in head and neck squamous cell carcinoma and patient survival. J Natl Cancer Inst 1998; 90(11): 824-32. [http://dx.doi.org/10.1093/jnci/90.11.824] [PMID: 9625170]

[19] Sabbah DA, Hajjo R, Sweidan K. Review on epidermal growth factor receptor (EGFR) structure, signaling pathways, interactions, and recent updates of EGFR inhibitors. Curr Top Med Chem 2020; 20(10): 815-34.

[http://dx.doi.org/10.2174/1568026620666200303123102] [PMID: 32124699]

[20] Quinlan M P, Settleman J. Isoform-specific ras functions in development and cancer 2009. [http://dx.doi.org/10.2217/14796694.5.1.105]

[21] Kuo MYP, Jeng JH, Chiang CP, Hahn LJ. Mutations of Ki- *ras* oncogene codon 12 in betel quid chewing-related human oral squamous cell carcinoma in Taiwan. J Oral Pathol Med 1994; 23(2): 70-4. [http://dx.doi.org/10.1111/j.1600-0714.1994.tb00259.x] [PMID: 8164156]

[22] Das N, Majumder J, DasGupta UB. ras Gene mutations in oral cancer in eastern India. Oral Oncol 2000; 36(1): 76-80. [http://dx.doi.org/10.1016/S1368-8375(99)00058-5] [PMID: 10889924]

[23] Aggarwal S, John S, Sapra L, Sharma SC, Das SN. Targeted disruption of PI3K/Akt/mTOR signaling pathway, *via* PI3K inhibitors, promotes growth inhibitory effects in oral cancer cells. Cancer Chemother Pharmacol 2019; 83(3): 451-61. [http://dx.doi.org/10.1007/s00280-018-3746-x] [PMID: 30519710]

[24] Lim YC, Han JH, Kang HJ, *et al.* Overexpression of C-Met promotes invasion and metastasis of small oral tongue carcinoma. Oral Oncol 2012; 48(11): 1114-9. [http://dx.doi.org/10.1016/j.oraloncology.2012.05.013] [PMID: 22704061]

[25] Chang KY, Tsai SY, Chen SH, *et al.* Dissecting the EGFR-PI3K-AKT pathway in oral cancer highlights the role of the EGFR variant III and its clinical relevance. J Biomed Sci 2013; 20(1): 43. [http://dx.doi.org/10.1186/1423-0127-20-43] [PMID: 23806066]

[26] Schmidt SM, Schag K, Müller MR, *et al.* Survivin is a shared tumor-associated antigen expressed in a broad variety of malignancies and recognized by specific cytotoxic T cells. Blood 2003; 102(2): 571-6. [http://dx.doi.org/10.1182/blood-2002-08-2554] [PMID: 12576330]

[27] Nisar S, Yousuf P, Masoodi T, *et al.* Chemokine-cytokine networks in the head and neck tumor microenvironment. Int J Mol Sci 2021; 22(9): 4584. [http://dx.doi.org/10.3390/ijms22094584] [PMID: 33925575]

[28] Darrasse-Jèze G, Bergot AS, Durgeau A, *et al.* Tumor emergence is sensed by self-specific CD44hi memory Tregs that create a dominant tolerogenic environment for tumors in mice. J Clin Invest 2009; 119(9): 2648-62. [http://dx.doi.org/10.1172/JCI36628] [PMID: 19652360]

[29] Hashimoto S, Hashimoto A, Muromoto R, Kitai Y, Oritani K, Matsuda T. Central roles of STAT3-mediated signals in onset and development of cancers: Tumorigenesis and immunosurveillance. Cells 2022; 11(16): 2618. [http://dx.doi.org/10.3390/cells11162618] [PMID: 36010693]

[30] Angelo LS, Kurzrock R. Vascular endothelial growth factor and its relationship to inflammatory mediators. Clin Cancer Res 2007; 13(10): 2825-30. [http://dx.doi.org/10.1158/1078-0432.CCR-06-2416] [PMID: 17504979]

[31] Johnson BF, Clay TM, Hobeika AC, Lyerly HK, Morse MA. Vascular endothelial growth factor and immunosuppression in cancer: Current knowledge and potential for new therapy. Expert Opin Biol Ther 2007; 7(4): 449-60. [http://dx.doi.org/10.1517/14712598.7.4.449] [PMID: 17373897]

[32] de Souza Malaspina TS, Gasparoto TH, Costa MRSN, *et al.* Enhanced programmed death 1 (PD-1) and PD-1 ligand (PD-L1) expression in patients with actinic cheilitis and oral squamous cell carcinoma. Cancer Immunol Immunother 2011; 60(7): 965-74. [http://dx.doi.org/10.1007/s00262-011-1007-5] [PMID: 21442435]

[33] Begg AC, Stewart FA, Vens C. Strategies to improve radiotherapy with targeted drugs. Nat Rev Cancer 2011; 11(4): 239-53. [http://dx.doi.org/10.1038/nrc3007] [PMID: 21430696]

[34] Gupta P, Sivasankari P. Specific role of targeted molecular therapy in treatment of oral squamous cell

carcinoma. Oncobiology and Targets 2017; 4: 1.
[http://dx.doi.org/10.18639/ONBT.2017.04.511575]

[35] Levin WP, Kooy H, Loeffler JS, DeLaney TF. Proton beam therapy. Br J Cancer 2005; 93(8): 849-54.
[http://dx.doi.org/10.1038/sj.bjc.6602754] [PMID: 16189526]

[36] Florea AM, Büsselberg D. Cisplatin as an anti-tumor drug: Cellular mechanisms of activity, drug resistance and induced side effects. Cancers 2011; 3(1): 1351-71.
[http://dx.doi.org/10.3390/cancers3011351] [PMID: 24212665]

[37] Cohen SS, Flaks JG, Barner HD, Loeb MR, Lichtenstein J. The mode of action of 5-fluorouracil and its derivatives. Proc Natl Acad Sci USA 1958; 44(10): 1004-12.
[http://dx.doi.org/10.1073/pnas.44.10.1004] [PMID: 16590300]

[38] Tjong E, Dimri M, Mohiuddin SS. Biochemistry, tetrahydrofolate.StatPearls. StatPearls Publishing 2021. Internet

[39] Rowinsky EK, Donehower RC. Paclitaxel. N Engl J Med 1995; 332(15): 1004-14.
[http://dx.doi.org/10.1056/NEJM199504133321507] [PMID: 7885406]

[40] Rock LD, Rosin MP, Zhang L, Chan B, Shariati B, Laronde DM. Characterization of epithelial oral dysplasia in non-smokers: First steps towards precision medicine. Oral Oncol 2018; 78: 119-25.
[http://dx.doi.org/10.1016/j.oraloncology.2018.01.028] [PMID: 29496039]

[41] Rao M, Thavarajah R, Joshua E, Ranganathan K. Loss of heterozygosity as a marker to predict progression of oral epithelial dysplasia to oral squamous cell carcinoma. J Oral Maxillofac Pathol 2018; 22(2): 155-60.
[http://dx.doi.org/10.4103/jomfp.JOMFP_151_18] [PMID: 30158764]

[42] Perry BJ, Zammit AP, Lewandowski AW, *et al.* Sites of origin of oral cavity cancer in nonsmokers vs smokers: Possible evidence of dental trauma carcinogenesis and its importance compared with human papillomavirus. JAMA Otolaryngol Head Neck Surg 2015; 141(1): 5-11.
[http://dx.doi.org/10.1001/jamaoto.2014.2620] [PMID: 25375930]

[43] Miller DL, Puricelli MD, Stack MS. Virology and molecular pathogenesis of HPV (human papillomavirus)associated oropharyngeal squamous cell carcinoma. Biochem J 2012; 443(2): 339-53.
[http://dx.doi.org/10.1042/BJ20112017] [PMID: 22452816]

[44] Fischer CA, Kampmann M, Zlobec I, *et al.* p16 expression in oropharyngeal cancer: Its impact on staging and prognosis compared with the conventional clinical staging parameters. Ann Oncol 2010; 21(10): 1961-6.
[http://dx.doi.org/10.1093/annonc/mdq210] [PMID: 20423915]

[45] Gilardi M, Wang Z, Proietto M, *et al.* Tipifarnib as a precision therapy for HRAS-mutant head and neck squamous cell carcinomas. Mol Cancer Ther 2020; 19(9): 1784-96.
[http://dx.doi.org/10.1158/1535-7163.MCT-19-0958] [PMID: 32727882]

[46] Corona SP, Generali D. Abemaciclib: A CDK4/6 inhibitor for the treatment of HR+/HER2– advanced breast cancer. Drug Des Devel Ther 2018; 12: 321-30.
[http://dx.doi.org/10.2147/DDDT.S137783] [PMID: 29497278]

[47] Laurent-Puig P, Cayre A, Manceau G, *et al.* Analysis of PTEN, BRAF, and EGFR status in determining benefit from cetuximab therapy in wild-type KRAS metastatic colon cancer. J Clin Oncol 2009; 27(35): 5924-30.
[http://dx.doi.org/10.1200/JCO.2008.21.6796] [PMID: 19884556]

[48] Stroh C, Reusch C, Schmidt J, Splittgerber J, Wesolowski JS Jr, Blaukat A. Pharmacological and immunological characteristics of the therapeutic anti-EGFR antibodies cetuximab, panitumumab, and nimotuzumab. J Clin Oncol 2010; 28: e13025-5.
[http://dx.doi.org/10.1200/jco.2010.28.15_suppl.e13025]

[49] Tiwari SR, Mishra P, Abraham J. Neratinib, a novel HER2-targeted tyrosine kinase inhibitor. Clin Breast Cancer 2016; 16(5): 344-8.

[http://dx.doi.org/10.1016/j.clbc.2016.05.016] [PMID: 27405796]

[50] Bellmunt J, Powles T, Vogelzang NJ. A review on the evolution of PD-1/PD-L1 immunotherapy for bladder cancer: The future is now. Cancer Treat Rev 2017; 54: 58-67. [http://dx.doi.org/10.1016/j.ctrv.2017.01.007] [PMID: 28214651]

CHAPTER 15

Therapeutic Potential of Phytoconstituents and Personalized Medicine

Baby Tabassum[1,*] and **Mohammad Hashim**[1,2]

[1] *Toxicology, Lab, Department of Zoology, Govt Raza P.G. College, Rampur- (U.P.) 244901, India*

[2] *Department of Biochemistry, Mohammad Ali Jauhar University, Rampur- (U.P.) 244901, India*

Abstract: India has a rich tradition of the use of herbal medicine since the time immemorial. The treatment using plant-based medicaments became possible owing to the rich medicinal plant biodiversity. Several spices used on a regular basis in food preparation offer protection from a variety of ailments. Further, food consumption in different parts of the country has evolved based on culture, tradition, weather, and availability of resource materials. In a rural set-up, generally, the food is cruder but natural and thus healthier. Food harnessing and garnishing have become a standard practice to enhance the taste and look. Some of the herbs are used directly as food whereas others as food additives. Simultaneously, a large number of phytoconstituents have been characterized for their medicinal properties. In this chapter, we report on Phytoconstituents used for herbal formulation and discuss their therapeutic potential in human diseases. It is envisaged that such information would be of great use for ameliorating diseases ensuring better health complementing the concept of personalized medicine.

Keywords: Food additives, Human diseases, Medicinal plants, Phytoconstituents, Personalized medicine.

INTRODUCTION

Natural remedies represent plant-derived compounds that have traditionally been used to prevent sickness maintaining the indigenous or regional therapeutic traditions. These plant-derived ingredients have undergone minimal or no major alteration. In the context of health care, traditional herbal medicines have attracted a great deal of attention. In the absence of doctors, clinicians, hospitals, and health centers, traditional medicines proved to be a lifeline for human civilization. Literature shows China's attempt to prevent or cure severe acute ailments through the traditional system [1]. Similarly, about eighty percent of the African popula-

* **Corresponding author Baby Tabassum:** Department of Zoology, Govt Raza P.G. College, Rampur- (U.P.) 244901, India; Tel: 9456677015; E-mail: dr.btabassum@gmail.com

Farzana Mahdi & Abbas Ali Mahdi (Eds.)

tion has used traditional herbal medicine [2]. From the ancient period till now, Indians have relied upon six well-articulated systems which are recognized as Ayurveda, Siddha, Unani, yoga, Naturopathy, and Homeopathy. Besides these, there are many folklore medicines in Indian homes which are not registered. However, in the past, limited studies have been conducted on several aspects of these systems [4].

Previous research on traditional herbal remedies has shown their potential for the well-being of the people world over. Traditional herbal studies have received significant financial support from several government bodies such as China, India, Nigeria, and the United States of America and the efforts of these countries have been endorsed by WHO [2]. Additionally, in search of herbal medicine, private sectors have spent millions of dollars on the exploration of new bioactive molecules from plants [3]. In this chapter, we elucidate the overall potential of herbal formulations particularly phytoconstituents, their active factors wherever possible and future prospects in the context of personalized medicine. The concept of personalized medicine is based on the fact that every individual is unique with respect to his/her genomic constitution, mutational landscape, metabolic activities, lifestyle, food habits, regions, religion, faith, and the choice of mating partners. All these attributes affect the body and therefore one single prescription works well for someone but the same prescription does not work for another person. In addition, the drug may have side effects in one person but the same drug does not affect the other person. This heterogeneous response of the patients towards a single drug, therefore, may be made more uniform if we are able to generate the consensus keeping in view all the variables. Since there are several sub-disciplines of personalized medicine, generating consensus will involve additional efforts in research and development. Many times, the drug needs to be titrated to be able to uncover the most effective dose for a patient. While drug titration may not be possible for every situation, past observation clearly suggests that drug titration must be taken seriously. A diabetic patient for example was found to have unstable glucose levels despite the correct medicine he was prescribed. Upon a careful investigation, the same drug was titrated and the quantity was increased. The result was very positive as his glucose level stabilized. This suggests that *one-size-fits-all* is not the correct approach. Since in this chapter we are dealing with herbal medicaments, we will remain confined to this realm only. Other chapters in the book will cover additional aspects of personalized medicine.

TRADITIONAL REMEDIES

Traditional medicine has its much deeper roots in India and has undergone a constant process of evolutionary transition since the Vedic age. A single drug or mixtures in crude shape are valued above multiple-fold preparations. Traditional Medicine has evolved into several systems because of which differences in the origins and historical development are found. However, they share a common background and their foundation is based on the plants and at times, some other additives such as (*Bhasma*). Medicinal plants have roots, shoots, leaves, bark, and flowers and fruits each one having a different property and potency. This warranted in-depth characterization to uncover their active factors and then monitor health potentials as therapeutic agents. Plants are important parts of our civilization and have been used extensively for a variety of fruits production, beautification, ornamentation, wine cheese, pickle, jam, and essential oil preparation. Plants have been used as traditional medicine since 2600 BCE as Mesopotamia recorded 1000 plant-based products. These include the use of extracted oils of *Cupressus arizonica* Greene, *Commiphora acuminata Mattick, Cedrus libani* A. Rich., *Glycyrrhiza glabra L.*, and *Papaver somniferum L.*, which are still used to treat common colds, coughs and swelling [5]. Egyptian pharmaceutical, which dates back to about 2900 BCE, claims to be the oldest form of modern medicine. The "Ebers Papyrus" is the best-known record from 1500 BCE, and lists more than 700 drugs, most of which were made from plants [6]. Over the course of many centuries, traditional Chinese medicine has gained widespread recognition, as evident from the record of around 2000 years ago (1100 BCE; Wu Shi Er Bing Fang; 52 medicines), followed by the herbal Shennong (100 BCE; 365 medicines) and the herbal Tang (659 CE; 850 medicines). On the other hand, records of traditional Indian medicine go back more than 5,000 years (Charaka and Sushruta Samhitas hold 341 and 395 herbal medicines separately 1,000 BCE ago) [7].

From across the globe, Romans and Greeks contributed a lot to the development of traditional medicine in the ancient Western world. Dioscorides, a Greek physician who lived around 100 BCE, wrote about how traditional medicine was collected, stored, and used in the "known world" at the time. About half of the top 50 drugs sold in European pharmacies are NPs (natural products) that are sold as herbal or food supplements. Although the modern pharmaceutical industry all over the world relies on synthetic drugs, however, close to about 25% of the drugs in the modern pharmacopeia come from plants. Several synthetic drugs are made using original formulations based on plants representing naturopathy (NPs) [8 - 10]. Thus, in the true sense, overall plant-based drug formulation would be more than 25%. Realizing the merit and potential of the plant-based drugs, the World Health Organization (WHO) has taken note of it. Thus, as per the WHO, "the entire understanding, abilities, and methods based on the hypotheses, convictions, and experiences of indigenous drugs used in different cultures, whether logical or not, actually provide substantial support to the human healthcare system. It may be noted that plant-based formulations have found their use for animals, particularly livestock species and other domestic animals. However, a comprehensive illustration of herbal formulation useful for animals is not the aim of this chapter. Thus, we would remain confined to the human system only. In addition, plant-based traditional medicine is helpful for the identification, improvement, treatment, and prevention, of physical and psychological instability [11, 12]. Incidentally, no large-scale trials of plant-based drugs are carried out assuming that the same is safe for the population. However, a systematic large-scale trial on the population and its subsequent follow-up will establish its scientific basis and usefulness across ethnicities under varying living conditions. This, in turn, will also detect if such drugs are effective uniformly or otherwise. Most of the time, such drugs do not have side effects and are thus considered to be compatible across a diverse group of populations. Nonetheless, their efficiency may vary amongst the heterogeneous population of the patients. Traditional Indian medicine is the world's oldest continuously practiced form of alternative medicine, and there are a large number of other traditional medical practices that share a wide range of beliefs and societal motivations [13, 14]. Ayurveda, the traditional Indian medicine, is the one that has been practiced the longest and has strong philosophical roots. Ayurveda also establishes the connectivity of the patients with nature because the greatest and the most efficient healer is none other than nature. Thus, the very root of Ayurveda is nature and its infinite bounties. Traditional medicine in India refers to the practice of medications that are either assumed to have originated in India or that were brought to India from other parts of the world and became ingrained in Indian culture. Like China, India is the only country in the world to have its own system of traditional medicine that is acknowledged internationally. These systems include Ayurveda, Siddha, Unani, Yoga, Naturopathy, and Homoeopathy. Despite the fact that Homoeopathy was introduced to India in the 18th century, it has been completely assimilated into Indian culture and has undergone development and improvement just like any other traditional system. As a result, it has been enriched and has become an integral component of Indian traditional medicine [15].

Ayurveda

Ayurveda uses natural resources for treatment through experimentation and daily life experiences. Ayurvedic medicine has two key rules. These help patients remember the cause of their condition. Ayurveda treats happy and miserable lives. It measures life expectancy and quality of life and discusses what is appropriate and inappropriate in life [16]. Thus, Ayurveda focuses on the entire body's makeup, and not just the symptoms of the disease. A person's bio-personality, bio-synthetic, and physiological characteristics, as well as their social and economic standing, are all factors that contribute to their susceptibility to developing a particular disease. Thus, during Ayurvedic treatment, all such aspects are taken into account by this drug delivery system. In addition, this paves the way to conduct additional research using cutting-edge modern experimental approaches to establish the efficacy of a medicine. Many common Ayurvedic remedies are complex combinations of multiple herbs, as well as other ingredients like metals and minerals. However, NPs are more common than the other derived compounds, as evidenced by both ancient manuscripts and the present Ayurvedic Pharmacopoeia [17]. Multidisciplinary platforms have boosted Ayurveda research in recent decades for the development of pharmacological lead compounds allowing uncovering the active factors. Ayurvedic medications are widespread worldwide due to their traditional acceptance, usefulness, socioeconomic advantage, and acceptability. Extensive research ensures ayurvedic medications' quality, safety, stability, and efficacy. The hunt for new therapeutic plant-derived medicines, especially bioactive chemicals, will continue to play a key role in India's healthcare development and administration.

Siddha

Siddha medicine dates back to 10,000–4000 BCE in India. Like Ayurveda, it uses natural resources to preserve health and is South India's oldest medical tradition. Saiva philosophy is one of the six Hindu religions. “Siddha” means “holy harmony,” “excellence,” or “known fact,” and “Siddhars” are super natural beings who gain intellectual powers by practicing this treatment. Thirumoolar, Ahappe, Agathiyar, Sunthara Ananthar, Bogar, Machchamuni, Konganar, Korakkar, Therayar, Karuvoorar, Nandi Devar, Idaikkadar, Iraamathevar, Sattamuni, Kuthampai, Paampaatti, Aluhanna, and Kahapusundar are said to have founded Siddha medicine. This therapeutic approach thinks human well-being is important to enjoy eternal bliss. Philosophical ideas include “food is medicine, and not medicine is food” and “the sound mind makes a sound body” [18 - 21]. Siddha system's philosophy and guiding principles of medicine are similar to Ayurveda. This system perceives the human body as a collection of three humors, waste products, and seven fundamental ingredients. The balance of humor indicates a healthy state of well-being, whereas its imbalance results in illness or disease. This is more like homeostasis prevalent in the allopathic system. Thus, a delicate balance is maintained in the human body with all the essential constituents needed for maintenance and survival. The human body is made up of 96 main components, which encompass its physical, physiological, moral, and intellectual attributes. Alteration causes the 96 principles to operate incorrectly, which results in the manifestation of disease [22]. Siddha's philosophy covers therapeutic, philosophical, and intellectual ones. It puts equal priority on the mind inside and outward body, especially finding ways of alchemy (changing base metals into gold), urine testing, and practice as mentioned in materia medica [23]. Siddha remedies are currently recognized as being acceptable to treat any condition, with the exception of emergency circumstances. In a similar vein, treatments made from herbo-metals or herbo-minerals, both of which probably include nanoparticles, are more successful in treating chronic illnesses [24].

Unani

The Unani medical system was developed in Greece and was transformed by Arabs into an elegant medical science based on the framework of the Greek philosopher and physician Hippocrates (Buqrat) (460-377 BCE), and Galen (Jalinoos). Greek and Arab scholars like Galen (131-212 CE), Raazes (850-925 CE), and Avicenna (980-1037 CE) significantly improved the system, which is now known as Greco-Arab Medicine [25]. Unani medicine is based on the four conditions of living, which are hot, sodden, frosty, and dry, as well as the four humours of Hippocratic theory, which are blood, yellow bile, dark bile, and mucus. Unani medicine was affected by Indian culture shaped by Mughal Emperors which is now used by a sizable part of the Indian population. The human body, according to Unani, is composed of seven standards: Mizaj (temperaments), Anza (organs), Quo (resources), Arkan (components), Arwah (spirits), Aklath (humours), and Afal (capacities). These standards monitor health prosperity and disease both [26 - 28]. Before making a diagnosis, and suggestion about treatment, a physician will take each of these factors into consideration. The NP medications that are utilized as a part of this framework are indicative of life, and their use does not result in any adverse effects. Before being used, these medicines, which are poisonous in their raw form, go through the processes of preparation and purification [29]. With the availability of modern equipment, this process has become more accurate and feasible.

In the Unani system of medicine, diet therapy, regimental treatment, and pharmaco-treatment are all types of medicine that are used. In the context of medicine, "diet treatment" refers to the organization of a specific diet together with the control plans for the treatment of various illnesses. In addition, routine regulation of both the quantity and nature of the food is monitored.

Regular treatment includes things like diaphoresis, diuresis, and Turkish shower, kneading of the body and body organs besides dry or oil massage. All these steps speed up the process of healing through natural means without putting undue pressure on the body.

INDIAN FOLK MEDICINES

Indian folk medicine offers excellent remedies for digestive and nervous system issues. This system has a rich history of therapeutic practices, many of which have evolved into distinct schools of thought reflecting distinctive regional emphases and philosophies. Realizing its significance, a planning commission was established after independence in 1951 to look into this aspect and prepare comprehensive lists of such folk medicines. Another division, the Department of Indian System of Medicine and Homoeopathy (ISM&H), was established in 1995. In 2003, ISM&H became a separate Department within India's Ministry of Health and Family Welfare, and now it has adopted the acronym AYUSH to represent its focus on traditional Indian medical practices such as Ayurveda, Yoga, Naturopathy, Unani, Siddha, and Homoeopathy. Thus, AYUSH provides an umbrella accommodating all these healthcare systems. Traditional Indian medicine is facing formidable challenges due to the dominance of modern pharmaceuticals, despite widespread faith and trust of the people in this system. There is a pressing need to consolidate and standardize traditional medical practices for more effective dissemination of our own medical heritage. For this reason, it is crucial to conduct both phytochemical and biochemical studies, with a focus on reviving and disseminating India's rich medical legacy for the greater good of society.

In the field of medicine, the use of home remedies for the symptom management of minor health concerns to this day has not been subjected to stringent levels of International scrutiny. In terms of the available literature, there is a great deal of information that is aimed at the general public, but the deep scientific literature is not available. According to recent surveys conducted in Germany for public opinion, approximately half of the population uses home remedies. Even in India, these days' people are looking towards naturopathy with the assumption that there will be no side effects [30, 31].

These are some simple foods that can be made with home-available ingredients. Such medicines are particularly efficient in treating realistic conditions such as cough, cold, fever, body ache, headache,dyspepsia, *etc*. For long-term conditions such as diabetes, joint stiffness, and skin infections, such remedies may be used with certain intoxicants. Thus, folk medicine has its own importance and is easily accessible even in the far-flung areas of the country.

Honey

Honey enjoys the status of both food and medicine and is acknowledged the world over for its divine qualities. This sweet and alluring divine gift is made by honeybees *(Apis mellifera*; Family: *Apidae*) [32] for which the never tiring insects suck nectars from the choice of flowers. It may be noted that the bees never ever visit poisonous flowers for nectars. Honey has been used by every civilization in the world for the last 5,500 years. Its nutritional value and medical benefits have been listed by all the ancient civilizations like the Greeks, the Chinese, the

Egyptians, the Romans, the Mayans, and the Babylonians. Besides food and medicine, it is used in the cosmetics and food industry to prepare a variety of items healthy for both men and women of all ages [33]. Honey does not need to be refrigerated because it does not spoil; it also can be stored unopened at ambient temperature [34]. Honey has a water activity of 0.56 to 0.62 and a pH of about 3.9. Due to the high level of fructose, it has been utilized as a sweetener and preservative. Indian Maharajas (rulers) are used to preserve ripe high-quality mangoes in a huge container of pure honey for their off-season use. This way, they used to have access to the mangoes throughout the year. Honey is twenty-five percent sweeter than tablet sugar [35, 36]. Moreover, Honey is also used extensively in beverages. Current electronic and print media provide information on using honey to treat many disorders, highlighting a broad range of undiscovered actions. Honey is a rich and reliable source of antioxidants, and has anti-inflammatory, antibacterial, hypoglycemic, respiratory, digestive, cardiac, and brain and nerve protection properties [37 - 39]. Thus, Honey is an unparalleled combination of natural food and medicine having far-reaching implications and health benefits.

Honey's Clinical Significance

Scientific proof from Dark Age paintings indicates that disease treatment with bee products such as honey and wax dates back to 8000 years. Honey was commonly deployed as a medicine throughout history, as proven by Sumerian clay tablets (6200 BC), Egyptian papyri (1900-1250 BC), the Veda (Hindu literature) dating back 5000 years, the Holy Quran, the Bible, and Hippocrates (460-357 BC) philosophy. The therapeutic efficacy of honey was clearly illustrated in the Qur'an [40 - 42]. Although several articles have been written about honey, the vast majority of them concentrated on biochemical assessment and its commercial applications. It was treated in traditional remedies for a wide range of medical issues, such as but not extended to: eye diseases, asthma, respiratory infections, TB, thirst, hiccups, exhaustion, dizziness, liver disease, diarrhea, worm infestation, piles, eczema, wound healing, and ulcers [43]. A spoonful of honey after dinner prior to bed helps maintain homeostasis improving the immune system. Thus, honey is a reliable immunomodulator, and works as an anti-aging agent. Despite the fact that it has a low glycemic index, people with diabetes are afraid to use it. This issue needs to be addressed by conducting research on a large number of diabetic patients. The uptake quantity of honey by these patients may be titrated and calibrated to uncover a range of safe doses. This will enable diabetic patients to shun the fear of honey and get its other several vital benefits.

Honey's Nutritional and Medicinal Qualities

Currently, around 300 varieties of honey have been reported [44]. These variants are linked with the various types of nectars collected by honeybees. The major component of honey is Carbohydrates accounting for 95–97% of the substance's dry weight. Most of these sugars are made when honey ripens and matures. The major organic acid in honey is gluconic acid, which itself is made when glucose breaks down. Small amounts of acetic, formic, and citric acid have also been found. Honey's acidic (pH 3.2- 4.5) quality is due to these organic acids. Furthermore, honey contains proteins, vitamins, amino acids, minerals, organic acids, flavonoids, polyphenols, reducing chemicals, alkaloids, glycosides, cardiac glycosides, anthrax-quinone, and volatile compounds [45, 46]. The primary protein components of honey are enzymes such as diastase, invertases, glucose oxidase, catalase, and acid phosphatase [47]. It would be of relevance for treating DNA with varying doses of honey to assess if the same has endonuclease activities, if yes, whether this activity is specific or a non-specific one. Similarly, honey may be used to assess its effect on different cancer cell lines using *in-vitro* cell culture. The biological effects of honey across the normal and abnormal cell systems may be explored to see if this approach helps delineate different cell types. It may seem out of the box idea to rub pure honey on the body of a patient suffering from leukoderma or vitiligo for different durations of time and assess its effect. Leukoderma or vitiligo do not have an easy cure. If this works and makes the skin normal, a large number of patients would be happy and indebted to honeybees. In an indirect experiment, the effect of honey can be monitored on the melanocytes. If the honey promotes the growth and development of melanocytes, that would surely work against white patches of the skin. The effects of pure honey on the microbes would be another fruitful study. If the harmful microbes are not allowed to flourish, honey will provide a cure for a large number of ailments.

Antioxidants, Organic Acids, and Polyphenols

Natural bioactive substances known as flavonoids, with a 15-carbon structure composed of double benzene rings linked by the heterocyclic pyrane ring, called "flavonoids" Quercetin, kaempferol, and pinobanksin are examples of flavonols. Similarly, luteolin, apigenin, and chrysin are flavones; naringenin, pinocembrin, and hesperetin are flavanones; genistein is an example of an isoflavone; and anthocyanidins are examples of flavonoid pigments. Genistein, chrysin, luteolin, and naringenin are only some of the flavonoids that have been associated with estrogenic activities. Chemical compositions exhibit honey's flavonoids and phenolic acids in Fig. (**1**) [48, 49]. Thus, honey has a large number of vital but complex molecules each harbouring a very special property.

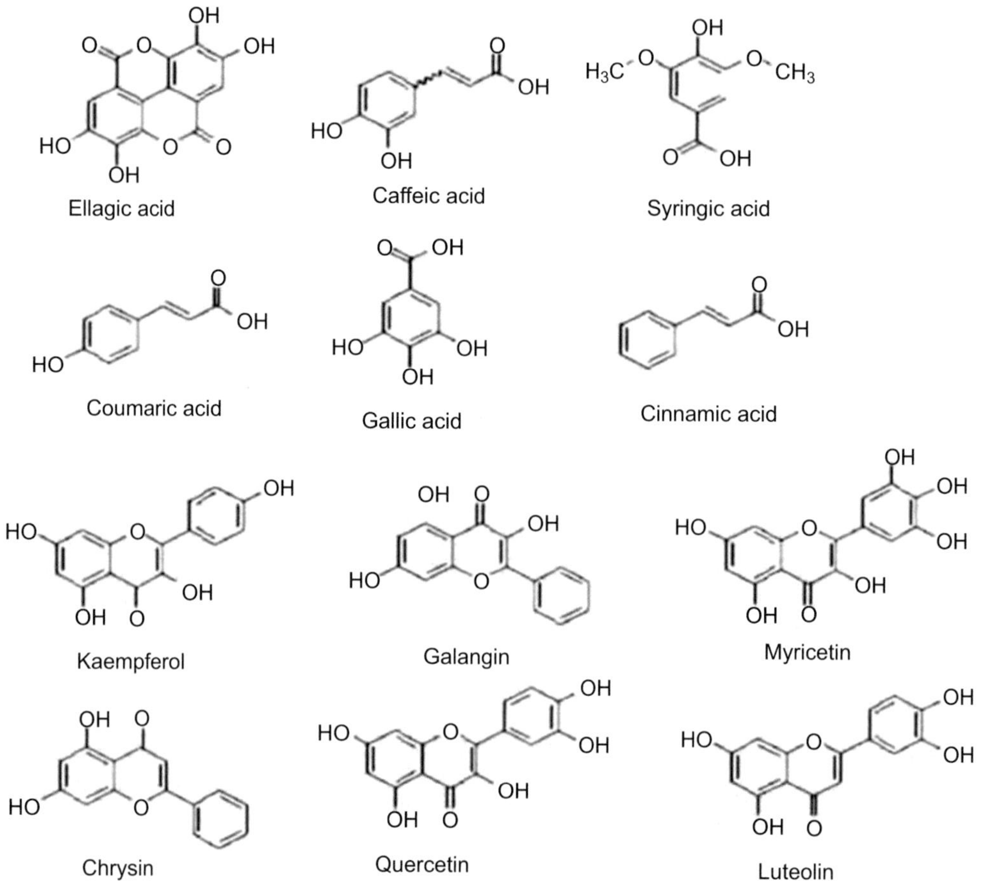

Fig. (1). The major bioactive compound of honey [46].

Biological Activities

Honey is safe to ingest and has no negative impacts like synthetic drugs. Its chemical ingredients, botanical origin, and types of nectar determine its biological activities and nutritional values (Fig. **2**).

Antibacterial Activity

Honey's ability to inhibit the growth of microorganisms is largely related to an enzymatic mechanism called glucose oxidation and some very specific elements of honey's physical abilities [50]. Due to its low water activity, honey is a strong antibacterial agent. Hydrogen peroxide, an effective antimicrobial, is generated by the action of glucose oxidase, but the capacity for this synthesis is sensitive on the honey's enzymatic activity as well. There are other, non-peroxide antibacterial chemicals that have a wide variety of chemical origins and mechanisms of activity. These include aromatic acids, unknown substances with different chemical properties, phenolic, and flavonoids. However, honey's antimicrobial activity can also be affected by a number of other factors, such as its hyperosmotic stress, pH values, climate, less protein concentration, carbon content to nitrogen level, under redox activity due to its high level of decline sugars, a viscosity that limits dissolved oxygen [51]. Furthermore, it is reported to inhibit Rubella virus, Leishmania parasite, and Echinococcus *in vitro*. Thus, natural pure honey has far too many qualities that have been discovered thus far. Regular use of honey in winter protects from colds, coughs, congestion, fatigue, and bouts of depression. It enhances the glow on the face, regulates the digestive system, helps balance homeostasis, and enhances longevity besides fighting cancer. During the early stages of oral cancer (leukoplakia), regular use of pure honey and keeping the honey in the mouth for a while before swallowing will result in the miraculous disappearance of the cancer cell. When a person has oral cancer, s/he is unable to swallow and speak because of fibrosis in the mouth. The effect of honey can easily be monitored by the patient without any medical test or instrument paraphernalia. The patient himself will feel the difference when the pain in the mouth disappears and new normal cells start proliferating.

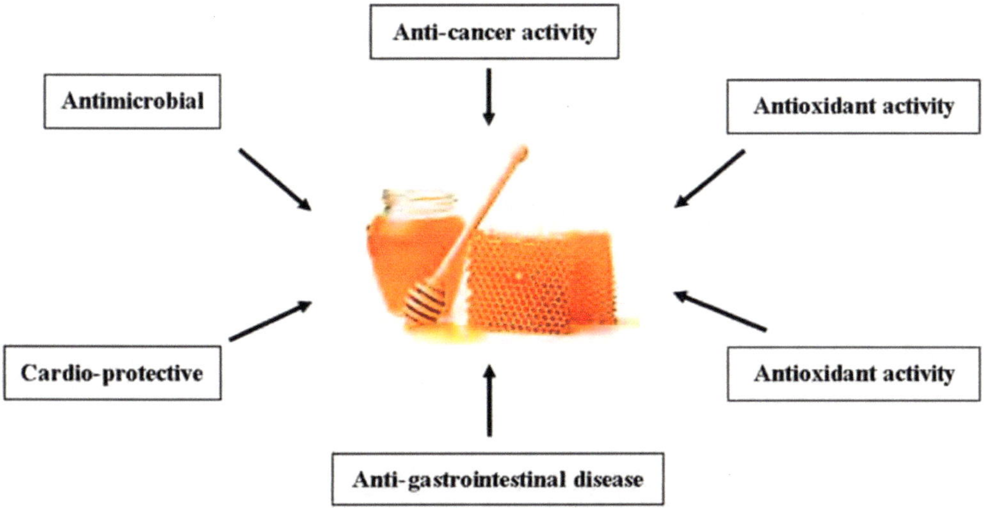

Fig. (2). The biological prowess of honey.

Anticancer Activity

Polyphenols, which are found in honey, have anticancer properties. Several polyphenolic compounds in honey, like Caffeic acid, Caffeic acid phenyl ester,

Chrysin, Galangin, Quercetin, Acacetin, Kaempferol, Pinocembrin, Pinobanksin, and Apigenin, are becoming great potential drugs for treating cancer. Furthermore, it was shown that combining alcohol with honey inhibits the injuries that might otherwise result from repeated exposure to the former [52, 53]. In case of urinary tract infection (UTI), bacterial vaginosis (it is a type of vaginal inflammation caused by the overgrowth of bacteria naturally found in the vagina, which upsets the natural balance), cervical cancer, vaginitis, pure honey applied topically is expected to provide relief. However, unequivocal experimental evidence on this line needs to be provided so that the patients, when using honey, have the patience to overcome the infection.

Antioxidant Activity

Antioxidants are molecules found in foods and in all the biological systems that neutralize oxidizing agents like oxygen [54]. However, studies have shown that pure honey had a role with an impact of senescence as well as activities involving strong oxidizing ingredients driven by O_2. Such free radicals and reactive oxygen species are generated by the body's metabolism. A number of these compounds have significant effects on enzymatic reactions, DNA, mRNA, cellular membrane proteins, and lipids. Such destructive responses cause a wide range of illnesses. Bioactive compounds stop oxidative stress from causing the diseases [55]. Literature show that honey may be a novel antioxidant that can be used individually or in combination with other therapies to help protect cell damage [56].

Anti-inflammatory Activity

As a result of the tissue damage it causes, chronic inflammation can inhibit the healing process. Previous research and clinical trials have demonstrated that honey can reduce the inflammatory response in animals [57, 58]. According to Schley and Field [59], the carbohydrates (*e.g.* Nigro oligos) in honey have the ability to improve the immune system [60].

Anti-gastrointestinal Activity

Bacteria attach to mucosal epithelial cells, producing gastroenteritis. Honey inhibits dangerous germs from interacting with intestinal cells, decreasing the chance of infection responsible for GI illnesses. Moreover, honey's antimicrobial qualities protect a person from microbial infection-induced diarrhea. The correct method to get honey's antimicrobial advantages is to combine a tablespoon of honey into a cup of warm water and drink it first in the morning. In addition to assisting the body’s natural detoxification, it reduces the incidence of different gastrointestinal illnesses. Further, the addition of a tablespoon of citrus juice to honey will enhance its flavor. Thus, in case of diarrhea or gastroenteritis, drinking water with honey would be a healthy option to hydrate the body and regain health [61]. Thus, several aspects of honey and its associated usefulness are still not known to us. This warrants more systematic research and innovation to uncover its bountiful and true benefits.

Ajwain (*Trachyspermum Ammi* L.)

Ajwain, *Trachyspermum ammi* (L.) Sprague, from the family Apiaceae, is a perennial plant that grows upright and contains a striated branch. This plant is native to the eastern parts of India and Persia. The plant *Trachyspermum ammi L.* comes from the 270 genus of the Apiaceae family. It is called Ajwain in Hindi, Bishop's weed in English, Yamini in Sanskrit, Lodhar Bengali in Punjabi, Ajma in Gujrati, Kath in Kashmiri, and Omam in Tamil, among many other names [62]. The part of ajwain that is used most commonly is the slight caraway-like tiny seed, which is popular in Indian scrumptious recipes, flavorful pastries, and snacks. It is utilized as a medicinal herb in the Ayurvedic medical system due to its anti-spasmodic, energetic, tonic, and carminative properties [63].

Phytoconstituents of Ajwain

Phytoconstituents, terpenoid, and their related compounds including alcohols, aldehydes, ketones, acids, and esters compose the majority of essential oils' volatile constituents. The majority of essential oils contain terpenes or thymol (50-60%), alpha-terpinene (-terpinene), and p-cymene that are extracted from the seeds. The other components include alpha- and beta-pinenes, alpha-thujene, myrcene, 1,8-cineole, and carvacrol. 11.9% fiber, 38.6% carbs, tannins, glycosides, 8.9% water, 15.4% protein, 18.1% fat, saponins, flavone, and 7.1% mineral (Fig. **3**), which exist in a series of important forms and participate in a number of biological activities [64 - 66].

Biological Activities of Ajwain

The volatile oil of Ajwain has significant antibacterial, antiviral, antifungal, antitussive, anti-inflammatory, analgesic, antioxidant, asthmatic, and anticancer properties [68, 69]. However, the dose of Ajwain should be carefully titrated to achieve its effectiveness. Systematic studies on this line on a sufficient number of patients encompassing all the properties have not been carried out. Thus, what needs to be done is to undertake all such properties of Ajwain as an independent attribute and then conduct research to establish its medicinal properties using an effective but titrated dose (Fig. **4**).

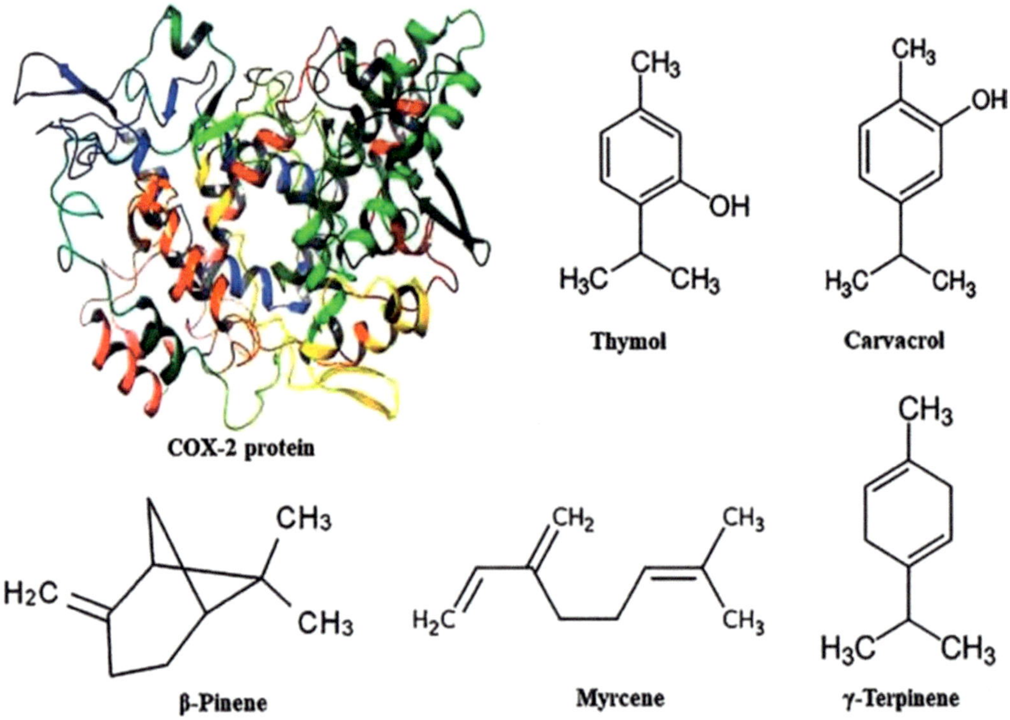

Fig. (3). The major bioactive compound of ajwain [67].

Antimicrobial Effects

Crude extract of Ajwain shows significant antibacterial activity *in vitro*. The ajwain oil was found to be protective against several species of bacteria, such as *Escherichia coli, Salmonella, Citrobacter, Hafnia alvei, Vibrio cholerae, Klebsiella, Pasteurella multocida, Bordetella bronchisepta, Acinetobacter baumanii, Stenotrophomonas maltophilia, Aeromonas hydrophila*. This was established by a diffusion method experiment using acetone and an aqueous extract of ajwain against bacteria [70]. It is possible that the presence of phenolic chemicals like thymol and carvacrol in ajwain is responsible for its antibacterial capabilities [71]. Thymol activity towards yeast and other microbes is largely unexplored but preliminary work suggested that its target is membrane envelope. In Candida strains, thymol affects vesicles and cell membranes and inhibits ergosterol production, affecting the permeability of the cell membrane [72].

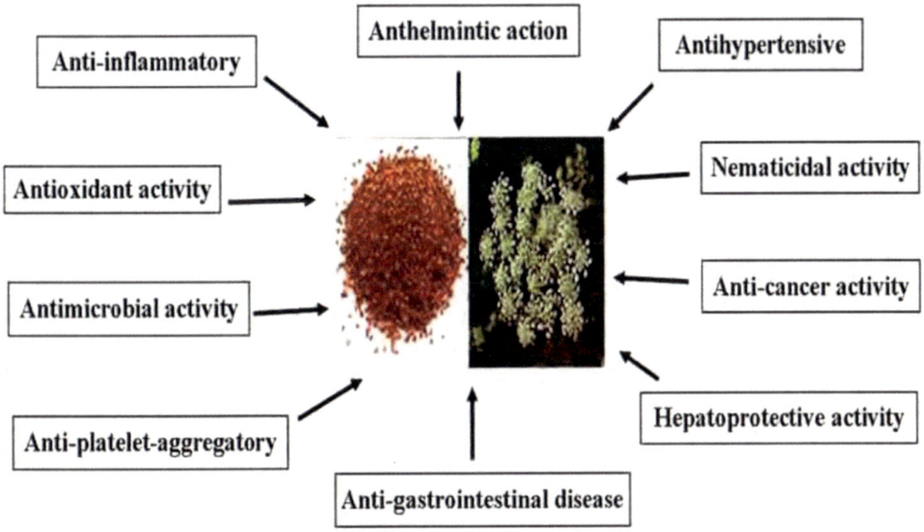

Fig. (4). Diagrammatic illustration of Ajwain showing multiple biological properties.

Antioxidant Activity

Ajwain is rich in vitamins, minerals, carotenoids (-carotene and lutein), and flavonoids, which give antioxidant properties. The antioxidant capacity of the ajwain seed extract mix was examined by H_2O_2 and NO radical scavenging tests. Ajwain extract inhibited hydrogen peroxide by 70.04% at 200g/ml. In nitric oxide radical scavenging experiment, it showed inhibition of nitric oxide radicals by 72.80% at 200g/ml, while ascorbic acid inhibited 94.96% [73]. The seed extracts prevented the injury to calf thymus DNA by the Reactive species. Thus, Ajwain seed extracts may be an important source of powerful antioxidants that can be used on a regular basis both as food additives and medicine [74].

Anti-inflammatory

In different studies, complete methanolic and total aqueous extracts of Ajwain seeds were analyzed for their potential anti-inflammatory effects. It showed anti-inflammatory efficacy with a statistical significance (P <0.001). There was a visible and substantial rise in the masses of the adrenal glands. However, extracts that come from ajwain seeds have a substantial possibility of relieving inflammatory symptoms [75].

Nematicidal Activity

The nematicidal activity of ajwain seed essential oil was shown to be effective against Bursaphelenchus xylophilus, Camphene, pinene, myrcene, limonene, terpinene, terpinen-4-ol, thymol, and carvacrol. These are the components of ajwain oil that have nematicidal action against pinewood nematode [76].

Antihypertensive, Anti-spasmodic, Bronchodilator

The anti-hypertensive impact of ajwain injected into the bloodstream *in vivo* and the anti-spasmodic and severe respiratory actions *in vitro* have shown that calcineurin inhibition mediates the spasmolytic effects of natural substances. It is believed that such a mechanism contributed to their observed result and supported the traditional use of ajwain in hyperactive intestine illnesses such as colic and flatulence, along with heart problems [77].

Hepato-protection

In animals, ajwain was 80% protective against a normally lethal dose of acetaminophen (1 g/kg). It stopped CCl_4 from making animals stay asleep longer when they were on pentobarbital, and it seemed to fix the high levels of hepatic enzymes in the blood that were caused by CCl_4-induced liver oxidative stress [78].

Antiplatelet-aggregatory

Many studies published *in vitro* using the blood of healthy volunteers reported that an ethereal extract of dry ajwain seeds reduced the aggregation of platelets produced by arachidonic acid, collagen, and adrenaline [78].

Anti-gastrointestinal Disease

Anti-ulcer activity of ajwain seed was demonstrated in several ulcer-producing animals. Different studies confirmed a significant reduction in the ulcer ratio and indicated that the extract and seeds provided a significant protective effect by decreasing the level of inflammatory ulcers [79].

Anthelmintic Action

The anthelmintic action of ajwain shows its impact on certain helminth parasites, including *Ascaris lumbricoides* in humans and *Haemonchus contortus* in sheep. Ajwain seems to have an antihelminthic effect by interfering with the way parasites use energy and making ATPase action more powerful, which causes them to use up their stored energy. It was also claimed that the plant possesses cholinergic activity with peristaltic movements of the gut, which helps get rid of parasitic infections inside the intestines [80].

Black Seeds (*Nigella sativa*)

Black Seed *Nigella sativa* (also known as black caraway, Roman coriander, kalonji) were discovered at a number of locations in Egyptian civilization, including that of Tutankhamun (Pharaoh) Tomb. Thus, this plant used to be cultivated at least 3,000 years ago. In Turkey, a Hittite bottle dating back to the second millennium before the Common Era was found to contain seed. It's possible that people in the Old World exploited black seed as a seasoning or condiment in their cuisine. In his book "Canon of Medicine," the Muslim Persian physician Avicenna outlined the use of black seeds as a therapy for dyspnea (breathing problem). In the Mideast, black seeds were traditionally employed in the practice of medicine [81, 82]. The black seed plant is an annual floral shrub that is native to Southern Europe, North Africa, and Southwest Asia. It is a member of the Ranunculaceae family of plants. The area surrounding the Mediterranean Sea in the Mideast, Southern Europe, Northern India, Pakistan, Syria, Turkey, Iran, and Saudi Arabia are a few of the places that grow black seed. Its seeds and the oil that is extracted from them are used both as nutrition and medicine in Indian and Arabian countries [83, 84].

Phytoconstituents of Black Seeds (Nagilla sativa)

The overall composition of *N. sativa* seeds contains oils ranging from 32 to 40%. *N. sativa* oil includes linoleic acid, oleic acid, palmitic acid, and trans-anethole, in addition to other minor ingredients such as nigellicine, nigellidine, nigellimine, and nigellimine N-oxide. Aromatics include thymoquinone, dihydrothymoquinone, p-cymene, carvacrol, a-thujene, thymol, -pinene, -pinene, and trans-anethole and different types of alkaloids, *i.e.* isoquinoline alkaloids (*e.g.* nigellicimine and nigellicimine-N-oxide) and pyrazole alkaloids (*e.g.* nigellidine and nigellicine) (Fig. **5**). The seeds include traces of protein in addition to a number of other alkaloids. Also contains a good amount of various vitamins and minerals like Cu, P, Zn, and Fe [85 - 87].

Biological Activity of Black Seeds

In multiple traditional herbal medicine systems, black cumin, also known as *Nigella sativa*, is used to treat a wide range of disease conditions. In traditional Moroccan therapy, the therapy for gestational diabetes often involves the use of black seeds. Many studies have also been performed to examine their potential effectiveness [87]. According to (Sahebkar, *et al* [88, 89], black seeds have a quick effect on decreasing arterial blood pressure and its different extracts may also decrease LDL, triglycerides, and total cholesterol. While the medicinal properties of this seed are all too well known to us, however, it has not been studied systematically focusing on one aspect of disease on a large number of people to establish its efficacy. Clearly, all such studies must titrate the quantity of the seed or its extracts to be used for a given diseased condition. The quantity of black seed used as a food additive will vary when the same is used as medicine. The following diagrammatic illustration highlights its overall application in different conditions (Fig. **6**).

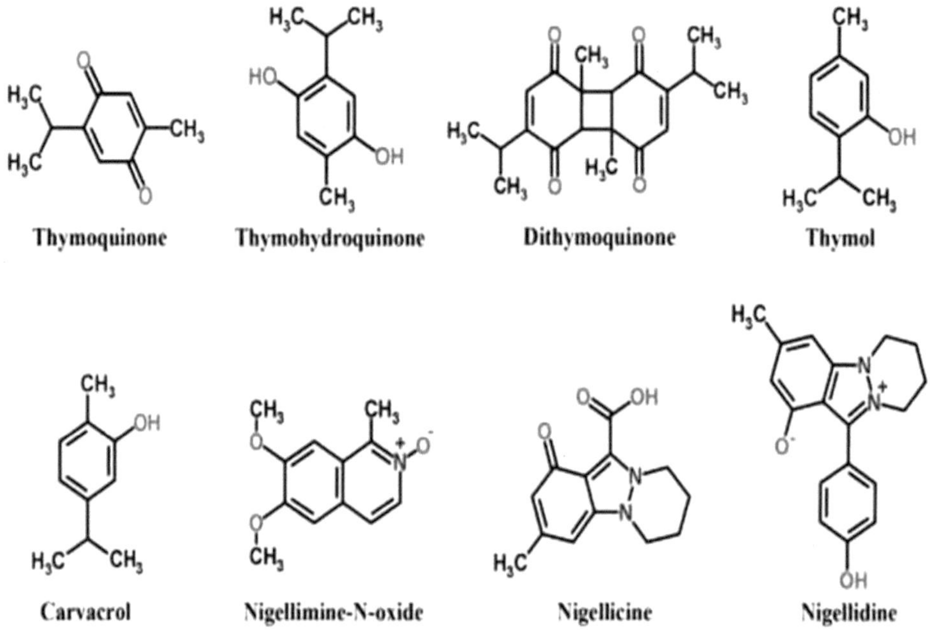

Fig. (5). The major bioactive compound of black seeds [67]

Anti-diabetic Effects

As part of indigenous herbal remedies, black seeds have long been used to control Type-1 diabetes. According to the report, defatted black seed extract increases glucose-induced insulin release from the isolated rat pancreatic cells *in-vitro* [90]. The anti-diabetic activities of *Nigella sativa* seeds may positively be predicted by the activation of insulin production, particularly by the basic sub-fraction of a seed. Over the course of two months, diabetic animals given *Nigella sativa* extracts by mouth had less lipid peroxidation, a stronger antioxidant defense system, and no liver disease caused by lipid peroxidation [91]. However, such observation has not been brought to the forefront to make it useful for humans in actual diabetic conditions. Thus, the actual success rate of using *Nigella sativa* seeds to cure type-1 diabetes needs to be fully established. This calls for some serious in-depth study to be able to bring it to a logical conclusion. In addition, persons suffering from kidney problems are advised to be careful using the *Nigella sativa* extracts. This aspect too needs to be researched before drawing a conclusion.

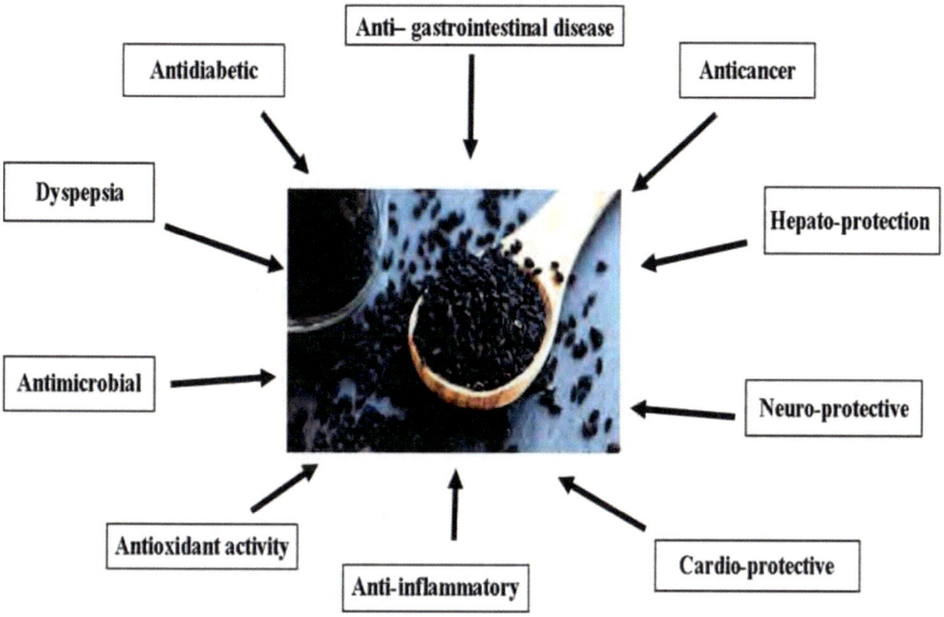

Fig. (6). Diagrammatic illustration showing medicinal properties of black seed.

Ameliorative Effects

It is well-established that dyslipidemia is a risk factor for ischemic heart disease. *Nigella sativa* has been used for the treatment of hypercholesterolemia and for a therapeutic target [92]. In clinical trials, the use of black seeds as a supplement to traditional hypo-lipidemic and hypoglycemic drugs was found to be more effective in addressing the aforementioned conditions. The lipid-lowering actions of seed extract can be attributed, in part, to a reduction of blood cholesterol absorption, a reduction in hepatic cholesterol production, and an up-regulation of LDL receptors. Therefore, clinical trials indicated that black seeds are an efficacious natural solution for those suffering from dyslipidemia [87].

Anti-inflammatory

The treatment of acetic acid, formalin, and mild tail flick tests revealed that the essential oil of black seeds caused a considerable analgesic effect. In a recent article, the anti-nociceptive and anti-inflammatory properties of black seeds provide credence to the general perception that these seeds are powerful analgesic and anti-inflammatory agents [93].

Antioxidant and Anti-cancer Activity

Antioxidants are plant-based substances that help in protecting the cells against damage from unstable radicals known as free radicals that are abundant in black seed oil. Antioxidants are essential for good wellness since they decrease inflammation and protect against cancer, Alzheimer's, and cardiovascular diseases. Specifically, black seed oil is rich in thymoquinone, a compound with powerful anti-oxidative and anti-inflammatory properties. Thus, research has shown that this substance may help the brain work better or help cure different kinds of tumors [94]. Several *in vitro* and *in vivo* models have examined the potential anti-cancer effects of black seeds. Slightly different cancer cells and cancer cell lines have been shown to be sensitive to the antioxidant, anti-mutagenic, cytotoxic, pro-apoptotic, anti-proliferative, and anti-metastatic properties of black seeds [95].

Gastro-protective Activity

Recently, *Nigella sativa* has been found to prevent and cure gastric ulcers [96]. Black seeds greatly improved stomach ulcers caused by chronic granulomatous substances by reducing the overall gastric wall mucus content and gastric mucosal non-protein sulfhydryl concentration. Its anti-ulcer activity is mediated by its anti-secretion and antioxidant actions [97]. Therefore, it decreased both the prevalence of diarrhea and body weight loss improving bleeding ulcer injury [98]. Further, it was discovered that glutathione concentrations increased while myeloperoxidase and malondialdehyde levels decreased significantly in the colon [99].

Nephro and Hepatoprotectivity

The liver is one of the most essential parts of the human body. It filters out toxins, breaks down substances, breaks down food, and makes protein molecules and chemical substances that are essential for health. A few potential animal research studies have discovered that black seed may help maintain the liver from damage [100]. In one investigation, a harmful substance was administered to rats with or without black seed. The black seed made the substance less dangerous and stopped it from hurting the kidneys and liver. The effects of black seed were due to its powerful antioxidants and its capacity to reduce inflammation and oxidative stress [87].

Anti-asthmatic Activity

Asthmatic patients frequently use natural remedies as one of the primary complementary and alternative medicine treatments [101]. Also, there isn't always enough evidence to prove that these medicines work for asthma. Studies in people with asthma have looked at the preventative effects of black seed extract (15 ml/kg of 0.1 g% boiling extract for 3 months). Therapy with black seed improved most measures of asthmatic symptoms, such as the prevalence of respiratory problems, chest coughing, *etc* [102]. Black seed therapy has been reported to decrease inflammatory pulmonary actions, leading researchers to believe that black seeds may have a protective impact on chronic respiratory system damage in animals following pulmonary aspiration [103]. If so, this approach may be used against lung fibrosis following COVID-19 infection. In COVID-19 patients, during follow-up studies, such lung fibrosis was dissolved by repurposing several anticancer drugs [104].

CONCLUSION

Home remedies like honey Ajwain, and black seeds have a long history of their use in Ayurveda and have been frequently used for treatment. Home remedies are an excellent source of water, protein, carbs, fat, minerals, fiber, calcium, phosphorus, iron, carotene, thiamine, riboflavin, and niacin are easily accessible. In addition, it has a high concentration of carotene. Natural compounds are responsible for a broad selection of biological activities, which are produced by both the chemical composition of the product and the existence of a number of different elements. Thus, the use of herbal drugs may be encouraged as an alternative source of the human health care system.

REFERENCES

[1] SARS: clinical trials on treatment using a combination of traditional Chinese medicine and western medicine. Geneva: WHO 2003; pp. 53-61.

[2] WHO traditional medicine strategy 2002–20052. Geneva: WHO 2002.

[3] Zamiska N. On the trail of ancient cures. Wall Str j 2006; B1-B12.

[4] Emanuel EJ, Wendler D, Killen J, Grady C. What makes clinical research in developing countries ethical? The benchmarks of ethical research. J Infect Dis 2004; 189(5): 930-7. [http://dx.doi.org/10.1086/381709] [PMID: 14976611]

[5] Atanasov AG, Waltenberger B, Pferschy-Wenzig EM, *et al.* Discovery and resupply of pharmacologically active plant-derived natural products: A review. Biotechnol Adv 2015; 33(8): 1582-614. [http://dx.doi.org/10.1016/j.biotechadv.2015.08.001] [PMID: 26281720]

[6] Nunn J. Ancient Egyptian Medicine. 2002.

[7] Unschuld P. Nature, Knowledge, Imagery in an Ancient Chinese Medical Text. University of California Press 2003; p. 286.

[8] Raphael S, Blunt W. The Illustrated herbal. London: Frances Lincoln 1994.

[9] Fahd T. Botany and agricultureEncyclopedia of the History of Arabic Science. Routledge 1996; p. 815.

[10] Anthony G, Glenn WM, Salvatore S. The Classical Tradition. Harvard University Press 2010.

[11] WHO Quality Control Methods for Herbal Materials. Geneva, Switzerland: World Health Organization 2011.

[12] Herbal medicinal products. European Medicines Agency 2011 .

[13] Kala CP. Preserving Ayurvedic herbal formulations by Vaidyas: The traditional healers of the Uttaranchal Himalaya region in India. HerbalGram 2006; 70: 42-50.

[14] Kala CP. Health traditions of Buddhist community and role of amchis in trans-Himalayan region of India. Curr Sci 2005; 89(8): 1331-8.

[15] Petrovska B. Historical review of medicinal plants' usage. Pharmacogn Rev 2012; 6(11): 1-5. [http://dx.doi.org/10.4103/0973-7847.95849] [PMID: 22654398]

[16] Semwal DK, Chauhan A, Mishra S, Semwal R. Ayurvedic research and methodology: Present status and future strategies. Ayu 2015; 36(4): 364-9. [http://dx.doi.org/10.4103/0974-8520.190699] [PMID: 27833362]

[17] Shilpa S, Venkatesha Murthy CG. Understanding personality from Ayurvedic perspective for psychological assessment: A case. Ayu 2011; 32(1): 12-9. [http://dx.doi.org/10.4103/0974-8520.85716] [PMID: 22131752]

[18] Semwal DK, Chauhan A, Mishra S, Semwal R. Ayurvedic research and methodology: Present status and future strategies. Ayu 2015; 36(4): 364-9. [http://dx.doi.org/10.4103/0974-8520.190699] [PMID: 27833362]

[19] Boslaugh S. The SAGE Encyclopedia of Pharmacology and Society. SAGE Publications 2015; p. 2492.

[20] National Institute of Siddha Chennai, India: NIS, Chennai. 2010.

[21] Britannica T. Siddha medicine. 2017. Available from: https://www.britannica.com/science/Siddha-medicine

[22] Jaiswal YS, Williams LL. A glimpse of Ayurveda – The forgotten history and principles of Indian traditional medicine. J Tradit Complement Med 2017; 7(1): 50-3. [http://dx.doi.org/10.1016/j.jtcme.2016.02.002] [PMID: 28053888]

[23] Joseph TJ. Siddha medicine--background and principles and the application for skin diseases. Clin Dermatol 2018; 26(1): 62-78. [http://dx.doi.org/10.1016/j.clindermatol.2007.11.010]

[24] Talwar S, Sood S, Kumar J, Chauhan R, Sharma M, Tuli HS. Ayurveda and allopathic therapeutic strategies in coronavirus pandemic treatment 2020. Curr Pharmacol Rep 2020; 6(6): 354-63. [http://dx.doi.org/10.1007/s40495-020-00245-2] [PMID: 33106765]

[25] Unani Medicine in India during 1901–1947 by Hakim Syed Zillur Rahman, Studies in History of Medicine and Science. IHMMR, New Delhi 1994; 8(1): 97-112.

[26] Alam Z. Herbal Medicines. APH 2008; pp. 13-5.

[27] Unani". Department of Ayurveda, Yoga and Naturopathy, Unani, Siddha and Homoeopathy, Govt. of India. 2007.

[28] Ahmad H, Sofi GD, Tajuddin T, Raman D, Kumar N. Unani system of medicine - introduction and challenges. Med J Islamic World Acad Sci 2010; 18(1): 27-30.

[29] Masic I, Miokovic M, Muhamedagic B. Evidence based medicine - new approaches and challenges. Acta Inform Med 2008; 16(4): 219-25. [http://dx.doi.org/10.5455/aim.2008.16.219-225] [PMID: 24109156]

[30] Frank R. Health in Europe. Nürnberg: GfK Nürnberg Gesellschaft für Konsumforschung e.v.: European Consumer Study 2007; 2: pp. 1-4.

[31] Parisius LM, Stock-Schröer B, Berger S, Hermann K, Joos S. Use of home remedies: A cross-sectional survey of patients in Germany. BMC Fam Pract 2014; 15(1): 116. [http://dx.doi.org/10.1186/1471-2296-15-116] [PMID: 24916173]

[32] Dashora N, Sodde V, Bhagat J, Kirti SP, Labo R. Antitumor activity of Dendrophoe falcate against Ehrlich ascites carcinoma in Swiss albino mice. Pharm Crop 2011; 2(1): 1-7. [http://dx.doi.org/10.2174/2210290601102010001]

[33] Bell SG. The therapeutic use of honey. Neonatal Netw 2007; 26(4): 247-51. [http://dx.doi.org/10.1891/0730-0832.26.4.247] [PMID: 17710959]

[34] Babacan S, Rand AG. Characterization of honey amylase. J Food Sci 2007; 72(1): C050-5. [http://dx.doi.org/10.1111/j.1750-3841.2006.00215.x] [PMID: 17995872]

[35] Hassapidou M, Fotiadou E, Maglara E, Papadopoulou SK. Energy intake, diet composition, energy expenditure, and body fatness of adolescents in Northern Greece. Obesity 2006; 14: 855-62. 8.. [http://dx.doi.org/10.1038/oby.2006.99]

[36] Pataca L, Neto W, Marcucci M, Poppi R. Determination of apparent reducing sugars, moisture and acidity in honey by attenuated total reflectance-Fourier transform infrared spectrometry. Talanta 2007; 71(5): 1926-31. [http://dx.doi.org/10.1016/j.talanta.2006.08.028] [PMID: 19071543]

[37] Samarghandian S, Farkhondeh T, Samini F. Honey and health: A review of recent clinical research. Pharmacognosy Res 2017; 9(2): 121-7. [PMID: 28539734]

[38] Abdulrhman M, El-Hefnawy M, Ali R, El-Goud AA. Honey and type 1 diabetes mellitus. In: Liu CP, Ed. Type 1 Diabetes – Complications, Pathogenesis, and Alternative Treatments Croatia: In Tech. 2008; p. 16.

[39] Ghosh S, Playford RJ. Bioactive natural compounds for the treatment of gastrointestinal disorders. Clin Sci 2003; 104(6): 547-56. [http://dx.doi.org/10.1042/CS20030067] [PMID: 12641494]

[40] Molan PC. The potential of honey to promote oral wellness. Gen Dent 2001; 49: 584-9.20.

[41] Samarghandian S, Farkhondeh T, Samini F. Honey and health: A review of recent clinical research. Pharmacognosy Res 2017; 9(2): 121-7. [PMID: 28539734]

[42] Bergman A, Yanai J, Weiss J, Bell D, David MP. Acceleration of wound healing by topical application of honey. Am J Surg 1983; 145(3): 374-6. [http://dx.doi.org/10.1016/0002-9610(83)90204-0] [PMID: 6837863]

[43] Irving TB, Ahmad K, Ahsan MM. The story of creation The Qur'an-Basic Teachings. Bath: Pitman Press 1987.

[44] Lay-flurrie K. Honey in wound care: Effects, clinical application and patient benefit. Br J Nurs 2008; 17(S5): S30-S36, S32-S36. [http://dx.doi.org/10.12968/bjon.2008.17.Sup5.29649] [PMID: 18773594]

[45] Betts J. The clinical application of honey in wound care. Nurs Times 2008; 104(14): 43-4.

[PMID: 18497240]

[46] Samarghandian S, Farkhondeh T, Samini F. Honey and health: A review of recent clinical research. Pharmacognosy Res 2017; 9(2): 121-7.
[PMID: 28539734]

[47] Iglesias MT, de Lorenzo C, Polo MC, Martín-Álvarez PJ, Pueyo E. Usefulness of amino acid composition to discriminate between honeydew and floral honeys. Application to honeys from a small geographic area. J Agric Food Chem 2004; 52(1): 84-9.
[http://dx.doi.org/10.1021/jf030454q] [PMID: 14709017]

[48] Zand RSR, Jenkins DJA, Diamandis EP. Steroid hormone activity of flavonoids and related compounds. Breast Cancer Res Treat 2000; 62(1): 35-49.
[http://dx.doi.org/10.1023/A:1006422302173] [PMID: 10989984]

[49] Kyselova Z. Toxicological aspects of the use of phenolic compounds in disease prevention. Interdiscip Toxicol 2011; 4(4): 173-83.
[http://dx.doi.org/10.2478/v10102-011-0027-5] [PMID: 22319251]

[50] Beretta G, Orioli M, Facino R. Antioxidant and radical scavenging activity of honey in endothelial cell cultures (EA.hy926). Planta Med 2007; 73(11): 1182-9.
[http://dx.doi.org/10.1055/s-2007-981598] [PMID: 17823875]

[51] Nisbet HO, Nisbet C, Yarim M, Guler A, Ozak A. Effects of three types of honey on cutaneous wound healing. Wounds 2010; 22(11): 275-83.
[PMID: 25901517]

[52] Helmy N, El-Soud A. Honey between traditional uses and recent medicine. Maced J Med Sci 2012; 5: 205-14.

[53] Pérez RA, Iglesias MT, Pueyo E, González M, de Lorenzo C. Amino acid composition and antioxidant capacity of Spanish honeys. J Agric Food Chem 2007; 55(2): 360-5.
[http://dx.doi.org/10.1021/jf062055b] [PMID: 17227066]

[54] Han DH, Denison MS, Tachibana H, Yamada K. Relationship between estrogen receptor-binding and estrogenic activities of environmental estrogens and suppression by flavonoids. Biosci Biotechnol Biochem 2002; 66(7): 1479-87.
[http://dx.doi.org/10.1271/bbb.66.1479] [PMID: 12224631]

[55] Pérez RA, Iglesias MT, Pueyo E, González M, de Lorenzo C. Amino acid composition and antioxidant capacity of Spanish honeys. J Agric Food Chem 2007; 55(2): 360-5.
[http://dx.doi.org/10.1021/jf062055b] [PMID: 17227066]

[56] Gheldof N, Wang XH, Engeseth NJ. Buckwheat honey increases serum antioxidant capacity in humans. J Agric Food Chem 2003; 51(5): 1500-5.
[http://dx.doi.org/10.1021/jf025897t] [PMID: 12590505]

[57] Candiracci M, Piatti E, Dominguez-Barragán M, *et al.* Anti-inflammatory activity of a honey flavonoid extract on lipopolysaccharide-activated N13 microglial cells. J Agric Food Chem 2012; 60(50): 12304-11.
[http://dx.doi.org/10.1021/jf302468h] [PMID: 23176387]

[58] Leong AG, Herst PM, Harper JL. Indigenous New Zealand honeys exhibit multiple anti-inflammatory activities. Innate Immun 2012; 18(3): 459-66.
[http://dx.doi.org/10.1177/1753425911422263] [PMID: 21978989]

[59] Schley PD, Field CJ. The immune-enhancing effects of dietary fibres and prebiotics. 2002; 87(S2): S221-30. 77.

[60] Chepulis LM. The effect of honey compared to sucrose, mixed sugars, and a sugar-free diet on weight gain in young rats. J Food Sci 2007; 72(3): S224-9.
[http://dx.doi.org/10.1111/j.1750-3841.2007.00286.x] [PMID: 17995819]

[61] Eteraf-Oskouei T, Najafi M. Traditional and modern uses of natural honey in human diseases: A review. Iran J Basic Med Sci 2013; 16(6): 731-42.
[PMID: 23997898]

[62] Chauhan B, Kumar G, Ali M. Composition of volatile oil of Carum copticum benth and hook fruits. Int J Res Ayurveda Pharm 2012; 3(7): 131-2.

[63] Singh G, Maurya S, Catalan C, de Lampasona MP. Chemical constituents, antifungal and antioxidative effects of ajwain essential oil and its acetone extract. J Agric Food Chem 2004; 52(11): 3292-6.
[http://dx.doi.org/10.1021/jf035211c] [PMID: 15161185]

[64] Süntar I, Küpeli Akkol E, Tosun A, Keleş H. Comparative pharmacological and phytochemical investigation on the wound-healing effects of the frequently used essential oils. J Essent Oil Res 2014; 26(1): 41-9.
[http://dx.doi.org/10.1080/10412905.2013.820672]

[65] Zule J, Tisler V, Zurej A, Torelli N. Isolation and characterization of essential oils from the cones of Norway Spruce (Picea abies Karst.), European Larch (Larix decidua Mill.) and Scots Pine (Pinus sylvestris). Zborniku Gozdarstva in Lesar 2003; 71: 159-72.

[66] Anwar S, Ahmed N, Sofiane H, Yousef A. Essential Oils in Food Preservation, Flavor and Safety || Ajwain (Trachyspermum ammi L). Oils 2016; pp. 181-92.
[http://dx.doi.org/10.1016/B978-0-12-416641-7.00019-5]

[67] Bahuguna A, Ramalingam S, Arumugam A, Natarajan D, Kim M. Molecular and in silico evidences explain the anti-inflammatory effect of Trachyspermum ammi essential oil in lipopolysaccharide induced macrophages. Process Biochem 2020; 96: 138-45.
[http://dx.doi.org/10.1016/j.procbio.2020.06.006]

[68] Singh G, Maurya S, Catalan C, de Lampasona MP. Chemical constituents, antifungal and antioxidative effects of ajwain essential oil and its acetone extract. J Agric Food Chem 2004; 52(11): 3292-6.
[http://dx.doi.org/10.1021/jf035211c] [PMID: 15161185]

[69] Zahin M, Ahmad I, Aqil F. Antioxidant and antimutagenic activity of Carum copticum fruit extracts. Toxicol In Vitro 2010; 24(4): 1243-9.
[http://dx.doi.org/10.1016/j.tiv.2010.02.004] [PMID: 20149861]

[70] Anwar S, Ahmed N, Sofiane H, Yousef A. Essential Oils in Food Preservation, Flavor and Safety || Ajwain (Trachyspermum ammi L). Oils 2016; pp. 181-92.
[http://dx.doi.org/10.1016/B978-0-12-416641-7.00019-5]

[71] Jafarpour M, Golparvar AR, Lotfi A. Antibacterial activity of essential oils from Thymus vulgaris, Trachyspermum ammi and Mentha aquatic against Erwinia carotovora *in vitro*. J Herb Drugs 2013; 4(3): 115-8.

[72] Ahmad A, Khan A, Akhtar F, *et al.* Fungicidal activity of thymol and carvacrol by disrupting ergosterol biosynthesis and membrane integrity against Candida. Eur J Clin Microbiol Infect Dis 2011; 30(1): 41-50.
[http://dx.doi.org/10.1007/s10096-010-1050-8] [PMID: 20835742]

[73] Bajpai KV, Agrawal P. Studies on phytochemicals, antioxidant, free radical scavenging and lipid peroxidation inhibitory effects of Trachyspermum ammi seeds. Pharm Res 2015; 49(1): 58-65.

[74] Goswami N, Chatterjee S. Assessment of free radical scavenging potential and oxidative DNA damage preventive activity of Trachyspermum ammi L. (carom) and Foeniculum vulgare Mill. (fennel) seed extracts. BioMed Res Int 2014; 2014: 1-8.
[http://dx.doi.org/10.1155/2014/582767] [PMID: 25143939]

[75] Bairwa R, Rajawat BS, Sodha RS. Trachyspermum ammi. Pharmacogn Rev 2012; 6(11): 56-60.
[http://dx.doi.org/10.4103/0973-7847.95871] [PMID: 22654405]

[76] Chahal KK, Dhaiwal K, Kumar A, Kataria D, Singla N. Chemical composition of Trachyspermum

ammi L. and its biological properties: A review. J Pharmacogn Phytochem 2017; 6(3): 131-40.

[77] Gilani AH, Jabeen Q, Ghayur MN, Janbaz KH, Akhtar MS. Studies on the antihypertensive, antispasmodic, bronchodilator and hepatoprotective activities of the Carum copticum seed extract. J Ethnopharmacol 2005; 98(1-2): 127-35. [http://dx.doi.org/10.1016/j.jep.2005.01.017] [PMID: 15763373]

[78] Bairwa R, Rajawat BS, Sodha RS. Trachyspermum ammi. Pharmacogn Rev 2012; 6(11): 56-60. [http://dx.doi.org/10.4103/0973-7847.95871] [PMID: 22654405]

[79] Ramaswamy S, Sengottuvelu S, Haja Sherief S, Jaikumar S, Saravanan R, Prasadkumar C. Gastroprotective activity of ethanolic extract of trachyspermum ammi fruit. Int J Pharm Biosci 2010; 1: 1-15.

[80] Jabbar A, Iqbal Z, Khan MN. *In vitro* anthelmintic activity of Trachyspermum ammi seeds. Pharmacogn Mag 2006; 2: 126-9.

[81] Salih B, Sipahi T, Dönmez EO. Ancient nigella seeds from Boyalı Höyük in north-central Turkey. J Ethnopharmacol 2009; 124(3): 416-20. [http://dx.doi.org/10.1016/j.jep.2009.05.039] [PMID: 19505557]

[82] Hassanien MMM, Abdel-Razek AG, Rudzińska M, Siger A, Ratusz K, Przybylski R. Phytochemical contents and oxidative stability of oils from non-traditional sources. Eur J Lipid Sci Technol 2014; 116(11): 1563-71. [http://dx.doi.org/10.1002/ejlt.201300475]

[83] Yarnell E, Abascal K. *Nigella sativa*: Holy herb of the Middle East. Altern Complement Ther 2011; 17(2): 99-105. [http://dx.doi.org/10.1089/act.2011.17203]

[84] Kalonji. Drugscom. 2011 .

[85] Boskabady MH, Shirmohammadi B. Effect of *Nigella sativa* on isolated guinea pig trachea. Arch Iran Med 2002; 5: 103-7.

[86] Nickavar B, Mojab F, Javidnia K, Amoli MAR. Chemical composition of the fixed and volatile oils of *Nigella sativa* L. from Iran. Z Naturforsch C J Biosci 2003; 58(9-10): 629-31. [http://dx.doi.org/10.1515/znc-2003-9-1004] [PMID: 14577620]

[87] Srinivasan K. Cumin (Cuminum cyminum) and black cumin (Nigella sativa) seeds: Traditional uses, chemical constituents, and nutraceutical effects. Food Quality Safety 2018; pp. 1-6. [http://dx.doi.org/10.1093/fqsafe/fyx031]

[88] Sahebkar A, Soranna D, Liu X, *et al.* A systematic review and meta-analysis of randomized controlled trials investigating the effects of supplementation with *Nigella sativa* (black seed) on blood pressure. J Hypertens 2016; 34(11): 2127-35. a [http://dx.doi.org/10.1097/HJH.0000000000001049] [PMID: 27512971]

[89] Sahebkar A, Beccuti G, Simental-Mendía LE, Nobili V, Bo S. *Nigella sativa* (black seed) effects on plasma lipid concentrations in humans: A systematic review and meta-analysis of randomized placebo-controlled trials. Pharmacol Res 2016; 106: 37-50. b [http://dx.doi.org/10.1016/j.phrs.2016.02.008] [PMID: 26875640]

[90] Rchid H, Chevassus H, Nmila R, *et al.* *Nigella sativa* seed extracts enhance glucose-induced insulin release from rat-isolated Langerhans islets. Fundam Clin Pharmacol 2004; 18(5): 525-9. [http://dx.doi.org/10.1111/j.1472-8206.2004.00275.x] [PMID: 15482373]

[91] Meral I, Yener Z, Kahraman T, Mert N. Effect of *Nigella sativa* on glucose concentration, lipid peroxidation, anti-oxidant defence system and liver damage in experimentally-induced diabetic rabbits. J Vet Med A Physiol Pathol Clin Med 2001; 48(10): 593-9. [http://dx.doi.org/10.1046/j.1439-0442.2001.00393.x] [PMID: 11848252]

[92] Asgary S, Sahebkar A, Goli-malekabadi N. Ameliorative effects of *Nigella sativa* on dyslipidemia. J

Endocrinol Invest 2015; 38(10): 1039-46.
[http://dx.doi.org/10.1007/s40618-015-0337-0] [PMID: 26134064]

[93] Amin B, Hosseinzadeh H. Black cumin (*Nigella sativa*) and its active constituent, thymoquinone: An overview on the analgesic and anti-inflammatory effects. Planta Med 2016; 82(1-2): 8-16.
[PMID: 26366755]

[94] Majdalawieh AF, Fayyad MW. Recent advances on the anti-cancer properties of *Nigella sativa*, a widely used food additive. J Ayurveda Integr Med 2016; 7(3): 173-80.
[http://dx.doi.org/10.1016/j.jaim.2016.07.004] [PMID: 27649635]

[95] Salim E. Cancer chemopreventive potential of volatile oil from black cumin seeds, *Nigella sativa* L., in a rat multi-organ carcinogenesis bioassay. Oncol Lett 2010; 1(5): 913-24.
[http://dx.doi.org/10.3892/ol_00000162] [PMID: 22966405]

[96] Khan SA, Khan AM, Karim S, Kamal MA, Damanhouri GA, Mirza Z. Panacea seed "Nigella": A review focusing on regenerative effects for gastric ailments. Saudi J Biol Sci 2016; 23(4): 542-53.
[http://dx.doi.org/10.1016/j.sjbs.2014.10.001] [PMID: 27298589]

[97] Al Mofleh I, Alhaider A, Mossa J, *et al.* Gastroprotective effect of an aqueous suspension of black cumin *Nigella sativa* on necrotizing agents-induced gastric injury in experimental animals. Saudi J Gastroenterol 2008; 14(3): 128-34.
[http://dx.doi.org/10.4103/1319-3767.41731] [PMID: 19568521]

[98] Lei X, Liu M, Yang Z, Ji M, Guo X, Dong W. Thymoquinone prevents and ameliorates dextran sulfate sodium-induced colitis in mice. Dig Dis Sci 2012; 57(9): 2296-303.
[http://dx.doi.org/10.1007/s10620-012-2156-x] [PMID: 22476588]

[99] Lei X, Lv X, Liu M, *et al.* Thymoquinone inhibits growth and augments 5-fluorouracil-induced apoptosis in gastric cancer cells both *in vitro* and *in vivo.* Biochem Biophys Res Commun 2012; 417(2): 864-8.
[http://dx.doi.org/10.1016/j.bbrc.2011.12.063] [PMID: 22206670]

[100] Saleem U, Ahmad B, Rehman K, Mahmood S, Alam M, Erum A. Nephro-protective effect of vitamin C and *Nigella sativa* oil on gentamicin associated nephrotoxicity in rabbits. Pak J Pharm Sci 2012; 25(4): 727-30.
[PMID: 23009987]

[101] Slader CA, Reddel HK, Jenkins CR, Armour CL, Bosnic-Anticevich SZ. Complementary and alternative medicine use in asthma: Who is using what? Respirology 2006; 11(4): 373-87.
[http://dx.doi.org/10.1111/j.1440-1843.2006.00861.x] [PMID: 16771907]

[102] Boskabady MH, Javan H, Sajady M, Rakhshandeh H. The possible prophylactic effect of *Nigella sativa* seed extract in asthmatic patients. Fundam Clin Pharmacol 2007; 21(5): 559-66.
[http://dx.doi.org/10.1111/j.1472-8206.2007.00509.x] [PMID: 17868210]

[103] Kanter M. Effects of *Nigella sativa* seed extract on ameliorating lung tissue damage in rats after experimental pulmonary aspirations. Acta Histochem 2009; 111(5): 393-403.
[http://dx.doi.org/10.1016/j.acthis.2008.10.008] [PMID: 19428057]

[104] Hangargekar CB, Quazi RS, Khan MS, Joshi A, Hangargekar PB. A Review on Kalonji (*Nigella Sativa*): A Seed Of Blessing. 2020; 4(9)

CHAPTER 16

Phytoconstituents and their Therapeutic Potential in Precision Medicine

Robeena Sarah[1], **Nida Idrees**[1] and **Baby Tabassum**[1,*]

[1] *Toxicology, Lab, Department of Zoology, Govt Raza P.G. College, Rampur- (U.P.) 244901, M.J.P. Rohilkhand University, Bareilly, (U.P.) 243005, India*

Abstract: Spices and herbs have been an integral part of Indian cuisine since ancient times. They are not only cherished for improving the flavor and taste of Indian food but also confer their health benefits. Instant herbal remedies prepared from spices and herbs found in the kitchens of Indian homes have been used to treat many ailments and infections in a natural way. Most of the spices and herbs have high nutritional and anti-oxidant properties responsible for their medicinal effects. This is because of the presence of phytochemicals in the plants. The emphasis of the current article is to provide an overview of the therapeutic potentials elucidating the phytochemical compositions of the key Indian plants. Many such plant products are used mainly as spices in Indian cuisine. In this review, we aim to highlight the chemical constituents and active factors of some of these spices and their pharmacological potential. We believe that in-depth molecular characterization of these spices for all their chemical constituents and their impact on cells, organs, and different organelles will provide a wealth of information useful for human health. These findings may further be chiseled in the form of personalized medicine.

Keywords: Indian Spices, nutritional values, personalized medicine, phytochemicals, therapeutic properties.

INTRODUCTION

Life without spices is dull and insecure because spices are known to regulate gut microbiomes. Spices are the aromatic components of plants, such as seeds, stalks, bark or flowers. They are hardly used in fresh form but frequently used in the dried form. Due to their exceptional medicinal value in traditional therapies, they are regarded as safe, reliable, affordable, and are efficient against a wide range of illnesses and ailments. Depending on their composition, different spices exhibit varying amounts of anti-bacterial and anti-oxidant activity, making them powerful scavengers of free radicals and fighters against microorganisms.

* **Corresponding author Baby Tabassum:** Toxicology Laboratory, Department of Zoology, Government Raza PG College, Rampur-244901 UP, India; Tel: 9456677015; E-mail: dr.btabassum@gmail.com

Farzana Mahdi & Abbas Ali Mahdi (Eds.)

As a result, they are referred to as "Potent therapeutic agents" [1, 2].

Flavonoids and phenols are known to act as primary anti-oxidants that can scavenge free radicals and strengthen the immune system. Alkaloids richly present in the spices are beneficial as they impart anti-rheumatic, anti-cancerous, and anti-spasmodic activity. While these properties are well documented in the context of human health, what still remains unknown is the precise quantity of these plant derivatives to be given to the patients. Since each patient is unique owing to genome heterogeneity, the herbal formulation needs to be adjusted and readjusted accordingly. This would fulfill the much desired aspirations of personalized medicine augmenting the human health care system in an affordable manner. India claims to have a large number of species in addition to an equally large number of medicinal plants. Some have been characterized whereas others still need to draw the attention of the researchers. Owing to the presence of tannins in the spices mainly in Clove and Ajwain, they exert anti-hemorrhoid and anti-diarrheal activity. The presence of terpenoids in large quantities particularly in Clove, Pepper and Cinnamon enhances the therapeutic properties. Hence they exert antiseptic, diuretic, analgesic, anti-rheumatic and anti-microbial activities [3] (Fig. **1**).

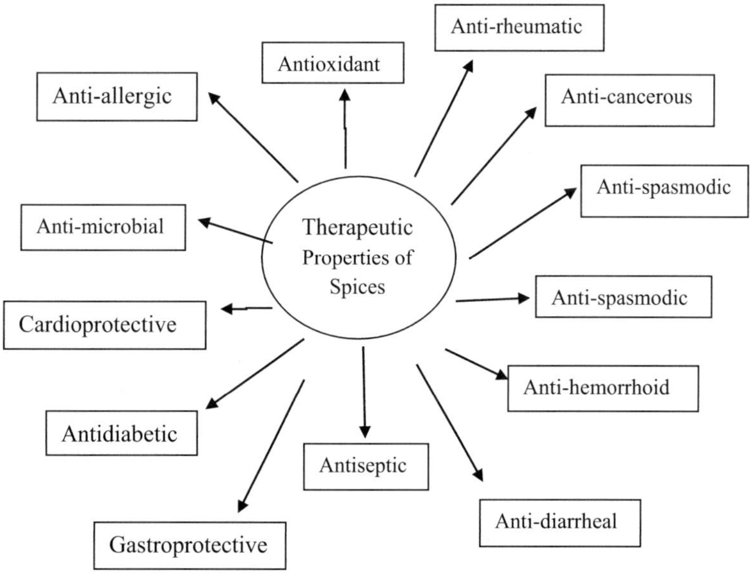

Fig. (1). Therapeutic properties of some common Spices used routinely for culinary preparation.

Consequently, phytochemicals derived from plants are crucial for maintaining human health and preventing disease. Due to the presence of such phytochemicals, spices and herbs have attracted a great deal of attention for their therapeutic and medicinal properties [4, 5] (Table **1**).

Table 1. Medicinal properties of some known spices and their chemical constituents.

S. No.	Name of the Spices	Part Used/ Common Name	Different Chemical constituents	Medicinal Properties	References
1	Turmeric (*Curcuma longa*)	Rhizome/ Haldi	Curcumin	anti-bacterial, anti-inflammatory, hypocholesteremic, anti-histaminic, anti-hepatotoxic, anti-fungal, and anti-arthritic	[6-7]
2	Black Cumin (*Nigella sativa* L.)	Seeds/ Kalonji	thymoquinone (TQ), thymohydroquinone, thymol, carvacrol, nigellidine, nigellicine, and –hederin	anti-oxidant, anti-inflammatory, immunomodulatory, anti-cancer, neuroprotective, anti-microbial, anti-hypertensive, cardioprotective, antidiabetic, gastroprotective, and nephroprotective and hepatoprotective	[8-9]
3	Fenugreek (*T. foenum-graecum*)	Leaves and Seeds/ Methi	Galactomannan,neutrallipids,Steroidalsaponins and alkaloids	Diuretic, galactogogue, anti-microbial, useful in heart diseases, Anti-diabetic, Gastroprotective and Hepatoprotective	[10-11]
4	Cumin (*Cuminumcyminum*)	Seeds/ Zeera	Cumaldehyde, vitamin A, vitamin C, cuminal, cuminicalcohol, γ-Terpinene, Safranal, p-Cymene, volatile oils, and β-Pinene.	Antispasmodic, carminative, digestive stimulant, anti-oxidant, hypocholesterolemic, anti-inflammatory.	[6, 12]
5	Cloves (*Syzgiumaromaticum*)	unopened flower buds/Laung	Caryophyllene, eugenol, salicyclic acid, tannin,, sterols, triterpenes, and flavonoids	Anti-inflammatory, anaesthetic, pain-relieving, anti-viral, anti-fungal, anti-microbial, anti-diabetic, anti-thrombotic, and anti-microbial effects.	[13-15]
6	Cinnamon (*Cinnamomumzylanicum*)	Bark/ Daalcheeni	Cinnamaldehyde, cinnamate, cinnamic acid, and a number of essential oils	Anti-inflammatory, anti-bacterial, anti-fungal, anti-oxidant, and antidiabetic properties and anti-cancer agent.	[16-17]

(Table 1) cont.....

S. No.	Name of the Spices	Part Used/ Common Name	Different Chemical constituents	Medicinal Properties	References
7	Bishop's weed (*Trachyspermumammi*)	Seeds/ Ajwain	Thimol, carvacrol, thymene, vitamin B, and volatile oils	Antispasmodic, anti-inflammatory, anti-diarrheal, stimulant, anticholerin, anti-bronchitis, anti-dyspepsia	[6, 18-20]
8	Fennel (*Foeniculumvulgare*)	Seeds/ Saunf	Anethol, fenchone and estragole	Anti-inflammatory, anti-stress, anti-oxidant, anti-allergic, analgesic, anti-bacterial, anti-cancer, and cytotoxic properties.	[21-23]
9	Garlic (*Allium sativum* L.)	Bulb/ Lehsun	Allcin, allicin, ajoenes, vinyldithiins, and sulfides	Indigestion, respiratory, urinary tract infections and cardiac disorders	[24-25]
10	Bay leaf (*Laurusnobilis*L.)	Leaves/ Tejpatta	1,8 cineole, sabinene, limonene, eugenol, and -pinene.	Anti-diabetic, anti-bacterial, insecticidal, anti-oxidant, and anti-convulsant	[26, 1, 6]
11	Black Pepper (*Piper nigrum*)	Dried seeds/ Kaalimirch	Phenolic compounds, alkaloids, flavonoids such as catechin, quercetin and myricetin, carotenoids, terpenoids	Anti-inflammatory, anti-bacterial, anti-fungal, anti-oxidant, anti-asthmatic effect, anticarcinogenic, gastroprotective	[27]
12	Onion (*Allium cepa*)	Bulb/ Pyaaz	Organosulfur compounds (OSCs), thiosulfinates, polyphenols, including flavonoids like anthocyanins,Kaempferol quercetin and fructooligosaccharides (FOS)	Anti-asthmatic effect, anticarcinogenic, hypocholesterolemic, antibiotic, anti-inflammatory, antiplatelet, antidiabetic, and cardioprotective agent	[28]
13	Nutmeg (*Myristicafragrans*)	fruit: nutmeg (jaiphal) from its seed and mace (javitri) from the covering of seed	Macelignan, carvacrol, myristicin, β-caryophyllene, β-pinene, α-pinene, p-cymene, and eugenol	anti-oxidant, anti-microbial, aphrodisiac, anti-cancer, hepatoprotective, anti-inflammatory, antidepressant, and cardioprotective activity	[29]
14	Cardamom (*Elettariacardamomum*)	capsules of dried fruits/ Elaichi	Flavonoids, terpenoids, anthocyanins, alkaloids and other phenolic constituents	anti-oxidant, antidiabetic, anti-bacterial, anti-cancer, gastro-protective and insecticidal activities	[30]

(Table 1) cont.....

S. No.	Name of the Spices	Part Used/ Common Name	Different Chemical constituents	Medicinal Properties	References
15	Coriander (*Coriandrumsativum*)	Leaves & seeds/ Dhania	Flavonoids, isocoumarins, fatty acids, sterols, and coriandrones, coumarins, catechins, polyphenolic compounds	anti-oxidant, anti-bacterial, anti-fungal, antidiabetic, hepatoprotective, and antihyperlipidemic activities	[31]
16	Sweet Neem (*Murrayakoenigii*)	Leaves/ curry patta	Carbazole alkaloids, essential oils, terpenoids,polyphenols and flavonoids	Anti-oxidative, hepatoprotective, anti-microbial, anti-fungal, anti-inflammatory, and nephroprotective activities	[32]
17	Lemon Grass (*Cymbopogoncitratus*)	Grass/Malabar grass	Limonene, citral, elemol, citronellal, 1,8 cineole, citronellol, linalool, geraniol, methylheptenone, b-carophyllene, geranylformate and geranyl acetic acid derivation	Anti-depressant, analgesic, anti-pyretic, bactericidal, anti-septic, carminative and astringent properties	[33]
18	Mustard seeds (*Brassica juncea*)	Seeds/ Rai, Sarso	Glucosinolates (and their degradation products), polyphenols and volatile components (allylisothiocyanate, 3-butyl isothiocyanate, *etc*.).	Anti-cancer, anti-oxidation, anti-inflammatory, anti-bacterial, anti-virus, anti- obesity, anti-depression, prevention, and treatment of diabetes and cataracts.	[34]
19	Poppy seeds (*Papaversomniferum*)	Seeds/ khash-khash	Alkaloids like morphine, codeine, the bain and porphyroxine, Papaverine, Xanthaline *etc*.	Antiallodynic activity, Analgesics, Antitussive activity, Anti-diarrheal, Antidepressant, Anti-Anxiety, Bronchodilator, anti-bacterial, Narcotic activity	[35]
20	Saffron (*Crocus sativus*)	Dried stigma of flower/ kesar, Zaafran	Safranal, picrocrocin, crocetin and its glycoside, crocins	Antiseptic, antidepressant, digestive, anti-cancer and anti-convulsant activity	[36]

IMPORTANT INDIAN SPICES AND THEIR MEDICINAL VALUES

There are many spices that are commonly used in Indian food and are known for their medicinal properties. Some of the important spices are as follows.

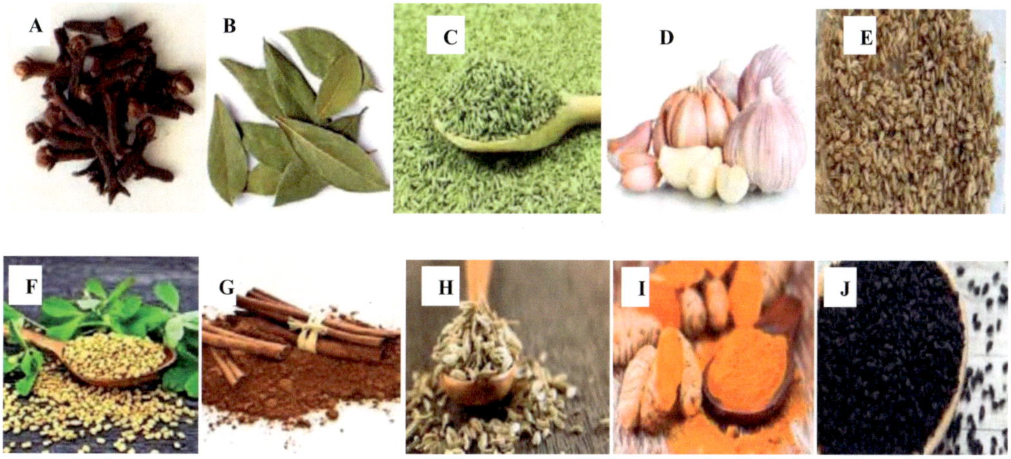

Fig. (2). Some commonly used indian spices: (A) Laung(B) Tejpatta(C) Saunf (D) Lehsun(E) Ajwain(F) Methi (G) Daalcheeni (H) Zeera (I) Haldi (J) Kalonji. It may be noted that these are some examples and they do not represent the entire list.
Fig A. https://bigapplecurry.files.wordpress.com/2012/07/photo-120.jpg?w=293
Fig B. https://m.media-amazon.com/images/I/41RwaQHI6GL.jpg
Fig C. https://ftborgano.b-cdn.net/media/yhcmp4la/green-fennel-saunf-500gm-199-price.jpg
Fig D. https://m.media-amazon.com/images/I/31TIJVPwpuS.jpg
Fig E. https://d36v5spmfzyapc.cloudfront.net/wp-content/uploads/2020/02/ajwain-848x424.png
Fig F. https://cf.organic bazar.net /wp -con tent/up loads/ 20 21/08/U ntit led-des ign- 2022-0 6-02 T1 60309.04 4.jpg
Fig G. https://www.organicherbals.in /wp-cont ent/uplo ads/2020/ 05/Dalchi ni-Daal cheeni-Cin namon-Sticks-Ci nnamomum-zey lanicum-520x574.jpg
Fig H. https://i.ndtvimg.com/i/2018-03/cumin_620x350_51521615731.jpg
Fig I. https://images.indianexpress.com/2020/04/haldi_759.jpg
Fig J. https:// new-img. patri ka.com /cdn-cgi /i mage /widt h=798, fit=cov er, gravity= auto ,forma t= webp,qua lity =100/ht tps: //new-img. patri ka.com/ uplo ad/20 22/02/ 20/kal onji.jpg

Cloves (*Syzgium aromaticum*)

The dried, fragrant, unopened flower buds of the medium-sized evergreen tree are referred to as "laung" in India (Fig. **2A**). It is a member of the Myrataceae family and is native to India, Indonesia, Zanzibar, Mauritius, and Ceylon [37]. The name comes from the words "Clov" and "Clout," both of which imply "nail," in French and English, respectively. The broad-headed nail is similar to cloves. Not only cloves are prized flavouring ingredients, but they are also utilized as scenting agents, oral hygiene products, and breath fresheners.

Due to its anti-bacterial properties, it is able to fight against illnesses including cholera and diarrhea. Cloves can be chewed to lessen nausea and vomiting. Flatulence and gastrointestinal spasms can be relieved by a decoction with water. When it comes to reducing cough, clove oil is a potent expectorant and stimulant. Clove is effective for ear and toothache since it is a "pain-killer spice." In the treatment of rheumatism and arthritis, it has anti-inflammatory properties. Asthma, ulcers, neurological problems, and hypertension can all be cured with cloves [38].

A drop of clove oil has 400 times more anti-oxidant potential per unit than blueberries. The therapeutic properties of cloves are strong, and it has a long tradition and history. Cloves are beneficial for mental, emotional, and physical health. They possess anti-inflammatory, anaesthetic, pain-relieving, anti-viral, anti-fungal, anti-microbial, anti-diabetic, antithrombotic, and anti-microbial effects. One of Mother Nature's most potent antiseptics is cloves. The primary ingredient in clove buds that gives them their therapeutic powers is eugenol. According to global trade, clove is the most significant spice in the world. Clove contains a small number of non-volatile substances, including tannins, sterols, triterpenes, and flavonoids [13]. Its plant contains caryophyllene, eugenol, salicyclic acid, tannin, and vitamin B among its active chemical components. Clove has been discovered to have pharmacological effects that include local anaesthetic, carminative, stimulant, aromatic, analgesic, anti-bacterial, anticonvulsion, and anticarcinogenic effects due to the presence of these active components [14, 15]. In order to evaluate the anti-oxidant ability, namely the protection of polyunsaturated fatty acids in the liver and retina throughout ageing, mice were given clove essential oil [39]. Due to its anti-oxidant capabilities, the clove's eugenol prevents food from getting spoiled. Cloves are utilized as dietary supplements and flavouring agents in meats and baked goods particularly because of their strong and warm pungent flavour. In both sweet and savoury foods, clove aroma can be used. It acts as a preservative owing to its anti-oxidant qualities. Betel nuts, pan masala, and chewing gum all contain it so often. Clove has been associated with a variety of other effects including antiparasitic, antidotal, anti-oxidant, antiperspirant, antiseptic, deodorant, gastrointestinal problems, rubefacient, and stomachic effects [40, 41]. Taking a single clove first in the morning and chewing it prior to eating anything will protect the heart from all the trouble.

Cinnamon (*Cinnamomum zylanicum*)

Cinnamon is essentially a spice made from the inner brown bark of specially chosen shoots, which is then preserved and dried. The bark becomes coiled cylinders or "quills" while drying. In addition to being warm, sweet, and aromatic, they offer a pleasant fragrance scent [42]. It is a member of the Lauraceae family and is indigenous to tropical Asia, including Sri Lanka, India, and other regions. The dried leaves and inner bark of cinnamon are used in incense, personal care products, fragrances, and other products outside medicine. They are also used to flavour pastries and desserts.

The two main components of cinnamon, cinnamaldehyde, and trans-cinnamaldehyde (Cin), are found in the essential oil and are responsible for the flavor and confer a range of biological effects [43]. Procyanidins and catechins are found in cinnamon bark [44]. Although this plant is mostly used as a spice, its essential oils and other components also have significant anti-bacterial, anti-fungal, anti-oxidant, and anti-diabetic properties. As an anti-inflammatory, anti-termite, nematicidal, mosquito larvicidal, insecticidal, antimycotic, and anti-cancer agent, cinnamon has been used for centuries [45]. Cinnamon is made up of several resinous substances, such as cinnamaldehyde, cinnamate, cinnamic acid, and a number of essential oils [46]. According to Singh *et al.* [47], cinnamaldehyde, present in Cinnamon, causes the spicy flavour and smell, which is brought on by oxygen absorption. The resinous components in cinnamon improve as it matures because of its darker hue [47]. Several essential oils, including trans-cinnamaldehyde, cinnamyl acetate, eugenol, L-borneol, caryophyllene oxide, b-caryophyllene, L-bornyl acetate, E-nerolidol, -cubebene, -terpineol, terpinolene, and -thujene, have been found in the Cinnamon [48, 49].

Fever, diarrhea, and irregularities of menstruation can all be effectively treated with cinnamon. It has a calming effect on the stomach in cases of indigestion, stomach ulcers, and bowel issues. Decoction helps to increase urine output and relieve flatulence. Cinnamon helps diabetics manage their blood sugar levels while also preventing genital and vaginal infections. Cinnamon is excellent against gum disease, toothaches, dental bacteria, skin infections and acne. The herb can be utilized as a natural birth control [50]. Given its natural and highly enticing properties, it would be appropriate to mix other herbs and synergize its effect focusing on ailments one after the other. This way, the complete potential of cinnamon may be realized.

Turmeric (*Curcuma longa*)

Turmeric is a frequently used and highly useful natural plant referred to as "Haldi" in India. It is a perennial plant found in Southeast Asia and a member of the Zingiberaceae family. The beneficial "turmeric" is made up of a short, thick rhizome [51]. It is mostly used as a daily spice. Turmeric possesses the ideal blend of special qualities for a flavorful spice, a vibrant yellow dye, a natural beauty aid, and an efficient home cure for a number of illnesses. When it comes to intestinal infections and worms, turmeric is a highly effective antiseptic. Vomiting during pregnancy can be effectively treated with fresh rhizome juice or decoction. It is a beneficial tonic and blood cleanser. For bronchial asthma, bronchitis, and tropical eosinophilia, turmeric is a reliable over-the-counter treatment. Turmeric is useful in treating anaemia since it is an excellent source of iron. Due to its anti-inflammatory qualities, the spice is helpful for rheumatism and arthritis. An effective expectorant, turmeric is helpful for throat discomfort and persistent coughing. Turmeric is helpful for oral diseases, skin infections, and skin improvement because of its anti-parasitic and anti-microbial characteristics [52].

Turmeric contains proteins, volatile oils, vitamin A, curcumin, and other chemically active substances [6]. It has significant anti-bacterial, anti-inflammatory, and hypocholesteremic, anti-histaminic, anti-hepatotoxic, anti-fungal, and antiarthritic effects [6, 7]. Curcumin has been demonstrated to have anti-oxidant, anti-inflammatory, anti-viral, anti-bacterial, anti-fungal, and anti-cancer properties and so has the potential to treat a number of chronic illnesses like diabetes, allergies, arthritis, Alzheimer's disease, and other malignant disorders [53]. The last two decades have proven the potency of curcumin as an immunomodulatory drug, with the ability to control the activation of T cells, B cells, macrophages, neutrophils, natural killer cells, and dendritic cells. This shows that curcumin's reported benefits for arthritic conditions, allergic reactions, asthma, atherosclerosis, heart disease, Alzheimer's disease, diabetes, and cancer may be entirely mediated by its capacity to influence the immune system [54]. Much research has been carried out to gain an insight on the effect of Curcumin on circadian rhythm. A moderate quantity of Curcumin can set the circadian clock back during trans-Atlantic travel when a person feels jet lag. However, such suggestive domains need to be carefully explored and systematically recorded before a conclusion can be drawn.

Seeds of Bishop's Weed (*Trachyspermum ammi*)

Bishop's weed seeds, known as "ajwain," are members of the Apiaceae family. Small and upright, the shrub only reaches a height of around one meter. The fragrant, crisp, peppery, and somewhat bitter dried seeds are used as a spice. According to the Unani medical system, it can be used to cure conditions including paralysis, chest pains, liver and spleen illnesses, hiccups, vomiting, dyspepsia, renal problems, inflammation, and more [55]. A quarter teaspoon of ajwain daily in the morning can provide maximum relief from prostate cancer. The fact that it is so very readily available for a negligible price, a common person does not find it reassuring. The weed has been growing in India since ancient times and is grown in Iran, Egypt, and Afghanistan. Seeds are used in pharmaceuticals as anti-oxidants, preservatives, and flavouring compounds. Ajwain has been discovered to have pharmacological characteristics *viz.* antispasmodic, anti-inflammatory, anti-diarrheal, stimulant, anticholerin, anti-bronchitis, anti-dyspepsia, and anti-colic [6, 18]. It is a glabrescent plant with linear, pinnately divided leaves and fusiform roots. The fruits are ovoid and mucricate, while the flowers are polygamous and white. In the Indian states of Punjab and West Bengal, ajwain is widely grown. Its fruits have long been used to treat inflammation, colic discomfort, anorexia, and flatulence [19]. Thimol, carvacrol, thymene, vitamin B, and volatile oils are among its active chemical components [7].

Since ancient times, Ajwain has been used as a carminative medication. The stimulating seeds can help with spasmodic conditions. The leaves are often used as a vermicide. Ajwain is effective in treating indigestion, gas, and other digestive issues. The seed paste can be used locally to reduce colic discomfort. Ajwain seeds can treat gastrointestinal illnesses that occur after childbirth. When it comes to colds and respiratory conditions, seeds are really helpful. Because it has anti-viral properties, inhaling it can effectively reduce nasal congestion. Rheumatic and neuralgic aches, as well as skin conditions including ringworm, scabies, urticaria, and psoriasis, can effectively be treated with ajwain oil. Its aphrodisiac qualities allow it to cure uterine prolapse and sexual adversity [56]. However, its effective dose and forms need to be standardized on sufficiently large number of patients who suffer from erectile dysfunction (ED), which incidentally has now become more common owing to unhealthy lifestyles and rampant use of junk food coupled with frequent intake of alcohol. Nature has always been kind to mankind; it is mankind who has been outrageously unkind to nature. A person may suffer from ED because of so many reasons. However, this aspect does not fall in the purview of this chapter and will be covered in another book where a comparative account of herbal formulation and allopathic medicine useful for addressing sexual anomalies will be presented.

Fenugreek (*Trigonellafoenum-graecum*)

Fenugreek (*Trigonellafoenum-graecum*) is a leguminous herb that is grown in India and North African nations. It belongs to the Fabaceae family. The seeds are used as seasonings, and the leaves are eaten as green leafy vegetables. Fenugreek seeds have a bitter flavour and have long been valued for their therapeutic properties. For more than 2,500 years, fenugreek seeds have been in use. Fenugreek is mostly produced in India, which also serves as a key market for both culinary and medical purposes. Fenugreek seeds are used in soups, pancakes, and in relatively higher amounts as a seasoning spice and flavouring enhancer. It is a stomach stimulant and is used in the Indian traditional medical system for treating anorexia [57, 58].

Fenugreek leaves and delicate stems can be eaten fresh or dry. The leaves are a wonderful source of several vitamins and minerals, but they are particularly high in choline. Fenugreek seeds can be consumed raw or cooked and are flavorful, bitter, carminative, galactagogue, and anti-microbial. The majority of the seed (50%) is made up of inaccessible carbohydrates. Oil, steroidal saponins, and alkaloids are the chief causes of bitterness. The soluble fraction (20%), which is mostly galactomannan, and the insoluble fraction (30%) make up the fibre component. The majority of the seed's 7.5% lipid content, or 6.3% triglycerides and 450 mg/100 g phospholipids, are neutral lipids [10]. Galactomannan obstructs glucose absorption in the intestine, as per animal testing. Water soluble fibre makes the intestines more viscous, which prevents glucose absorption. Natural sources of iron, silicon, salt, and thiamine could be present in fenugreek. Mucilaginous compounds found in fenugreek are known to calm and relax inflammatory tissues. Alkaloids found in fenugreek seeds include trigonelline, gentianine, and carpine compounds. The seeds also include fenugreekine, a substance that may have hypoglycemic properties, fibre, and 4-hydroxyisoleucine. The process is believed to reduce carbohydrate absorption, postpone stomach emptying, and prevent glucose transport. Fenugreek may also boost peripheral tissue glucose consumption and the amount of insulin receptors in red blood cells, suggesting possible anti-diabetic benefits on the pancreas as well as other organs [11]. While fenugreek seeds are used as spice, the leaves are used as leafy vegetables especially during winter across the country. This healthy tradition of fenugreek uptake in the form of food ensures nutrition for a healthy body and a cure for hyperglycemia.

Cumin (*Cuminum cyminum*)

In India, *Cuminum cyminum* Linn, a member of the Umbelliferae family, is frequently used as the spice jeerak. It is a slender, glabrous, annual plant with compound, linear leaves, belonging to the Apiaceae family. The fruits are cylindrical, with dorsally compressed seeds and constricted apex and base. It is mostly grown in Punjab and Southern India. Its seeds have long been used to treat worm infestation, insufficient breastfeeding, piles, colic pain, and stomach discomfort [19]. Some of the key chemical components of this plant are cumaldehyde, vitamin A, vitamin C, cuminal, cuminic alcohol, γ-Terpinene, Safranal, p-cymene, volatile oils, and β-Pinene [7]. Using GC and GC-MS to describe the essential oils extracted by hydrodistillation of *Cuminum cyminum*, it was discovered that the main components were pinene (29.1%), 1,8-cineole (17.9%), and linalool (10.4%). *C. cyminum* oil has shown potent anti-bacterial properties against *E. coli*, *S. aureus*, and *L. monocytogenes* [12]. Pharmaceutical studies have revealed the carminative, stimulant, anti-cancer, and anti-oxidant effects of cumin [6]. Cumin seeds have an exceptional anti-diabetic effect showing a decrease in hyperglycemia and glucosuria in streptozotocin-induced diabetic rats. These rats were given an eight-week diet plan that included cumin powder (1.25%). As evidenced by diabetic rats' decreased excretions of urea and creatinine as well as lower blood urea levels, dietary cumin also prevented other metabolic changes [59]. An astringent and fragrant plant, cumin is good for the digestive system. It has been used as a carminative, eupeptic, astringent, cough suppressant, and analgesic in the treatment of moderate digestive ailments [60].

Cumin contains vitamins including thiamine, riboflavin, and niacin along with carbohydrates, proteins, fats, and soluble dietary fibres. Cumin is a good source of iron and minerals, with Fe^{2+} (6.0) and Zn^{2+} (6.5) (mg/100 g), which are helpful for boosting the immune system, treating skin conditions, and generating energy. Cumin has demonstrated a variety of effects in both general usage and pharmaceutical settings. Cumin has some negative effects that warrant its medicinal use with caution, although it is widely used as a nutrient-rich spice today [61].

Black Cumin (*Nigella sativa*)

Black Cumin *N. sativa* is popularly known as black cumin or black seed belongs to the family Ranunculaceae, which is a valuable traditional medicine and is well-known for its culinary use. Black cumin is grown in several countries including Egypt, Iran, Greece, Syria, Albania, Turkey, Saudi Arabia, India, and Pakistan. It is native to a large area of the eastern Mediterranean, northern Africa, the Indian subcontinent, and Southwest Asia. Black cumin is an elixir that has been recommended in traditional medicine in the forms of essential oil, paste, powder, and extract for a variety of illnesses and disorders, including eczema, anorexia, amenorrhea, paralysis, rheumatism, headaches, back pain, and hypertension, to name a few [62]. Due to their extensive range of therapeutic benefits, *N. sativa* seeds have long been used as an anti-oxidant, anti-inflammatory, immunomodulatory, anti-cancer, neuroprotective, anti-microbial, anti-hyper-tensive, cardio-protective, antidiabetic, gastroprotective, nephroprotective and hepatoprotective agents [8]. The main compound in black cumin seed is its essential oil, which has pharmacological effects and therapeutic properties. This includes thymoquinone (TQ), thymohydroquinone, thymol, carvacrol, nigellidine, nigellicine, and hederin [9]. Despite receiving less attention in scientific literature, black cumin has a considerable amount of protein and fat and an important amount of vital fatty acids, amino acids, vitamins, and minerals [63]. Black cumin is a significant source of nutraceuticals since it contains both active phytochemicals and essential elements that support the immune system and overall health of the human body [64].

Fennel (*Foeniculum vulgare*)

Fennel, or *Foeniculum vulgare*, is a medicinal herb used to cure a number of illnesses. This plant is a fragrant and medicinal representative of the Umbelliferae family that was first discovered close to banks along the Mediterranean Sea coast. Argentina, Bulgaria, Germany, Greece, India, and Lebanon are the countries with significant distribution of *Foeniculum vulgare* [65]. The leaves may reach a length of 40 cm, and the plant can reach a height of 2.5 m with a hollow stem. Fruit consists of 4–10 mm long dry seeds [19]. The herb *Foeniculum vulgare* comprises saponins, flavonoids, cardiac glycosides, steroids, triterpenes, coumarin, proteins, essential oils, and vitamins [22]. This plant offers a variety of medicinal benefits, including anti-inflammatory, anti-stress, anti-oxidant, anti-allergic, analgesic, anti-bacterial, and anti-cancer, and has cytotoxic properties [66]. Animal studies have indicated that fennel seed extracts may be useful as a diuretic, and a possible medication for treating hypertension, and glaucoma. It has been used as a galactagogue to increase a nursing mother's milk production [67].

The mature seeds, leaves, and roots are frequently utilised in home medicines, targeting the digestive tract [68]. Additionally, it is also used in cosmetics. Essential oil of *F. vulgare* seed contains a nethole, estragole, and fenchone [21 - 23]. According to preliminary phytochemical research, the plant's composition included protein, fat, fibre, and carbohydrates in addition to saponins, flavonoids, cardiac glycosides, sterols, triterpenes, and coumarins. The fennel seeds contain the volatile oil. The two primary ingredients are fenchone and trans-anethole. In addition, limonene, camphene, and pinene are found in essential oils [69]. According to Al Snafi [22], the essential oil of *Foeniculum vulgare* contains 74.8% anethole, 11.1% limonene, 4.7% methyl chavicol, 2.5% fenchone, and 1.3% -pinene. Majority of fennel comprises anethole (40–70%), fenchone (1-20%), and estragole (2–9%) [70]. This has been popular amongst the ancient remedies and has great significance for the food industry. It offers a notable base for pharmaceutical operations to develop/formulate novel medications useful for future clinical applications.

Bay leaf (*Laurus nobilis*)

Laurus nobilis L. (Tejpatta) belongs to the Lauraceae family, which has 32 genera and around 2,000 to 2,500 species. According to [71], Laurus is also known as the sweet bay, bay laurel, Grecian laurel, real bay, and bay tree. It can be found in India in Sikkim, Assam, Mizoram, Meghalaya, Uttarakhand, and Himachal Pradesh along the Western Himalaya. At an elevation of 900 to 2500 meters, the tropical and subtropical Himalayas are its natural environment [72]. Tejpatta is used in a variety of dishes to add a distinctive flavour. It imparts to meals a warm, peppery, clove-cinnamon taste. The main elements found in bay seed essential oil comprised 1,8 cineole, sabinene, limonene, eugenol, and -pinene. There are several pharmacological uses of bay leaf essential oil, including anti-bacterial, insecticidal, and anti-oxidant ones, and it has anti-convulsant properties. Bay leaf essential oil may contain a range of different components [26].

Tejpatta, which is high in anti-oxidants and possesses gastroprotective effects, may also help prevent stomach ulcers by lowering the free radical damage done to stomach cells. Due to the carminative properties of its leaves, its addition to food helps in digestion and reduces gas and flatulence.

Tejpatta oil is beneficial for treating rheumatoid arthritis because of its anti-inflammatory and anti-oxidant characteristics. Massages with Tejpatta oil on the joints might help ease pain and swelling. Since it has anti-bacterial and anti-microbial properties, it may be used topically to the skin to cure boils and guard against wound infections [1].

Tejpatta improves insulin secretion while protecting pancreatic beta cells from harm. Consequently, it reduces blood sugar levels [6]. Additionally, beneficial to heart health, it lowers bad cholesterol and regulates blood pressure by flushing out excess salt owing to its diuretic properties.

According to Ayurveda, the cause of diabetes, also known as Madhumeha, is an aggravation of Vata and a problem with digestion. Improper digestion causes harmful waste products to build up in the body and in the pancreatic cells, which inhibits insulin's ability to operate. Tejpatta, used in many diets, aids in lowering blood sugar levels which is due to its Ushna (hot) potency, which supports healthy digestive fire while lowering Ama.

Tejpatta may help manage common colds, according to a study [2], but more data is required to provide enough evidence to recommend its use in treating common colds. It stops coughing, eliminates mucus, and opens up the airways, enabling the patient to breathe freely. It also reduces chronic wheezing. This is a result of its ability to balance Kapha. From an Ayurvedic perspective, Tejpatta helps to regulate asthma symptoms and provides relief in cases of breathlessness. However, to substantiate this point, a detailed study must be conducted on a large number of people showing Tejpatta's involvement in the cure of asthma. The primary doshas associated with asthma, according to Ayurveda, are Vata and Kapha. The lungs' Kaphadosha is unbalanced by an elevated Vatadosha. Breathing becomes challenging as a result of the blockage in the airways. The name of this condition is Swas-Roga (asthma). Tejpatta aids in achieving Vatadosha and Kapha balance. Due to its Ushna (hot) nature, it assists in removing excessive mucus from the lungs by melting it. This contributes to lowering the symptoms of asthma.

Garlic (*Allium sativum*)

One of the oldest and most significant herbs that have been utilised as traditional medicine since ancient times is garlic (*Allium sativum* L.; Family:

Amaryllidaceae), an aromatic annual spice [73, 74]. It is regarded as the second most widely used species of Allium after onion (*Allium cepa* L.). This is used for treating a number of common ailments such as cold, flu, snake bites, and hypertension [75]. Allium species and their active ingredients have been shown to lower the risk of diabetes and cardiovascular disease, protect against infections by boosting immune function, and have anti-microbial, anti-fungal, anti-aging, and anti-cancer properties, which have been supported by epidemiological data from the human clinical studies [76]. Sulfur-containing compounds such as alliin, allicin, ajoenes, vinyldithiins, and sulfides, are the main constituents isolated from *A. sativum* extracts [25].

Garlic is used to flavour meals, and for several therapeutic purposes. It is used for the treatment of lung disorders, whooping cough, stomach disorders, cold, and earaches, and assists in preventing cardiovascular diseases [74]. Moreover, garlic has been used in traditional medicine to treat indigestion, respiratory and urinary tract infections, and cardiac disorders and it is known for its carminative, anti-pyretic, sedative, aphrodisiac, and diuretic effects [24].

CONCLUSION

The purpose of the current study was to collect, collate, and critically evaluate some common spices and elucidate their medical, and therapeutic applications. In several instances, hard-core scientific evidence is needed to draw an unequivocal conclusion. However, besides, their use in culinary and cuisine, they offer much promise as medical alternatives. What now needs to be done is to identify different compounds from these species at the molecular level. This in turn would enable to uncover their biological and therapeutic activities. Since several spices have overlapping properties, the purified compound may be mixed to synergize their effects. Finally, these compounds may be assessed for their biological, biomedical therapeutic and immunogenic potentials. This would enable undertaking a systematic trial of such medicinal formulations across the spectrum of ethnic groups and establish their broader application in ameliorating a variety of ailments.

ACKNOWLEDGMENTS

The authors are thankful to the Research Council, Department of Higher Education, Uttar Pradesh Government for providing financial assistance, Government Raza PG College, Rampur for infrastructure and Professor Sher Ali, Era University, Lucknow, for his constructive comments.

REFERENCES

[1] Husain N, Pandey B. Ethno-medicinal use and Pharmacological actions of some of the domestically

used Indian Spices- A Review. Indo Ame Jour Pharmacu Res 2015; 5(12): 3892-5.

[2] Radha krishnan K, Babuskin S, Azhagu Saravana Babu P, *et al.* anti-microbial and anti-oxidant effects of spice extracts on the shelf life extension of raw chicken meat. Int J Food Microbiol 2014; 171(3): 32-40.
[http://dx.doi.org/10.1016/j.ijfoodmicro.2013.11.011]

[3] Tacouri DD, Ramful-Baboolall D, Puchooa D. *In vitro* bioactivity and phytochemical screening of selected spices used in Mauritian foods. Asian Pac J Trop Dis 2013; 3(4): 253-61.
[http://dx.doi.org/10.1016/S2222-1808(13)60066-3]

[4] Apak R, Güçlü K, Demirata B, *et al.* Comparative evaluation of various total anti-oxidant capacity assays applied to phenolic compounds with the CUPRAC assay. Molecules 2007; 12(7): 1496-547.
[http://dx.doi.org/10.3390/12071496] [PMID: 17909504]

[5] Ahmad I, Beg AZ. anti-microbial and phytochemical studies on 45 Indian medicinal plants against multi-drug resistant human pathogens. J Ethnopharmacol 2001; 74(2): 113-23.
[http://dx.doi.org/10.1016/S0378-8741(00)00335-4] [PMID: 11167029]

[6] Sharma PC, Yelne MB, Dennis TJ. Database on medicinal plants used in Ayurveda. 2001.

[7] Chatterjee A, Pakrashi SC, Eds. Volume 1 to 5. The Treatise on Indian Medicinal Plants. New Delhi: Publications and Information Directorate; 1995–1997.

[8] Yimer EM, Tuem KB, Karim A, Ur-Rehman N, Anwar F. *Nigella sativa* L. (Black Cumin): A promising natural remedy for wide range of illnesses. Evid Based Complement Alternat Med 2019; 2019: 1-16.
[http://dx.doi.org/10.1155/2019/1528635] [PMID: 31214267]

[9] Kooti W, Hasanzadeh-Noohi Z, Sharafi-Ahvazi N, Asadi-Samani M, Ashtary-Larky D. Phytochemistry, pharmacology, and therapeutic uses of black seed (Nigella sativa). Chin J Nat Med 2016; 14(10): 732-45.
[http://dx.doi.org/10.1016/S1875-5364(16)30088-7] [PMID: 28236403]

[10] Shankaracharya NB, Anandaraman S, Natarajan CP. Chemical composition of raw androasted fenugreek. J Food Sci Technol 1973; 10: 179-81.

[11] Kor NM, Didarshetaban MB, Pour HRS. Fenugreek (Trigonellafoenum-graecum L.) As a Valuable Medicinal Plant. Int J Adv Biol Biomed Res 2013; 1(8): 922-31.

[12] Gachkar L, Yadegari D, Rezaei M, Taghizadeh M, Astaneh S, Rasooli I. Chemical and biological characteristics of *Cuminum cyminum* and *Rosmarinus officinalis* essential oils. Food Chem 2007; 102(3): 898-904.
[http://dx.doi.org/10.1016/j.foodchem.2006.06.035]

[13] Parle M, Khanna D. Clove: A Champion Spice. IJRAP 2011; 2(1): 47-54.

[14] Sharma PC, Yelne MB, Dennis TJ. Database on medicinal plants used in Ayurveda. Department of Indian system of medicine Govt of India, New Delhi. 2011; 90: pp. 213-404.

[15] Chatterjee A, Pakrashi SC, Eds. Volume 1 to 5. The Treatise on Indian Medicinal Plants. New Delhi: Publications and Information Directorate: 1995–1997.

[16] Rao PV, Gan SH. Cinnamon: A Multifaceted Medicinal Plant Volume 2014, 2014; 2014 Article ID 642942, 12 pages.
[http://dx.doi.org/10.1155/2014/642942]

[17] Senanayake UM, Lee TH, Wills RBH. Volatile constituents of cinnamon (Cinnamomum zeylanicum) oils. J Agric Food Chem 1978; 26(4): 822-4.
[http://dx.doi.org/10.1021/jf60218a031]

[18] Thangam C, Dhananjayan R. Anti-inflammatory potential of the seeds of Carumcopticum Linn. Indian J Pharm 2003; 35(6): 388-91.

[19] Sharma PV, Dravyaguna V. ChaukhambaBharati Academy: Varanasi, India. 1995; 69, 72, 138, 152, 162, 246, 250, 314, 331, 332, 350, 362, 365, 394, 401, 458, 494, 596, 642, 719, 729, 823..

[20] Chatterjee A, Pakrashi SC, Eds. The treatise on indian medicinal plants. Publications and Information Directorate. 1995-7.

[21] Gani HO, Hoq O, Tamanna T. Pharmacological and phytochemical analysis of Foeniculum vulgare Mill. RE:view 2019; 3: 13-8.

[22] Al-Snafi AE. The chemical constituents and pharmacological effects of Foeniculum vulgare-A review. IOSR J Pharm 2018; 8: 81-96.

[23] Kooti W, Moradi M, Ali-Akbari S, Sharafi-Ahvazi N, Asadi-Samani M, Ashtray-Larky D. Therapeutic and pharmacological potential of Foeniculum vulgare Mill: a review. J HerbMedPharmacol 2015; 4: 1-9.

[24] Souza GA, Ebaid GX, Seiva FR, *et al.* N-acetylcysteinean Allium plant compound improves high-sucrose diet-induced obesity and related effects. Evid.Based Complement. AlternMed 2011; 643269.

[25] El-Saber Batiha G, Magdy Beshbishy A, G Wasef L, *et al.* Chemical constituents and pharmacological activities of garlic (*allium sativum* l.): A review. Nutrients 2020; 12(3): 872.
[http://dx.doi.org/10.3390/nu12030872] [PMID: 32213941]

[26] Chahal KK, Kaur M, Bhardwaj U, Singla N, Kaur A. A review on chemistry and biological activities of Laurus nobilis L. essential oil. J Pharmacogn Phytochem 2017; 6(4): 1153-61.

[27] Ashokkumar K, Murugan M, Dhanya MK, Pandian A, Warkentin TD. Phytochemistry and therapeutic potential of black pepper [Piper nigrum (L.)] essential oil and piperine: a review. Clinical Phytoscience 2021; 7(1): 52.
[http://dx.doi.org/10.1186/s40816-021-00292-2]

[28] Sagar NA, Pareek S, Benkeblia N, Xiao J. Onion (*Allium cepa* L.) bioactives: Chemistry, pharmacotherapeutic functions, and industrial applications. Food Front 2022; 3(3): 380-412.
[http://dx.doi.org/10.1002/fft2.135]

[29] Gupta E. Elucidating the Phytochemical and Pharmacological Potential of Myristicafragrans. 2020.
[http://dx.doi.org/10.4018/978-1-7998-2524-1.ch004]

[30] Ashokkumar K, Murugan M, Dhanya MK, Warkentin TD. Botany, traditional uses, phytochemistry and biological activities of cardamom [Elettaria cardamomum (L.) Maton] – A critical review. Journal of Ethnopharmacology 2020; 246
[http://dx.doi.org/10.1016/j.jep.2019.112244]

[31] Asgarpanah J, Kazemivash N. Phytochemistry, pharmacology and medicinal properties of Coriandrum sativum L. Afr J Pharm Pharmacol 2012; 6(31)
[http://dx.doi.org/10.5897/AJPP12.901]

[32] Balakrishnan R, Vijayraja D, Jo SH, Ganesan P, Su-Kim I, Choi DK. Medicinal profile, phytochemistry, and pharmacological activities of murraya koenigii and its primary bioactive compounds. anti-oxidants 2020; 9(2): 101.
[http://dx.doi.org/10.3390/antiox9020101] [PMID: 31991665]

[33] Wifek A, Saeed A, Rehman R, Nisar S. Lemongrass: A review on its botany, properties, applications and active components. International Journal of Chemical and Biochemical Sciences 2016; (9): 79-84.

[34] Tian Y, Deng F. Phytochemistry and biological activity of mustard (*Brassica juncea*): a review. CYTA J Food 2020; 18(1): 704-18.
[http://dx.doi.org/10.1080/19476337.2020.1833988]

[35] Masihuddin, Jafri MA, Siddiqui A, Chaudhary S. Traditional uses, phytochemistry and pharmacological activities of Papaver somniferum with special reference of Unani medicine: an updated review, Journal of Drug Delivery and Therapeutics. 2018; 8(5-s).
[http://dx.doi.org/10.22270/jddt.v8i5-s.2069]

[36] Akowuah GA, Htar TT. Therapeutic properties of saffron and its chemical constituents. Journal of Natural Products 2014; (7): 5-13.

[37] Parle M, Khanna D. Clove: A Champion Spice. Intern Jour of Res in Ayu and Phar 2011; 2(1): 47-54.

[38] Cortés-Rojas DF, de Souza CRF, Oliveira WP. Clove (Syzygium aromaticum): A precious spice. Asian Pac J Trop Biomed 2014; 4(2): 90-6.
[http://dx.doi.org/10.1016/S2221-1691(14)60215-X] [PMID: 25182278]

[39] Deans SG, Noble RC, Hiltunen R, Wuryani W, Pénzes LG. anti-microbial and anti-oxidant properties of *Syzygium aromaticum* (L.) Merr. & Perry: Impact upon bacteria, fungi and fatty acid levels in ageing mice. Flavour Fragrance J 1995; 10(5): 323-8.
[http://dx.doi.org/10.1002/ffj.2730100507]

[40] Bhat KS, Vivek K. Biocidal potential of clove oils against Aedealbopictus – A comparative study. African Journal of Biotechnology 2009; 8(24): 6933-7.

[41] Delaquis P, Stanich K, Girard B, Mazza G. anti-microbial activity of individual and mixed fractions of dill, cilantro, coriander and eucalyptus essential oils. Int J Food Microbiol 2002; 74(1-2): 101-9.
[http://dx.doi.org/10.1016/S0168-1605(01)00734-6] [PMID: 11929164]

[42] Debjit B, Sampath KP, Akhilesh Y, Shweta S, Shravan P, Amit SD. Trends in indian traditional herbs syzygiumaromaticum and its health benefits. J Pharmacogn Phytochem 2012; 1(1): 13-22.

[43] Yeh HF, Luo CY, Lin CY, Cheng SS, Hsu YR, Chang ST. Methods for thermal stability enhancement of leaf essential oils and their main constituents from indigenous cinnamon (Cinnamomum osmophloeum). J Agric Food Chem 2013; 61(26): 6293-8.
[http://dx.doi.org/10.1021/jf401536y] [PMID: 23738884]

[44] Nonaka G, Morimoto S, Nishioka I. Tannins and related compounds. Part 13. Isolation and structures of trimeric, tetrameric, and pentameric proanthicyanidins from cinnamon. J Chem Soc, Perkin Trans 1 1983; (1): 2139-45.
[http://dx.doi.org/10.1039/p19830002139]

[45] Rao PV, Gan SH. Cinnamon: A Multifaceted Medicinal Plant 2014; 12.
[http://dx.doi.org/10.1155/2014/642942]

[46] Senanayake UM, Lee TH, Wills RBH. Volatile constituents of cinnamon (Cinnamomum zeylanicum) oils. J Agric Food Chem 1978; 26(4): 822-4.
[http://dx.doi.org/10.1021/jf60218a031]

[47] Singh G, Maurya S, deLampasona MP, Catalan CAN. A comparison of chemical, anti-oxidant and anti-microbial studies of cinnamon leaf and bark volatile oils, oleoresins and their constituents. Food Chem Toxicol 2007; 45(9): 1650-61.
[http://dx.doi.org/10.1016/j.fct.2007.02.031] [PMID: 17408833]

[48] Tung YT, Chua MT, Wang SY, Chang ST. Anti-inflammation activities of essential oil and its constituents from indigenous cinnamon (Cinnamomum osmophloeum) twigs. Bioresour Technol 2008; 99(9): 3908-13.
[http://dx.doi.org/10.1016/j.biortech.2007.07.050] [PMID: 17826984]

[49] Tung YT, Yen PL, Lin CY, Chang ST. Anti-inflammatory activities of essential oils and their constituents from different provenances of indigenous cinnamon (*Cinnamomum osmophloeum*) leaves. Pharm Biol 2010; 48(10): 1130-6.
[http://dx.doi.org/10.3109/13880200903527728] [PMID: 20815702]

[50] Zafar R. Medicinal Plants of India. CBS Publis and Distrib 2009; pp. 1-15.

[51] Roshan PY, Gaur T. Versatility of turmeric: A review the golden spice of life. J Pharmacogn Phytochem 2017; 6(1): 41-6.

[52] Deepika Y, Shiv KY, Roop KK, Mohammad M, Mohammad A. Turmeric (Curcuma longa L): A promising spice for phytochemical and pharmacological activities, Review article. Intern Jour of

Green Pharm 2013; pp. 85-9.

[53] Gupta M. Pharmacological properties and traditional therapeutic uses of important indian spices: A review. Int J Food Prop 2010; 13(5): 1092-116. [http://dx.doi.org/10.1080/10942910902963271]

[54] Jagetia GC, Aggarwal BB. "Spicing up" of the immune system by curcumin. J Clin Immunol 2007; 27(1): 19-35. [http://dx.doi.org/10.1007/s10875-006-9066-7] [PMID: 17211725]

[55] Rashmi Y, Chandan KP, Deepika G, Rahul K. Health Benefits Of Indian Aromatic Plant Ajwain (TrachycpermumAmmi). Intern Jour of Phar &Techn 2011; 3(3): 1356-66.

[56] Mohammad MZ, Mahmoodreza M, Soliman MS, Peyman P. An Overview on Ajwain (Trachyspermumammi) Pharmacological Effects; Modern and Traditional. J Nat Rem 2014; 14(1): 98-105.

[57] Chopra RN, Nayar SL, Chopra IC, Eds. Glossary of Indian Medicinal Plants. New Delhi: Council of Scientific and Industrial Research 1986.

[58] Fillips R, Foy N. Herbs. London: Pan Books Ltd. 1990.

[59] Willatgamuwa SA, Platel K, Saraswathi G, Srinivasan K. Antidiabetic influence of dietary cumin seeds () in streptozotocin induced diabetic rats. Nutr Res 1998; 18(1): 131-42. [http://dx.doi.org/10.1016/S0271-5317(97)00207-8]

[60] De M, De AK, Mukhopadhvay R, Banerjee AB, Micro M. anti-microbial activity of Cuminumcyminum L. ArsPharmaceutica 2003; 44: 257-69.

[61] Singh RP, Gangadharappa HV, Mruthunjaya K. Cuminumcyminum – A Popular Spice: An Updated Review. Pharmacogn J 2017; 9(3): 292-301. [http://dx.doi.org/10.5530/pj.2017.3.51]

[62] Chaudhry Z, Khera RA, Hanif MA, Ayub MA, Sumrra SH. Cumin. In: Hanif MA, Nawaz H, Khan MM, Byrne HJ, Eds. Medicinal Plants of South Asia. Amsterdam, The Netherlands: Elsevier 2020; pp. 165-78. [http://dx.doi.org/10.1016/B978-0-08-102659-5.00013-6]

[63] Kabir Y, Shirakawa H, Komai M. Nutritional composition of the indigenous cultivar of black cumin seeds from Bangladesh. Prog Nutr 2019; (21): 428-34.

[64] Hannan MA, Rahman MA, Sohag AAM, *et al.* Black Cumin (*Nigella sativa* L.): A Comprehensive Review on Phytochemistry, Health Benefits, Molecular Pharmacology, and Safety. Nutrients 2021; 13(6): 1784. [http://dx.doi.org/10.3390/nu13061784] [PMID: 34073784]

[65] Jamwal NS, Kumar S, Rana A. Phytochemical and Pharmacological Review on FoeniculumVulgare. PharmaSciMonit 2013; 4: 327-41.

[66] Kooti W, Moradi M, Ali-Akbari S, Sharafi-Ahvazi N, Asadi-Samani M, Ashtray-Larky D. Therapeutic and pharmacological potential of Foeniculumvulgare Mill: a review. J HerbMedPharmacol 2015; 4: 1-9.

[67] Rather MA, Dar BA, Sofi SN, Bhat BA, Qurishi MA. Foeniculum vulgare: A comprehensive review of its traditional use, phytochemistry, pharmacology, and safety. Arab J Chem 2016; 9: S1574-83. [http://dx.doi.org/10.1016/j.arabjc.2012.04.011]

[68] Barros L, Carvalho AM, Ferreira ICFR. The nutritional composition of fennel (Foeniculum vulgare): Shoots, leaves, stems and inflorescences. Lebensm Wiss Technol 2010; 43(5): 814-8. [http://dx.doi.org/10.1016/j.lwt.2010.01.010]

[69] Afify AEMMR, El-Beltagi HS, Hammama AAEA, Sidky MM, Mostafa OFA. Distribution of trans-anethole and estragole in fennel (Foeniculumvulgare Mill) of callus induced from different seedling parts and fruits. Not Sci Biol 2011; 3(1): 79-86.

[http://dx.doi.org/10.15835/nsb315422]

[70] Anubhuti P, Rahul S, Kant KC. Standardization of fennel (Foeniculumvulgare), its oleoresin and marketed ayurvedic dosage forms. Int J Pharm Sci Drug Res 2011; 3: 265-9.

[71] Garg SN, Siddiqui MS, Agarwal SK. New fatty acidesters and hydroxyl ketones from fruits of *Laurusnobilis.* J Nat Prod 1992; 55(9): 1315-9.
[http://dx.doi.org/10.1021/np50087a023]

[72] Dighe VV, Gursale AA, Sane RT, Menon S, Patel PH. Quantitative determination of eugenol from *Cinnamomum tamala* Nees and Eberm. Leaf powder andpolyherbal formulation using reverse phase liquidchromatography. Chromatographia 2005; 61(9-10): 443-6.
[http://dx.doi.org/10.1365/s10337-005-0527-6]

[73] Ayaz E, Alpsoy HC. [Garlic (*Allium sativum*) and traditional medicine]. Turkiye Parazitol Derg 2007; 31(2): 145-9.
[PMID: 17594659]

[74] Badal DS, Dwivedi AK, Kumar V, *et al.* Effect of organic manuresand inorganic fertilizers on growth, yield and its attributing traits in garlic (*Allium sativum* L.). J Pharmacogn Phytochem 2019; (8): 587-90.

[75] Barnes J, Anderson LA, Phillipson JD. Herbal Medicines. 2nd ed. London, UK: Pharmaceutical Press 2002; p. 14.

[76] Rahman K. Historical perspective on garlic and cardiovascular disease. J Nutr 2001; 131(3): 977S-9S.
[http://dx.doi.org/10.1093/jn/131.3.977S] [PMID: 11238800]

[77] Fig A. Available from: https://bigapplecurry.files.wordpress.com/2012/07/photo-120.jpg?w=293

[78] Fig B. Available from: https://m.media-amazon.com/images/I/41RwaQHI6GL.jpg

[79] Fig C. Available from: https://ftborgano.b-cdn.net/media/yhcmp4la/green-fennel-saunf-500g--199-price.jpg

[80] Fig D. Available from: https://m.media-amazon.com/images/I/31TIJVPwpuS.jpg

[81] Fig E. Available from: https://d36v5spmfzyapc.cloudfront.net/wp-content/uploads/2020/02/ajwai--848x424.png

[82] Fig F. Available from: https://cf.organicbazar.net/wp-content/uploads/2021/08/Untitled-design-2-22-06-02T160309.044.jpg

[83] Fig G. Available from: https://www.organicherbals.in/wp-content/uploads/2020/05/Dalchin--Daalcheeni-Cinnamon-Sticks-Cinnamomum-zeylanicum-520x574.jpg

[84] Fig H. Available from: https://i.ndtvimg.com/i/2018-03/cumin_620x350_51521615731.jpg

[85] Fig I. Available from: https://images.indianexpress.com/2020/04/haldi_759.jpg

[86] Fig J. Available from: https://new-img.patrika.com/cdn-cgi/image/width=798,fit=cover,gravity=auto,format=webp,quality=100/https://new-img.patrika.com/upload/2022/02/20/kalonji.jpg

CHAPTER 17

High Altitude Hypoxia Stressor Associated Diseases and Precision Medicine

Subhojit Paul[1], **Anamika Gangwar**[1], **Swaraj Mohanthy**[1] and **Yasmin Ahmad**[1,*]

[1] *Defence Institute of Physiology & Allied Sciences (DIPAS), Defence R & D Organization (DRDO), Timarpur, New Delhi-110054, India*

Abstract: Hypoxia is a condition wherein an organism, a cell or a region of an organ does not receive adequate levels of oxygen to carry out normal life processes. The ability to sense oxygen levels and respond appropriately is termed "oxygen sensing" which might be used in certain cases to describe the biological effects of hypoxia. Hypoxia is an important facet involved in multiple diseases. Ranging from high-altitude pulmonary edema to cancer, oxygen-sensing molecular networks are crucial for survival and have a notable impact on human health systems. The type, duration, and intensity of hypoxic episodes have been found to have a multitude of effects ranging from beneficial to harmful in diverse conditions like obesity, type 2 diabetes and obstructive sleep apnea. A very important niche of hypoxia is the study of environmental stressors also called high-altitude hypoxia. High-altitude hypoxia holds multiple molecular similarities with diabetes, cancer, obesity, and other diseases like COPD. In addition, unregulated exposure to hypobaric hypoxia is known to directly cause high-altitude illnesses like HAPE/HACE. An interesting facet of high-altitude hypoxia is the ability of the molecular and physiological systems to acclimatize to the high altitude. This acclimatization is known to prevent the occurrence of high-altitude illnesses. This review highlights the previous studies to build a framework that elucidates the occurrence of hypobaric hypoxia, its socio-economic impact, molecular underpinnings, and correlation with inflammation, cancer, diabetes, obesity and possible therapeutic approaches to these diseases.

Keywords: Disease, Hypobaric hypoxia, High altitude acclimatization, Inflammation, Therapeutics.

INTRODUCTION

Human life revolves around genetics and the environment. Genetics contributes only about 10% whereas environment plays major roles.

* **Corresponding author Yasmin Ahmad:** Peptide & Proteomics Division, DIPAS, DRDO, New Delhi-110054, India, E-mail: yasminchem@gmail.com

Farzana Mahdi & Abbas Ali Mahdi (Eds.)

There are several aspects of environment that include our lifestyle, food habits, ethnicity, choice of mating partner, social and religious practices, demography, epidemiology, social interactions, genetic susceptibility and resistance, and environmental living condition. A large number of environmental conditions tend to affect our physiology and immune system. Lack of exercise, and the use of substances (marijuana, heroin, cocaine, or methamphetamine and alcohol) invariably affect our health and often result in comorbidity. Living at higher altitudes is part of the environment that causes stress and affects our body although the body tries to acclimatize with its surrounding.

Table 1. List of major high altitude cities worldwide and their populations.

Average height	Country	Population	Est. year
4,150 m	El Alto, Bolivia	1,184,942	2014
4,090 m	Potosi, Bolivia	170,000	2007
3,836 m	Shigatse, China	117,000	2013
3,825 m	Juliaca, Peru	225, 146	2007
3,819 m	Puno, Peru	120, 229	2007
3,706 m	Oruro, Bolivia	250,700	2011
3,658 m	Lhasa, China	373,000	2009
3,640 m	La Paz, Bolivia	845,480	2010
3, 399 m	Cusco, Peru	358,052	2011
3,053 m	Huancayo, Peru	425,000	2012
3,050 m	Huaraz, Peru	135,000	2011

ENVIRONMENTAL-INDUCED STRESS AND ITS EFFECTS ON HUMANS

A change in the environmental factors/conditions either natural or man-made causes undesirable impact on the organismal fitness and performance of essential tasks. This may result in endangering the survival of the organism in that particular environment. The stress caused due to any environment becomes an environmental stressor and the effects are termed environmental stress [1]. Environmental stress has several forms that include everyday air and noise pollution observed in urbanized areas, high pressure at depths of 30 m or more in oceans, and low visibility combined with treacherous roads at high altitude areas. The WHO, in line with multiple human studies [2 - 7], recognized environmental stress and stressors as a significant cause of many diseases like diabetes, cardiovascular diseases, and cancer [8]. Cardiovascular diseases, according to WHO, are the leading cause of deaths globally (https://www.who.int/news-room/fact-sheets/detail/cardiovascular-diseases-(cvds); accessed on 17th January 2019). A majority of environmental stressors activate the hypothalamic-pituitary-adrenocortical axis and the sympathetic nervous system subsequently cause the onset of inflammation and oxidative stress leading to disease and mortality [9 - 11]. Environmental stressors and their significant effect on health and quality of life have been a focus of research since the late 70s. Thus, irrespective of the types of environmental exposure, the management of stressors present in that environment is of prime importance. It becomes all the more important when the environment happens to be of a very high altitude.

The environmental stressors at high altitudes consist of rough uneven terrain, cold temperature, UV radiation, low humidity levels, and risk of avalanches and landslides. However, the most pertinent stressor is hypobaric hypoxia. Hypobaric hypoxia refers to the decline in partial pressure of oxygen in the atmosphere owing to the decline in barometric pressure. All known high altitude illnesses (HAIs) are purported to be patho-physiological responses to hypobaric hypoxia. These include acute mountain sickness (AMS), high altitude pulmonary edema (HAPE), and high altitude cerebral edema (HACE).

SOCIO-ECONOMIC ASPECTS OF HIGH-ALTITUDE AREAS

High altitude has no precise definition but any geographical entity with an elevation of at least 8,000 ft (~2438 m) is termed a high altitude area. In India, as per Army order No. 110/80, high altitude is considered to be an elevation of 2700 m (8859 ft) or above. Extreme altitude may be defined as one exceeding 5800 m (19028 ft) where permanent residence is practically not feasible (Army orders No.110/80, New Delhi, 1980). The highest permanent human settlement is La Rinconada, Peru at 16,700 ft (5100 m) [12]. Only a handful of urbanized places exist at such elevations and interestingly most of them lie in the South American countries like Bolivia, Peru and Ecuador. In Asia, only Lhasa (in Tibet) is a major city at high altitude. Even though countries like India, China, Nepal and Bhutan are well-documented to have multiple native populations in their high-altitude regions [13, 14]. The highest percentage of the world's high altitude native populations [15] lack major cities point and live in remote and difficult areas. The names and populations of some high-altitude cities are shown below in Table **1**.

According to Moore *et al*, till 1983, there were 140 million people living permanently above 2500 m (~8,000 ft) constituting about 2% of the world's population then [16]. In 1998, a study published by Cohen and Small reported that about 33% of the world population lived within 100 m (328 ft) of mean sea level and the median altitude of residence worldwide was 194 m (636 ft) above the sea level [16]. They further determined a greater than an exponential decline in population with an increase in altitude [17]. Considering the rate of population growth that varied from 1.8-1.07% between 1980-2019 (http://www.worldometers .info/world-population/ accessed on 16th January 2019), assuming that only 2% of the world's population is currently inhabiting high altitude areas, and at least 152 million people (world population being approximated as 7.6 billion) are currently residing above 2500 m (8200 ft). Coupled with the robust growth in high-altitude infrastructure and subsequent tourism, even in difficult places like Tibet, there is now an increased incidence of HAIs and consequently increased medical and associated costs for their treatment [18]. Since most of the visitors consist of non-acclimatized individuals, there are ever growing possibilities of HAIs. HAIs typically affect only non-acclimatized climbers upon acute entry into the high altitude environment [19]. HAIs may damage the daily life and charm of the native populations by placing them with unwanted socioeconomic burdens when visitors suffer. Even natural calamities at high altitudes require far greater resources particularly manpower when compared to similar calamities in lowland areas. During the high altitude earthquake in Yushu, Qinghai, it was observed that a great number of rescue workers immediately flown into high altitude suffered from HAIs, with deaths due to HAPE and HACE and nearly 80% incidence of AMS being reported by Wu [20]. Thus, there is an urgent need for research and development in high altitude molecular omics (altitudeomics) for the better management of HAIs and to provide rapid induction strategies in high altitude areas during emergencies.

PATHOPHYSIOLOGICAL CONSEQUENCES AT HIGH ALTITUDE

Some important physiological parameters often utilized in high altitude studies are summarized in Table **2**.

The initial line of investigation for high altitude hypoxia is focused on the physiological aspects. The effect of hypobaric hypoxia on human physiology is manifested by various beneficial/harmful changes. When these changes are orchestrated in a controlled manner, they favor acclimatization. However, when allowed to manifest in an uncontrolled fashion, they lead to patho-physiological entities like acute mountain sickness (AMS), high altitude pulmonary edema (HAPE) and high altitude cerebral edema (HACE). A gradual ascent with enough rest factored as one moves further above 3000 m (9842 ft) is considered the best approach to prevent or reduce the incidence of AMS, HACE and HAPE. Based on the above mentioned basic principles of the rise, a few "golden rules" have been formulated as standard protocols for high altitude travel (Table **3**).

Table 2 (a). Different physiological terms are used in the context of hypoxia. (**b**). Approximate barometric pressure, inspired partial pressure of oxygen, and partial pressure of arterial oxygen and carbon dioxide at various altitudes for acclimatized people. Adapted from Grissom, C. "High-altitude diseases (HACE/HAPE)" Respiratory emergencies. London: Hodder Arnold (2006): 253-267.

Symbol	Term
P_B	Barometric pressure (mm Hg)
Po_2	Partial pressure of Oxygen
Pio_2	Inspired Po_2 = [0.21* (P_B-47 mm Hg*)]
P_Ao_2	Po2 in alveolous
$Paco_2$	Partial pressure of carbon dioxide in arterial blood
Pao_2	Po_2 in arterial blood
$Sao_{2\%}$	Arterial oxygen saturation percentage (Hbo_2/Total Hb *100)
R	Respiratory quotient (Co_2 produced/O_2 consumed)
$P_Ao_2 = Pio_2 - Paco_2/R$	Alveolar gas equation

*Vapor pressure of H_2O at 37^{0}C

(b).

Altitude (in Meters; feet)	Barometric pressure (mm Hg)	Pio_2 (mm Hg)	Pao_2 (mm Hg)	$Paco_2$ (mm Hg)
Sea Level	760	150	90	40
1524; 5,000	635	124	75	36
2743; 9,000	550	106	60	33
4572; 15,000	430	80	52	25
6000; 19,700	355	64	41	20
8000; 26,250	280	49	37	13
8848; 29,030	253	43	30	11

At high altitudes, within minutes of exposure, hyperventilation begins which is the first physiological adjustment to the altitude. This process occurs due to the carotid bodies signaling a deficiency of oxygen levels in the blood (arterial pO_2) linked with the respiration center in the medulla. This is termed hypoxic ventilatory response (HVR). Pulmonary artery pressure (PAP) also facilitates a greater exchange of gases in the alveoli [21]. Hyperventilation alone is usually not capable of meeting the systemic requirement of oxygen. Thus, breathing rate and breathing depth increase simultaneously, termed hyperpnea, which is the first sign of acute acclimatization. Additionally, there is also a decrease in water content at high altitudes resulting in highly viscous blood owing to the increased density of red blood cells. Consequently, there is respiratory alkalosis due to the above factors [22]. Respiratory alkalosis inhibits hyperventilation [23]. This event sometimes leads to an increased mis-match in ventilation-perfusion ratio as the pulmonary artery pressure and that may not have decreased proportionately to the decrease in hyperpnea. A gravely mis-matched ventilation-perfusion ratio is attributed to the onset of HAPE [24, 25]. To counter alkalosis and stabilize the pH of blood and cerebrospinal fluid, the kidneys excrete excess bicarbonate ions [26]. Oxygen dissociation curve, a measure of oxyhemoglobin percentage at a given pO_2, has been reported since long by many authors to shift slightly to the right upon acclimatization to hypobaric hypoxia [27]. Also, there is lowered oxygen saturation of blood as there is low pO_2. To ensure the already limited oxygen which is effectively distributed among tissues, the cardiovascular system functions harder. There is an increased heart rate leading to an increased cardiac output eventually turning into tachycardia. Hemoglobin levels also increase, initially due to the increased concentration of erythrocytes *via* loss of fluids (due to increased diuresis) followed by the increased production of erythrocytes (due to erythropoiesis) [28, 29]. However, the thickened blood due to water loss and more red blood cells increase the strain on the cardiovascular system. When this remains uncontrolled, Monge's disease or chronic mountain sickness (CMS) develops in the long term. This aspect is also associated with thrombosis. The tissues also show marked alterations to augment oxygen retrieval and energy efficiency. They have increased angiogenesis (due to HIF1a and VEGF), increased myoglobin levels, and higher mitochondrial concentration per unit area of tissue [26]. The above processes have the conjugated effect of suppressing metabolic activity while increasing energy demands leading to weight loss [30]. Since the central nervous system is primarily dependent upon aerobic respiration for energy, hypobaric hypoxia causes poor cognitive performance in addition to poor physical performance for the same tasks at higher altitudes. The patho-physiological aspects are summarized in Fig. (**1**). All these changes are reversed, at least partially in the short-term by altitude acclimatization. Residence at high-altitude over generations leads to multiple permanent phenotypic and genotypic alterations collectively called altitude adaptation. Both acclimatization and adaptation are discussed below prior to a brief description of HAIs, particularly HAPE.

ACCLIMATIZATION TO ALTITUDE ZONES

Acclimatization is a process by which an individual becomes tolerant of adverse environmental conditions. During high altitude exposure, the individual must acclimatize so as to survive the associated harsh environmental conditions like cold, UV, low humidity and, most importantly, hypobaric hypoxia. Acclimatization to altitude is in essence a spectrum of physiological and molecular processes that provide increased oxygen influx to the organism mainly by modifying oxygen transport system, reducing oxygen consumption, heart rate and stroke volume [31]. A cardinal physiological sign of successful acclimatization to a particular altitude zone (Fig. **2**) is considered the blood oxygen saturation being similar to sea-level values for the given individual [32]. However, these studies also hint at the acclimatization towards all concomitant reductions of cellular energy turnover and oxygen demand. This is achieved partly by down-regulating energy-intensive cellular mechanisms like ion-pumps and protein turnover [33]. However, studies on the molecular signature as well as the signaling events of acclimatization are conspicuous by their absence. Apart from acute HAIs, even chronic ones like Monge's disease (Chronic mountain sickness; CMS) are also linked to the loss of acclimatization [34 - 36]. Thus, the molecular processes causing altitude acclimatization become more pertinent. An interesting aspect overlooked by many workers is that of acclimatization related omics studies. Although several reports are there showing physiological effects of varying exposures to HH of different durations (*e.g.* reduced plasma volume, increased vascularization, a decrease in albumin content, decreased SpO_2, decreased muscle mass, increased aerobic capacity during exercise and reduced spatial cognitive ability/confusion) [37 - 43]. The molecular events conferring altitude acclimatization during various acclimatization protocols include (graded ascent; climb high, sleep low; train low, sleep high; train high, sleep low *etc.*) [39, 41, 44 - 46]. However, the effects of various altitude zones (varying intensity of HH) for a fixed duration of HH remain largely unattended except for a few reports [47, 48]. Thus, there needs to be a consolidated investigation into both the molecular events that confer acclimatization as well as betterment of the protocol for altitude acclimatization.

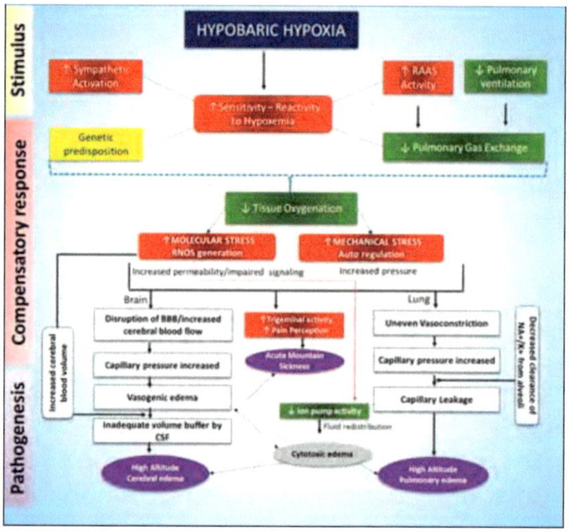

Fig. (1). Summary of hypobaric hypoxia induced pathophysiological changes owing to elevation.

While some individuals' short stay at altitude lasting a few months is made possible by undergoing acclimatization, longer stays lasting a lifetime or generations involving a population require more extensive changes not only to physiology but also to the genetic constitution.

ADAPTATION TO ALTITUDE

Adaptation may be termed the destination of extremely long-term acclimatization. The main factor differentiating the two homologous processes is the involvement of the temporal scale. Acclimatization requires weeks and months while adaptation occurs over generations and involves changes to the genotypic and phenotypic constitution of a population. Hence, acclimatization and adaptation to altitude depend on two factors: the given altitude zone and the time spent at the given altitude zone. Adaptation to altitude involves lowered basal energy demands; improved oxygenation but without a strong hypoxic ventilatory response; improved vasculature with dense capillary network and absence of pulmonary artery hypertension. Adaptation has been well documented among various high-altitude native populations like Andeans, Ethiopians and Tibetans. In these sub-populations, instead of a common route to high altitude adaptation, varying changes in different genes and signaling patterns were observed. Hemoglobin levels and oxygen saturation of hemoglobin were observed to be divergent in these three populations, even though Tibetans and Andeans live at similar altitudes [49]. However, there is a final convergence in these three populations leading to similar outcomes, which include adaptation *via* improved angiogenesis, circulation and more efficient oxygen transport [50]. Andean population is the most studied as it has the highest proportion of mal-adapted individuals indicated by the high number of CMS patients [50, 51]. Beall reported that Tibetans have higher resting ventilation, exhaled NOx levels and arterial oxygen but lower hemoglobin concentration and % oxygen saturation as compared to Andeans while mitochondrial volume was found to be similar in both [52]. Further, in addition to populations exhibiting arterial hypoxemia+ erythrocytosis (Andeans) and arterial hypoxemia+normal venous hemoglobin concentration (Tibetans), Beall and co-workers also identified a third route of high-altitude adaptation in Ethiopians of the Semien plateau. In the Ethiopian model, both hemoglobin concentration and arterial oxygen saturation were near sea-level values [53]. A multitude of genome studies have been instrumental in determining the genes and signaling involved in altitude adaptation. The Tibetan population is reportedly still undergoing strong selective currents and is evolving with higher variation [52]. Genetic interaction networks pertaining to the development of the nervous system, immune mediators, cardiovascular system and cell growth, death and survival were found to be associated with altitude adaptation [50]. The important genes and their prospective functions, exclusively limited to humans, are listed below (Table **4**).

HIGH ALTITUDE ILLNESSES

The high altitude environment and its associated hypobaric hypoxia adversely affect human biology. Altitude sickness finds the first mention in the words of Tseen Hanshoo, some 2000 years ago, when he described the "Great and Little headaches" from high altitude areas [54]. Further notable progress was observed during the late 19th century when Europeans took note of the adverse effects of rapid ascent to high altitude during hot-air ballooning [26]. High altitude hypoxia causes acute as well as chronic illnesses, collectively termed high altitude illnesses (HAIs). CMS is the sole chronic HAI while acute HAIs consist of AMS, HACE, and HAPE.

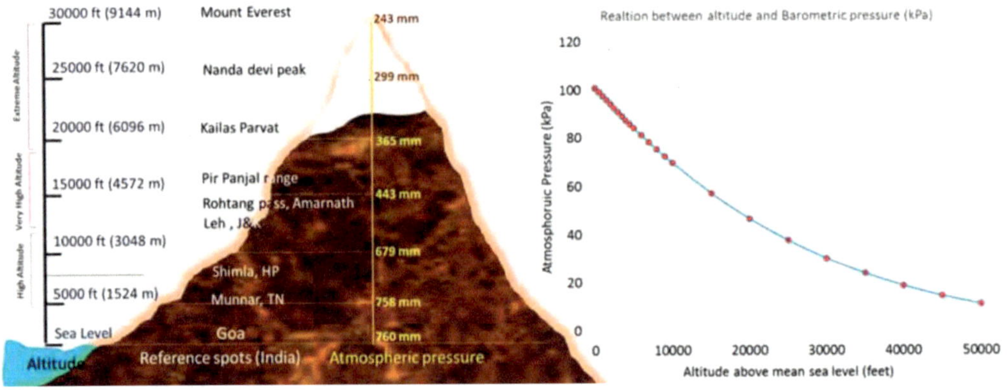

Fig. (2). Altitude zones and changes in relative atmospheric pressure. High altitude zone: 5000-11,500 feet (1500-3500 m); Very high altitude zone: 11500 ft – 18000 ft (3500-5500 m) and Extreme altitude zone: above 18000 feet (>5500 m) (Famous locations of India for reference). Death zone begins above 25,000 feet (7620 m). The decline in barometric pressure with increased altitude is shown in right panel. (Modified from Radak *et al.*, 2004).

CHRONIC MOUNTAIN SICKNESS (CMS)

CMS occurs in individuals who have adapted or acclimatized for a long period of time to high altitude. Being old and an overweight male with <85% pulse oximetry predicted FVC <80% and was said to be predisposed to CMS [55 - 57]. The cardinal signs of CMS are excessive erythropoiesis leading to very high hematocrits (≥21 g/dL in males; ≥19 g/dL in females) due to inefficient ventilation and hypoxic pulmonary vasoconstriction [58]. The extremely viscous nature of blood in CMS patients leads to Cor Pulmonale (Right-sided heart failure) or congestive heart failure as the heart, particularly the right ventricle is overburdened [59]. It is the sole HAI that affects native populations or life-long residents living at a particular altitude. Headache, dizziness, breathlessness, palpitations, perturbed sleep, exhaustion, cyanosis, palms of hands and soles of feet showing a burning sensation, dilated veins, muscle and joint pain, lack of appetite, depleted mental concentration, tinnitus and memory problems are symptoms of CMS [34]. The severity of CMS increases with advancing age [60]. In 2013, Sahota and Pawar reported CMS prevalence to be between ~6-13% in Himachal Pradesh, India [61]. Various studies have pegged CMS rates to range from 0% in Ethiopia; ~18% in Peru to ~29% in India [62 - 68]. A scoring system for CMS diagnosis (Qinghai score) and its accuracy, has been the subject of a crisp article by Leon-Velarde [69]. Currently, CMS has no direct treatments clinically as descent as exercise which is considered the safest option. This is so because safety and efficacy of pharmacological agents like enalapril have not been substantiated [34, 70]. However, a trial with acetazolamide administration in CMS patients proved successful [71].

ACUTE MOUNTAIN SICKNESS (AMS) AND HIGH ALTITUDE CEREBRAL EDEMA (HACE)

AMS has been the most frequently reported HAI, yet its symptoms and diagnosis are non-specific. AMS is not life-threatening if further ascent is prevented till its resolution. AMS is very common in lowlanders who ascend from the sea level to altitudes greater than 2600 m (8530 ft) and typically affects 30-50% of mountain climbers around the world when ascending above 9,000 ft (~2800 m) [72]. Following ascent, AMS symptoms begin in 2-3 hours. The condition is generally, but not always, self-limiting with most symptoms disappearing after 2-3 days, although insomnia may persist [73]. AMS must be treated as an emergency situation. The illness will resolve if no further altitude is gained. However, in some cases, descent to a lower altitude may be necessary in order to reverse the condition. AMS will present mostly on the first night at a new altitude as a stout headache (a minuscule minority do not report headache but have other symptoms of altitude sickness), loss of appetite/nausea, dizziness, fatigue at rest, insomnia and lassitude [74]. These symptoms are mostly non-specific and thus, classification, rather diagnosis of AMS is mostly dependent on self-scoring done using the Lake Louise questionnaire [75]. Non-responsive AMS where antiemetics (a drug that prevents or alleviates nausea and vomiting) and analgesics fail to abrogate nausea and headache usually is indicative of the progression of AMS into HACE. AMS and HACE are mutually associated disorders as both constitute two ends of the same spectrum of cerebral effects at high altitude. HACE is the more aggressive and lethal form mandating emergency medical services. Symptoms of HACE include ataxia, swelling of the face, confusion and coma [74, 76, 77]. HACE, a rarity considering AMS dissuades most individuals from further ascent, is reportedly caused by the disruption of the blood-brain barrier but a coherent explanation for the patho-physiological aspects of HACE are still lacking. Since HACE is characterized by increased intracranial pressures and visible edema in MRI, multiple factors like cerebral venous outflow, pain thresholds in the large cerebral vessels and meninges, compensatory capacity of cerebrospinal fluid *etc.* may be involved in the progression of MS into HACE [74, 77]. VEGF (vascular endothelial growth factor), a protein involved in hypoxia signaling downstream of HIF-1 [78, 79] and previously known to promote angiogenesis [80, 81] has emerged as prominent causative agent involved in the exacerbation of vasogenic edema leading to HACE [82]. An interesting aspect is the concomitance of AMS, HACE and HAPE in patients with one HAI leading to another [83].

HIGH ALTITUDE PULMONARY EDEMA (HAPE)

AMS is also recognized to occasionally develop into HAPE [74, 84], although most cases of HAPE do not coincide with AMS. HAPE incidence ranges from <0.2% to 7% depending upon ascent rate, individual susceptibility and altitude attained [74]. The HAPE incidence among Indian soldiers ascending by road (N=1003) or air (N=4178) to 3400 m (11,150 ft) was observed to be about ~0.3-0.4% [85]. However, for an unselected population of Indian Soldiers, airlift to an altitude of 5500 m (18044 ft) was associated with an HAPE incidence of up to 15% [86].

Table 3. Rules that have been laid down to acclimatize to cope up with the hypoxia.

Rule 1:	**If you are ill at altitude, your symptoms are due to the altitude until proven otherwise.**
Rule 2:	If you have altitude symptoms, do not go any higher.
Rule3:	If you are feeling very ill or are getting worse, or if you cannot walk heel-to-toe in a straight line, or have shortness of breath at rest, descend immediately.
Rule 4:	A person ill with altitude illness must always be accompanied by a responsible companion

The rules of altitude sickness were taken from Basnyat, Buddha. "High altitude cerebral and pulmonary edema." *Travel medicine and infectious disease* 3, no. 4 (2005): 199-211.

Symptoms of HAPE include non-productive cough, dyspnea during exertion, difficulty breathing at rest, mild to excessive frothy cough, chest tightness, crackles (upon auscultation of chest), cyanosis and tachycardia with clinical confirmation relying on a chest radiological/CT scan showing cloudy regions in the lungs indicative of edematous fluid accumulation [74, 87, 88]. HAPE is primarily a sequence of events where there is a ventilation-perfusion mis-match in the lungs due to higher pulmonary artery pressures, capillary stress failure, the inability to clear excess fluid accumulating in the alveolar space and most importantly lower pO_2. These events ultimately cause the cessation of lung function due to the disruption of alveolar air space owing to an exudate rich in proteins and inflammatory cells/molecules accumulating within the alveoli. The lung is also damaged by inflammatory events that occur during HAPE. Higher pulmonary artery pressures have long been held accountable for susceptibility to HAPE [89] but no cut-off values have emerged that can differentiate individuals into HAPE susceptible or tolerant based on the degree of hypoxic pulmonary vasoconstriction observed [74, 90]. Inflammation is also linked with HAPE. Bronchoalveolar lavage fluid from HAPE patient's blood and urine samples have shown increased inflammation in HAPE patients [91 - 94]. However, it was observed that inflammation occurs after the accumulation of fluid within alveoli and most of the volunteers developing HAPE suffered initially from viral upper respiratory tract infection [95, 96]. The role of alveolar epithelial sodium transporters in fluid clearance, and the inability to do so during HAPE have been discussed in many articles [97 - 101]. A major step towards understanding the molecular events associated with HAPE was the creation of a radiologically validated HAPE rat model which indicated pulmonary edema and inflammation synergistic events, and not the cause and effect [102]. Other studies have established potential HAPE markers in human patients [103, 104].

All HAIs are usually recoverable by following established guidelines for treatment. The most common protocol for the treatment of HAIs is descent and oxygen. HAPE and HACE involve emergency medical services [105]. They require treatment in the intensive care unit while AMS is usually cured by the administration of acetazolamide and rest [106]. For prevention of HAIs also, dexamethasone, acetazolamide, nifedipine, salmeterol and emergent pharmaceuticals like tadalafil, sildenafil are being used [74, 107 - 110].

THE UNDERLYING MOLECULAR EVENTS RESPONSIBLE FOR PHYSIOLOGICAL AND PATHO-PHYSIOLOGICAL OUTCOMES

As more and more investigations of the physiological effects of high-altitude associated hypoxia were unearthed, it was observed that there are a lot of underlying similarities in those individuals suffering from HAIs. The same is true for acclimatized and adapted individuals. Acclimatized or adapted individuals have a greater ability to use the full spectrum of aerobic metabolism even with reduced oxygen supply as compared to those newly inducted to a high-altitude environment. Although the symptoms of HAIs vary, they all ultimately cause increased inflammation and edema while stressing either the cardiopulmonary or cerebrovascular systems. Even end-stage co-associations between HAIs wherein one HAI (say AMS) leads to other HAIs (say HAPE) during its progression hint at shared molecular mechanisms unifying the ultimate causal event for different HAIs.

Hypoxia at the molecular level challenges the mitochondrial respiratory process leading to the excessive formation of oxygen radicals. During hypoxia, since mitochondrial function is solely dependent on oxygen levels, Complex III of the mitochondrial respiratory complex mal-functions lead to excess generation of reactive oxygen species [111, 112]. This in turn is thought to provide impetus for hypoxic signaling at large [113]. Mitochondria are known to require the biggest share of oxygen (~90%) in a cell to empower the process of oxidative phosphorylation (OXPHOS). OXPHOS is known to provide adequate ATP supply to the cell during normal resting condition. However, during hypoxia, due to insufficient oxygen levels, OXPHOS and resultant ATP production are down-regulated. If this lowered ATP count is not managed or is very severe, then cell death might occur. To manage this shortfall of oxygen derived ATP, glycolytic pathways are activated (*via* AMP-activated protein kinase pathway) [114]. However, glycolysis is effective only in the short-term. For longer durations of hypoxia, HIF-1 is activated. The activation of HIF-1 is dependent upon HIF-1a subunit stabilization. HIF-1a in normoxic conditions is marked for proteasomal degradation (polyubiquitinylation) by von Hippel Lindau protein (of E3 ubiquitin ligase complex). This occurs due to HIF-1a being hydroxylated by prolyl hydroxylases using oxygen [115, 116]. However, during hypoxic conditions, this hydroxylation is down-regulated, its extent being proportional to the degree of hypoxia encountered [116, 117]. Thus, HIF-1 complex becomes functional and over 200 genes are transcriptionally altered [118, 119].Various factors like mitochondrial products, citric acid cycle intermediates and free radicals apart from oxygen levels play important inter-related roles that affect HIF-1a hydroxylation/stabilization [120 - 122]. Hence, chronic durations of hypoxic exposure are usually associated with metabolic perturbations. In this regard, the interconnected nature of calcium and mitochondria needs to be highlighted. Calcium levels are known to rise intracellularly during the glycolytic switch occurring in hypoxia [123]. In a fantastic special issue edited by E.C. Toescu (Cell Calcium, Volume 36, Issues 3–4, Pages 181-348 (September–October 2004), various aspects related to calcium, mitochondrial energy homeostasis, and hypoxia-ischemia have been elaborated. Intracellular calcium ions, their channels/transporters and their differential levels have all been implicated in some way to various aspects of hypoxia. This includes oxygen sensing, vascular tone, pulmonary circulation, glial metabolism, ion channel regulation, gene expression and neuronal activity [123 - 134]. Sadly, in the context of hypobaric hypoxia, calcium signaling and calcium associated processes have received much less investigation, even though calpain (a calcium associated protein) was implicated in high altitude cases of thrombosis [135].

Another important linker to mitochondrial energy homeostasis and calcium is nitric oxide. Many reports show the interplay between calcium and nitric oxide levels. Both are induced by hypoxia exposure and tend to have a positive effect on each other's expression [136 - 138]. Calmodulin is the linker between calcium and nitric oxide [137, 139]. Nitric oxide has proven to be highly effective in subsiding the deleterious effects of hypobaric hypoxia (*e.g.* HAPE), mainly by vasorelaxation [24, 140 - 143]. However, nitric oxide is also known to cause certain adverse effects [144, 145] and post-translational modifications like nitrosylation and nitration [146 - 150] whose effects are yet to be fully comprehended at the organismal level. A recent *in vitro* study observed nitrosylation to be responsible for inhibiting carbonylation of proteins, thus providing insight towards cross-talk between PTMs and the protective role of nitric oxide [151].

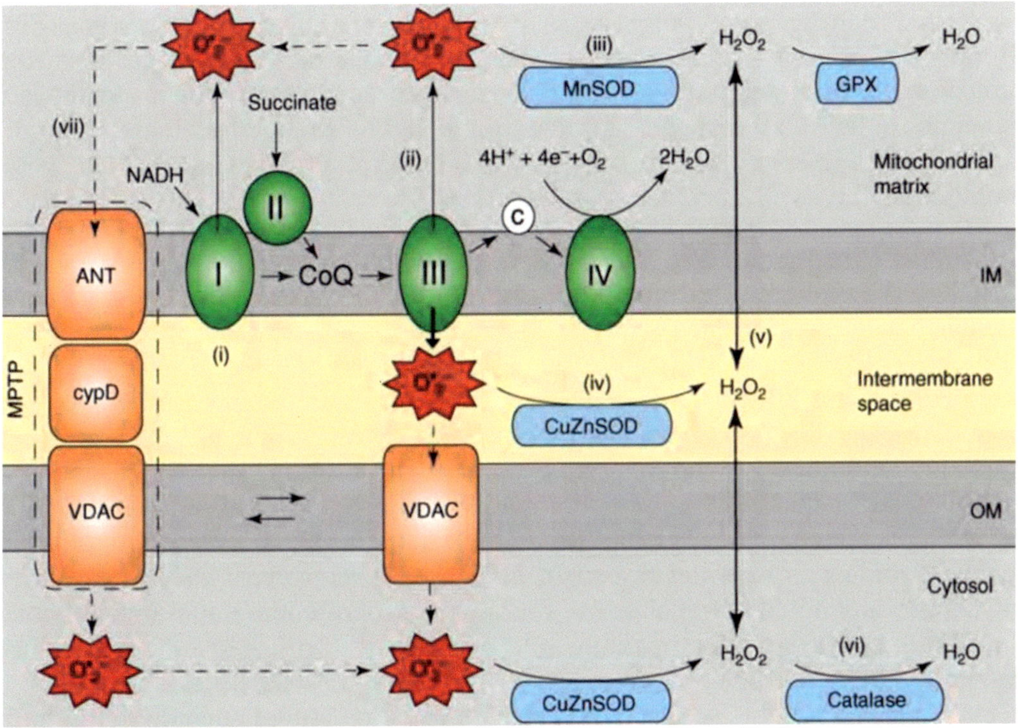

Fig. (3). Production of oxygen radicals at Complex III during OXPHOS and their subsequent neutralization by anti-oxidants like SOD, Catalase and GPX (Adapted from Poyton, R. O., Ball, K. A., & Castello, P. R. (2009). Mitochondrial generation of free radicals and hypoxic signaling. Trends in Endocrinology & Metabolism, 20(7), 332–340.)

It is widely known that reactive oxygen and nitrogen radicals (RONS) are generated in excess during high altitude hypoxia exposure by xanthine oxidase, mitochondrial respiratory chain and nitric oxide synthase [152]. These mechanisms of excessive RONs production are obviously related to calcium signaling, nitric oxide levels and deficient oxygen levels. To counter these, the organism possesses certain anti-oxidants molecules. Regressing and addressing the issue of excess radicals being generated during hypoxic exposure, it was observed that although basal radical levels are necessary for cell signaling events [153, 154], excessive free radical production causes damage to cellular components leading to inflammation, diseases and cell death in extreme cases [155 - 159]. Oxidative stress has also been linked to AMS severity in a recent study [160]. Other authors have also indicated increased oxidative stress to be a causal factor for acute HAIs and involving trigemino-vascular system [161 - 164]. Thus, preservation and exacerbation of anti-oxidants reserves in their functional state are of prime importance to manage high altitude hypoxia induced redox stress. Catalase, superoxide dismutase, thioredoxin, glutathione and their associated reductases and peroxidases are the central anti-oxidants reserves (Fig. **3**) naturally present within the organism [165]. Since these are all proteins, the proteome becomes the first line of defense against redox stress. The proteome is a dynamic 'ome' that responds almost immediately to environmental stimuli, particularly stressors through complex mechanistic procedures and has been highlighted for its diagnostic capabilities [166].

Proteomic investigations in the context of hypobaric hypoxia have revealed differential expression and notable perturbations in multiple proteins. Proteins involved in the anti-inflammatory response [167], anti-oxidant response [168], thrombotic tendencies [135] and neuronal functioning [169], apart from other niches have been identified in these proteome investigations. However, an important lacuna in these investigations is the confined contours of the hypobaric hypoxic conditions instead of broad ranges. In addition, there is a specific organism and a specific tissue proteome under investigation (plasma proteome is usually considered to be a 'global' proteome). SD rats have been used in multiple hypoxia studies as a model organism [170 - 175]. However, very few studies [176] have attempted to translate the findings in rat proteome into humans. Since wet lab experiments encompassing all these factors will lead to confounding results even if logistical limitations are overcome, dry lab techniques offer a convenient and reliable solution to create an *in silico* model encompassing both model organisms (rat and human) [177]. Also, using the composite data from previous proteomic investigations, potential therapeutic targets can be selected based on their functional relevance. These proteins can then be further evaluated for their roles in hypoxic adaptation by exogenously manipulating their levels. Exogenous administration of synthetic proteins or peptide mimetics (which mimic their unique structural features and/or downstream effects) is a strategy that augments bio-availability, does not induce side-effects upon controlled dosing and does not require extravagant formulations. However, it does not perform every function of the protein. The classification of peptide mimetics is A-D. A and B class mimetics have protein-like structural scaffolds, thus closely resemble the protein. C and D class mimetics have no such resemblance structurally. They are small molecules that only mechanistically resemble the protein. This should not be confused with L- and D- peptide mimetics, which are based on chirality of peptides. L-form amino acids form the structural backbone of L-peptide mimetics while the same backbone for D-peptide mimetics is courtesy of D-amino acids. L-amino acids occur naturally. These are subject to easy digestion, proteolysis and other associated biological regulations *in vivo*. D-amino acids, although just mirror images of L-amino acids, are more resistant to excretion and proteolysis due to their structure but have similar molecular effects without high immunogenicity *in vivo*. Thus, therapeutic peptide mimetics are generally D-peptides for the purpose of stability and enhanced activity [178, 179].

Reverting back to the anti-oxidants present in the organism, it has been widely observed that hypobaric hypoxia exposure decimates anti-oxidants reserves as per the degree and time of exposure [180, 181] and anti-oxidants supplementation in diet and/or increases in the natural anti-oxidants reserves *via* pre-conditioning and other related physical strategies, which is a crucial advantage during hypoxic exposures [182 - 188] and in diseases, like diabetes [189]. Thus, oral supplementation with anti-oxidants substances will help in attenuating many deleterious effects of hypobaric hypoxia. The oral anti-oxidants should be low-dosage, free of prescription, have negligible side-effects and easy availability. Sadly, not much work has been done in this direction except a few studies on plant extracts like *Rhodiola* [190 - 193] and silymarin [194].

HYPOXIA IS A FACET OF MULTIPLE DISEASES

Hypoxia, also termed oxygen sensing/availability, has been the crux of the Nobel Prize in Medicine and Physiology (2019) dedicated to hypoxia researchers Dr. Kaelin Jr, Dr. Ratcliffe and Dr. Semenza. This is due to the last decade's research realizing hypoxia is a crucial molecular event in multiple diseases like cancer, diabetes, obesity and lung diseases (*e.g.* chronic obstructive lung disease). Molecular processes like inflammation, as shown in the previous sections, are inextricably linked to hypoxia. Previous reviews state an intricate interconnected cascade between HIFs and inflammatory molecules like NF-kb, TLRs (innate immunity) along with T-cell sub-populations (adaptive immunity) which may have clinical relevance in treating diverse diseases like acute lung injury, myocardial ischemia and inflammatory bowel disease [195]. This review will focus only cancer and metabolic diseases as lung diseases, *e.g.* COPD, and their association with hypoxia are self-evident.

Multiple studies have shown hypoxia as an extremely important aspect in tumor biology/cancer, especially its relevance to cancer progression and treatment resistance in the past decade and a half [196 - 198]. More recent studies have revealed a greater therapeutic relevance of targeting HIFs in cancer, indicating plausible effects on cancer types, metabolism and ion channel operation caused by hypoxia, with one article claiming HIFs as the master regulator of cancer progression [199 - 204]. An extensive study by Bhandari *et al.* in 2019 on >8,000 tumors and 19 tumor types revealed hypoxia was associated with genomic instability, characteristic driver-mutation signatures, allelic loss of specific genes and shorter telomeres. They also identified mi-R133a-3p as a hypoxia modulated microRNA in hypoxic tumors [205].

Table 4. High altitude studies on humans have shown the mechanism of function of the genes involved in adaptation. Adapted from Azad, P., Stobdan, T., Zhou, D., Hartley, I., Akbari, A., Bafna, V., & Haddad, G. G. (2017). High-altitude adaptation in humans: From genomics to integrative physiology. Journal of Molecular Medicine, 95(12), 1269-1282.

Gene(s)	Population	Phenotype measured in human
EGLN1	Tibetan	Excessive erythrocytosis
SENP1	Andean	Excessive erythrocytosis
EPAS1	Tibetan	Repression and activation of EPAS1 targets
HMOX2	Tibetan	Binding of transcription factor Sp1
GUCY1A3	Kyrgyz	NO sensitivity

Initial research in the first decade of 21st century revealed a complex relationship between hyperglycemia and hypoxia. Researchers observed a loss of hypoxia signaling and HIF-1a function in diabetes [206] as well as impaired hypoxic endothelial progenitor cell-mediated blood vessel formation [207] and vasodilation [208]. More recent studies have been even more complex and contradictory. Gerber and Rutter had stated pancreatic beta cell dysfunction and loss at the onset of type 2 diabetes which are a result of excess oxidative stress due to hypoxia caused by enhanced mitochondrial respiration (triggered by hyperglycemia) [209]. A clinical study on eight adults with confirmed type 2 diabetes who were not taking medications, had no history of altitude sickness/sleep apnea/cardiovascular disease, and had a BMI of 55 kg/m^{2}or lower, showed moderate hypoxia (15% O_2) and it helped improved insulin sensitivity and glucose homeostasis [210]. Although the sample size is very small, in view of the two studies, it is clear that dose, duration and type of hypoxia are extremely important in deciding a beneficial or harmful effect of hypoxia in type 2 diabetes. Obesity too has been linked to hypoxia signaling. Adipocytes, after hyperplasia and hypertrophy owing to increased lipid storage, are known to become hypoxic.

HIF-1a is known to be an upstream modulator of multiple adipose tissue genes like leptin, GLUT1, MMPs (2&9), ILs (4&6) and PAI-1 [211]. Considering the close association of HIFs to other inflammatory molecules like NF-kb discussed above, the links between hypoxic signaling and chronic inflammation characteristic of obese individuals become self-evident. Seo *et al.* and Leake separately established adenine nucleotide translocase 2 (ANT2) as a focal protein connecting the paradigms of obesity, hypoxia and inflammation [212, 213]. The therapeutic relevance of HIFs association with obesity is shown by Xie *et al.* who established links between hepatic steatosis and intestinal HIF-2a in obesity [214]. Song *et al.* demonstrated a direct relevance between chronic high-altitude hypoxia exposure and obesity outcomes. They showed improved mitochondrial function and AMPK signaling in mice exposed to high-altitude hypoxia and fed a high fat diet for 8 weeks which resulted in increased lipolysis and decreased lipid accumulation. They have hypothesized that this may be a new treatment strategy for non-alcoholic fatty liver disease [215]. Obesity induced hypoxia also has epigenetic effects. Hypoxia during obesity has recently been implicated in aberrant methylation of genes involved in vascular function and inflammation [216]. Recent reviews have deeply dealt with the interlinks between obesity and cancer [217]. Thus, it is evident from the abovementioned studies that a large gamut of non-communicable diseases (*e.g.* cancer, metabolic diseases), which together make up the largest proportion of affected individuals, are all linked to hypoxia signaling. In the study of these diseases, high altitude hypoxia serves as an easy to implement, large cohort friendly, healthy population control group which may help elucidate the interactomes of these diseases if we are diligent and discerning in examining the molecular similarities between them.

CONCLUSION

This chapter has been finalized in the context of precision medicine and human health. Studies on Hypoxia have highlighted several aspects of the human system such as changes in the "omics" of the body and enhanced susceptibility to diseases or resistance. In view of the available data, the search may be mounted to uncover under what hypoxia conditions, genes and their expression, regulation and mutations are affected across the spectrum of population. Clearly, the high altitude study may prove to be a control compared to non-altitude population. Finally, it would be a rewarding proposition if herbal formulations are explored as a remedy not only to ameliorate the ill effect of hypoxia but also to provide a cure for the diseases caused due to hypoxia. Thus, we can learn a lot more from the studies on hypoxia than that we have learnt so far and then correlate the outcome with precision medicine.

LIST OF ABBREVIATIONS

COPD	Chronic obstructive pulmonary disease
HAPE	High altitude pulmonary edema
HACE	High altitude cerebral edema
WHO	World Health Organization
UV	Ultraviolet
HAI	High altitude illness
AMS	Acute mountain sickness
HVR	Hypoxic ventilatory response
PAP	Pulmonary artery pressure
pH	Potential of hydrogen
CMS	Chronic mountain sickness
HIF	Hypoxia-inducing factor
VEGF	Vascular endothelial growth factor
HH	Hypobaric hypoxia
SpO_2	Oxygen saturation
AMPK	Adenosine monophosphate kinase
ANT2	Adenine nucleotide transferase
PAI	Plasminogen activator inhibitor
MMP	Matrix metalloproteases
NF-kB	Nuclear factor kappa B
GLUT1	Glucose transporter 1
BMI	Body mass index
TLR's	Toll like receptors
SD	*Sprague Dawley*
RONS	Reactive oxygen and nitrogen radicals
ATP	Adenosine triphosphate
AMP	Adenosine monophosphate
OXPHOS	Oxidative phosphorylation
MRI	Magnetic resonance imaging
MS	Mountain sickness
FVC	Forced vital capacity
pO_2	Partial pressure of oxygen

AUTHOR CONTRIBUTIONS

YA developed the whole conception of the review and substantially contributed to the editing of the final version. SP and AG wrote the review.

REFERENCES

[1] Schulte PM. What is environmental stress? Insights from fish living in a variable environment. J Exp Biol 2014; 217(1): 23-34. [http://dx.doi.org/10.1242/jeb.089722] [PMID: 24353201]

[2] Münzel T, Sørensen M, Gori T, *et al.* Environmental stressors and cardio-metabolic disease: part I-epidemiologic evidence supporting a role for noise and air pollution and effects of mitigation strategies. Eur Heart J 2017; 38(8): 550-6. [PMID: 27460892]

[3] Münzel T, Sørensen M, Gori T, *et al.* Environmental stressors and cardio-metabolic disease: Part II-mechanistic insights. Eur Heart J 2017; 38(8): 557-64. [PMID: 27460891]

[4] Agyemang C, van Hooijdonk C, Wendel-Vos W, *et al.* Ethnic differences in the effect of environmental stressors on blood pressure and hypertension in the Netherlands. BMC Public Health 2007; 7(1): 118. [http://dx.doi.org/10.1186/1471-2458-7-118] [PMID: 17587458]

[5] Kristensen TS. Cardiovascular diseases and the work environment. A critical review of the epidemiologic literature on nonchemical factors. Scand J Work Environ Health 1989; 15(3): 165-79. [http://dx.doi.org/10.5271/sjweh.1864] [PMID: 2675305]

[6] Sexton K. Cumulative risk assessment: An overview of methodological approaches for evaluating combined health effects from exposure to multiple environmental stressors. Int J Environ Res Public Health 2012; 9(2): 370-90. [http://dx.doi.org/10.3390/ijerph9020370] [PMID: 22470298]

[7] Walston JD, Matteini AM, Nievergelt C, *et al.* Inflammation and stress-related candidate genes, plasma interleukin-6 levels, and longevity in older adults. Exp Gerontol 2009; 44(5): 350-5. [http://dx.doi.org/10.1016/j.exger.2009.02.004] [PMID: 19249341]

[8] Organization WH. *The world health report 2002: reducing risks, promoting healthy life.* World Health Organization 2002.

[9] Miller GE, Chen E, Zhou ES. If it goes up, must it come down? Chronic stress and the hypothalamic-pituitary-adrenocortical axis in humans. Psychol Bull 2007; 133(1): 25-45. [http://dx.doi.org/10.1037/0033-2909.133.1.25] [PMID: 17201569]

[10] Pacák K. Stressor-specific activation of the hypothalamic-pituitary-adrenocortical axis. Physiol Res 2000; 49 (1): S11-7. [PMID: 10984067]

[11] Cutolo M, Sulli A, Pizzorni C, Craviotto C, Straub RH. Hypothalamic-pituitary-adrenocortical and gonadal functions in rheumatoid arthritis. Ann N Y Acad Sci 2003; 992(1): 107-17. [http://dx.doi.org/10.1111/j.1749-6632.2003.tb03142.x] [PMID: 12794051]

[12] West JB. Highest permanent human habitation. High Alt Med Biol 2002; 3(4): 401-7. [http://dx.doi.org/10.1089/15270290260512882] [PMID: 12631426]

[13] Karan PP, Jenkins WM. The Himalayan Kingdoms: Bhutan, Sikkim, and Nepal. New Jersey: D. Van Nostrand Company 1963.

[14] Rai AK, Palni U, Tamang JP. Traditional knowledge of the Himalayan people on production of indigenous meat products 2009.

[15] Moore LG, *et al.* Comparative Aspects of High-Altitude Adaptation in Human Populations. In: Lahiri S, Prabhakar NR, Forster RE, Eds. Oxygen Sensing: Molecule to Man. Boston, MA: Springer US 2002; pp. 45-62. [http://dx.doi.org/10.1007/0-306-46825-5_6]

[16] Moore LG, Niermeyer S, Zamudio S. Human adaptation to high altitude: Regional and life-cycle perspectives. Am J Phys Anthropol 1998; 107(S27) (27): 25-64. [http://dx.doi.org/10.1002/(SICI)1096-8644(1998)107:27+<25::AID-AJPA3>3.0.CO;2-L] [PMID: 9881522]

[17] Cohen JE, Small C. Hypsographic demography: The distribution of human population by altitude. Proc Natl Acad Sci USA 1998; 95(24): 14009-14. [http://dx.doi.org/10.1073/pnas.95.24.14009] [PMID: 9826643]

[18] Gonggalanzi , *et al.* Acute mountain sickness among tourists visiting the high-altitude city of Lhasa at 3658 m above sea level: A cross-sectional study. Archives of public health = Archives belges de sante publique 2016; 74: 23-3. [http://dx.doi.org/10.1186/s13690-016-0134-z]

[19] Hackett P, Roach R, Sutton J. High-altitude medicine. Wilderness medicine 1995; 2.

[20] Wu T. Mountain rescue: the highest earthquake in Yushu. High Alt Med Biol 2011; 12(1): 93-5. [http://dx.doi.org/10.1089/ham.2010.1082] [PMID: 21452971]

[21] Kronenberg RS, Safar P, Lee J, *et al.* Pulmonary artery pressure and alveolar gas exchange in man during acclimatization to 12,470 ft. J Clin Invest 1971; 50(4): 827-37. [http://dx.doi.org/10.1172/JCI106554] [PMID: 5547278]

[22] Weil JV. Sleep at high altitude. High Alt Med Biol 2004; 5(2): 180-9. [http://dx.doi.org/10.1089/1527029041352162] [PMID: 15265339]

[23] Foster GT, Vaziri ND, Sassoon CS. Respiratory alkalosis. Respir Care 2001; 46(4): 384-91. [PMID: 11262557]

[24] Scherrer U, Vollenweider L, Delabays A, *et al.* Inhaled nitric oxide for high-altitude pulmonary edema. N Engl J Med 1996; 334(10): 624-30. [http://dx.doi.org/10.1056/NEJM199603073341003] [PMID: 8592525]

[25] Hopkins SR, Garg J, Bolar DS, Balouch J, Levin DL. Pulmonary blood flow heterogeneity during hypoxia and high-altitude pulmonary edema. Am J Respir Crit Care Med 2005; 171(1): 83-7. [http://dx.doi.org/10.1164/rccm.200406-707OC] [PMID: 15486339]

[26] Paralikar S, Paralikar J. High-altitude medicine. Indian J Occup Environ Med 2010; 14(1): 6-12. [http://dx.doi.org/10.4103/0019-5278.64608] [PMID: 20808661]

[27] Chiodi H. Respiratory adaptations to chronic high altitude hypoxia. J Appl Physiol 1957; 10(1): 81-7. [http://dx.doi.org/10.1152/jappl.1957.10.1.81] [PMID: 13405834]

[28] Viault F. On the large increase in the number of red cells in the blood of the inhabitants of the high plateaus of South America. High altitude physiology Stroudsburg, PA: Hutchinson Ross 1981; 333-4.

[29] Auerbach PS, Auerbach PS. Wilderness medicine. USA: Mosby Elsevier Philadelphia 2007.

[30] Butterfield GE, Gates J, Fleming S, Brooks GA, Sutton JR, Reeves JT. Increased energy intake minimizes weight loss in men at high altitude. J Appl Physiol 1992; 72(5): 1741-8. [http://dx.doi.org/10.1152/jappl.1992.72.5.1741] [PMID: 1601781]

[31] Sutton J, Reeves J, Groves B, *et al.* Oxygen transport and cardiovascular function at extreme altitude: Lessons from Operation Everest II. Int J Sports Med 1992; 13(S 1): S13-8. [http://dx.doi.org/10.1055/s-2007-1024580] [PMID: 1483751]

[32] Calbet JAL, Boushel R, Rådegran G, Søndergaard H, Wagner PD, Saltin B. Why is $\dot{V}O_{2\,max}$ after altitude acclimatization still reduced despite normalization of arterial O_2 content? Am J Physiol Regul

Integr Comp Physiol 2003; 284(2): R304-16.
[http://dx.doi.org/10.1152/ajpregu.00156.2002] [PMID: 12388462]

[33] Grocott M, Montgomery H, Vercueil A. High-altitude physiology and pathophysiology: Implications and relevance for intensive care medicine. Crit Care 2007; 11(1): 203-3.
[http://dx.doi.org/10.1186/cc5142] [PMID: 17291330]

[34] Villafuerte FC, Corante N. Chronic mountain sickness: Clinical aspects, etiology, management, and treatment. High Alt Med Biol 2016; 17(2): 61-9.
[http://dx.doi.org/10.1089/ham.2016.0031] [PMID: 27218284]

[35] Arias-Stella J, Krüger H, Recavarren S. Pathology of chronic mountain sickness. Thorax 1973; 28(6): 701-8.
[http://dx.doi.org/10.1136/thx.28.6.701] [PMID: 4787982]

[36] Peñaloza D, Sime F. Chronic cor pulmonale due to loss of altitude acclimatization (chronic mountain sickness). Am J Med 1971; 50(6): 728-43.
[http://dx.doi.org/10.1016/0002-9343(71)90181-1] [PMID: 4253583]

[37] Barcroft J, *et al.* Observations upon the effect of high altitude on the physiological processes of the human body, carried out in the Peruvian Andes, chiefly at Cerro de Pasco. Philos Trans R Soc Lond, B Contain Pap Biol Character 1923; 351-480.

[38] Dent C. Physiological effects of high altitudes. Geogr J 1893; 1(1): 46-8.
[http://dx.doi.org/10.2307/1774202]

[39] Lundby C, Calbet JAL, Sander M, *et al.* Exercise economy does not change after acclimatization to moderate to very high altitude. Scand J Med Sci Sports 2007; 17(3): 281-91.
[http://dx.doi.org/10.1111/j.1600-0838.2006.00530.x] [PMID: 17501869]

[40] McFarland RA. Psycho-physiological studies at high altitude in the Andes. I. The effect of rapid ascents by aeroplane and train. J Comp Psychol 1937; 23(1): 191-225.
[http://dx.doi.org/10.1037/h0058262]

[41] Naeije R. Physiological adaptation of the cardiovascular system to high altitude. Prog Cardiovasc Dis 2010; 52(6): 456-66.
[http://dx.doi.org/10.1016/j.pcad.2010.03.004] [PMID: 20417339]

[42] Wagner PD, Araoz M, Boushel R, *et al.* Pulmonary gas exchange and acid-base state at 5,260 m in high-altitude Bolivians and acclimatized lowlanders. J Appl Physiol 2002; 92(4): 1393-400.
[http://dx.doi.org/10.1152/japplphysiol.00093.2001] [PMID: 11896002]

[43] Westerterp-Plantenga MS, Westerterp KR, Rubbens M, Verwegen CRT, Richelet JP, Gardette B. Appetite at "high altitude" [Operation Everest III (Comex-'97)]: a simulated ascent of Mount Everest. J Appl Physiol 1999; 87(1): 391-9.
[http://dx.doi.org/10.1152/jappl.1999.87.1.391] [PMID: 10409600]

[44] Benoit H, *et al.* Pre-acclimatization to high altitude using exercise with normobaric hypoxic gas mixtures. International journal of sports medicine 1992; 13(1): 213-6.
[http://dx.doi.org/10.1055/s-2007-1024643]

[45] Levine BD, Stray-Gundersen J. "Living high-training low": effect of moderate-altitude acclimatization with low-altitude training on performance. J Appl Physiol 1997; 83(1): 102-12.
[http://dx.doi.org/10.1152/jappl.1997.83.1.102] [PMID: 9216951]

[46] Muza SR. Military applications of hypoxic training for high-altitude operations. DTIC Document 2007.
[http://dx.doi.org/10.1249/mss.0b013e3180de49fe]

[47] Paul S, Gangwar A, Bhargava K, Ahmad Y. STAT3-RXR-Nrf2 activates systemic redox and energy homeostasis upon steep decline in pO_2 gradient. Redox Biol 2018; 14: 423-38.
[http://dx.doi.org/10.1016/j.redox.2017.10.013] [PMID: 29078168]

[48] Paul S, Gangwar A, Bhargava K, Khan N, Khurana P, Ahmad Y. Plasma protein(s)–based conceptual diagnostic tool for assessing high-altitude acclimation in humans. Funct Integr Genomics 2020; 20(2): 191-200.
[http://dx.doi.org/10.1007/s10142-019-00712-0] [PMID: 31444657]

[49] Beall CM. Andean, Tibetan, and Ethiopian patterns of adaptation to high-altitude hypoxia. Integr Comp Biol 2006; 46(1): 18-24.
[http://dx.doi.org/10.1093/icb/icj004] [PMID: 21672719]

[50] Azad P, Stobdan T, Zhou D, *et al.* High-altitude adaptation in humans: from genomics to integrative physiology. J Mol Med (Berl) 2017; 95(12): 1269-82.
[http://dx.doi.org/10.1007/s00109-017-1584-7] [PMID: 28951950]

[51] Monge C, León-Velarde F, Arregui A. Increasing prevalence of excessive erythrocytosis with age among healthy high-altitude miners. N Engl J Med 1989; 321(18): 1271.
[http://dx.doi.org/10.1056/NEJM198911023211817] [PMID: 2797095]

[52] Beall CM. Two routes to functional adaptation: Tibetan and Andean high-altitude natives. Proc Natl Acad Sci USA 2007; 104: 8655-60.
[http://dx.doi.org/10.1073/pnas.0701985104] [PMID: 17494744]

[53] Beall CM, Decker MJ, Brittenham GM, Kushner I, Gebremedhin A, Strohl KP. An Ethiopian pattern of human adaptation to high-altitude hypoxia. Proc Natl Acad Sci 2002; 99(26): 17215-8.
[http://dx.doi.org/10.1073/pnas.252649199] [PMID: 12471159]

[54] Krieger BP, de la Hoz RE. Altitude-related pulmonary disorders. Crit Care Clin 1999; 15(2): 265-280, 8.
[http://dx.doi.org/10.1016/S0749-0704(05)70054-3] [PMID: 10331128]

[55] Sime F, Monge C, Whittembury J. Age as a cause of chronic mountain sickness (Monge's disease). Int J Biometeorol 1975; 19(2): 93-8.
[http://dx.doi.org/10.1007/BF01463864] [PMID: 1165128]

[56] Moore LG, Niermeyer S, Vargas E. Does chronic mountain sickness (CMS) have perinatal origins? Respir Physiol Neurobiol 2007; 158(2-3): 180-9.
[http://dx.doi.org/10.1016/j.resp.2007.06.016] [PMID: 17706469]

[57] De Ferrari A, Miranda JJ, Gilman RH, *et al.* Prevalence, clinical profile, iron status, and subject-specific traits for excessive erythrocytosis in andean adults living permanently at 3,825 meters above sea level. Chest 2014; 146(5): 1327-36.
[http://dx.doi.org/10.1378/chest.14-0298] [PMID: 24874587]

[58] León-Velarde F, Maggiorini M, Reeves JT, *et al.* Consensus statement on chronic and subacute high altitude diseases. High Alt Med Biol 2005; 6(2): 147-57.
[http://dx.doi.org/10.1089/ham.2005.6.147] [PMID: 16060849]

[59] León-Velarde F, Villafuerte FC, Richalet JP. Chronic mountain sickness and the heart. Prog Cardiovasc Dis 2010; 52(6): 540-9.
[http://dx.doi.org/10.1016/j.pcad.2010.02.012] [PMID: 20417348]

[60] Moore LG. Human genetic adaptation to high altitude. High Alt Med Biol 2001; 2(2): 257-79.
[http://dx.doi.org/10.1089/152702901750265341] [PMID: 11443005]

[61] Sahota I, Panwar N. Prevalence of Chronic Mountain Sickness in high altitude districts of Himachal Pradesh. Indian J Occup Environ Med 2013; 17(3): 94-100.
[http://dx.doi.org/10.4103/0019-5278.130839] [PMID: 24872667]

[62] Pasha MAQ, Newman JH. High-altitude disorders: pulmonary hypertension: pulmonary vascular disease: the global perspective. Chest 2010; 137(6) (Suppl.): 13S-9S.
[http://dx.doi.org/10.1378/chest.09-2445] [PMID: 20522576]

[63] Jiang C, Chen J, Liu F, *et al.* Chronic mountain sickness in Chinese Han males who migrated to the

Qinghai-Tibetan plateau: application and evaluation of diagnostic criteria for chronic mountain sickness. BMC Public Health 2014; 14(1): 701.
[http://dx.doi.org/10.1186/1471-2458-14-701] [PMID: 25007716]

[64] Penaloza D, Arias-Stella J. The heart and pulmonary circulation at high altitudes: healthy highlanders and chronic mountain sickness. Circulation 2007; 115(9): 1132-46.
[http://dx.doi.org/10.1161/CIRCULATIONAHA.106.624544] [PMID: 17339571]

[65] Negi PC, Asotra S, v RK, *et al.* Epidemiological study of chronic mountain sickness in natives of Spiti Valley in the Greater Himalayas. High Alt Med Biol 2013; 14(3): 220-9.
[http://dx.doi.org/10.1089/ham.2012.1127] [PMID: 24067183]

[66] Monge C, León-Velarde F, Arregui A. Increasing prevalence of excessive erythrocytosis with age among healthy high-altitude miners. N Engl J Med 1989; 321(18): 1271.
[http://dx.doi.org/10.1056/NEJM198911023211817] [PMID: 2797095]

[67] Richalet JP, Rivera M, Bouchet P, *et al.* Acetazolamide. Am J Respir Crit Care Med 2005; 172(11): 1427-33.
[http://dx.doi.org/10.1164/rccm.200505-807OC] [PMID: 16126936]

[68] Appenzeller O, Claydon VE, Gulli G, *et al.* Cerebral vasodilatation to exogenous NO is a measure of fitness for life at altitude. Stroke 2006; 37(7): 1754-8.
[http://dx.doi.org/10.1161/01.STR.0000226973.97858.0b] [PMID: 16763189]

[69] León-Velarde F, *et al.* Proposal for scoring severity in chronic mountain sickness (CMS), in Hypoxia. 2003, Springer. 2003; pp. 339-54.

[70] Plata R, Cornejo A, Arratia C, *et al.* Angiotensin-converting-enzyme inhibition therapy in altitude polycythaemia: a prospective randomised trial. Lancet 2002; 359(9307): 663-6.
[http://dx.doi.org/10.1016/S0140-6736(02)07812-1] [PMID: 11879862]

[71] Richalet JP, Rivera-Ch M, Maignan M, *et al.* Acetazolamide for Monge's disease: Efficiency and tolerance of 6-month treatment. Am J Respir Crit Care Med 2008; 177(12): 1370-6.
[http://dx.doi.org/10.1164/rccm.200802-196OC] [PMID: 18388356]

[72] Chawla A. Incidence of Acute Mountain Sickness in patients of high altitude pulmonary edema: Is the Lake Louise scoring accurate. Int J Aerosp Med 2009; 53(1): 1-5.

[73] West JB. The physiologic basis of high-altitude diseases. Ann Intern Med 2004; 141(10): 789-800.
[http://dx.doi.org/10.7326/0003-4819-141-10-200411160-00010] [PMID: 15545679]

[74] Luks AM, Swenson ER, Bärtsch P. Acute high-altitude sickness. Eur Respir Rev 2017; 26(143): 160096.
[http://dx.doi.org/10.1183/16000617.0096-2016] [PMID: 28143879]

[75] Roach R, *et al.* The Lake Louise acute mountain sickness scoring system. Hypoxia and molecular medicine 1993; 272(4)

[76] Yarnell PR, Heit J, Hackett PH. High-altitude cerebral edema (HACE): the Denver/Front Range experience. in Seminars in neurology. Inc: Thieme Medical Publishers 2000.

[77] Hackett PH, Roach RC. High altitude cerebral edema. High Alt Med Biol 2004; 5(2): 136-46.
[http://dx.doi.org/10.1089/1527029041352054] [PMID: 15265335]

[78] Matsumura A, Kubota T, Taiyoh H, *et al.* HGF regulates VEGF expression via the c-Met receptor downstream pathways, PI3K/Akt, MAPK and STAT3, in CT26 murine cells. Int J Oncol 2013; 42(2): 535-42.
[http://dx.doi.org/10.3892/ijo.2012.1728] [PMID: 23233163]

[79] Gray MJ, Zhang J, Ellis LM, *et al.* HIF-1α, STAT3, CBP/p300 and Ref-1/APE are components of a transcriptional complex that regulates Src-dependent hypoxia-induced expression of VEGF in pancreatic and prostate carcinomas. Oncogene 2005; 24(19): 3110-20.
[http://dx.doi.org/10.1038/sj.onc.1208513] [PMID: 15735682]

[80] Koukourakis M, Papazoglou D, Giatromanolaki A, Bougioukas G, Maltezos E, Sivridis E. VEGF gene sequence variation defines VEGF gene expression status and angiogenic activity in non-small cell lung cancer. Lung Cancer 2004; 46(3): 293-8.
[http://dx.doi.org/10.1016/j.lungcan.2004.04.037] [PMID: 15541813]

[81] Chen MC, Hsu WL, Hwang PA, Chou TC. Low molecular weight fucoidan inhibits tumor angiogenesis through downregulation of HIF-1/VEGF signaling under hypoxia. Mar Drugs 2015; 13(7): 4436-51.
[http://dx.doi.org/10.3390/md13074436] [PMID: 26193287]

[82] Schoch HJ, Fischer S, Marti HH. Hypoxia-induced vascular endothelial growth factor expression causes vascular leakage in the brain. Brain 2002; 125(11): 2549-57.
[http://dx.doi.org/10.1093/brain/awf257] [PMID: 12390979]

[83] Grissom CK. Medical therapy of high altitude illness. Amer Alpine J 1993; 35: 118-23.

[84] Grissom CK, Zimmerman GA, Whatley RE. Endothelial selectins in acute mountain sickness and high-altitude pulmonary edema. Chest 1997; 112(6): 1572-8.
[http://dx.doi.org/10.1378/chest.112.6.1572] [PMID: 9404756]

[85] Apte CV, Tomar RKS, Sharma D. Incidence of high altitude pulmonary edema in low-landers during re-exposure to high altitude after a sojourn in the plains. Med J Armed Forces India 2015; 71(3): 214-20.
[http://dx.doi.org/10.1016/j.mjafi.2013.03.009] [PMID: 26288488]

[86] Singh I, Roy SB. High altitude pulmonary edema: Clinical, hemodynamic, and pathologic studies. Biomedicine of high terrestrial elevation problems 1969; 108-20.

[87] Hultgren HN. High altitude pulmonary edema. Biomedicine of high terrestrial elevations, 1969; 131-41.

[88] Hultgren HN, Honigman B, Theis K, Nicholas D. High-altitude pulmonary edema at a ski resort. West J Med 1996; 164(3): 222-7.
[PMID: 8775933]

[89] Bärtsch P, Mairbäurl H, Maggiorini M, Swenson ER. Physiological aspects of high-altitude pulmonary edema. J Appl Physiol 2005; 98(3): 1101-10.
[http://dx.doi.org/10.1152/japplphysiol.01167.2004] [PMID: 15703168]

[90] Dehnert C, Mereles D, Greiner S, *et al.* Exaggerated hypoxic pulmonary vasoconstriction without susceptibility to high altitude pulmonary edema. High Alt Med Biol 2015; 16(1): 11-7.
[http://dx.doi.org/10.1089/ham.2014.1117] [PMID: 25803140]

[91] Kaminsky DA, Jones K, Schoene RB, Voelkel NF. Urinary leukotriene E4 levels in high-altitude pulmonary edema. A possible role for inflammation. Chest 1996; 110(4): 939-45.
[http://dx.doi.org/10.1378/chest.110.4.939] [PMID: 8874249]

[92] Hackett P, Rennie D. High-altitude pulmonary edema. JAMA 2002; 287(17): 2275-8.
[http://dx.doi.org/10.1001/jama.287.17.2275] [PMID: 11980529]

[93] Durmowicz AG, Noordeweir E, Nicholas R, Reeves JT. Inflammatory processes may predispose children to high-altitude pulmonary edema. J Pediatr 1997; 130(5): 838-40.
[http://dx.doi.org/10.1016/S0022-3476(97)80033-9] [PMID: 9152300]

[94] Duplain H, Sartori C, Lepori M, *et al.* Exhaled nitric oxide in high-altitude pulmonary edema: role in the regulation of pulmonary vascular tone and evidence for a role against inflammation. Am J Respir Crit Care Med 2000; 162(1): 221-4.
[http://dx.doi.org/10.1164/ajrccm.162.1.9908039] [PMID: 10903245]

[95] Schoene RB, Hultgren H, Swenson E. High-altitude pulmonary edema. Lung Biology in Health and Disease 2001; 161: 777-814.

[96] Swenson ER, Maggiorini M, Mongovin S, *et al.* Pathogenesis of high-altitude pulmonary edema:

inflammation is not an etiologic factor. JAMA 2002; 287(17): 2228-35. [http://dx.doi.org/10.1001/jama.287.17.2228] [PMID: 11980523]

[97] Mairbäurl H. Role of alveolar epithelial sodium transport in high altitude pulmonary edema (HAPE). Respir Physiol Neurobiol 2006; 151(2-3): 178-91. [http://dx.doi.org/10.1016/j.resp.2005.11.001] [PMID: 16337225]

[98] Nagyova B, O'Neill M, Dorrington KL. Inhibition of active sodium absorption leads to a net liquid secretion into in vivo rabbit lung at two levels of alveolar hypoxia. Br J Anaesth 2001; 87(6): 897-904. [http://dx.doi.org/10.1093/bja/87.6.897] [PMID: 11878694]

[99] Mairbäurl H, Schwöbel F, Höschele S, *et al.* Altered ion transporter expression in bronchial epithelium in mountaineers with high-altitude pulmonary edema. J Appl Physiol 2003; 95(5): 1843-50. [http://dx.doi.org/10.1152/japplphysiol.01156.2002] [PMID: 14555664]

[100] Zhou G, Dada LA, Sznajder JI. Regulation of alveolar epithelial function by hypoxia. Eur Respir J 2008; 31(5): 1107-13. [http://dx.doi.org/10.1183/09031936.00155507] [PMID: 18448505]

[101] Matthay MA, Folkesson HG, Clerici C. Lung epithelial fluid transport and the resolution of pulmonary edema. Physiol Rev 2002; 82(3): 569-600. [http://dx.doi.org/10.1152/physrev.00003.2002] [PMID: 12087129]

[102] Paul S, Gangwar A, Patir H, Bhargava K, Ahmad Y. Reverse translating SULT1A1, a potential biomarker in roentgenographically tested rat model of rapid HAPE induction. Life Sci 2019; 229: 132-8. [http://dx.doi.org/10.1016/j.lfs.2019.05.035] [PMID: 31100325]

[103] Ahmad Y, Shukla D, Garg I, *et al.* Identification of haptoglobin and apolipoprotein A-I as biomarkers for high altitude pulmonary edema. Funct Integr Genomics 2011; 11(3): 407-17. [http://dx.doi.org/10.1007/s10142-011-0234-3] [PMID: 21755356]

[104] Saxena S, Kumar R, Madan T, Gupta V, Muralidhar K, Sarma PU. Association of polymorphisms in pulmonary surfactant protein A1 and A2 genes with high-altitude pulmonary edema. Chest 2005; 128(3): 1611-9. [http://dx.doi.org/10.1378/chest.128.3.1611] [PMID: 16162765]

[105] Luks AM, McIntosh SE, Grissom CK, *et al.* Wilderness Medical Society consensus guidelines for the prevention and treatment of acute altitude illness. Wilderness Environ Med 2010; 21(2): 146-55. [http://dx.doi.org/10.1016/j.wem.2010.03.002] [PMID: 20591379]

[106] Luks AM, Swenson ER. Medication and dosage considerations in the prophylaxis and treatment of high-altitude illness. Chest 2008; 133(3): 744-55. [http://dx.doi.org/10.1378/chest.07-1417] [PMID: 18321903]

[107] Gallagher SA, Hackett PH. High-altitude illness. Emerg Med Clin North Am 2004; 22(2): 329-355, 8. [http://dx.doi.org/10.1016/j.emc.2004.02.001] [PMID: 15163571]

[108] Rodway GW, Hoffman LA, Sanders MH. High-altitude-related disorders—part I: Pathophysiology, differential diagnosis, and treatment. Heart Lung 2003; 32(6): 353-9. [http://dx.doi.org/10.1016/j.hrtlng.2003.08.002] [PMID: 14652526]

[109] Fiore DC, Hall S, Shoja P. Altitude illness: risk factors, prevention, presentation, and treatment. Am Fam Physician 2010; 82(9): 1103-10. [PMID: 21121556]

[110] Luks AM, McIntosh SE, Grissom CK, *et al.* Wilderness Medical Society practice guidelines for the prevention and treatment of acute altitude illness: 2014 update. Wilderness Environ Med 2014; 25(4) (Suppl.): S4-S14. [http://dx.doi.org/10.1016/j.wem.2014.06.017] [PMID: 25498261]

[111] Guzy RD, Schumacker PT. Oxygen sensing by mitochondria at complex III: The paradox of increased reactive oxygen species during hypoxia. Exp Physiol 2006; 91(5): 807-19.

[http://dx.doi.org/10.1113/expphysiol.2006.033506] [PMID: 16857720]

[112] de Groot H, Littauer A. Hypoxia, reactive oxygen, and cell injury. Free Radic Biol Med 1989; 6(5): 541-51.
[http://dx.doi.org/10.1016/0891-5849(89)90047-6] [PMID: 2663666]

[113] Bell EL, Klimova TA, Eisenbart J, *et al.* The Qo site of the mitochondrial complex III is required for the transduction of hypoxic signaling via reactive oxygen species production. J Cell Biol 2007; 177(6): 1029-36.
[http://dx.doi.org/10.1083/jcb.200609074] [PMID: 17562787]

[114] Santore MT, McClintock DS, Lee VY, Budinger GRS, Chandel NS. Anoxia-induced apoptosis occurs through a mitochondria-dependent pathway in lung epithelial cells. Am J Physiol Lung Cell Mol Physiol 2002; 282(4): L727-34.
[http://dx.doi.org/10.1152/ajplung.00281.2001] [PMID: 11880298]

[115] Vasco Ferreira J, Rosa Soares A, Silva Ramalho J, Pereira P, Girao H. K63 linked ubiquitin chain formation is a signal for HIF1A degradation by Chaperone-Mediated Autophagy. Sci Rep 2015; 5(1): 10210.
[http://dx.doi.org/10.1038/srep10210] [PMID: 25958982]

[116] Semenza GL. Hydroxylation of HIF-1: Oxygen sensing at the molecular level. Physiology 2004; 19(4): 176-82.
[http://dx.doi.org/10.1152/physiol.00001.2004] [PMID: 15304631]

[117] Ollerenshaw M, Page T, Hammonds J, Demaine A. Polymorphisms in the hypoxia inducible factor-1α gene (HIF1A) are associated with the renal cell carcinoma phenotype. Cancer Genet Cytogenet 2004; 153(2): 122-6.
[http://dx.doi.org/10.1016/j.cancergencyto.2004.01.014] [PMID: 15350301]

[118] Semenza GL. Targeting HIF-1 for cancer therapy. Nat Rev Cancer 2003; 3(10): 721-32.
[http://dx.doi.org/10.1038/nrc1187] [PMID: 13130303]

[119] Kaluz S, Kaluzová M, Stanbridge EJ. Rational design of minimal hypoxia-inducible enhancers. Biochem Biophys Res Commun 2008; 370(4): 613-8.
[http://dx.doi.org/10.1016/j.bbrc.2008.03.147] [PMID: 18402769]

[120] Solaini G, Baracca A, Lenaz G, Sgarbi G. Hypoxia and mitochondrial oxidative metabolism. Biochim Biophys Acta Bioenerg 2010; 1797(6-7): 1171-7.
[http://dx.doi.org/10.1016/j.bbabio.2010.02.011]

[121] Pan Y, Mansfield KD, Bertozzi CC, *et al.* Multiple factors affecting cellular redox status and energy metabolism modulate hypoxia-inducible factor prolyl hydroxylase activity in vivo and in vitro. Mol Cell Biol 2007; 27(3): 912-25.
[http://dx.doi.org/10.1128/MCB.01223-06] [PMID: 17101781]

[122] Lin X, David CA, Donnelly JB, *et al.* A chemical genomics screen highlights the essential role of mitochondria in HIF-1 regulation. Proc Natl Acad Sci 2008; 105(1): 174-9.
[http://dx.doi.org/10.1073/pnas.0706585104] [PMID: 18172210]

[123] Kristián T. Metabolic stages, mitochondria and calcium in hypoxic/ischemic brain damage. Cell Calcium 2004; 36(3-4): 221-33.
[http://dx.doi.org/10.1016/j.ceca.2004.02.016] [PMID: 15261478]

[124] Kahlert S, Reiser G. Glial perspectives of metabolic states during cerebral hypoxia—calcium regulation and metabolic energy. Cell Calcium 2004; 36(3-4): 295-302.
[http://dx.doi.org/10.1016/j.ceca.2004.02.009] [PMID: 15261485]

[125] Ouyang YB, Giffard RG. Cellular neuroprotective mechanisms in cerebral ischemia: Bcl-2 family proteins and protection of mitochondrial function. Cell Calcium 2004; 36(3-4): 303-11.
[http://dx.doi.org/10.1016/j.ceca.2004.02.015] [PMID: 15261486]

[126] Peers C, Kemp PJ. Ion channel regulation by chronic hypoxia in models of acute oxygen sensing. Cell

Calcium 2004; 36(3-4): 341-8.
[http://dx.doi.org/10.1016/j.ceca.2004.02.005] [PMID: 15261490]

[127] Seta KA, Yuan Y, Spicer Z, *et al.* The role of calcium in hypoxia-induced signal transduction and gene expression. Cell Calcium 2004; 36(3-4): 331-40.
[http://dx.doi.org/10.1016/j.ceca.2004.02.006] [PMID: 15261489]

[128] Starkov AA, Chinopoulos C, Fiskum G. Mitochondrial calcium and oxidative stress as mediators of ischemic brain injury. Cell Calcium 2004; 36(3-4): 257-64.
[http://dx.doi.org/10.1016/j.ceca.2004.02.012] [PMID: 15261481]

[129] Tauskela JS, Morley P. On the role of Ca^{2+} in cerebral ischemic preconditioning. Cell Calcium 2004; 36(3-4): 313-22.
[http://dx.doi.org/10.1016/j.ceca.2004.02.008] [PMID: 15261487]

[130] Thorne GD, Ishida Y, Paul RJ. Hypoxic vasorelaxation: Ca^{2+}-dependent and Ca^{2+}-independent mechanisms. Cell Calcium 2004; 36(3-4): 201-8.
[http://dx.doi.org/10.1016/j.ceca.2004.02.018] [PMID: 15261476]

[131] Toescu EC. Hypoxia sensing and pathways of cytosolic Ca^{2+} increases. Cell Calcium 2004; 36(3-4): 187-99.
[http://dx.doi.org/10.1016/j.ceca.2004.02.019] [PMID: 15261475]

[132] Ward JPT, Snetkov VA, Aaronson PI. Calcium, mitochondria and oxygen sensing in the pulmonary circulation. Cell Calcium 2004; 36(3-4): 209-20.
[http://dx.doi.org/10.1016/j.ceca.2004.02.017] [PMID: 15261477]

[133] Yamashima T. Ca^{2+}-dependent proteases in ischemic neuronal death. Cell Calcium 2004; 36(3-4): 285-93.
[http://dx.doi.org/10.1016/j.ceca.2004.03.001] [PMID: 15261484]

[134] Yao H, Haddad GG. Calcium and pH homeostasis in neurons during hypoxia and ischemia. Cell Calcium 2004; 36(3-4): 247-55.
[http://dx.doi.org/10.1016/j.ceca.2004.02.013] [PMID: 15261480]

[135] Tyagi T, Ahmad S, Gupta N, *et al.* Altered expression of platelet proteins and calpain activity mediate hypoxia-induced prothrombotic phenotype. Blood 2014; 123(8): 1250-60.
[http://dx.doi.org/10.1182/blood-2013-05-501924] [PMID: 24297866]

[136] Hampl V, Cornfield DN, Cowan NJ, Archer SL. Hypoxia potentiates nitric oxide synthesis and transiently increases cytosolic calcium levels in pulmonary artery endothelial cells. Eur Respir J 1995; 8(4): 515-22.
[http://dx.doi.org/10.1183/09031936.95.08040515] [PMID: 7664847]

[137] Busse R, Mülsch A. Calcium-dependent nitric oxide synthesis in endothelial cytosol is mediated by calmodulin. FEBS Lett 1990; 265(1-2): 133-6.
[http://dx.doi.org/10.1016/0014-5793(90)80902-U] [PMID: 1694782]

[138] Tjong YW, Li M, Hung MW, Wang K, Fung ML. Nitric oxide deficit in chronic intermittent hypoxia impairs large conductance calcium-activated potassium channel activity in rat hippocampal neurons. Free Radic Biol Med 2008; 44(4): 547-57.
[http://dx.doi.org/10.1016/j.freeradbiomed.2007.10.033] [PMID: 17996205]

[139] Zubrow AB, Delivoria-Papadopoulos M, Ashraf QM, Fritz KI, Mishra OP. Nitric oxide-mediated Ca^{2+}/calmodulin-dependent protein kinase IV activity during hypoxia in neuronal nuclei from newborn piglets. Neurosci Lett 2002; 335(1): 5-8.
[http://dx.doi.org/10.1016/S0304-3940(02)01138-2] [PMID: 12457729]

[140] Tuder RM, Flook BE, Voelkel NF. Increased gene expression for VEGF and the VEGF receptors KDR/Flk and Flt in lungs exposed to acute or to chronic hypoxia. Modulation of gene expression by nitric oxide. J Clin Invest 1995; 95(4): 1798-807.
[http://dx.doi.org/10.1172/JCI117858] [PMID: 7706486]

[141] Haynes WG, Noon JP, Walker BR, Webb DJ. Inhibition of nitric oxide synthesis increases blood pressure in healthy humans. J Hypertens 1993; 11(12): 1375-80. [http://dx.doi.org/10.1097/00004872-199312000-00009] [PMID: 7510736]

[142] Joannides R, Haefeli WE, Linder L, *et al.* Nitric oxide is responsible for flow-dependent dilatation of human peripheral conduit arteries in vivo. Circulation 1995; 91(5): 1314-9. [http://dx.doi.org/10.1161/01.CIR.91.5.1314] [PMID: 7867167]

[143] Umans JG, Levi R. Nitric oxide in the regulation of blood flow and arterial pressure. Annu Rev Physiol 1995; 57(1): 771-90. [http://dx.doi.org/10.1146/annurev.ph.57.030195.004011] [PMID: 7539996]

[144] Udayabanu M, Kumaran D, Nair RU, *et al.* Nitric oxide associated with iNOS expression inhibits acetylcholinesterase activity and induces memory impairment during acute hypobaric hypoxia. Brain Res 2008; 1230: 138-49. [http://dx.doi.org/10.1016/j.brainres.2008.06.081] [PMID: 18639532]

[145] Fagan KA, Morrissey B, Fouty BW, *et al.* Upregulation of nitric oxide synthase in mice with severe hypoxia-induced pulmonary hypertension. Respir Res 2001; 2(5): 306-13. [http://dx.doi.org/10.1186/rr74] [PMID: 11686901]

[146] Serrano J, Manuel Encinas J, Salas E, *et al.* Hypobaric hypoxia modifies constitutive nitric oxide synthase activity and protein nitration in the rat cerebellum. Brain Res 2003; 976(1): 109-19. [http://dx.doi.org/10.1016/S0006-8993(03)02691-X] [PMID: 12763628]

[147] Swamy M, Salleh MJM, Sirajudeen KNS, Yusof WRW, Chandran G. Nitric oxide (no), citrulline - no cycle enzymes, glutamine synthetase and oxidative stress in anoxia (hypobaric hypoxia) and reperfusion in rat brain. Int J Med Sci 2010; 7(3): 147-54. [http://dx.doi.org/10.7150/ijms.7.147] [PMID: 20567615]

[148] Peinado MÁ, Hernández R, Peragón J, Ovelleiro D, Pedrosa JÁ, Blanco S. Proteomic characterization of nitrated cell targets after hypobaric hypoxia and reoxygenation in rat brain. J Proteomics 2014; 109: 309-21. [http://dx.doi.org/10.1016/j.jprot.2014.07.015] [PMID: 25064252]

[149] Alonso D, Serrano J, Rodríguez I, *et al.* Effects of oxygen and glucose deprivation on the expression and distribution of neuronal and inducible nitric oxide synthases and on protein nitration in rat cerebral cortex. J Comp Neurol 2002; 443(2): 183-200. [http://dx.doi.org/10.1002/cne.10111] [PMID: 11793355]

[150] McMahon TJ, Doctor A. Extrapulmonary effects of inhaled nitric oxide: role of reversible S-nitrosylation of erythrocytic hemoglobin. Proc Am Thorac Soc 2006; 3(2): 153-60. [http://dx.doi.org/10.1513/pats.200507-066BG] [PMID: 16565424]

[151] Gangwar A, Paul S, Ahmad Y, Bhargava K. Competing trends of ROS and RNS-mediated protein modifications during hypoxia as an alternate mechanism of NO benefits. Biochimie 2018; 148: 127-38. [http://dx.doi.org/10.1016/j.biochi.2018.03.009] [PMID: 29571702]

[152] Dosek A, Ohno H, Acs Z, Taylor AW, Radak Z. High altitude and oxidative stress. Respir Physiol Neurobiol 2007; 158(2-3): 128-31. [http://dx.doi.org/10.1016/j.resp.2007.03.013] [PMID: 17482529]

[153] Lander HM. An essential role for free radicals and derived species in signal transduction. FASEB J 1997; 11(2): 118-24. [http://dx.doi.org/10.1096/fasebj.11.2.9039953] [PMID: 9039953]

[154] Schieber M, Chandel NS. ROS function in redox signaling and oxidative stress. Curr Biol 2014; 24(10): R453-62. [http://dx.doi.org/10.1016/j.cub.2014.03.034] [PMID: 24845678]

[155] Wu D, Cederbaum AI. Alcohol, oxidative stress, and free radical damage. Alcohol Res Health 2003;

27(4): 277-84.
[PMID: 15540798]

[156] Cadenas E, Davies KJA. Mitochondrial free radical generation, oxidative stress, and aging11This article is dedicated to the memory of our dear friend, colleague, and mentor Lars Ernster (1920–1998), in gratitude for all he gave to us. Free Radic Biol Med 2000; 29(3-4): 222-30.
[http://dx.doi.org/10.1016/S0891-5849(00)00317-8] [PMID: 11035250]

[157] Floyd RA, Carney JM. Free radical damage to protein and DNA: Mechanisms involved and relevant observations on brain undergoing oxidative stress. Ann Neurol 1992; 32(S1) (Suppl.): S22-7.
[http://dx.doi.org/10.1002/ana.410320706] [PMID: 1510377]

[158] Baynes JW. Role of oxidative stress in development of complications in diabetes. Diabetes 1991; 40(4): 405-12.
[http://dx.doi.org/10.2337/diab.40.4.405] [PMID: 2010041]

[159] Aruoma OI. Free radicals, oxidative stress, and anti-oxidants in human health and disease. J Am Oil Chem Soc 1998; 75(2): 199-212.
[http://dx.doi.org/10.1007/s11746-998-0032-9] [PMID: 32287334]

[160] Irarrázaval S, Allard C, Campodónico J, *et al.* Oxidative stress in acute hypobaric hypoxia. High Alt Med Biol 2017; 18(2): 128-34.
[http://dx.doi.org/10.1089/ham.2016.0119] [PMID: 28326844]

[161] Dosek A, Ohno H, Acs Z, Taylor AW, Radak Z. High altitude and oxidative stress. Respir Physiol Neurobiol 2007; 158(2-3): 128-31.
[http://dx.doi.org/10.1016/j.resp.2007.03.013] [PMID: 17482529]

[162] Bakonyi T, Radak Z. High altitude and free radicals. J Sports Sci Med 2004; 3(2): 64-9.
[PMID: 24482580]

[163] Vij AG, Dutta R, Satija NK. Acclimatization to oxidative stress at high altitude. High Alt Med Biol 2005; 6(4): 301-10.
[http://dx.doi.org/10.1089/ham.2005.6.301] [PMID: 16351564]

[164] Bailey DM, Bärtsch P, Knauth M, Baumgartner RW. Emerging concepts in acute mountain sickness and high-altitude cerebral edema: From the molecular to the morphological. Cell Mol Life Sci 2009; 66(22): 3583-94.
[http://dx.doi.org/10.1007/s00018-009-0145-9] [PMID: 19763397]

[165] Irshad M, Chaudhuri P. Oxidant-anti-oxidants system: role and significance in human body 2002.

[166] Anderson NL, Anderson NG. The human plasma proteome: history, character, and diagnostic prospects. Mol Cell Proteomics 2002; 1(11): 845-67.
[http://dx.doi.org/10.1074/mcp.R200007-MCP200] [PMID: 12488461]

[167] Ahmad Y, Sharma NK, Garg I, Ahmad MF, Sharma M, Bhargava K. An insight into the changes in human plasma proteome on adaptation to hypobaric hypoxia. PLoS One 2013; 8(7): e67548.
[http://dx.doi.org/10.1371/journal.pone.0067548] [PMID: 23844025]

[168] Ahmad Y, Sharma NK, Ahmad MF, Sharma M, Garg I, Bhargava K. Proteomic identification of novel differentiation plasma protein markers in hypobaric hypoxia-induced rat model. PLoS One 2014; 9(5): e98027.
[http://dx.doi.org/10.1371/journal.pone.0098027] [PMID: 24842778]

[169] Kumar G, Chhabra A, Mishra S, *et al.* H 2 S Regulates hypobaric hypoxia-induced early glio-vascular dysfunction and neuro-pathophysiological effects. EBioMedicine 2016; 6: 171-89.
[http://dx.doi.org/10.1016/j.ebiom.2016.03.002] [PMID: 27211559]

[170] Fletcher EC, Lesske J, Qian W, Miller CC III, Unger T. Repetitive, episodic hypoxia causes diurnal elevation of blood pressure in rats. Hypertension 1992; 19(6_pt_1): 555-61.
[http://dx.doi.org/10.1161/01.HYP.19.6.555] [PMID: 1592450]

[171] Gozal D, Daniel JM, Dohanich GP. Behavioral and anatomical correlates of chronic episodic hypoxia during sleep in the rat. J Neurosci 2001; 21(7): 2442-50. [http://dx.doi.org/10.1523/JNEUROSCI.21-07-02442.2001] [PMID: 11264318]

[172] Kumar GK, Rai V, Sharma SD, *et al.* Chronic intermittent hypoxia induces hypoxia-evoked catecholamine efflux in adult rat adrenal medulla via oxidative stress. J Physiol 2006; 575(1): 229-39. [http://dx.doi.org/10.1113/jphysiol.2006.112524] [PMID: 16777938]

[173] Mirand EA, Prentice TC. Presence of plasma erythropoietin in hypoxic rats with or without kidney (s) and/or spleen. Exp Biol Med (Maywood) 1957; 96(1): 49-51. [http://dx.doi.org/10.3181/00379727-96-23390] [PMID: 13485015]

[174] Karcher L, Zagermann P, Krieglstein J. Effect of an extract of Ginkgo biloba on rat brain energy metabolism in hypoxia. Naunyn Schmiedebergs Arch Pharmacol 1984; 327(1): 31-5. [http://dx.doi.org/10.1007/BF00504988] [PMID: 6493348]

[175] Chen L, Einbinder E, Zhang Q, Hasday J, Balke CW, Scharf SM. Oxidative stress and left ventricular function with chronic intermittent hypoxia in rats. Am J Respir Crit Care Med 2005; 172(7): 915-20. [http://dx.doi.org/10.1164/rccm.200504-560OC] [PMID: 15976378]

[176] Ahmad Y, Sharma NK, Ahmad MF, *et al.* The proteome of hypobaric induced hypoxic lung: insights from temporal proteomic profiling for biomarker discovery. Sci Rep 2015; 5(1): 10681. [http://dx.doi.org/10.1038/srep10681] [PMID: 26022216]

[177] Paul S, Bhargava K, Ahmad Y. The meta-analytical paradigm in an in silico hybrid: Pathways and networks perturbed during exposure to varying degrees of hypobaric hypoxia. Proteomics Clin Appl 2017; 11(7-8): 1600160. [http://dx.doi.org/10.1002/prca.201600160] [PMID: 28155252]

[178] Welch BD, VanDemark AP, Heroux A, Hill CP, Kay MS. Potent D-peptide inhibitors of HIV-1 entry. Proc Natl Acad Sci USA 2007; 104(43): 16828-33. [http://dx.doi.org/10.1073/pnas.0708109104] [PMID: 17942675]

[179] Weinstock MT, Francis JN, Redman JS, Kay MS. Protease-resistant peptide design—empowering nature's fragile warriors against HIV. Biopolymers 2012; 98(5): 431-42. [http://dx.doi.org/10.1002/bip.22073] [PMID: 23203688]

[180] Nakanishi K, Tajima F, Nakamura A, *et al.* Effects of hypobaric hypoxia on anti-oxidants enzymes in rats. J Physiol 1995; 489(3): 869-76. [http://dx.doi.org/10.1113/jphysiol.1995.sp021099] [PMID: 8788950]

[181] Joanny P, Steinberg J, Robach P, *et al.* Operation Everest III (Comex'97): the effect of simulated severe hypobaric hypoxia on lipid peroxidation and anti-oxidants defence systems in human blood at rest and after maximal exercise. Resuscitation 2001; 49(3): 307-14. [http://dx.doi.org/10.1016/S0300-9572(00)00373-7] [PMID: 11723998]

[182] Guo H, Zhang Z, Zhang L, *et al.* Chronic intermittent hypobaric hypoxia protects the heart against ischemia/reperfusion injury through upregulation of anti-oxidants enzymes in adult guinea pigs. Acta Pharmacol Sin 2009; 30(7): 947-55. [http://dx.doi.org/10.1038/aps.2009.57] [PMID: 19543301]

[183] Stroev SA, Gluschenko TS, Tjulkova EI, *et al.* Preconditioning enhances the expression of mitochondrial anti-oxidants thioredoxin-2 in the forebrain of rats exposed to severe hypobaric hypoxia. J Neurosci Res 2004; 78(4): 563-9. [http://dx.doi.org/10.1002/jnr.20282] [PMID: 15468176]

[184] Asha Devi S, Subramanyam MVV, Vani R, Jeevaratnam K. Adaptations of the anti-oxidants system in erythrocytes of trained adult rats: Impact of intermittent hypobaric-hypoxia at two altitudes. Comp Biochem Physiol C Toxicol Pharmacol 2005; 140(1): 59-67. [http://dx.doi.org/10.1016/j.cca.2005.01.003] [PMID: 15792624]

[185] Singh M, Arya A, Kumar R, Bhargava K, Sethy NK. Dietary nitrite attenuates oxidative stress and

activates anti-oxidants genes in rat heart during hypobaric hypoxia. Nitric Oxide 2012; 26(1): 61-73. [http://dx.doi.org/10.1016/j.niox.2011.12.002] [PMID: 22197744]

[186] Bailey DM, Davies B. Acute mountain sickness; prophylactic benefits of anti-oxidants vitamin supplementation at high altitude. High Alt Med Biol 2001; 2(1): 21-9. [http://dx.doi.org/10.1089/152702901750067882] [PMID: 11252695]

[187] Bautista-Ortega J, Ruiz-Feria CA. l-Arginine and anti-oxidants vitamins E and C improve the cardiovascular performance of broiler chickens grown under chronic hypobaric hypoxia. Poult Sci 2010; 89(10): 2141-6. [http://dx.doi.org/10.3382/ps.2010-00764] [PMID: 20852105]

[188] Pialoux V, Mounier R, Ponsot E, *et al.* Effects of exercise and training in hypoxia on anti-oxidants/pro-oxidant balance. Eur J Clin Nutr 2006; 60(12): 1345-54. [http://dx.doi.org/10.1038/sj.ejcn.1602462] [PMID: 16788711]

[189] Norouzirad R, González-Muniesa P, Ghasemi A. Hypoxia in obesity and diabetes: potential therapeutic effects of hyperoxia and nitrate. Oxidative medicine and cellular longevity 2017; 2017 [http://dx.doi.org/10.1155/2017/5350267]

[190] Lee S-Y, *et al.* Rhodiola crenulata extract alleviates hypoxic pulmonary edema in rats. Evidence-Based Complementary and Alternative Medicine 2013; 2013

[191] Lee S-Y, *et al.* Rhodiola crenulata and its bioactive components, salidroside and tyrosol, reverse the hypoxia-induced reduction of plasma-membrane-associated Na, K-ATPase expression via inhibition of ROS-AMPK-PKCζ pathway. Evidence-Based Complementary and Alternative Medicine, 2013; 2013.

[192] Ip SP, Che CT, Leung PS. Association of free radicals and the tissue renin-angiotensin system: prospective effects of Rhodiola, a genus of Chinese herb, on hypoxia-induced pancreatic injury 2001; 2(1): 16-25.

[193] WANG, L.-j., et al., N-butanol extract of Potentilla anserina L. inhibited injury resulted by acute hypobaric hypoxia in mice [J]. Acta Academiae Medicinae CPAF, 2011. 3(002).

[194] Paul S, Arya A, Gangwar A, Bhargava K, Ahmad Y. Size restricted silymarin suspension evokes integrated adaptive response against acute hypoxia exposure in rat lung. Free Radic Biol Med 2016; 96: 139-51. [http://dx.doi.org/10.1016/j.freeradbiomed.2016.04.020] [PMID: 27105952]

[195] Eltzschig HK, Carmeliet P. Hypoxia and Inflammation. N Engl J Med 2011; 364(7): 656-65. [http://dx.doi.org/10.1056/NEJMra0910283] [PMID: 21323543]

[196] Brown JM, Wilson WR. Exploiting tumour hypoxia in cancer treatment. Nat Rev Cancer 2004; 4(6): 437-47. [http://dx.doi.org/10.1038/nrc1367] [PMID: 15170446]

[197] Wilson WR, Hay MP. Targeting hypoxia in cancer therapy. Nat Rev Cancer 2011; 11(6): 393-410. [http://dx.doi.org/10.1038/nrc3064] [PMID: 21606941]

[198] Vaupel P, Mayer A. Hypoxia in cancer: Significance and impact on clinical outcome. Cancer Metastasis Rev 2007; 26(2): 225-39. [http://dx.doi.org/10.1007/s10555-007-9055-1] [PMID: 17440684]

[199] Eales KL, Hollinshead KER, Tennant DA. Hypoxia and metabolic adaptation of cancer cells. Oncogenesis 2016; 5(1): e190-0. [http://dx.doi.org/10.1038/oncsis.2015.50] [PMID: 26807645]

[200] Schito L, Semenza GL. Hypoxia-inducible factors: Master regulators of cancer progression. Trends Cancer 2016; 2(12): 758-70. [http://dx.doi.org/10.1016/j.trecan.2016.10.016] [PMID: 28741521]

[201] Wigerup C, Påhlman S, Bexell D. Therapeutic targeting of hypoxia and hypoxia-inducible factors in cancer. Pharmacol Ther 2016; 164: 152-69.

[http://dx.doi.org/10.1016/j.pharmthera.2016.04.009] [PMID: 27139518]

[202] Marchiq I, Pouysségur J. Hypoxia, cancer metabolism and the therapeutic benefit of targeting lactate/H+ symporters. J Mol Med (Berl) 2016; 94(2): 155-71. [http://dx.doi.org/10.1007/s00109-015-1307-x] [PMID: 26099350]

[203] Jun JC, Rathore A, Younas H, Gilkes D, Polotsky VY. Hypoxia-inducible factors and cancer. Curr Sleep Med Rep 2017; 3(1): 1-10. [http://dx.doi.org/10.1007/s40675-017-0062-7] [PMID: 28944164]

[204] Al Tameemi W, Dale TP, Al-Jumaily RMK, Forsyth NR. Hypoxia-modified cancer cell metabolism. Front Cell Dev Biol 2019; 7: 4. [http://dx.doi.org/10.3389/fcell.2019.00004] [PMID: 30761299]

[205] Bhandari V, Hoey C, Liu LY, *et al.* Molecular landmarks of tumor hypoxia across cancer types. Nat Genet 2019; 51(2): 308-18. [http://dx.doi.org/10.1038/s41588-018-0318-2] [PMID: 30643250]

[206] Bento CF, Pereira P. Regulation of hypoxia-inducible factor 1 and the loss of the cellular response to hypoxia in diabetes. Diabetologia 2011; 54(8): 1946-56. [http://dx.doi.org/10.1007/s00125-011-2191-8] [PMID: 21614571]

[207] Capla JM, Grogan RH, Callaghan MJ, *et al.* Diabetes impairs endothelial progenitor cell-mediated blood vessel formation in response to hypoxia. Plast Reconstr Surg 2007; 119(1): 59-70. [http://dx.doi.org/10.1097/01.prs.0000244830.16906.3f] [PMID: 17255657]

[208] Miura H, Wachtel RE, Loberiza FR Jr, *et al.* Diabetes mellitus impairs vasodilation to hypoxia in human coronary arterioles: Reduced activity of ATP-sensitive potassium channels. Circ Res 2003; 92(2): 151-8. [http://dx.doi.org/10.1161/01.RES.0000052671.53256.49] [PMID: 12574142]

[209] Gerber PA, Rutter GA. The role of oxidative stress and hypoxia in pancreatic beta-cell dysfunction in diabetes mellitus. Antioxid Redox Signal 2017; 26(10): 501-18. [http://dx.doi.org/10.1089/ars.2016.6755] [PMID: 27225690]

[210] Marlatt KL, Greenway FL, Kyle Schwab J, Ravussin E. Two weeks of moderate hypoxia improves glucose tolerance in individuals with type 2 diabetes. Int J Obes 2020; 44(3): 744-7. [http://dx.doi.org/10.1038/s41366-019-0422-0] [PMID: 31324880]

[211] Foti DP, Brunetti A. Editorial: "Linking Hypoxia to Obesity". Front Endocrinol 2017; 8: 34. [http://dx.doi.org/10.3389/fendo.2017.00034] [PMID: 28275368]

[212] Leake I. ANT2 mediates hypoxia and inflammation in obesity. Nat Rev Endocrinol 2019; 15(2): 64-4. [http://dx.doi.org/10.1038/s41574-018-0140-z] [PMID: 30531919]

[213] Seo JB, Riopel M, Cabrales P, *et al.* Knockdown of ANT2 reduces adipocyte hypoxia and improves insulin resistance in obesity. Nat Metab 2018; 1(1): 86-97. [http://dx.doi.org/10.1038/s42255-018-0003-x] [PMID: 31528845]

[214] Xie C, Yagai T, Luo Y, *et al.* Activation of intestinal hypoxia-inducible factor 2α during obesity contributes to hepatic steatosis. Nat Med 2017; 23(11): 1298-308. [http://dx.doi.org/10.1038/nm.4412] [PMID: 29035368]

[215] Song K, Zhang Y, Ga Q, Bai Z, Ge RL. High-altitude chronic hypoxia ameliorates obesity-induced non-alcoholic fatty liver disease in mice by regulating mitochondrial and AMPK signaling. Life Sci 2020; 252: 117633. [http://dx.doi.org/10.1016/j.lfs.2020.117633] [PMID: 32289432]

[216] Ali MM, Naquiallah D, Hassan C, *et al.* Obesity-associated hypoxia contributes to aberrant methylation of genes implicated in inflammation and vascular function. FASEB J 2020; 34(S1): 1-1. [http://dx.doi.org/10.1096/fasebj.2020.34.s1.08921]

[217] Almendros I, Martinez-Garcia MA, Farré R, Gozal D. Obesity, sleep apnea, and cancer. Int J Obes

2020; 44(8): 1653-67.
[http://dx.doi.org/10.1038/s41366-020-0549-z] [PMID: 32071426]

CHAPTER 18

Nanomaterials in Precision Medicine

Radhika Chaurasia[1], **Akshay A. Jain**[2] and **Monalisa Mukherjee**[1,*]

[1] *Amity Institute of Click Chemistry Research and Studies, Amity University, Noida, Uttar Pradesh - 201313, India*

[2] *Metropolis Healthcare Ltd., Wankhede House T Point, Congress Nagar, Nagpur, Maharashtra - 440012, India*

Abstract: The exigency for the most accurate form of diagnosis and treatment to challenge the failure of evidence-based medicine unlocked new avenues for tailored treatment. Precision Medicine encompasses the novel techniques and methods of therapy considering the genetic complexity, variations, and mutations in the human population. Recent advances in nanotechnology have paved a new path in therapeutics. The fusion of Precision Medicine with cutting-edge nanotechnology has offered unique headways into the healthcare management system. Novel approaches of nanoparticle synthesis and drug delivery techniques to cure heterogeneous populations with varied genetic alterations is now possible through precision medicine. This chapter highlights the promising role of nanomaterials in precision oncology where conventional therapy dwindles. Moreover, we discuss the emerging scope of precision medicine in dentistry to cure genetic diseases. Cystic fibrosis, which was once a nightmare, is now completely curable with the boon of Precision Nanomedicine. Precision medicine has revolutionized the medical world with a ray of hope to achieve the pinnacle of human health.

Keywords: Cystic Fibrosis, Human Health, Nanomedicine, Precision Dentistry, Precision Medicine, Precision Oncology.

INTRODUCTION

Healthcare practitioners have long been concerned with making their therapies as efficient and suitable for the particular patient as possible. The traditional one-size-fits-all paradigm involves identical treatment to patients presenting with a similar array of symptoms. The quest for a more precise diagnosis and therapy to overcome the shortcomings of evidence-based medicine resulted in new possibilities for tailored and personalized treatment. Precision Medicine (PM) is synonymically referred to as personalized medicine in certain arenas of therapeutics [1]. However, the United States National Research Council, expr-

* **Corresponding author Monalisa Mukherjee:** Amity Institute of Click Chemistry Research and Studies, Amity University, Noida, Uttar Pradesh - 201313, India; Tel: 9873279964; E-mail: mmukherjee@amity.edu

esses a broader concept that, while it may not be feasible to design therapies explicitly for individual patients on an individual level, subsets of patients should be able to be demarcated and treated [2]. Precision medicine does not indicate the development of drugs or medical devices tailored to the needs of a specific patient. Instead, it refers to the segregation of people into sub-groups, depending on their vulnerability to a specific disease, the biology of the disease and their responses to a specific treatment [3]. The concept of PM has existed for the past 2500 years since the time of Greek philosopher Hippocrates, but now it has gained momentum. Several Scientists have contributed to this field with the passage of time. Archibald E. Garrod (1857-1936) is the most prominent name who is considered as the father of precision medicine. He demonstrated genetic variations as the fundamental source of diseases such as alkaptonuria, albinism, cystinuria, and pentosuria. He suggested that all individuals differ from one another, even the uniovular twins are genetically distinct warranting the requirement of precise treatment for each person [4]. In 2015, the Precision Medicine Initiative was launched by President Barack Obama, for "providing the right treatment at the right time to the right person and taking into account patients' health history, genes, environments, and lifestyles" [5].

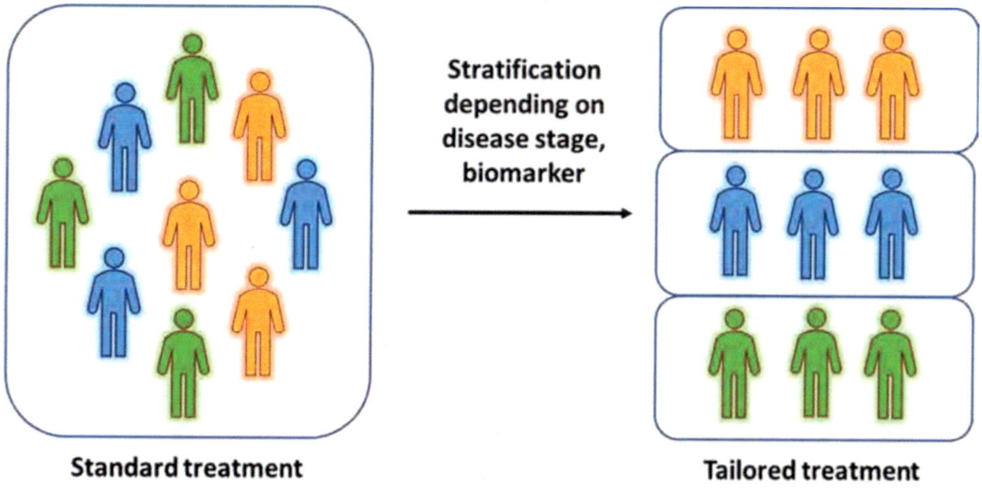

Fig. (1). Schematic representation showing stratification of the patients useful for precision medicine deviating from *one-size-fits-all* conventional treatment [45].

Precision public health (PPH) is a contemporary approach that accompanies the growth of precision medicine by harnessing improved newer technology and information available through big data to effectively aim public health initiatives for the communities. A vital function of PPH is the utilization of population-level data to create a larger group of individuals who may be subjected to precision medicine. This can be achieved by a surge in the understanding of the biochemical processes involved in various illnesses [6].

PRECISION NANOPARTICLES

Nanomaterials have a promising role in disease diagnosis and treatment. To maximize safety and efficacy, nanomaterials enhance the stability and bioavailability of encapsulated cargos, facilitating transport across the biological membranes, and extending the circulation time [7]. However, the paucity of knowledge of the pathophysiological variations in animals and humans nanomaterials especially with the way these differences impact the activity and effectiveness of nanomedicine is not clear. Individual heterogeneity potentially hinders the efficacy of nanomedicine. Moreover, there is an inadequate study on the interplay of nanomedicine with stratified patient groups [8]. Consequently, a limited number of nanomedicines is suggested as first-line therapy choices, although several benefits have been demonstrated only in a minor proportion of the patients. The reason is that the diseased tissue exhibits altered proliferation, morphology, and physiology affecting the pharmacokinetic properties of the NPs. Advancements in the synthesis strategy and design of nanoparticles, incorporating bio-responsive molecules possessing intricate structures and targeting agents offer great hopes. The rising pre-dominance of PM can be linked in particular to the development of NPs to circumvent biological barriers unique to patient sub-groups or pathological conditions [9].

Types of Nanoparticles

Lipid-based Nanoparticles

Lipid-based NPs are FDA-approved drug delivery vehicles, having several benefits including the ease of fabrication, self-assembly, excellent bioavailability, and biocompatibility and having the potential to bear substantial payloads. Moreover, a variety of physical and chemical properties may be tuned to regulate their biological character [10]. Liposomes are lipid-based structures composed of one or more phospholipid bilayers, capable of encapsulating drugs along with aqueous media. The stability of the lipid bilayer and the therapeutic material contained are determined by the lipid content and cholesterol concentrations. Their size range from 25 to 100 nm and these are regulated by the maximum amount of drug retained inside the bilayer retaining their flexibility [11].

Inorganic Nanoparticles

Reducing the size to the nanometer range, inorganic nanoparticles frequently display unique physical features [12]. Inorganic materials including gold, cadmium, zinc, iron, and silica have been employed to create nanoparticles for biomedical applications [13]. The most extensively researched nanoparticles (AuNPs) are employed in a variety of shapes that include nanospheres, nanorods, nanostars, nanoshells, and nanocages [14]. In the last 20 years, several physical, chemical, and biological methods have been established for the synthesis of nanoparticles with diverse size ranges, morphologies, and compositions. This has been done to fulfill the escalating requirement for both metallic and nonmetallic nanoparticles [15]. Physical approaches include high-energy irradiation, laser ablation, and lithography. The physical approach employs industrial machineries that works at high pressure and temperature and demands a large amount of space for their setup [16]. Electrochemistry, chemical reduction, and photochemical reduction are the most prominent chemical methods for producing nanomaterials. However, these methods require hazardous chemicals for the synthesis [17]. Biogenic and plant-mediated synthesis of nanoparticles aids in economical, biodegradable, and sustainable alternative to the traditional NPs synthesis. Nanoparticles of various shapes and sizes can be synthesized from a variety of plant extracts and microorganisms [18]. Synthesis of NPs from fungi, bacteria, yeast, and algae surmounts the use of hazardous chemicals [19]. In comparison to other microbes, bacterial synthesis of NPs is preferred owing to their ability to grow in a short time with the ease of recovery of NPs [20].

Quantum Dots

Quantum Dots (QDs) are semiconductor nanostructures with size-dependent tunable optical and electronic properties [21]. They are usually spherical in shape with sizes ranging from 1-10 nm. They can be synthesized in other shapes as well such as rods and tetrapods, however, for medical applications, spherical QDs are usually preferred [22]. The quantum confinement effect, which is accountable for the distinctive size-dependent photo-physical features of QDs, is produced by limiting the mobility of charge carriers (electrons and holes) within nanoscale dimensions [23]. It has been observed that the properties of QDs are influenced by the particle size, especially the fluorescence emission wavelength. Fluorescence emission may be modulated from the near ultraviolet to the visible and into the near-infrared (NIR) spectrum by varying QDs size and chemical composition, encompassing a wide wavelength range of 400-2000 nm. This is essential for deep tissue imaging in living organisms [24 - 26]. Due to broad excitation profiles and narrow emission peaks; with a single light source, multicolored QDs could be simultaneously excited, with minimal spectral overlapping. This property of QDs proves beneficial for the multiplexed detection of molecular targets. To be used in biomedical applications, QDs must possess hydrophilic property to assimilate in aqueous buffers therefore surface modifications on QDs are required [27].

Polymeric Nanoparticles

These are colloidal molecules which possess the properties of a solid structure. Depending on the fabrication methods, they can form two types of shapes namely nanospheres or nanocapsules. Nanospheres are composed of a solid matrix system where the therapeutic agent can be adsorbed or co-precipitated with the polymer. Nanocapsules are membrane-bound vesicular systems where the drug is present in a cavity, enveloped by a unique polymeric membrane. Their further subdivision depends on their shape which includes polymersomes, micelles, and dendrimers [28]. Polymers that are from a natural origin for instance carbohydrate and protein base polymers can be hydrophilic, hydrophobic or amphiphilic. Conversely, synthetic polymers are predominantly hydrophilic in nature and can exist in a pre-polymerized form or can be polymerized during the fabrication procedure. However, depending on the nature of the synthesized product, they can be biodegradable and non-biodegradable. Synthetic polymers, for example, Poly Lactic Acid (PLA), Poly Glycolic Acid (PGA) and Polylactic-co-glycolic acid (PLGA) are biodegradable; hence, utilized in drug delivery systems [29].

PRECISION NANOPARTICLES AND PUBLIC HEALTH

Precision Oncology

When DNA sequences are damaged, cells either start their repair process or, if the damage is severe enough, the cells undergo apoptosis. Healthy cells transform into tumor cells, as a result of variation (mutation) in DNA. The mutations induced are usually caused by the environmental stimuli that trigger genetic alterations. Tumors formed from a single transformed cell begin to multiply abnormally as a result of unrepaired DNA alterations [30]. Tumor growth is considered as a cascade of events including cell mutation and selection with gradually increased proliferative, survival, and invasion capabilities. The accelerated progression of tumors, resulting in low oxygen rates, is one of the characteristics of cancer [31]. Cancer involves unregulated cell proliferation due to anomalous somatic mutations in oncogenes and tumor suppressor genes [32]. According to the World Health Organization (WHO) statistics, it is the second leading cause of mortality around the globe, with an estimated 9.6 million deaths in the year 2018 which means one in six. It has been observed that men are more prone to lung, colorectal, stomach liver, and prostate cancers whereas breast, colorectal, lung, cervical, and thyroid cancer are typical among women [33]. In principle, mutational variations in specific genes are the key factors for carcinogenesis. Firstly, the activation of Proto-oncogenes (Cancer-promoting oncogenes) confers additional attributes to cancer cells for instance hyperactive division and proliferation, and resistance to normal programmed cell death, secondly, the inactivation of antioncogenes (tumor suppressor genes). Mutations among both types of genes have been widely reported resulting in the formation of a malignant neoplasm.

Cancer Diagnosis

Cancer detection, particularly in its early stages, is critical for successful disease prevention. Timely detection of cancer enhances the odds of effective treatment, resulting in lower fatalities and improved longevity of patients. However, the seemingly low sensitivity and accuracy, and lack of early diagnosis of cancer have been a roadblock [34]. In the preliminary phase of detection of malignancy such as in colorectal cancer, the 5-year survival rate is 91% while in the advanced stages, average 5-year survival rate is 26% [35]. The disease prognosis typically involves surgical biopsy for the identification of histopathological variables such as the tumor size, lymph node, distal metastases and differentiation grade [36]. Patients exhibiting indistinguishable clinical manifestations may have extremely diverse outcomes due to biological variability, leading either to absolute cure or death. Conventional anticancer drugs work on the mechanism to arrest the neoplastic cell cycle, disrupting the process of cell division which eventually leads to apoptosis [37]. Chemotherapy not only kills tumor cells but also the normal cells. To avoid these adverse effects, attempts to enhance chemotherapy treatment have aimed to develop compounds that are more selective and specific against malignancies [38]. Moreover, depending on the possibility of recurrence and metastasis, stratifying patients will expose only the high-risk patients to receive more intensive therapy while avoiding excessive overtreatment of low-risk patients [45].

Emerging technological advancements are often used to extend population-level knowledge of the human genome, epigenome, metabolome, transcriptome, and proteome which offer alternative strategies to interpret biochemical processes implicated in illness [39]. The advent of the Human Genome Project spurred the dawn of the Era of Precision Medicine (PM) [40]. Single nucleotide variations (SNVs), minor insertions and deletions (INDELs), and structural variants (SVs), all such variations in the nucleotide sequences may lead to the development of malignancy [41]. "Genomics" is the study of the structure and function of human chromosomes at the gene level along with its evolution and mapping [42]. Sequencing technologies for instance the Sanger sequencing and Next-Generation Sequencing (NGS) methods can identify single as well as multi-gene disorders [43, 44]. Considering the amount of information collected by these approaches, genomic signatures uniquely distinguish a particular tumor. The investigation of gene expression utilizing transcriptome approaches is extremely relevant to assess differential expression between the cases and controls or in various tumor sub-groups.

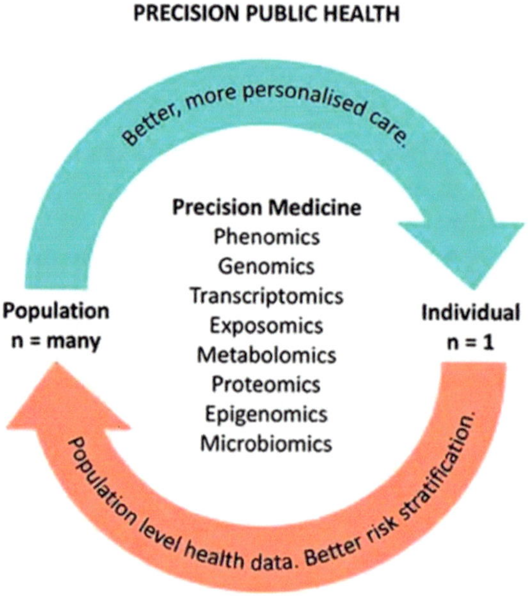

Fig. (2). A precision medicine research strategy (As outlined in the 2011 Institute of Medicines National Research Council report entitled Toward Precision Medicine) [45]

Biomarkers as Diagnostic Agents

Biomarkers play a crucial role in the accurate identification of cancer. The National Institutes of Health Biomarkers Definitions Working Group defined a biomarker as "a characteristic that is objectively measured and evaluated as an indicator of normal biological processes, pathogenic processes, or pharmacologic responses to a therapeutic intervention" [46]. Tumor biomarkers are distinct units formed by the malignant cells that are present in the tumor tissue and biofluid of the affected individual. Variations in the concentrations of a diverse array of biological entities, including cells, proteins, peptides, DNA, post-translational modifications, metabolites, and genetic variations, can signify the existence of carcinoma in a person as well as assist in personalized risk factor assessments, prognostics, and therapy response prediction. For cancer diagnosis, nanomaterials can be an effective tool. For example, iron oxide nanoparticles have been used as contrasting agent in MRI imaging though these experiments are in their pre-clinical stage [47].

Precision Oncotherapeutics

Doxorubicin is the drug of choice for a variety of cancers; however, free doxorubicin exhibits cardiotoxicity [38]. Vascular defects are caused by neoangiogenesis phenomena induced by the neoplastic cells through which the liposomal drug carrier should essentially enter the tumor site. Usually, the smaller-sized particles can readily enter the cancer tissue. However, larger liposomes while still remaining in the tumor vasculature release the drug at the neoplastic tissues [48]. In this way, nanostructures remain in the blood circulatory system for an extended length of time, allowing medication to be released at the prescribed dose. As a result, they induce lesser plasma fluctuations with minimal negative repercussions [49].

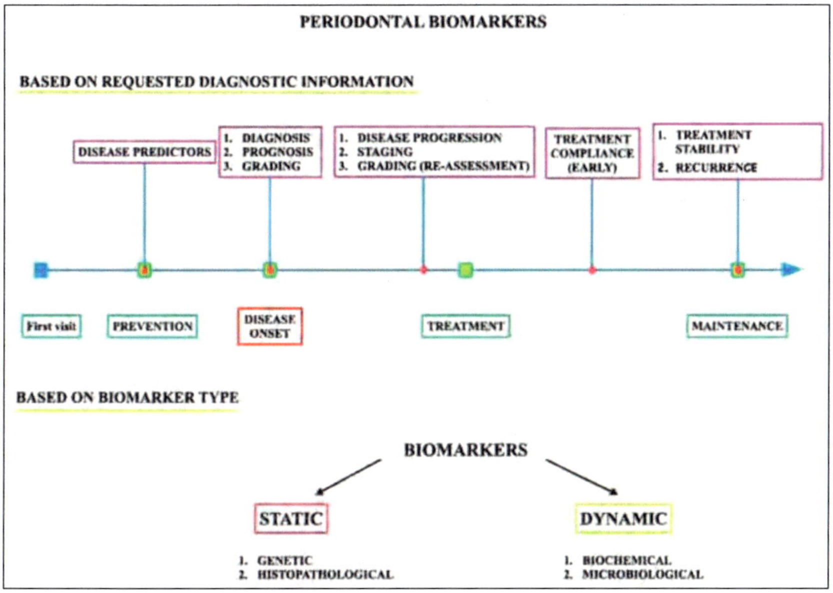

Fig. (3). Details of Biomarkers used in periodontology [67].

During the lifespan, genetic defects in the BRCA tumor suppressor genes raise the likelihood of acquiring breast cancer by 45-65% and ovarian cancer by 45–60% women [50]. Recently, Ibnat *et al.* [51] have reported the restoration of BRCA1 and BRCA2 tumor suppressor activities through the intracellular delivery of BRCA1 and BRCA2 genes with the aid of inorganic carbonate apatite nanoparticles [51]. Tyrosine kinase overexpression has been reported in chronic myelogenous leukemia (CML), and gastrointestinal stromal tumours (GISTs) [52]. Imatinib mesylate inhibits the tyrosine kinase activity of the BCR-Abl mutated gene. Moreover, imatinib mesylate also inhibits KIT and PDGFR receptors which are expressed in normal cells and play significant roles in the formation of blood, vascular development, and its maintenance [53, 54]. Administration of free imatinib mesylate *in-vivo* reported the presence of cardiac lesions, characterized by cytoplasmic vacuolization and myofibrillar loss. Imatinib mesylate-induced cardiotoxicity is greatly reduced by PLGA nano-encapsulation [55].

Precision Dentistry

For generations, oral and dental care like dental caries or periodontitis has been managed in a uniform fashion for all patients and disease conditions based on a limited knowledge of the complexity of dental diseases [56]. Precision dentistry is a modern, multidisciplinary, data-driven strategy to oral health care that stratifies identical patients into phenotypic groups based on individual variables. The intention is to offer caregivers the knowledge that will enable them to enhance therapeutic intervention and individual response to therapy. Precision oral healthcare practitioners would shift from offering an "identical treatment" for all patients to a specified diagnosis and toward more precise therapies for people within each diagnostic sub-group [57]. Periodontitis is a chronic inflammatory oral disease marked by periodontal tissue deterioration. It is medically shown to have clinical attachment loss (CAL), periodontal pocketing, gingival bleeding, and radiological indications of alveolar bone loss [58, 59]. Technological advancements in biomedical science, notably in high-throughput methods, highly sensitive diagnostic strategies, and artificial intelligence algorithms, have transformed the nature of periodontal pathogenesis and have also revealed the shortcomings of the routine medical methodology in delivering highly accurate and patient-specific prognostic details [60, 61]. The latest periodontal disease classification recommendations issued in 2018 embrace evaluation methodology based on stage and grade classification. Stage classification is based on disease severity and its complexity in disease management whereas, grade classification is based on the rate of disease advancement and the degree of risk involvement [62]. The idea of P4 medicine is combined with prediction, prevention, personalization, and participation as the four components of clinical patient care by Bartold *et al.* for the therapy of periodontitis [63]. Studies have revealed that the key genes related to periodontal disease were IL1A, IL1B, IL4, IL6, IL10, TNFA, FcγR, VDR, TLR2, TLR4, and MMP1 [64, 65]. Especially the IL-1 gene cluster has been studied from the early days of periodontal genetics research, and single nucleotide polymorphism (SNPs) in the IL-1 genes are proposed to be utilized for genotyping of the periodontal patients. Hence, stratification of individuals on the basis of genotype for the early detection and treatment of disease is the need of the hour. Emerging innovations have revealed efforts to produce photosensitive nanoparticles for more effective drug delivery [66].

Methylene blue-loaded polylactic-co glycolic acid (PLGA) nanoparticles, curcumin-silica nanoparticles, copper sulphide nanoparticles along with indocyanine green (ICG), chlorin e6, coumarin 6 in Fe_3O_4 nanoparticles and numerous other nanoparticles have been developed. These nanomaterials target the oral bacteria to produce an antibacterial effect. However, further enhancement in the treatment strategy is required for a precise treatment.

Precision Medicine in Other Diseases

Cystic Fibrosis (CF) is an autosomal, monogenic, recessive disease caused by a genetic defect in the CFTR gene which encodes for cystic fibrosis transmembrane conductance regulator (CFTR) protein. The disease is inherited from one generation to another and is the most common disease among the white population [68]. This life-threatening disease condition previously had no treatment, however being a monogenic disorder, it is now managed by gene therapy. The CFTR gene can be restored or carefully repaired *in vitro*. However, owing to issues with gene expression and transport, gene therapy for cystic fibrosis has been mainly ineffective *in vivo.* Nonetheless, nanoparticles are competent to surmount such delivery hurdles. Several inhalable NP formulations have been synthesized, which are successfully delivering genetic materials such as mRNA to targeted cells. Cystic fibrosis damages the cells that secrete mucus, causing it to thicken. This is the primary symptom of the condition, but it is also a major obstacle to drug delivery. NPs with better much-penetrating characteristics have now been designed for application in cystic fibrosis lung delivery as well as oral delivery [69]. Similar to inert hydrophilic coatings such as PEG or polyethylene oxide, NPs having a size smaller than the mucous bed, have a better ability to penetrate through the mucous. PEGylation was demonstrated to increase penetration into the cystic fibrosis mucus [70]. Unfortunately, mucus can vary greatly amongst patients, and current mouse models may not adequately simulate the thicker airway mucus generated by cystic fibrosis patients. Muco-penetrating lipoplexes, mucolytic proteins, thiolated hyaluronic acid coatings, and N-acetylcysteine are among the other current techniques for enhancing mucosal delivery. Each of these approaches aims at promoting mucosal barrier penetration by modifying surface characteristics of NPs.

CONCLUSION

The use of NPs in precision medicine-based applications empowers enhanced targeting of specific cells, reduced imprecise target effects and more accurate therapies. All of these are possible by tailoring NPs for the desired purpose, enhancing concentration at the targeted site and incorporating responsiveness for drug release whenever required, which reduces undesirable risks and enables a broader spectrum of doses or combinatorial therapies. By enhancing the specificity and target site activity of NP systems, the impacts of precision medicine therapies can be augmented, broadening the sub-groups of patients served and improving the quality of patient care altogether. Smart NP design may enhance precision medicine with a holistic approach. Moreover, the insights into precision medicine, for instance, the patient stratification and genetic profiling, can drive judicious selection of a NP platform, culminating in optimal NP-based precision treatment.

ABBREVIATIONS

PM Precision Medicine

PPH Precision Public Health

NPs Nanoparticles

FDA Food and Drug Administration

AuNPs Gold Nanoparticles

QDs Quantum Dots

NIR Near-infrared

DNA Deoxyribonucleic acid

WHO World Health Organization

SNVs Single Nucleotide Variations

INDELs Insertions and deletions

NGS Next-Generation Sequencing

BRCA BReast CAncer gene

CML Chronic myelogenous leukaemia

GISTs gastrointestinal stromal tumours

CAL clinical attachment loss

PLGA polylactic-coglycolic acid

ACKNOWLEDGEMENT

MM thank University Grants Commission (UGC DAE CSR) CRS/2021-22/04/642 for their funding. MM and RC thank the Department of Science and Technology DST/WOS-A/CS-106/2021 for their funds.

REFERENCES

[1] Akhoon N. Precision medicine: A new paradigm in therapeutics. 2021.

[2] Council NR. Committee on A Framework for Developing a New Taxonomy of Disease Toward precision medicine: building a knowledge network for biomedical research and a new taxonomy of disease. Washington, DC: National Academies Press 2011.

[3] Singla P, Musyuni P, Aggarwal G, Singh H. Precision Medicine: An emerging paradigm for improved diagnosis and safe therapy in pediatric oncology. Cureus 2021; 13(7): e16489. [http://dx.doi.org/10.7759/cureus.16489] [PMID: 34430104]

[4] Perlman RL, Govindaraju DR. Archibald E. Garrod: the father of precision medicine. Genet Med 2016; 18(11): 1088-9. [http://dx.doi.org/10.1038/gim.2016.5] [PMID: 26963281]

[5] STONE A. Precision medicine: Health care tailored to you. The White House Blog. Available from: https://obamawhitehouse.archives.gov/blog/2016/02/25/precision-medicine-health-care-tailored-you

[6] Bilkey GA, Burns BL, Coles EP, Mahede T, Baynam G, Nowak KJ. Optimizing precision medicine for public health. Front Public Health 2019; 7: 42. [http://dx.doi.org/10.3389/fpubh.2019.00042] [PMID: 30899755]

[7] Blanco E, Shen H, Ferrari M. Principles of nanoparticle design for overcoming biological barriers to drug delivery. Nat Biotechnol 2015; 33(9): 941-51. [http://dx.doi.org/10.1038/nbt.3330] [PMID: 26348965]

[8] Hua S, de Matos MBC, Metselaar JM, Storm G. Current Trends and Challenges in the Clinical Translation of Nanoparticulate Nanomedicines: Pathways for Translational Development and Commercialization. Front Pharmacol 2018; 9: 790. [http://dx.doi.org/10.3389/fphar.2018.00790] [PMID: 30065653]

[9] Gao P, Chang X, Zhang D, *et al.* Synergistic integration of metal nanoclusters and biomolecules as hybrid systems for therapeutic applications. Acta Pharm Sin B 2021; 11(5): 1175-99. [http://dx.doi.org/10.1016/j.apsb.2020.12.004] [PMID: 34094827]

[10] Zhang C, Ma Y, Zhang J, *et al.* Modification of Lipid-Based Nanoparticles: An Efficient Delivery System for Nucleic Acid-Based Immunotherapy. Molecules 2022; 27(6): 1943. [http://dx.doi.org/10.3390/molecules27061943] [PMID: 35335310]

[11] Akbarzadeh A, Rezaei-Sadabady R, Davaran S, *et al.* Liposome: classification, preparation, and applications. Nanoscale Res Lett 2013; 8(1): 102. [http://dx.doi.org/10.1186/1556-276X-8-102] [PMID: 23432972]

[12] Khan I, Saeed K, Khan I. Nanoparticles: Properties, applications and toxicities. Arab J Chem 2019; 12(7): 908-31. [http://dx.doi.org/10.1016/j.arabjc.2017.05.011]

[13] Spirescu VA, Chircov C, Grumezescu AM, Vasile BȘ, Andronescu E. Inorganic nanoparticles and composite films for antimicrobial therapies. Int J Mol Sci 2021; 22(9): 4595. [http://dx.doi.org/10.3390/ijms22094595] [PMID: 33925617]

[14] Li W, Cao Z, Liu R, *et al.* AuNPs as an important inorganic nanoparticle applied in drug carrier systems. Artif Cells Nanomed Biotechnol 2019; 47(1): 4222-33. [http://dx.doi.org/10.1080/21691401.2019.1687501] [PMID: 31713452]

[15] Augustine R, Hasan A. Multimodal applications of phytonanoparticles. Phytonanotechnology: Challenges and Prospects 2020; (Jan): 195-219. [http://dx.doi.org/10.1016/B978-0-12-822348-2.00011-5]

[16] Baig N, Kammakakam I, Falath W. Nanomaterials: A review of synthesis methods, properties, recent progress, and challenges. Materials Advances 2021; 2(6): 1821-71. [http://dx.doi.org/10.1039/D0MA00807A]

[17] Ramanathan S, Gopinath SCB, Arshad MKM, Poopalan P, Perumal V. Nanoparticle synthetic methods: strength and limitations. Nanoparticles in Analytical and Medical Devices 2021; (Jan): 31-43. [http://dx.doi.org/10.1016/B978-0-12-821163-2.00002-9]

[18] Singh J, Dutta T, Kim KH, Rawat M, Samddar P, Kumar P. 'Green' synthesis of metals and their

oxide nanoparticles: Applications for environmental remediation. J Nanobiotechnology 2018; 16(1): 84.
[http://dx.doi.org/10.1186/s12951-018-0408-4] [PMID: 30373622]

[19] Boroumand Moghaddam A, Namvar F, Moniri M, Md Tahir P, Azizi S, Mohamad R. Nanoparticles Biosynthesized by Fungi and Yeast: A Review of Their Preparation, Properties, and Medical Applications. Molecules 2015; 20(9): 16540-65.
[http://dx.doi.org/10.3390/molecules200916540] [PMID: 26378513]

[20] Mohd Yusof H, Mohamad R, Zaidan UH, Abdul Rahman NA. Microbial synthesis of zinc oxide nanoparticles and their potential application as an antimicrobial agent and a feed supplement in animal industry: A review. J Anim Sci Biotechnol 2019; 10(1): 57.
[http://dx.doi.org/10.1186/s40104-019-0368-z] [PMID: 31321032]

[21] Singh S, Dhawan A, Karhana S, Bhat M, Dinda AK. Quantum Dots: An Emerging Tool for Point-o--Care Testing. Micromachines 2020; 11(12): 1058.
[http://dx.doi.org/10.3390/mi11121058] [PMID: 33260478]

[22] Bailey RE, Smith AM, Nie S. Quantum dots in biology and medicine. Physica E 2004; 25(1): 1-12.
[http://dx.doi.org/10.1016/j.physe.2004.07.013]

[23] Smith AM, Gao X, Nie S. Quantum dot nanocrystals for in vivo molecular and cellular imaging. Photochem Photobiol 2004; 80(3): 377-85.
[http://dx.doi.org/10.1111/j.1751-1097.2004.tb00102.x] [PMID: 15623319]

[24] Bailey RE, Nie S. Alloyed semiconductor quantum dots: Tuning the optical properties without changing the particle size. J Am Chem Soc 2003; 125(23): 7100-6.
[http://dx.doi.org/10.1021/ja035000o] [PMID: 12783563]

[25] Wehrenberg BL, Wang C, Guyot-Sionnest P. Interband and Intraband Optical Studies of PbSe Colloidal Quantum Dots. J Phys Chem B 2002; 106(41): 10634-40.
[http://dx.doi.org/10.1021/jp021187e]

[26] Lim YT, Kim S, Nakayama A, Stott NE, Bawendi MG, Frangioni JV. Selection of quantum dot wavelengths for biomedical assays and imaging. Mol Imaging 2003; 2(1): 50-64.
[http://dx.doi.org/10.1162/153535003765276282] [PMID: 12926237]

[27] Wu X, Liu H, Liu J, *et al.* Immunofluorescent labeling of cancer marker Her2 and other cellular targets with semiconductor quantum dots. Nat Biotechnol 2003; 21(1): 41-6.
[http://dx.doi.org/10.1038/nbt764] [PMID: 12459735]

[28] Nagaich U. Polymeric nanocapsules: An emerging drug delivery system. J Adv Pharm Technol Res 2018; 9(3): 65.
[http://dx.doi.org/10.4103/japtr.JAPTR_325_18] [PMID: 30338230]

[29] Zabihi F, Xin N, Jia J, Chen T, Zhao Y. High Yield and High Loading Preparation of Curcumin–PLGA Nanoparticles Using a Modified Supercritical Antisolvent Technique. Ind Eng Chem Res 2014; 53(15): 6569-74.
[http://dx.doi.org/10.1021/ie404215h]

[30] Merlin F. Evolutionary Chance Mutation: A Defense of the Modern Synthesis' Consensus View. Philosophy and Theory in Biology 2010; 2(20170609)
[http://dx.doi.org/10.3998/ptb.6959004.0002.003]

[31] Blazejczyk A, Papiernik D, Porshneva K, Sadowska J, Wietrzyk J. Endothelium and cancer metastasis: Perspectives for antimetastatic therapy. Pharmacol Rep 2015; 67(4): 711-8.
[http://dx.doi.org/10.1016/j.pharep.2015.05.014] [PMID: 26321272]

[32] Chandrashekar P, Ahmadinejad N, Wang J, *et al.* Somatic selection distinguishes oncogenes and tumor suppressor genes. Bioinformatics 2020; 36(6): 1712-7.
[http://dx.doi.org/10.1093/bioinformatics/btz851] [PMID: 32176769]

[33] Available from: https://www.who.int/health-topics/cancer#tab=tab_1

[34] Loud JT, Murphy J. Cancer Screening and Early Detection in the 21 st Century. Semin Oncol Nurs 2017; 33(2): 121-8.
[http://dx.doi.org/10.1016/j.soncn.2017.02.002] [PMID: 28343835]

[35] Chen X, Gole J, Gore A, *et al.* Non-invasive early detection of cancer four years before conventional diagnosis using a blood test. Nat Commun 2020; 11(1): 3475.
[http://dx.doi.org/10.1038/s41467-020-17316-z] [PMID: 32694610]

[36] Gurcan MN, Boucheron LE, Can A, Madabhushi A, Rajpoot NM, Yener B. Histopathological image analysis: A review. IEEE Rev Biomed Eng 2009; 2: 147-71.
[http://dx.doi.org/10.1109/RBME.2009.2034865] [PMID: 20671804]

[37] Pistritto G, Trisciuoglio D, Ceci C, Garufi A, D'Orazi G. Apoptosis as anticancer mechanism: function and dysfunction of its modulators and targeted therapeutic strategies. Aging 2016; 8(4): 603-19.
[http://dx.doi.org/10.18632/aging.100934] [PMID: 27019364]

[38] Lao J, Madani J, Puértolas T, *et al.* Liposomal Doxorubicin in the treatment of breast cancer patients: A review. J Drug Deliv 2013; 2013: 1-12.
[http://dx.doi.org/10.1155/2013/456409] [PMID: 23634302]

[39] Manzoni C, Kia DA, Vandrovcova J, *et al.* Genome, transcriptome and proteome: the rise of omics data and their integration in biomedical sciences. Brief Bioinform 2018; 19(2): 286-302.
[http://dx.doi.org/10.1093/bib/bbw114] [PMID: 27881428]

[40] Carrasco-Ramiro F, Peiró-Pastor R, Aguado B. Human genomics projects and precision medicine. Gene Ther 2017; 24(9): 551-61.
[http://dx.doi.org/10.1038/gt.2017.77] [PMID: 28805797]

[41] Mullaney JM, Mills RE, Pittard WS, Devine SE. Small insertions and deletions (INDELs) in human genomes. Hum Mol Genet 2010; 19(R2): R131-6.
[http://dx.doi.org/10.1093/hmg/ddq400] [PMID: 20858594]

[42] Capps B. New Technologies: Ethics of Genomics.International Encyclopedia of Public Health. Elsevier 2017; pp. 240-7.
[http://dx.doi.org/10.1016/B978-0-12-803678-5.00300-3]

[43] Behjati S, Tarpey PS. What is next generation sequencing? Arch Dis Child Educ Pract Ed 2013; 98(6): 236-8.
[http://dx.doi.org/10.1136/archdischild-2013-304340] [PMID: 23986538]

[44] Wei X, Ju X, Yi X, *et al.* Identification of sequence variants in genetic disease-causing genes using targeted next-generation sequencing. PLoS One 2011; 6(12): e29500.
[http://dx.doi.org/10.1371/journal.pone.0029500] [PMID: 22216297]

[45] Vargas AJ, Harris CC. Biomarker development in the precision medicine era: lung cancer as a case study. Nat Rev Cancer 2016; 16(8): 525-37.
[http://dx.doi.org/10.1038/nrc.2016.56] [PMID: 27388699]

[46] Strimbu K, Tavel JA. What are biomarkers? Curr Opin HIV AIDS 2010; 5(6): 463-6.
[http://dx.doi.org/10.1097/COH.0b013e32833ed177] [PMID: 20978388]

[47] Canese R, Vurro F, Marzola P. Iron oxide nanoparticles as theranostic agents in cancer immunotherapy. Nanomaterials 2021; 11(8): 1950.
[http://dx.doi.org/10.3390/nano11081950] [PMID: 34443781]

[48] Maeda H, Wu J, Sawa T, Matsumura Y, Hori K. Tumor vascular permeability and the EPR effect in macromolecular therapeutics: A review. J Control Release 2000; 65(1-2): 271-84.
[http://dx.doi.org/10.1016/S0168-3659(99)00248-5] [PMID: 10699287]

[49] Patra JK, Das G, Fraceto LF, *et al.* Nano based drug delivery systems: Recent developments and future prospects. J Nanobiotechnology 2018; 16(1): 71.
[http://dx.doi.org/10.1186/s12951-018-0392-8] [PMID: 30231877]

[50] Paul A, Paul S. The breast cancer susceptibility genes (BRCA) in breast and ovarian cancers. Front Biosci 2014; 19(4): 605-18.
[http://dx.doi.org/10.2741/4230] [PMID: 24389207]

[51] Ibnat N, Chowdhury EH. Retarding breast tumor growth with nanoparticle-facilitated intravenous delivery of BRCA1 and BRCA2 tumor suppressor genes. Sci Rep 2023; 13(1): 536.
[http://dx.doi.org/10.1038/s41598-022-25511-9] [PMID: 36631481]

[52] Paul MK, Mukhopadhyay AK. Tyrosine kinase : Role and significance in Cancer. Int J Med Sci 2004; 1(2): 101-15.
[http://dx.doi.org/10.7150/ijms.1.101] [PMID: 15912202]

[53] Andrae J, Gallini R, Betsholtz C. Role of platelet-derived growth factors in physiology and medicine. Genes Dev 2008; 22(10): 1276-312.
[http://dx.doi.org/10.1101/gad.1653708] [PMID: 18483217]

[54] Lennartsson J, Rönnstrand L. Stem cell factor receptor/c-Kit: From basic science to clinical implications. Physiol Rev 2012; 92(4): 1619-49.
[http://dx.doi.org/10.1152/physrev.00046.2011] [PMID: 23073628]

[55] Sheeba CJ, Marslin G, Revina AM, *et al.* Delivery as nanoparticles reduces imatinib mesylate-induced cardiotoxicity and improves anticancer activity. Int J Nanomedicine 2015; 10(Apr): 3163-70.
[http://dx.doi.org/10.2147/IJN.S75962] [PMID: 25995626]

[56] Innes NPT, Chu CH, Fontana M, *et al.* A century of change towards prevention and minimal intervention in cariology. J Dent Res 2019; 98(6): 611-7.
[http://dx.doi.org/10.1177/0022034519837252] [PMID: 31107140]

[57] Beck JD, Philips K, Moss K, Divaris K, Morelli T, Offenbacher S. Advances in precision oral health. Periodontol 2020; 82(1): 268-85.
[http://dx.doi.org/10.1111/prd.12314] [PMID: 31850630]

[58] Könönen E, Gursoy M, Gursoy U. Periodontitis: A Multifaceted Disease of Tooth-Supporting Tissues. J Clin Med 2019; 8(8): 1135.
[http://dx.doi.org/10.3390/jcm8081135] [PMID: 31370168]

[59] Pihlstrom BL, Michalowicz BS, Johnson NW. Periodontal diseases. Lancet 2005; 366(9499): 1809-20.
[http://dx.doi.org/10.1016/S0140-6736(05)67728-8] [PMID: 16298220]

[60] Highfield J. Diagnosis and classification of periodontal disease. Aust Dent J 2009; 54(s1) (1): S11-26.
[http://dx.doi.org/10.1111/j.1834-7819.2009.01140.x] [PMID: 19737262]

[61] Fatima A, Shafi I, Afzal H, *et al.* Advancements in Dentistry with Artificial Intelligence: Current Clinical Applications and Future Perspectives. Healthcare 2022; 10(11): 2188.
[http://dx.doi.org/10.3390/healthcare10112188] [PMID: 36360529]

[62] Tonetti MS, Greenwell H, Kornman KS. Staging and grading of periodontitis: Framework and proposal of a new classification and case definition. J Periodontol 2018; 89(S1) (1): S159-72.
[http://dx.doi.org/10.1002/JPER.18-0006] [PMID: 29926952]

[63] Bartold PM, Ivanovski S. P4 Medicine as a model for precision periodontal care. Clin Oral Investig 2022; 26(9): 5517-33.
[http://dx.doi.org/10.1007/s00784-022-04469-y] [PMID: 35344104]

[64] Martínez-García M, Hernández-Lemus E. Periodontal Inflammation and Systemic Diseases: An Overview. Front Physiol 2021; 12: 709438.
[http://dx.doi.org/10.3389/fphys.2021.709438] [PMID: 34776994]

[65] Folwaczny M, Glas J, Török H-P, Limbersky O, Folwaczny C. Toll-like receptor (TLR) 2 and 4 mutations in periodontal disease. Clin Exp Immunol 2004; 135(2): 330-5.
[http://dx.doi.org/10.1111/j.1365-2249.2004.02383.x] [PMID: 14738464]

[66] Kikuchi T, Hayashi J, Mitani A. Next-generation examination, diagnosis, and personalized medicine

in periodontal disease. J Pers Med 2022; 12(10): 1743.
[http://dx.doi.org/10.3390/jpm12101743] [PMID: 36294882]

[67] Rakic M, Pejcic N, Perunovic N, Vojvodic D. A Roadmap towards Precision Periodontics. Medicina 2021; 57(3): 233.
[http://dx.doi.org/10.3390/medicina57030233] [PMID: 33802358]

[68] Chen Q, Shen Y, Zheng J. A review of cystic fibrosis: Basic and clinical aspects. Animal Model Exp Med 2021; 4(3): 220-32.
[http://dx.doi.org/10.1002/ame2.12180] [PMID: 34557648]

[69] Ong V, Mei V, Cao L, Lee K, Chung EJ. Nanomedicine for Cystic Fibrosis. SLAS Technol 2019; 24(2): 169-80.
[http://dx.doi.org/10.1177/2472630318824334] [PMID: 30707858]

[70] Suk JS, Lai SK, Wang YY, *et al.* The penetration of fresh undiluted sputum expectorated by cystic fibrosis patients by non-adhesive polymer nanoparticles. Biomaterials 2009; 30(13): 2591-7.
[http://dx.doi.org/10.1016/j.biomaterials.2008.12.076] [PMID: 19176245]

CHAPTER 19

Nanotechnology, Drug Delivery and Prospects in Precision Medicine

Rafat Ali[1,2], **Mohd Adil**[1], **Armiya Sultan**[3], **Nida Jamil Khan**[2] and **Romana Ishrat**[1,*]

[1] *Centre for Interdisciplinary Research in Basic Sciences, Jamia Millia Islamia, New Delhi, India*

[2] *Department of Biosciences, Jamia Millia Islamia, New Delhi, India*

[3] *Department of Biotechnology, Jamia Millia Islamia, New Delhi, India*

Abstract: Nanotechnology has the potential to revolutionize the field of drug delivery by enabling targeted and controlled release of drugs within the body. This article provides an overview of the current state of the art in nanotechnology-based drug delivery systems and their potential applications. It discusses the various types of nanoparticles that are currently being used or developed for drug delivery, including liposomes, dendrimers, and polymeric nanoparticles, and highlights their advantages and disadvantages. It also covers some of the key challenges and risks associated with the use of nanotechnology in drug delivery, such as toxicity and regulatory issues. Finally, the article explores the future prospects of nanotechnology in drug delivery and highlights some of the areas where further research and development are needed. Overall, the article demonstrates that nanotechnology-based drug delivery systems hold great promise for improving the efficacy and safety of drug treatments and that on-going research in this field has the potential to transform the way we approach drug delivery in the future. Finally, it's envisaged that this technology will facilitate the augmentation of precision medicine for better human health care across the spectrum of diseases.

Keywords: Dendrimers, Drug delivery, Liposomes, Nanoparticles, Nanotechnology, Precision medicine, Polymeric nanoparticles, Stimuli-responsive micelles.

INTRODUCTION

Nanotechnology is the study and application of very small particles or structures, typically those that are smaller than 100 nanometers in size [1]. A nanometer is one billionth of a meter, or about 1/100,000th the width of a human hair. Nano-

* **Corresponding author Romana Ishrat:** Centre for Interdisciplinary Research in Basic Sciences, Jamia Millia Islamia, Jamia Nagar- 110025, New Delhi, India; E-mail: romana05@gmail.com

Farzana Mahdi & Abbas Ali Mahdi (Eds.)

technology has applications in a wide range of fields, including electronics, medicine, energy, and materials science [2].

For example, nanotechnology is being used to develop more efficient solar cells, drug delivery systems that can target specific cells in the body, and stronger and more durable materials for use in construction and manufacturing [3]. Nanotechnology also poses some potential risks, such as the possibility of toxicity or environmental harm if nanoparticles are not properly handled or disposed of [2]. As a result, there is ongoing research and discussion about the ethical, social, and environmental implications of nanotechnology. Nanotechnology involves manipulating and engineering materials at the atomic or molecular level, often using specialized tools and techniques such as scanning probe microscopes, electron microscopes, and other sophisticated instrumentation [4]. This allows researchers to create materials and devices with unique properties and characteristics, such as increased strength, conductivity, or reactivity.

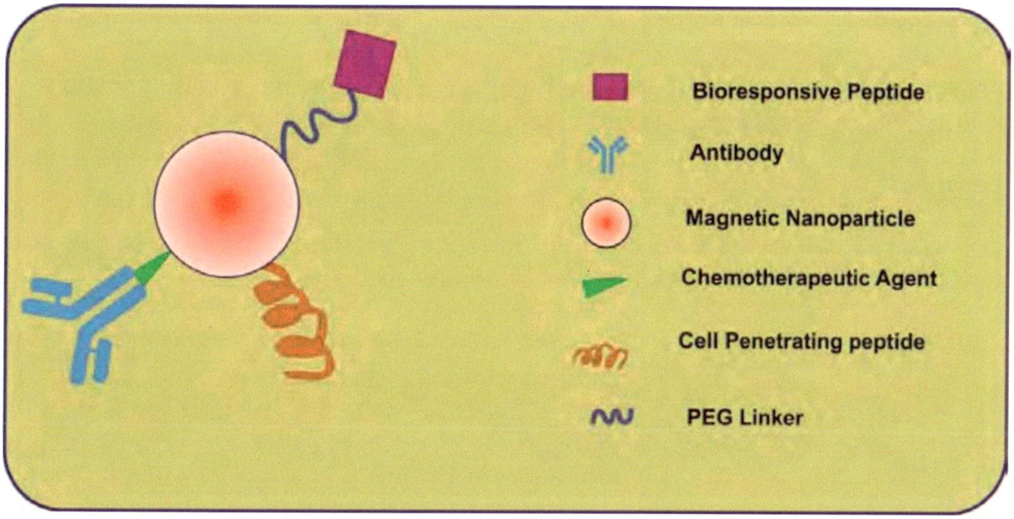

Fig. (1). Schematic diagram showing the functionalization of magnetic nanoparticles with bio responsive peptide, chemotherapeutic agent, PEG linker, antibody, and cell-penetrating peptide [34].

NANOTECHNOLOGY IN MEDICINE

Nanotechnology has the potential to revolutionize medicine by enabling the development of new diagnostic and therapeutic tools with unprecedented precision and efficiency [1 - 4]. Some potential applications of nanotechnology in medicine include:

Drug Delivery

Nanoparticles can be engineered to carry drugs and target specific cells or tissues in the body, which can increase the effectiveness of the treatment while minimizing side effects.

Imaging

Nanoparticles can be used as contrast agents to enhance the resolution and sensitivity of medical imaging techniques such as MRI and CT scans.

Tissue Engineering

Nanotechnology can be used to create scaffolds or matrices that mimic the structure and function of natural tissues, which can be used to repair or replace damaged or diseased tissues.

Diagnostics

Nanoparticles can be used to develop highly sensitive and specific diagnostic tests that can detect diseases at an early stage.

Therapeutics

Nanoparticles can be used to develop new therapies that target specific disease pathways or cellular processes, such as cancer or viral infections.

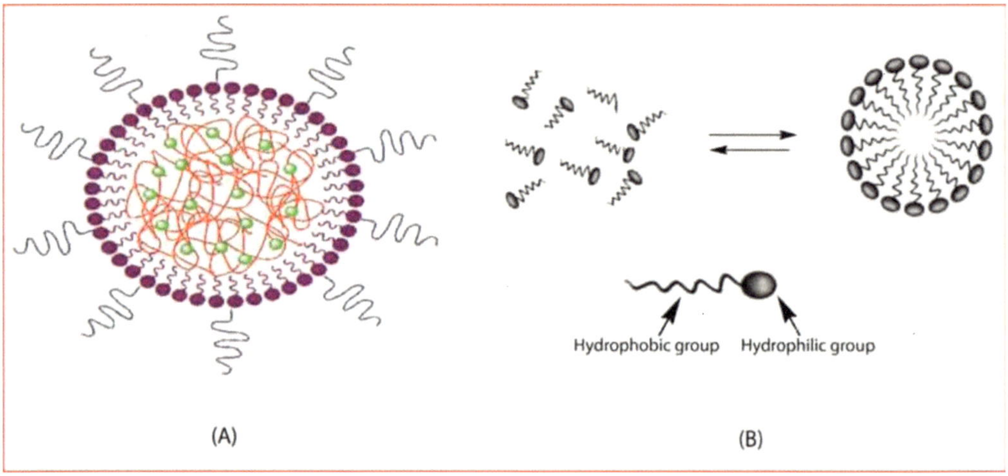

Fig. (2). Schematic diagram showing; (A) the structure of polymeric nanoparticle, and (B) the structure and reversible formation of micelles [54].

However, there are also some challenges and risks associated with the use of nanotechnology in medicine, such as the potential toxicity of nanoparticles, the need to ensure that nanoparticles can be safely eliminated from the body, and the ethical and regulatory issues surrounding the use of new and innovative technologies. As a result, ongoing research and development in this area are needed to ensure that the benefits of nanotechnology in medicine can be realized in a safe and effective manner.

NANOTECHNOLOGY IN DRUG DELIVERY

Nanotechnology has the potential to significantly improve drug delivery by enabling targeted and controlled release of drugs within the body. Drug delivery refers to the process of administering medications or therapeutic agents to a patient using various methods such as oral, topical, transdermal, inhalation, injection, or implantation. The goal of drug delivery is to optimize the drug's efficacy and safety by delivering it to the targeted site in the body while minimizing side effects and reducing the required dosage. Some examples of nanoparticle-based drug delivery systems that are currently being developed include liposomes, dendrimers, and polymeric nanoparticles. While these systems show great promise, there are also challenges and risks associated with their use, such as potential toxicity, difficulty in large-scale manufacturing, and regulatory issues. As a result, ongoing research and development are needed to ensure that the benefits of nanotechnology in drug delivery can be realized in a safe and effective manner.

The delivery can be performed by conventional or novel drug delivery systems. Conventional drug delivery systems are the traditional methods of drug delivery, such as oral pills, capsules, injections, and topical creams, among others. These systems have been widely used and are relatively inexpensive. However, they may have limitations such as poor solubility, low bio-availability, and lack of targeted delivery. Novel drug delivery systems refer to advanced technologies that have been developed to overcome the limitations of conventional drug delivery. Examples of novel drug delivery systems include liposomes, polymeric nanoparticles, hydrogels, and implantable devices, among others. These systems can improve drug solubility, bio-availability, and targeted delivery to specific tissues or cells, resulting in enhanced therapeutic efficacy and reduced side effects. Advanced drug delivery systems such as nanotechnology-based drug delivery, are being developed to improve drug delivery efficiency and therapeutic outcomes. Nanoparticles can act as colloidal drug carriers with 10-1000 nm in size to deliver drugs to their target sites [1].

Nanotechnology refers to the study and manipulation of matter at the nanoscale, which is the scale of atoms and molecules. This field involves the design, production, and application of materials, devices, and systems with novel properties and functions that are unique to the nanoscale. At the nanosized scale, atoms or molecules function in different manners and offer a variety of uses with astonishing and interested facts. Nanotechnology has broad applications in various fields, such as electronics, energy, medicine, and materials science. Examples of nanotechnology-based products and processes include computer chips, solar cells, drug delivery systems, and water purification systems. The unique properties of nanomaterials, such as high surface area, quantum effects, and size-dependent behaviour, enable the development of new technologies with enhanced performance and efficiency. However, the use of nanotechnology also raises concerns about potential health and environmental risks, which require careful evaluation and regulation. Basically nanotechnology appears to be like more of a 'catch-all' term for the science that is promoting a whole array of areas, from environmental to health care systems as well as commercial products [2, 3].

Important Characteristics of Nanoparticles for Drug Delivery

Nanoparticles are being developed for drug delivery due to their unique physicochemical properties that enable targeted delivery of drugs. The important characteristics of nanoparticles for drug delivery include:

Particle Size

Nanoparticles should have a size range of 1-100 nanometers to achieve a high surface area-to-volume ratio, which increases drug loading capacity and enhances cellular uptake. Presently, photon-correlation spectroscopy or dynamic light scattering are the fastest and most routine methods that are used to determine the nanoparticle size. For these spectroscopic methods, the viscosity of the medium should be known. By using Brownian motion and light scattering properties of particles, the diameter of the particle can be calculated [4]. Usually, the results obtained by photon-correlation spectroscopy can be verified by scanning electron microscopy or transmission electron microscopy (SEM or TEM). The most important characteristics of nanoparticles are their particle size and size distribution. These properties basically determine the *in vivo* distribution, toxicity and biological fate, and the targeting ability for such delivery systems. Moreover, they can show a better impact on drug loading and release, and nanoparticles' stability. It has been demonstrated by many studies that nanoparticles offer several advantages over micro particles [5]. Generally, the cell uptake by nanoparticles is relatively high in comparison to micro particles and their availability for a broader range of cellular and intra-cellular targets is because of their size and mobility. Due to minute size, nanoparticles can easily cross the blood-brain barrier with the use of hyperosmotic mannitol on the opening of the endothelial tight junctions, which helps in providing a sustained delivery of some therapeutic agents and bioactive drugs for some hard-to-treat diseases like cervical tumours [6]. It is reported that blood-brain barrier has been crossed by Tween 80-coated nanoparticles as well [7]. Also the sub-micron nanoparticles have been shown in good contact with cells, but larger micro particles, are not taken up by most of the cell types [8]. Certainly, the uptake rate for 100 nm nanoparticles was 2.5-fold greater in comparison to 1 μm micro particles, and 6-times greater uptake as compared to 10 μm micro particles by Caco-2 cells [9]. In an analogous study, effective penetration has been shown by nanoparticles all over the sub-mucosal layers of rat intestinal loop model, although micro particles' location in sub-mucosal layers is predominant in the epithelial lining [10]. This gives an indication that the distribution of particle can be tuned by controlling the size of particle. Particle size similarly affects the drug release. As smaller particles are having a larger surface area-to-volume ratio; so therefore, small particles would have most of the drugs associated with them on or near the surface of the particle, which leads to quick drug release. While, the bigger particles having large cores, allow large drug quantity or size to get encapsulated in a single particle and thus result in slower drug release [10]. Hence, controlling the particle size is measured as an important means of fine-tuning the drug release rates.

Surface Characteristics of Nanoparticles

The surface charge of nanoparticles can influence their stability, interaction with biological membranes, and cellular uptake. Nanoparticles with a neutral or slightly negative charge are preferred for drug delivery. There might be a modification of the drug bio-distribution profile when the drug is associated with conventional carriers. The host immune system can recognize nanoparticles when intravenously administered and clear them from the circulation by phagocytes [11]. Other than nanoparticles' size, the hydrophobicity of nanoparticles assists in determining the level of blood components (like, opsonin's) which bind to the surface of these particles. Henceforth, the *in vivo* fate is well influenced by hydrophobicity of nanoparticles [12]. When the surface unmodified nanoparticles or say conventional nanoparticles reach the blood stream, they are rapidly opsonized and massively cleared by the mononuclear phagocyte system (MPS) [13]. For the characterization of surface charge property of the nanoparticles, commonly, zeta potential of a nanoparticle is used. This shows that the electrical potential of the particles is affected by both the particle composition and dispersive medium [14].

Bio-compatibility and Stability

Nanoparticles should be biocompatible and non-toxic to avoid immune system activation or adverse reactions in the body. Nanoparticles should be stable in biological fluids to avoid aggregation or degradation, which can lead to reduced drug delivery efficiency.

Drug Loading

A successful Nano delivery system is the one which has an efficient drug-loading capacity, thus aids in reducing matrix materials quantity required for administration. The process of drug loading can be achieved mainly by two methods which include the incorporation and adsorption methods. Incorporation method needs the drug to be merged during the period of formulation of nanoparticles. The adsorption/absorption approaches call for the absorption of drug after the nanoparticle has been formed and this is accomplished by incubation of the Nano-carrier with concentrated drug solution. The efficiency of drug loading and incorporation depends on drug solubility in the excipient matrix material (liquid dispersion agent or a solid polymer), matrix composition, drug-polymer interactions, molecular weight, and the end functional groups present *i.e.* carboxyl or ester either in the matrix or the drug [15]. PEG polymer is a choice for many nanoparticle formulations since it has slight or no effect on drug-loading and the interactions involved [16]. Moreover, drugs, macromolecules, or the protein that gets encapsulated in nanoparticles display the highest loading efficiency when they are loaded at or near their isoelectric point (pI) [17]. Specifically, for small molecules, studies demonstrate that the use of ionic interaction between the drug and matrix materials can be very effective in increasing drug-loading capacity [18].

Controlled Drug Release

Nanoparticles should allow controlled release of drugs to avoid toxicity and maximize therapeutic efficacy. This can be achieved through stimuli-responsive, time-controlled, or site-specific drug release mechanisms. While developing a Nano particulate delivery system, it is important to consider both drug release and biodegradation of polymers. In general, the drug release rate depends on: (1) solubility of drugs; (2) drug diffusion through the matrix of nanoparticle; (3) desorption of the adsorbed or surface-bound drug; (4) nanoparticle matrix degradation or erosion; and (5) the combination of diffusion and erosion processes. Hence, the release process is governed by solubility, diffusion, and particle matrix biodegradation. In case of Nanospheres, where the distribution of drug is uniform, drug release occurs by either diffusion or erosion of the matrix. Diffusion process is largely a controlling factor for the mechanism of release if the diffusion of the drug is faster than matrix erosion. The rapid, 'burst' or initial release, is primarily accredited to weakly adsorbed or bound drug to relatively bulky surface of nanoparticles [19]. The incorporation method influences the release profile. So, the system shows comparatively a slight burst effect and sustained release characteristic, if loading of drug molecules is achieved through the incorporation method [20]. On the other hand, if the nanoparticle is coated *i.e.* by polymer, then release is measured by the diffusion of the drug molecules from the membrane of the polymer. As membrane coating acts as a barrier for drug release; thus, solubility and diffusion of drug in or across the polymeric membrane becomes an aspect of determination in drug release. Furthermore, ionic interactions between the drug and auxiliary ingredients also influence the release rate. When the auxiliary ingredients interact with entrapped drug, the formation of hydrophobic complexes can result, that can slow the release of drug – with no burst release effect [18]. However, if the auxiliary ingredients' addition, *e.g.*, ethylene oxide propylene oxide block copolymer (PEO-PPO) to chitosan, it leads to a reduction in the interaction of the drug with its matrix material because of competitive electrostatic interactions of PEO-PPO with chitosan, that results in the surge in drug release [17].

Targeting Ability

Nanoparticles can be engineered to target specific cells or tissues in the body, which enhances drug delivery efficiency and reduces side effects. This can be achieved through surface modifications or functionalization with targeting moieties.

By optimizing these characteristics, nanoparticles can improve drug delivery efficiency, reduce side effects, and enhance therapeutic efficacy, leading to improved patient outcomes.

ADVANTAGES OF NANOPARTICLES

Nanoparticles have several advantages in various fields, including medicine, electronics, energy, and materials science. Some of the advantages of nanoparticles are:

High Surface Area-to-volume Ratio

Nanoparticles have a high surface area-to-volume ratio, which makes them more reactive than bulk materials. This property is useful in catalysis, chemical sensing, and drug delivery, where high surface area enables increased drug loading and targeted delivery.

Size-dependent Properties

Nanoparticles have size-dependent physical and chemical properties that differ from bulk materials, such as optical, magnetic, and electronic properties. These unique properties are useful in developing new materials and devices with enhanced performance.

Targeted Drug Delivery

Nanoparticles can be designed to deliver drugs to specific cells or tissues in the body, improving drug efficacy and reducing side effects.

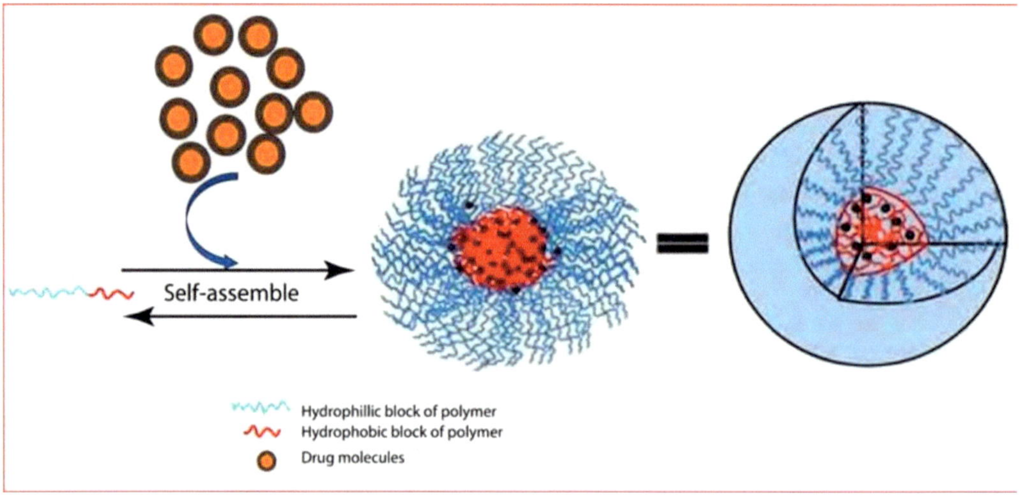

Fig. (3). Illustrating the formation and drug loading of polymeric micelles by self-assembly of amphiphilic block copolymers in aqueous solution [58].

Improved Drug Solubility

Nanoparticles can improve drug solubility, which can enhance drug absorption and bio-availability, leading to better therapeutic outcomes.

Sustained Drug Release

Nanoparticles can be engineered to release drugs at a controlled rate, leading to sustained drug release, reduced toxicity, and improved therapeutic efficacy.

Diagnostic Capabilities

Nanoparticles can be functionalized with biomolecules for diagnostic purposes, such as imaging and biosensing, enabling the detection of diseases at an early stage.

Overall, the unique physicochemical properties of nanoparticles enable the development of new technologies with enhanced performance and functionality, leading to improved outcomes in various fields.

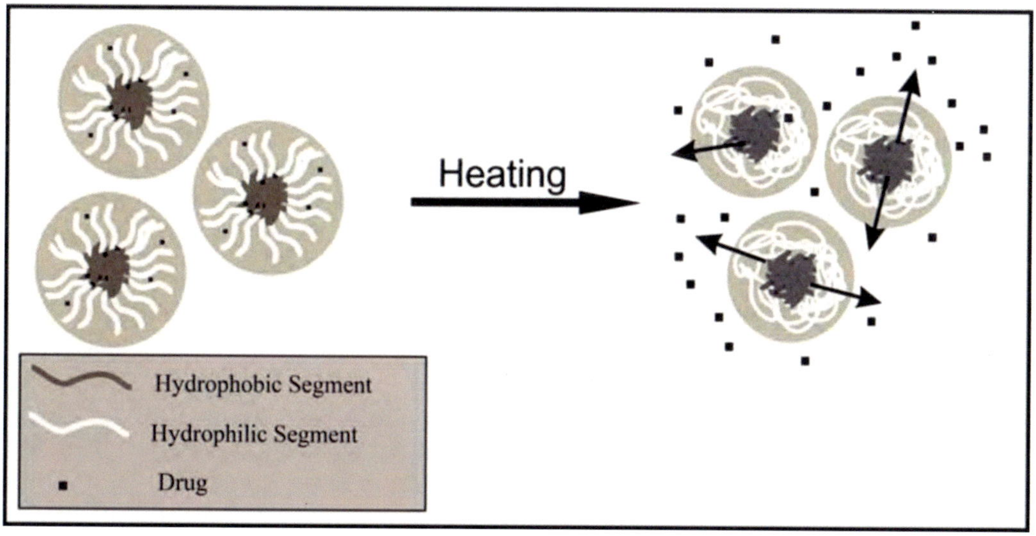

Fig. (4). Schematic diagram showing the release mechanism of DexAc from thermo- responsive PHBHV-PNIPAAm nanoparticles. When the temperature goes above the LCST (lower critical solution temperature) of the PNIPAAm, the expended form of the PNIPAAm in the shell part gets converted into the compact one and this leads to the ejection of drug [66].

TYPES OF NANOPARTICLES IN DRUG DELIVERY SYSTEM

Inorganic Nanoparticles

These are nanoparticles made up of inorganic materials, such as gold, silver, and iron oxide. Inorganic nanoparticles have unique properties that make them useful for drug delivery, such as their magnetic or optical properties, which can be used for imaging and targeted drug delivery. These are basically the particles of metal oxide which possess minimum one length scale in the Nano-meter range. Such particles have unique physio-chemical and biological properties. Because of their Nano size, they have gained ample attention. Several challenges are faced in the preparation of the nanoparticles because there are no a one-size-fits-all kinds of nanoparticles production mechanism and mostly the processes will vary largely between diverse research centres and large-scale laboratories [21, 22].

Metal Nanoparticles

Metal nanoparticles are a type of inorganic nanoparticles composed of metallic elements, such as gold, silver, platinum, and iron. Metal nanoparticles have unique optical, electronic, and magnetic properties that make them useful in various fields, including medicine, electronics, and materials science. In medicine, metal nanoparticles have been used in drug delivery, imaging, and therapeutics due to their bio-compatibility, stability, and targeting ability. Over a hundred of years, scientists have been fascinated by metallic nanoparticles because of their unique characteristics and applications over other materials. Today, a number of methods are available for the synthesis of these particles and modification *via* various functional groups. This makes them to be conjugated to different antibodies, ligands and drugs and many other biologically important biomolecules. So far, several imaging techniques have been developed such as PET, SERS, MRI, CT and optical imaging that aid in imaging of various disease states. These imaging facilities differ in both technological and instrumental sense and demand for a contrasting agent having unique physiochemical properties. This warrants the development of several contrasting agents in the nanoparticles' range for their application in these imaging techniques. The most commonly used metallic nanoparticles are gold, silver, magnetic, iron oxide, zinc oxide and gadolinium titanium oxide [23]. Magnetic nanoparticles can be functionalized with a number of bioactive agents (Fig. **1**). The large surface area provided by these particles enable the drugs to be incorporated in large doses [24 - 26]. Gold nanoparticles provide good utility in human cancer cells and in xenograft tumor cells as demonstrated by Qian et al. Non-toxic and biocompatible PEG-gold nanoparticles used for *in vitro* targeting were detected spectroscopically using Surface Enhanced Raman Scattering (SARS) [27]. For cancer imaging, the AuNPs provide good utility by selectively transporting AuNPs into the nucleus of a cancerous cell. The conjugation of arginine-glycine-aspartic acid peptide (RGD) and a nuclear localization signal peptide (NLS) was done to a 30-nm AuNP *via* PEG for the selective transport of the AuNPs into the cancer cell nucleus [28]. RGD interacts with the $\alpha_v\beta_6$ integrin's receptors which are present on the surface of the cell, whereas NLS having lysine-lysine-lysine-arginine-lysine(KKKRK) sequence targets karyopherin (importins) which are present in the cytoplasm enabling translocation into the nucleus [29, 30, 31]. So, RGD aids cancer cell specific targeting whereas NLS will exhibit the targeting specific for cancer cell nucleus. Instead of non-toxicity and bio-compatibility of these particles, a significant fraction of these can be retained and finally get accumulated in the body after the drug has been administered, which can result in toxicity [32]. The use of silver as a potent anti-microbial agent is known since ancient times. These nano agents have been used usually to counter the broad-spectrum microbes. Also these are used in medicines that reduce the chances of infection in burnt tissues and arthroplasties [33].

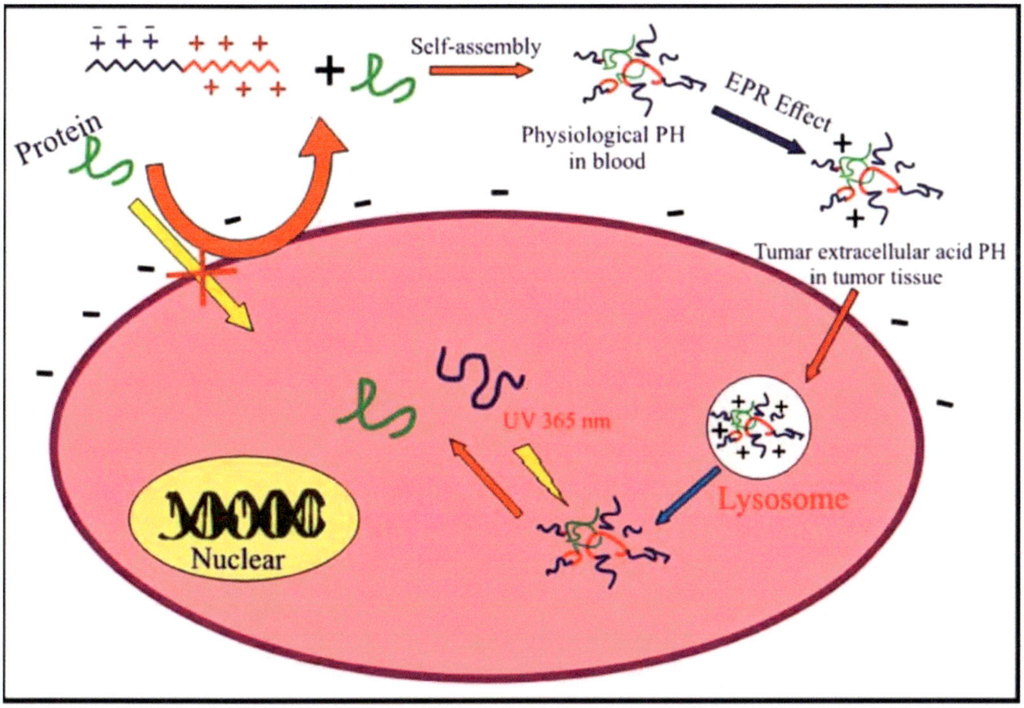

Fig. (5). Showing Light-responsive polyion complex micelles with a switchable surface charge for efficient and effective delivery of protein [74].

Overall, metal nanoparticles have unique properties that make them useful in various biomedical applications. With continued research and development, metal nanoparticles hold promise for improving drug delivery, imaging, and therapeutics in medicine.

MESOPOROUS SILICA SYSTEMS

Mesoporous silica systems are a type of nanoparticles composed of this silica, which is a porous material with a regular pore size distribution and a large surface area. Mesoporous silica nanoparticles (MSNs) can be synthesized with various shapes, such as spheres, rods, and discs, and can be functionalized with targeting moieties, drugs, and imaging agents for drug delivery and imaging applications.

The mesoporous structure of MSNs provides several advantages for drug delivery. First, the large surface area and pore volume allow for high drug loading, leading to increased drug efficacy. Second, the pores can be used to control drug release kinetics, enabling sustained drug release over an extended period. Third, the surface of MSNs can be functionalized with targeting moieties, such as antibodies, enabling specific targeting of cancer cells.

MSNs have been used in various biomedical applications, such as cancer therapy and imaging. In cancer therapy, MSNs can be loaded with anti-cancer drugs and targeted to cancer cells, leading to improved therapeutic efficacy and reduced toxicity. In imaging, MSNs can be functionalized with imaging agents, such as fluorescent dyes or magnetic nanoparticles, enabling visualization of cancer cells and tissues.

From the last few years, the synthesis as well as applications of mesoporous particles have gained a vast attention owing to the unique properties such as structures which are highly ordered, have a large pore size and considerable surface area [35]. Because of these properties, the mesoporous materials appear to be an ideal choice for the incorporation of biologically important pharmaceutical agents, proteins, and other biogenic compounds. So, the strategy employing the hosting and then the delivery of a variety of pharmaceutically important particles by mesoporous systems have been appeared and in great use [36]. Several mesoporous materials were used and important of them are MSU, M415, SBA and MMS in drug delivery. The important characteristics for synthesized MSNs and for their biomedical and biotechnological applications are the control of their structure, size and surface properties. For example, for the gene to be transfected or carriers for the intracellular delivery of pharmaceuticals, the microsphere materials cannot be the preferred agent because cell-engulfing of large particles *via* endocytosis is rather inefficient. Moreover, microspheres of mesoporous silica are in the size range of bacteria and thus can potentially result in triggering a serious immune response *in vivo*. To overcome such problems, a synthetic method/approach has been developed by researchers for the preparation of the mesoporous silica nanoparticles [37].

Following are some of the interesting properties of MSNs

• MSN have a tunable size with a range of 50-300 nm that allows easy endocytosis by living cells either plant or animal without causing any significant cytotoxicity.

• In comparison to other polymer-based drug carriers, MSNs have been proven to be more stable towards temperature, pH, mechanical stress, and degradations induced in hydrolytic environment.

• MSN offers a huge surface area (>900 m2/g) with a large pore volume (>0.9 cm3); hence allowing drug molecules to be loaded in high amounts [38].

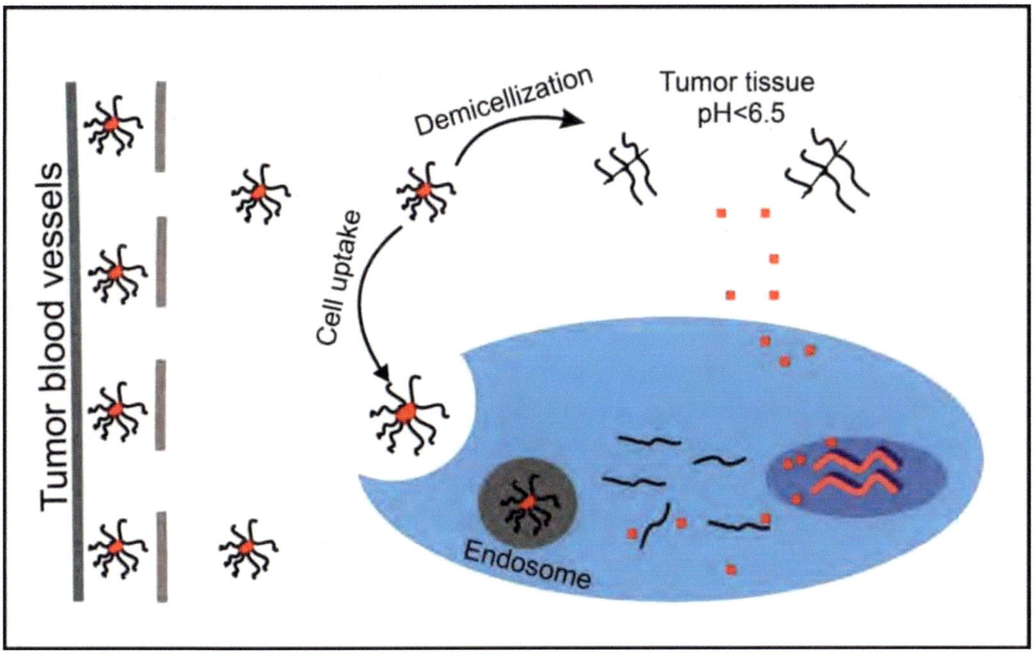

Fig. (6). Illustration of DOX-loaded PAE-graft-ADPC (12-acryloyl oxy dodecyl phosphorylcholine) micelles responding to the extracellular pH [80].

• MSNs have an internal as well as external surface that corresponds to cylindrical pores and external particle surface, respectively. This important property allows both the interior and exterior surface of MSN selectively functionalized with diverse moieties.

• It is well known that the interconnecting porous structure is the basic structural property of many drug delivery materials; for example, dendrimers having branched porous structure and liposomes with a huge interior core (void) and outer porous shell. The unique porous structure of MSN marks it suitable for drug delivery [39].

Preparation of MSNs is generally carried out under all the three conditions *i.e.*, basic, acidic, or neutral. Both the particle size (Nano-scale) and the morphology of MSNs are controllable under basic conditions [40]. However, under the basic conditions, the pore size tuning on MSNs is rather difficult and encountered many problems, thus restricting their bio applications to load and deliver nanocrystals or quantum dots and huge molecules like DNA, SiRNA, enzymes and proteins. Here, MSNs being Nano scaled particles with a large pore diameter are desired much. In case of acidic conditions, the pore size is controllable in a wide range especially non-ionic surfactant-templated MS like SBA-15 series MS. It's also easy to synthesize MS with various shapes and different surface patterns but control of the particle size is mostly done in micro scale. However, this is not that easy in the nanoscale due to the difficulties that are faced in the regulation of dimensions of micelles [40]. Under neutral conditions, the synthesis of MSNs is also efficient and worth noting. The synthesis of organic and inorganic hybrid MSNs forms organically esterified or amidated silica precursors and within their cores, they have mononuclear inclusion compounds that can get hydrolyzed easily under either acidic or basic conditions. But, like in acidic conditions, again the MS particle size is not controlled in nanoscale [41]. The synthesis of MSNs is done by the reaction of tetraethyl orthosilicate with a template made of micellar rods. The collection of nano-sized spheres or rods is achieved and further these structures are filled with pores arranged in a regular manner. Then by washing with a solvent of proper pH, the template can be removed easily [42]. There is another technique, a simple sol-gel method that can be used to synthesize MSNs or a spray drying method is also productive [43].

For various nano-medical applications, another category of MSNs *i.e.*, hollow MSNs (HMSNs) carrying a large void in the core have been successful owing to their inimitable characteristics such as large specific surface areas, low density, efficient loading capacity and the reduction potential in the number of carriers used. Soft and hard templating method is a general synthetic strategy for these special HMSNs and that basically includes the formation and surface functionalization of uniform soft/hard templates, which is followed by the desired shell deposition [44]. The soft templates are present in different forms; these can be the Emulsion drops, PVP aggregates, or micellar aggregates [45]. On the other hand, Fe_3O_4 nanocrystals, Au nanoparticles, polystyrene spheres or carbon spheres [46] represent hard templates. Although, great success has been achieved for the fabrication HMSNs by a variety of templates, but the actual use of these as Nano drug delivery systems (Nano-DDS) *in vivo* is yet to be known. This is mainly due to difficulty in obtaining HMSNs with properties like high dispersity, controlled size of particles and pores and thickness of shell etc [47].

Overall, mesoporous silica systems provide a versatile platform for drug delivery and imaging, with potential for improving cancer therapy and diagnostics.

POLYMERS IN DRUG DELIVERY SYSTEMS OR POLYMER THERAPEUTICS

Polymer therapeutics include several biologically important polymeric compounds such as conjugates of polymer protein and polymeric micelles where the drug is expected to bound covalently. Polymers provide the biggest advantage over others carrying the possibility of manipulating their properties such as molecular weight, linkers etc. so that they can adapt to the requirements of dry delivery. Conjugation of nano-ranged particles and materials to polyethylene glycol (PEG), referred to as PEGylation, offers a bunch of advantages viz, increased protein solubility and stability, immunogenicity reduction, resistance to the clearance effect by reticuloendothelial system (RES) [48].

Polymer-based Nanoparticles

These are nanoparticles made up of synthetic or natural polymers, such as poly(lactic-co-glycolic acid) (PLGA) and chitosan. These nanoparticles can be formulated to have different properties, such as particle size, surface charge, and drug release kinetics. These particles are made of biodegradable or bios table polymers or copolymers having size (<1000). Polymeric nanoparticles have a core shell structure that can be altered by making changes in hydrophilic and hydrophobic blocks on the polymeric chains (Fig. **3.1 A**). For the delivery of DNA, protein, oligonucleotides and drugs, naturally occurring polymers like chitosan and heparin are materials of choice. A nanoparticle formulation of anti-cancer drug, Paclitaxel, also having an included serum albumin as a carrier *i.e.* nanomaterial sized albumin-bound paclitaxel (Abraxane: protein bound paclitaxel), has been used for metastatic breast cancer treatment.[57] Apart from metastatic breast cancer, they have been effective in clinical trials that involve many other cancers including non-small-cell lung carcinoma and advanced non-hematologic malignancies [49]. In conjugate synthesis of pharmaceuticals, poly -L-glutamic acid was used for conjugate synthesis as the first biodegradable polymer, others being the N-(2-hydroxypropyl)-meth acrylamide copolymer (HPMA), polystyrene-maleic anhydride copolymer, and polyethylene glycol (PEG). Several chemotherapeutics that are used broadly in the clinic are being used with PGA as conjugates both *in vivo* and *in vitro*. They have shown that these polymers have got the potential to evade the limitations of their free drug counterparts [50]. A few of them are Xyotax (PGA paclitaxel) and CT-2106 (PGA-camptothecin) that are now in clinical uses [51].

Polymeric Micelles (amphiphilic block copolymers)

These are the amphiphilic nanoscale (>1000nm) block copolymers having a core-shell structure. Biodegradable hydrophobic nanoparticles make up the core which is protected by an amphiphilic block copolymer which helps in their dispersion stabilization in aqueous media (Fig. **2**). The hydrophobic core and hydrophilic shell region serve different functions *i.e.* the hydrophobic core is responsible for holding the drug within it while the hydrophilic shell region helps in stabilizing the hydrophobic core and also renders the polymer water-soluble, thus making the particle a suitable candidate for administration. The formation and loading of drug into polymeric micelles are shown in Fig. (**3**) [52]. Loading of drugs within the polymeric micelle can be achieved by two ways: physical encapsulation or chemical covalent liking [53].

Polymeric micelles have attained much attention over surfactant micelles because polymeric micelles have larger cores which lead to increased solubilisation capacity of the pharmaceuticals than regular micelles [55]. Polymeric micelles have blocks made up of polyethylene oxide, which are stabilized sterically. They can undergo opsonisation and uptake to a lesser extent by the macrophages of RES by which the circulation time of micelles increases in the blood [56]. A lot of study and investigation have been carried out on polymeric micelles and nanoparticles in drug delivery systems. Polymeric micelles can be observed as a unique system where there is a dynamic equilibrium between aggregated copolymers and the universe. Although a polymeric nanoparticle has the same core-shell structure as micelles, they are solid colloidal and matrix type, therefore, generally show greater stability than micelles. There is also the size difference between polymeric nanoparticles and polymeric micelles *i.e.*, 100-500 nm and 10-100 nm respectively. Thus, polymeric nanoparticles are larger and may show more polydisperse size distribution. Solubilisation of poorly soluble drugs by micelles which are formed from amphiphilic copolymers has got much attention [57].

If there is a considerable solubility difference between the hydrophobic and hydrophilic parts of the amphiphilic block copolymers, then they show a great tendency to self-assemble into micelles. In an aqueous solution, micelle formation takes place with typical core-shells structure through the segregation of insoluble hydrophobic blocks towards the core, surrounded by a shell made of hydrophilic blocks. Thus, this core-shell structure enables the use of these polymers, which is dependable on the polarity or the nature of the drug molecule that can be entrapped in: (a) the core (hydrophobic or non-polar molecule), (b) the shell (polar or hydrophilic molecule) and (c) between the two *i.e.* core and shell or palisade layer (intermediate polarity) [59, 60]. Polymeric micelles offer some unique characteristics, such as the nanoscale size, being relatively more stable due to low critical micelle concentration (CMC) and most importantly, the arrangement of a core-shell. These properties make them a true candidate for drug delivery systems for clinical applications, particularly for hydrophobic drugs to increase their solubility [61].

STIMULI- RESPONSIVE MICELLES

For the first time in 1970s, the concept of stimuli responsive micelles was introduced for drug delivery and that too came with the use of modified liposomes (thermosensitive) for the release of drugs out of hyperthermia [62]. From then onwards, in the past decade, stimuli responsive molecules have been a topic of research for efficient drug delivery. Their drug delivery is typically based on their design with application as Nano carriers [63]. Stimuli responsive copolymers basically contain two parts *i.e.*, a permanently hydrophilic part and a stimuli-responsive block that is sensitive to a number of factors. The stimuli segment can undergo a specific protonation, a hydrolytic cleavage or a conformational change of molecule in response to specific physical stimulation. This property promotes the self-assembly of such block copolymers into micellar-like structures having a core-shell structure. The hydrophobic segments can be sequestered in these amphiphilic structures and can be released under conditions which stimulate the stimuli-responsive block [37]. The sensitivity of nanoscale stimuli-responsive devices is attributed to a number of specific endogenous stimuli including a higher concentration of glutathione or an increased level of specific enzymes like matrix metalloproteinases, a lowered intestinal pH, etc. At the cellular level, two fates can be possible for a drug sensitive to pH; it can either result in causing the release of the transported drug into lysosomes or late endosomes or the escape of Nano carriers to the cell cytoplasm from lysosomes. Specific micro environmental changes that are associated with neoplastic diseases and other pathological conditions such as ischemia, inflammatory disease or infection can be of great use at the tissue level. The treatment of these diseases is the emphasis of research effort done on stimuli responsive Nano carriers. Extracorporeal physical stimuli can also be applicable for example; the targeted and sustained delivery of drugs can be achieved by magnetic, ultrasound, light, thermo-sensitive nanoparticle systems. Moreover, there is a possibility of different routes for administration *i.e.* Intravenous, mucosal or oral [63]. There are two types of stimuli responsive drug delivery:

EXOGENOUS

The delivery that takes advantage of externally applied stimuli.

Thermo-responsive Systems / Response to Temperature

Thermo-responsive drug delivery is one of the most studied stimuli-responsive strategies. It has also been explored extensively in the field of oncology. The property of thermo-responsiveness is generally governed by the nonlinear sharp variation in the properties of stimuli responsive block component of SRM. So, this sharp change is responsible for the discharge of the drug afterward a variation in the surrounding temperature. Ideally, the thermosensitive Nano carriers should not be sensitive to the normal body temperature *i.e.* they should retain their load at body temperature (37°C) and then rapid delivery of the drug within a locally heated tumor (40-40°). After delivery it should counteract the fast blood passage time and then washout from tumor. Temperature sensitivity is an interesting property in stimuli responsive polymers. These smart polymeric systems can stimulate a number of changes such as physical, chemical or mechanical with small temperature variations. These changes can be noticed as soon as the systems cross the relevant transition temperature. Or say, local heating or cooling through a particular period can be used to control the release of drug. The broadly studied temperature-sensitive polymer is the Poly (N-isopropyl acrylamide) (PNIPAAm) [64]. Fig. (**4**) shows the release mechanism of DexAc from thermo-responsive PHBHV-PNIPAAm nanoparticles) and others being poly (ethylene oxide)–poly (propylene oxide)– poly (ethylene oxide) triblock (PEO–PPO–PEO), multiblocks and poly (ethylene glycol) poly (lactic acid)–poly (ethylene glycol) triblock (PEG–PLA–PEG). For on–off control, the local hyperthermia has been used successfully as the stimulus for the activity of cell-penetrating peptides (CPP). Here, the temperature-activated assembly of the diblock-copolymer elastin-like polypeptides permit the arginine residues to be demonstrated at the periphery of micelles. This leads to more than 8-fold hike in the uptake of HeLa-cells [65].

The phenomenon of thermo-responsiveness can also be responsive with a small temperature decrease *i.e.*, also known as cold shock or 'cryotherapy'. Here, the nano carriers would experience a thermally reversible swelling or de-swelling which results in free dispersion of the encapsulated drug molecules because of increased porosity. For example, for the efficient delivery of the SiRNA into cytosol followed by the subsequent silencing of target mRNA, Pluronic F127–polyethyleneimine (PEI) Nano capsules are used [67].

Magnetically responsive Nano systems

The main advantage of utilizing magnetic field relies on the altered nature, which is achieved by a magnetic response, that can be a magnetic control under a permanent magnetic field, an increase in temperature with the application of an alternative magnetic field or both when they are used alternatively. Therefore, their responsive system allows for the variety within the drug delivery pathways. Moreover, it provides the opportunity to perform magnetic resonance imaging (MRI) and so helps in a single system to associate diagnostics and therapy in it *i.e.* theragnostic approach [68]. Typically, magnetic guidance is obtained by focusing an extracorporeal magnetic field on the biological target while a magnetically responsive Nano carrier is being injected. This concept has delivered a great potential in experimental cancer therapy because of increased drug accumulation inside the solid-tumor models. Various candidate Nano systems that can be of value for such a productive therapeutic approach are: core–shell nanoparticles (a magnetic core composed of magnetite (Fe_3O_4) coated with silica or polymer) magneto-liposomes (liposomes encapsulating Fe_3O_4 or maghemite (Fe_2O_3) nanocrystals) and porous metallic Nano capsules [69]. The results shown *in vitro*, by most core-shell nanoparticles are found promising, but improved tumour accumulation and anti-cancer pharmacological efficacy are demonstrated by only some of them. Though, with no normalized benchmark experiments, the comparison has been a difficult task between such systems. The drugs and Nano carriers can be linked covalently with various formulations to evade limitations that are related to the entrapment of drugs by the physical process (for example, the uncontrolled burst release or an inefficient drug loading). For example, the absence of burst release, significant therapeutic efficacy and enhancement of the MRI contrast in the targeted L1210 solid tumor node have been demonstrated by Fe_3O_4 nanocrystals that were loaded in squalene-gemcitabine conjugate nanoparticles [70]. Also, magnetically guided Nano-carriers have found a great role in nucleic acids delivery that include SiRNA and genes. Generally, these types of magneto faction experiments are performed using Nano assemblies with cationic coatings to condense nucleic acids which lead to higher transfection efficiencies under a permanent magnetic field. For instance, this technique has resulted in improved effectiveness in transfecting SiRNA *in vitro* and/or *in vivo* when applied against prostate and breast cancers, and also in gene transfer to oligonucleotide precursors for neural repair [71].

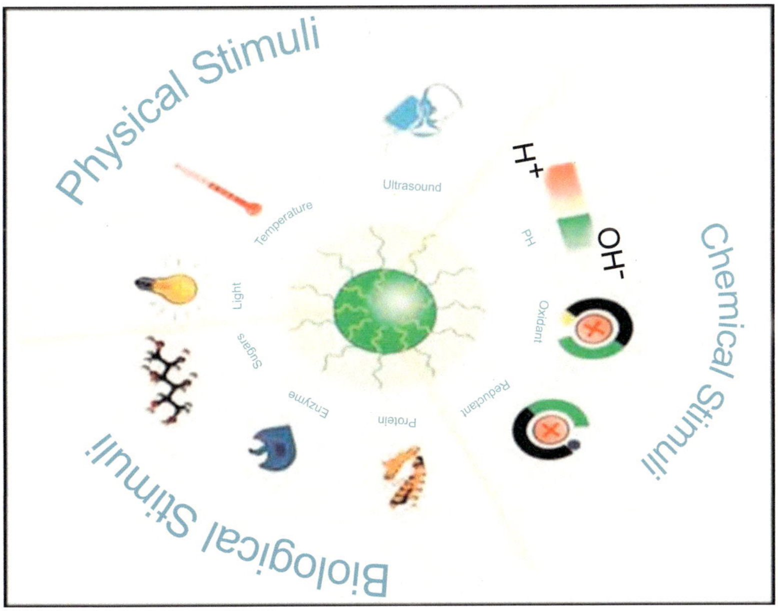

Fig. (7). Illustration of various physical, chemical and biological stimuli [98].

Ultrasound-triggered drug delivery

To attain spatio-temporal control over the drug release at the specific site and avert negative side effects to healthy tissues, ultrasound acts as an effective method of choice. The use of ultrasound is appealing because of some of its unique properties, such as the absence of ionizing radiation. Their non-invasiveness, facile governance, and control of the tissue penetration are achieved by tuning the frequency, duty cycles and exposure time. The waves formed by ultrasound can prompt the release of a drug molecule from several nanocarriers through either thermal or mechanical effectors. These effectors are produced by the cavitation phenomenon or radiation forces. Indeed, it is reported that Nano carrier destabilization, drug release and transient surge in vessel permeability can be induced by physical forces associated with cavitation, which leads to the cellular uptake of therapeutic agents [72]. A cavitation threshold can be achieved effortlessly when low threshold frequencies (kHz range) are utilised. Nevertheless, enhancement in vessel permeability mediated by ultrasound may lead to various possible shortcomings; for example, metastatic diffusion. Thus, microbubbles or other different agents carrying the ability to interact with ultrasonic waves are effectively being used at diagnostic frequencies so that the required threshold for cavitation can be reduced. Although the use of microbubbles for tissue targeting can be limited by their short lifespan and absence of extravasation, this difficulty can be circumvented by the development of perfluorocarbon (PFC) Nano emulsions, which, under the action of therapeutic ultrasounds, convert into microbubbles. The formation of bubbles takes place through the process of acoustic droplet vaporization. After their formation, they are exposed to cavitation. Cavitation promotes the cellular uptake and discharge of the encapsulated drugs into the tumor site. It has been successful in the suppression of metastatic dissemination and also with significant therapeutic efficacy [73].

Light-activated drug delivery

Photo-responsive systems are found to be non-invasiveness. They show the possibility of remote spatio-temporal control. Several photo-responsive systems have been engineered in the past decade to attain the on-demand drug release. This on-demand release of drug molecules is in response to the illumination of a wavelength (in ultraviolet, visible or near-infrared (NIR) regions) (Fig. **5**).

The available strategies depend on either a one-time or repeatable on–off drug-release event triggered by photosensitivity-induced structural modifications of Nanocarriers. For example, the reversible photoisomerization of the azobenzene group and its derivatives induced by ultraviolet visible waves, from cis to trans by the shining light in the visible region and from trans to cis by irradiating at 300–380 nm, enabling controlled drug release by photo regulation. It is possible through azobenzene functionalization of the core interior of MSNPs [75], through azo-modified DNA valves at the mouth of the pore and also through the light-controlled host–guest recognition between the cavity of cyclodextrin and azobenzene derivatives [76]. The hydrophobic-hydrophilic transition that accompanies trans-cis photo isomerization can also be used. For instance, the cationic micelles of azo-modified surfactants are disassembled at the UV light of 350 nm and can initiate a quick release of intracellular DNA [77]. Nanoparticles with photo-switchable drug release properties in illuminated cells can also be obtained by taking the benefit from the ultraviolet light-triggered spiropyran–merocyanine isomerization. Reversible shrinkage in lipid nanoparticles (spiropyran–PEGylated) can also be activated by UV light that enables deeper tissue penetration [78].

ENDOGENOUS

The systems take advantage of the variations of redox potential, pH, or concentrations of definite analytes or enzymes. The polymeric drug carriers that have pH-sensitive (pH-cleavable) bonds are utilized to produce stimuli-responsive drug delivery systems. Such drug carriers should be stable in circulation or within normal tissues. However, they attain the ability to be degraded and release the entrapped drug molecules in body areas or within cell compartments of lowered pH, such as infarcts, inflammation zones of tumor or endosomes and cell cytoplasm. Fig. (**6**) illustrates DOX-loaded PAE-graft-ADPC micelles) [79].

Two main strategies exist for the release of the entrapped drug: the utilization of polymers (either poly acids or polybases) having ionisable groups that can undergo conformational changes and/or solubility changes. These changes are in response to dissimilarity in the environmental pH and the design of polymeric systems having acid-sensitive bond cleavage. This leads to the release of molecules anchored at the backbone of the polymer and modification of the polymeric charge or the exposure of targeting ligands. A plethora of anti-cancer drug-delivery systems exist that basically take advantage of the slight difference in pH existing between healthy tissues (~7.4) and the extracellular environment of solid tumors (6.5–7.2). This results from irregular angiogenesis in fast-growing tumors, which causes a rapid decrease of both nutrients and oxygen. Thus, a shift towards a glycolytic metabolism subsequently leads to the production of acidic metabolites in tumor interstitials. Hence, for an elusive change of pH in the tumor extracellular microenvironment, efficient pH-sensitive systems must show a sharp response. For example, the release of encapsulated tumor necrosis factor-alpha (TNFα) in the local acidic environment of tumor tissues through chitosan swelling induced on amino-group protonation (pKa ~6.3) [81]. Sudden disassembly of PEG–poly (β-amino ester) micelles at pH 6.4–6.8 resulted in the leakage of encapsulated camptothecin [82]. pH-variation activated the delivery of proteins into ischemic areas. The delivery is achieved through piperidine and imidazole-modified PEG–poly (β-aminoester) micelles [83]. Bacterial infections are usually characterized by very low pH values due to the anaerobic fermentation and subsequent inflammation presence. In this regard, systemic antibiotic therapy has been attained by the incorporation of polyhistidine segment (ionisable) in a block copolymer. The incorporation was done to make PLGA-b-poly histidine-b-PEG triblock copolymer nanoparticles. The interactions were promoted by the presence of a charged switch at the sites of localized acidity with the negatively charged bacterial cell wall. That leads to an increased uptake of nanoparticles in Gram-positive as well as in Gram-negative bacteria [84]. The gastrointestinal (GI) tract has a broad range of pH. So, for oral drug delivery, the pH-responsive systems have been designed in a way that the drugs are protected from the harsh conditions found in the gastric environment. Hence, it improves the absorption of drugs in the intestine [85]. Poly (methacrylic acid)-based copolymers are used as pH-sensitive coatings at the surface of porous silica nanoparticles; also they are used to prepare copolymer micelles that are able to be applied to MSNPs [86]. Thus, the electrostatic interactions are used for drug release, which can be achieved at a neutral pH and also for chitosan nanoparticles for intestinal delivery [87].

Response to Reductive Environment

As there exists the redox potential difference (100–1000 fold) between the extracellular and intracellular space, it is established that the extracellular and intracellular spaces act in oxidative and reductive modes, respectively. This feature is strongly related to the concentration of glutathione in intra- and extracellular components. On this basis, the redox-sensitive systems are expected to be a promising and effective method for intracellular delivery, particularly for genes or SiRNA delivery. The glutathione pathway that controls the intracellular redox potential is expressively involved in these kinds of stimuli-sensitive mechanisms [88]. Apart from this, a drug molecule or a gene fragment can be conjugated or encapsulated to redox-sensitive nano carriers having the disulfide bonds. If there is an excess of glutathione inside the cell, the disulfide bonds get reduced, and the drug or gene in the Nano carrier gets released. This is successfully achieved with the use of reductively degradable micelles formed by self-assembled amphiphilic copolymers that have disulfide links in the hydrophobic backbone [89]. The use of two polymer blocks that contain a single disulfide bond at their connection also plays the same role [90]. Other routes that use the GSH-sensitive crosslinking agents, which are incorporated either in the core or in the shell of the micelles, lead to the quick disassembling of micelles and, subsequently the specific intracellular releasing the hydrophobic drugs [91]. Systems that are Redox-sensitive can use a number of other formulations for drug delivery, such as the capped mesoporous material, conjugates of dendrimer and drugs which contain thiol-cleavable bonds, liposomes formed from a Quinone-lipid conjugate or Nano gels cross-linked with disulfide [92]. For the activated release of drugs in inflammatory tissues also, oxidation responsiveness has been explored, which is characterized by the accumulation of reactive oxygen species (ROS). For example, the formulation of thioketal-based nanoparticles with a polymer sensitive to ROS exhibited the competence of specific TNFα–siRNA delivery in the intestinal inflammation sites hence after being administrated orally, they provide the therapeutic levels of gene silencing [93].

Multi Stimuli-responsive Drug Delivery

Drug delivery can be further improved by sensitivity to more than one stimuli *i.e.*, the systems that respond to multiple concurrently applied stimuli (Fig. **7**). Because a pH gradient and oxidative environment can co-exist in several pathological conditions, or in many cases a combination of pH and redox responsiveness may be used that enhances the efficiency of drug delivery (Fig. **8**), showing dual response to acidic pH of tumor tissue and reductive environment of GSH). Also, the conjugation of doxorubicin and antisense-bcl 2 oligonucleotides to a four-arm PEG having redox-reducible and acid-cleavable linkers resulted in the proficient apoptosis of cancer cells [94]. pH-sensitive polypeptide micelles containing a redox-sensitive cross-linked interlayer triggered the disassembly of Nanocarriers and a burst of doxorubicin release, leading to their enhanced therapeutic efficacy *in vivo* [95]. Liposomes and ionically self-assembled nanoparticles have shown improved drug delivery for being responsive to temperature as well as pH [96]. The pH responsiveness can be associated with light sensitivity by exploitation of the resonance surface properties of silver and palladium [97].

Dendrimers

Dendrimers have a unique shape and structure, being highly branched and having a three-dimensional appearance resembling the architecture of a tree [102]. Typically, a dendrimer consists of mainly three-structure components: 1) a focal core, (2) building blocks containing numerous interior layers that are made of repeating units, and (3) multiple functional groups present on the periphery (Fig. **9**).

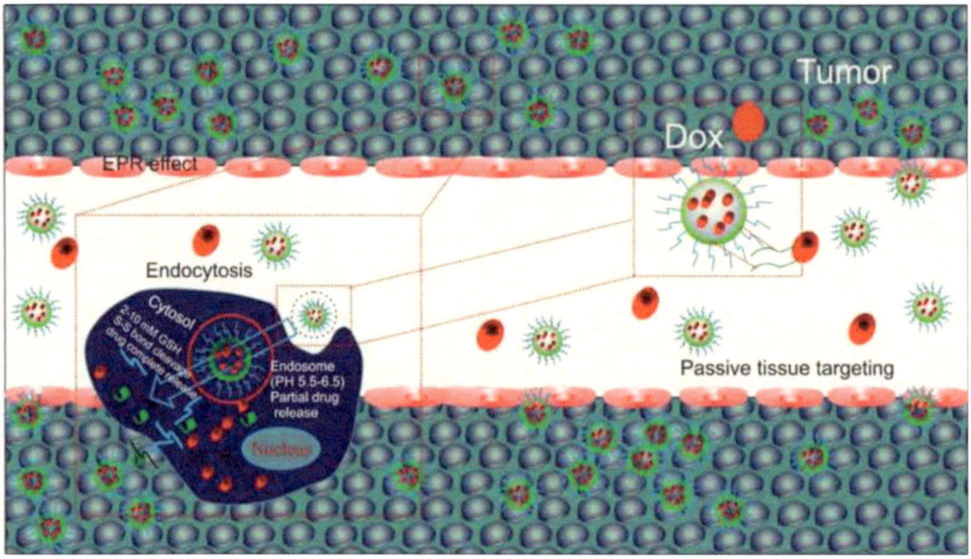

Fig. (8). Schematics of the complete process of DOX-loaded mPEG-SS-PNLG micelles uptake by tumor cells and intracellular release of DOX *via* dual responsiveness *i.e.*, response to acidic pH of tumor tissue and then to GSH breaking disulphide bonds which lead to the release of drugs [99]. Moreover, a great response has been displayed by other systems to temperature or magnetic field for the delivery of methotrexate to skeletal muscle [100]. The response has also been noted towards light and the reducing environment with the purpose of controlling the release kinetics of the block copolymer micelles [59] and to ultrasounds and enzymes for the enhancement of drug release from bubble liposomes [101].

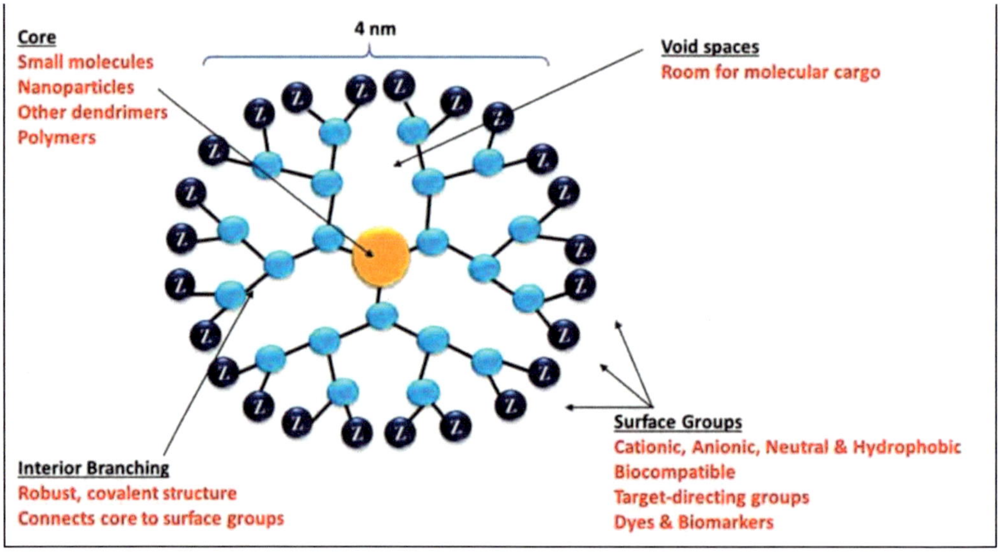

Fig. (9). General structure of dendrimer (a third-generation dendrimer). "Generations" correspond to the layers in which the branched units are established", and that represent the repeating monomer unit of these Macromolecules [103].

Cascade Reactions: the Foundation of Dendrimer Synthesis

Chemists were aware much earlier of the basic iterative methods that are presently employed in the synthesis of dendrimers. For example, solid-phase peptide synthesis is based on similar schemes. In turn, similar iterative strategies in biochemical synthetic pathways have long been exploited by biological studies; an example is the fatty acid bio-synthesis [104].

Synthesis of Dendrimers: a Divergent or Convergent Approach

For the synthesis of dendrimers, there are two main approaches available (Fig. **10**). The Divergent approach, used earlier, where the synthesis starts from the core of a dendrimer with attached arms that are supported by building blocks in a comprehensive and stepwise order. Second is the convergent approach, where the synthesis is initiated from the exterior, which begins with the molecular structure, which eventually turns to be the outermost arm of the final structure (dendrimer). In this approach, pre-determination is required for the final generation number, which demands the synthesis of the branches of a variety of sizes in advance for each generation [105].

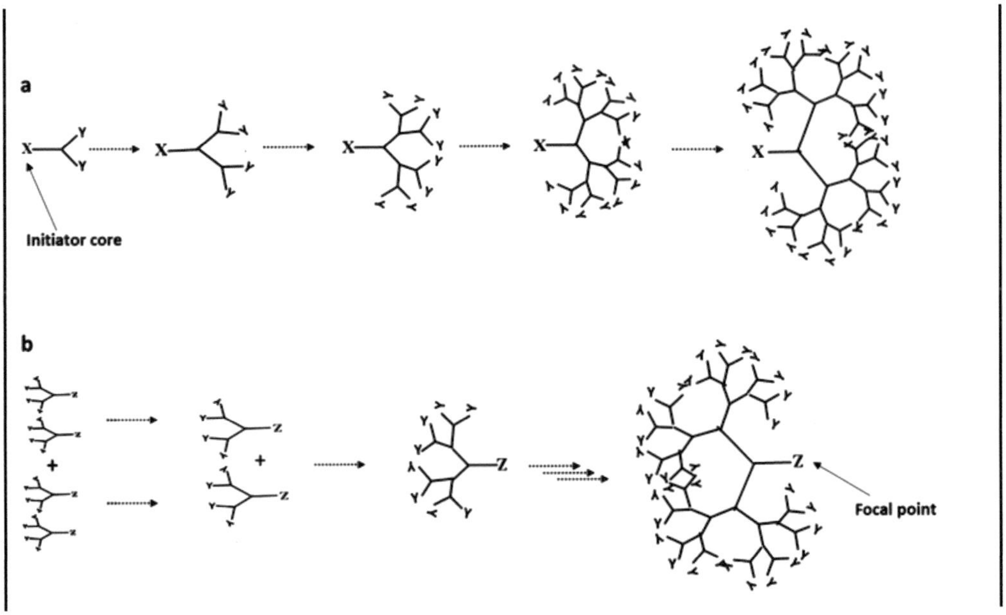

Fig. (10). Dendrimer synthesis methods (a) divergent approach: the dendrimer is assembled from a multifunctional core, that is extended outward through a series of reactions, usually a Michael reaction (b) convergent approach: the dendrimers are formed from small molecules which end up at the surface of the sphere, and reactions proceed inward building and are eventually attached to a core [106].

The last two decades of scientific research have led to the development of dendrimers as a potential drug delivery vehicle and have become most fascinating active areas of research in biomed and pharmaceutical science. As drug carrier candidates, dendrimers offer several featured advantages. That include:

• High density and reactivity shown by the functional groups that are present on the peripheral side of dendrimers that help in facile modification of the multifarious bioactive molecules onto the surface [107, 108].

• Properties like predictable molecular weight, distinct globular structure, and the monodispersity of the dendrimers ensure the reproductive pharmacokinetics [13].

• Various biomedical applications are satisfied by the generation-dependent controllable size of dendrimers [109].

• There is an increased cellular uptake level of drugs, which are conjugated to dendrimers through the cell membrane because of the high penetration ability shown by dendritic structures.

• Dendrimers are much safer choices than synthesized peptide carriers and other natural protein carriers because they lack immunogenicity [110].

• Dendrimers show an enhanced permeability and retention (EPR) effect that offers the cancer tissue the preferential uptake of the materials [111].

• There are well-defined methodologies for the construction of the Nanodevices with several functional moieties that are based on dendrimers. Such devices have provided various biomedical and biotechnological applications with promising effects, for example, cancer targeting therapy, photodynamic therapy, magnetic response imaging (MRI), and neutron capture therapy [112].

• Reduced toxicity, a simplified dosing schedule and increased bio-availability due to perfectly programmed release of the drug molecules or other bioactive agents from dendrimers [113].

• Other potential advantages of dendrimer architecture are prolonged residence time of drugs in blood and the protection of bioactive from their environment with improved stability [114].

Different types of dendrimers are utilized as hosts for both the hydrophobic and hydrophilic drugs, including polyamidoamine (PAMAM), polylysine dendrimers, polypropylene imine (PPI), *etc.* A model dendritic drug carrier should satisfy these conditions *i.e.*, it should be non-toxic, preferably biodegradable, not immunogenic, should present an adequate bio-distribution and thus allow tissue targeting efficiently [115].

LIPID-BASED DRUG CARRIERS

Liposomes as Drug Carriers

Prof. A.D. Bangham of the United Kingdom, demonstrated, for the first time in an article, the preparation of the liposomes with entrapped solutes. Since the inception of liposomes, they have been explored as carriers for many drug molecules and pharmaceuticals of biological interest [116, 117]. A well-studied drug carrier class is presented by liposomes with a general characteristic of having a lipid bilayer, primarily composed of amphipathic phospholipids (Fig. **11**) that enclose an interior aqueous space. Presently, to combat deadly cancer and infectious diseases, there are a number of liposome formulations in clinical use. It is noteworthy to mention that Doxil®/caylex (a formulation base on liposomes in anti-cancer drug doxorubicin, Ortho-Biotech) was the first approved formulation for application in clinic use. Thus, this may be considered an honorary nanoparticle for the care of a patient [118].

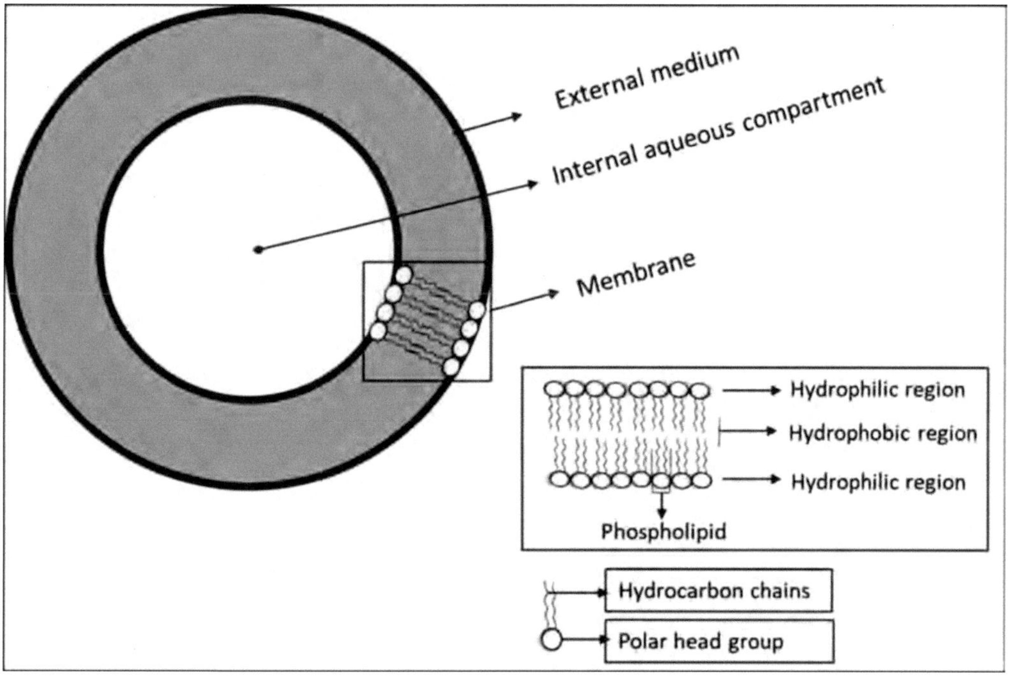

Fig. (11). Showing the basic structure and composition of liposomes [119].

The main constituents of liposomes are phospholipids (phosphatidylcholines, generally referred "lecithins"). They usually form concentric bilayers (A.D. Bangham primarily called them "bangosomes") because of their amphipathic properties. Several protocols and techniques are available for these multilamellar lipid dispersions to transfer them into single bilayer structures (referred to as unilamellar vesicles or liposomes). Laboratory methods that are used commonly include reverse-phase evaporation, extrusion, sonication and solvent injection [120]. The advantage of using 100–200 nm sized liposomes as Nano carriers for the delivery of anti-cancer agents to tumor cells has been studied extensively [121]. So, for the therapy of carcinoma, this approach involves "passive targeting" of drug-loaded Nanocarriers. These particles are expected to accumulate in the tumor area. The accumulation is because they show leaky vasculature and EPR *i.e.* the enhanced permeability and retention effect of tumor cells. Generally, the structural differences between normal and cancerous tissue are represented by this effect because of the increased permeability of capillaries in the tumor area. The consequences of passive targeting are largely dependent on several characteristics that include the vascularization degree of tumor, angiogenesis, porosity and the tumor vessel pore size. The pore size and porosity differ with the tumor type and its status [122]. The mentioned factors directly affect the bio-division and pharmacokinetics of any liposome. There are also other additional issues that are related to "passive targeting" along with the kinetics of drug discharge, tumor retention and efflux of the released drug into tumor cells. These are some important factors that also show a positive impact on the likely outcome of any effective treatment. For example, due to the EPR effect, liposomes (100-150 nm) are reported to accumulate preferentially in the tumors [123]. A number of candidates' ligands have been examined for targeting liposomes on lumps that are intended to exploit the overexpressed receptors; which comprise antibodies, affibodies, and also small ligands like lectins, folate, peptides, and aptamers [120].

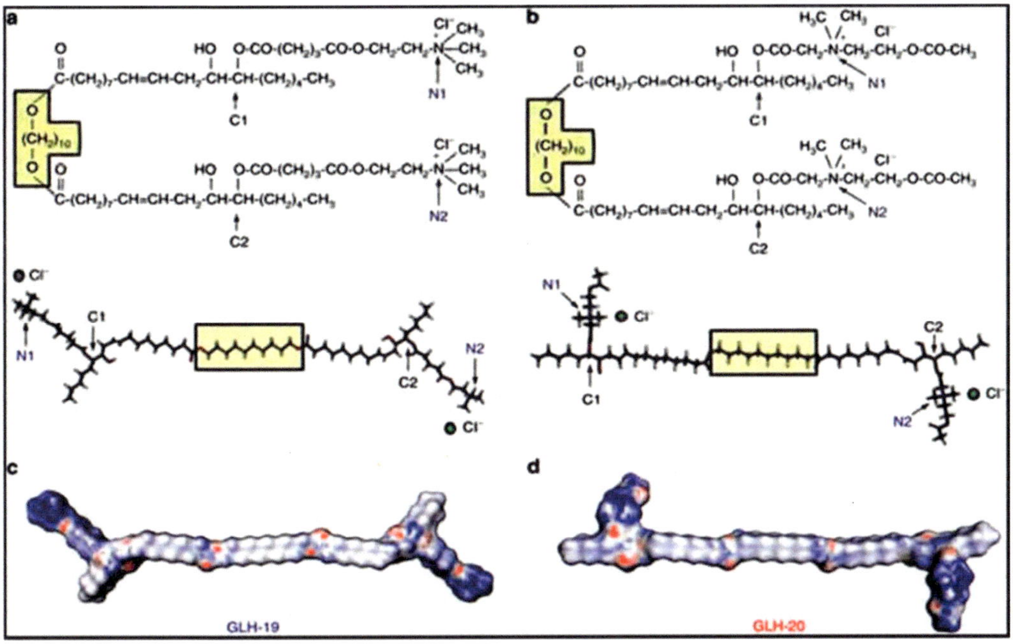

Fig. (12). Molecular structures of bola amphiphiles (a) GLH-19 and (b) GLH-20. For an indication of the correspondence to the 3D illustrative presented in the lower half, a fragment that is common to both bola amphiphiles (O-$(CH_2)_{10}$-O) was placed in the yellow box [124]. Electrostatic surface potential maps of (**c**) GLH-19 and (**d**) GLH-20. Red, blue, and white colours correspond to negatively charged, positively charged, and neutral regions, respectively.

Monolayer Membrane from Bola Amphiphiles

Bola amphiphiles, also called bola lipids, are an exclusive class of lipids that have two hydrophilic head groups attached to the hydrophobic domain on both ends Fig. (**12**), showing a structure of bola amphiphiles (a) GLH-19 and (b) GLH-20.

In comparison to the single-hydrophilic headed amphiphiles, for example, phospholipids, whose characteristic feature is the formation of bilayer membranes, bola amphiphiles may form monolayer membranes [125]. There are reports that demonstrate that the membranes made from bola amphiphiles show less permeability and are more durable than those composed of monopolar lipids [126]. The unique combination provided by these properties has developed an interest in the productive and potential use of bola amphiphiles. They can be used as membrane-stabilizing agents in various applications, such as membrane-protein-based biosensors and drug delivery [127].

Bola amphiphiles bear two different hydrophilic head groups called unsymmetrical bola amphiphiles. These bola amphiphiles are attracting considerable attention in the Nano- and biotechnological field because of encountering water; they can self-assemble to form unsymmetrical monolayer lipid membranes. These unsymmetrical membranes display parallel molecular packing, resulting in specific nanostructures possessing diverse inner and outer surfaces that are covered with either head group. These nano-structures can be highly applicable for medical diagnosis and delivery systems. The basic principle of their selection is the selective and effective encapsulation of biomolecules and functional nanomaterials are selected for these biomolecules for sufficient inner space [128, 129]. Liposomes made up of phospholipid amphiphiles undergo aggregation to result in bilayer membranes. These agents are now widely studied and investigated as potent drug-delivery systems [130, 131]. However, in various cases, there is a rapid clearing of liposomes from the system when injected into the bloodstream, and thus, only a fraction of them reach the target site. Even when liposomes are PEG-coated, the effect is not much different. To overcome this, promising alternatives are being employed, which include the monolayer membranes composed of vesicles formed from bola amphiphiles. These vesicles are effectively more stable than the classical bilayer liposomes. Hence, due to a reduction in lipid exchange, they are not likely expected to fuse with each other or with cell membranes [132].

TARGETED DRUG DELIVERY

There are two ways to achieve targeted delivery, *i.e.*, active or passive. In active targeting, the pharmaceutical agent or the carrier system is conjugated to a cell-specific ligand [133]. While passive targeting is comparatively achieved through the incorporation of the therapeutic agent into a macromolecule or a nanoparticle. The drug molecule then reaches the target organ passively. Tumors or lumps may be passively targeted by drugs that are encapsulated in nanoparticles, or the macromolecule coupled drugs can act through the EPR effect. Alternatively, for the infusion of nanoparticles into the target organ or tissues, catheters can also be used. For instance, the localized delivery of nanoparticles bearing drug to the vascular restenosis sites can be suitable to provide a sustained release of drug at definite locations on the arterial wall [134]. Basically, nanoparticle entrapment of drugs is based on two aims *i.e.*, either for the improved delivery to target cells or to bring a decrease in the toxic effects of the free drug that can affect to other than target organs. Both conditions will lead to an amplified therapeutic index, *i.e.*, the dose margins that can lead to therapeutic efficacy (*e.g.*, death of a tumor cell) and toxicity to other organ systems. For these purposes, the creation of target-specific and long-lived nanoparticles is needed. Most of the compounds are biodegradable polymers that lead to drug release following degradation. The use of particulate drug carriers, which also include nanomaterials, faces a problem, *i.e.*, the drug carrier gets entrapped in the phagocytic system, which is present in the spleen or liver [8, 135]. This could be circumvented by surface modification with polyethylene glycol (PEG), which results in the increased circulation time of nanoparticles by the inhibition of recognition and phagocytosis by the mononuclear phagocytic system [136]. Apart from alteration of the distribution, the PEG modification, it also results in reducing *in vitro* toxicity when gold Nanorods are modified by using PEG. Nanoparticles need to be coated to avert agglomeration. Various coatings have been reported to avoid agglomeration and to retain the particles in colloidal suspension that include several polymers *e.g.*, polyethylene glycol (PEG), polyvinylpyrrolidone) (PVP) etc., other natural polymers like pullulan, chitosan, dextran etc., and surfactants like oleic acid, sodium salt, dodecyl amine etc [137]. For successful delivery of drugs, other than organ or cellular level targeting is of significance, but also the Nano carriers' fate within the cells is of importance. Particles usually end up intracellularly in lysosomes or endosomes, which is followed by their degradation. To encapsulate drugs, their release into the cytosol is required. Nevertheless, cellular uptake has also been demonstrated for nanoparticles sized 20 nm without contributions from the endocytic mechanisms [138]. The fate of nanoparticles in cells can also be determined by chemical characteristics such as the surface charge. Gold nanoparticles were surface functionalized with PEG, which resulted in their efficient internalization in endosomes and cytosol, and localization in the nuclear region. Poly(DL-lactide-co-glycolide) nanoparticles are found to be ingested by cells and then by lysosomes through the process of endocytosis [139]. It has been suggested that a change in surface charge causes the escape from these endosomes into the cellular cytoplasm. A change in the surface charge of the PLGA nanoparticles from negative to positive leads to cytoplasmic delivery of the combined drugs. The hypothesis that the transition of surface charge from negative to positive influences the escape from the endosomes has been supported by the data that was obtained with negatively charged nanoparticles of polystyrene that could not reach the cytosol. These nanoparticles were assumed to remain in the endosomal compartments of smooth muscle cells (used in this study), whichhindered their reach to the cytosol [140]. It may also be possible to achieve specific targeting to retinal pigment epithelium cells present in the eyes [141]. For specific targeting, very small quantum dots (<10 nm) have been used for the peptide-coated dots to the vasculature of tumors and lungs [142]. Moreover, the polymer shells that are on quantum dots can be allied to targeting molecules. For instance, an increase in the half-life was reported by using hydrophilic polyethylene glycol (PEG) for the coating of quantum dots cores. However, it was also demonstrated that quantum dots taken up by lymph nodes could be observed for up to 4 months, so the accumulation appears likely [143]. Surface modifications of nanoparticles reflect opportunities for various medical applications, such as drug targeting in terms of cellular binding, uptake, and intracellular transport. On the surface of biocompatible and biodegradable PLGA or *poly* (lactic-*co*-glycolic acid) Nanospheres, carbohydrate binding ligands are reported to surge cellular binding [144]. Such an increased adherence may result in an enhancement in the drug activity that is entrapped in nanoparticles. Coupling of the specific proteins, such as antibodies with nanoparticles' surface may help in specific and effective immunologically directed targeting of particles [145].

THE BRAIN – THE ULTIMATE TARGET FOR DRUG DELIVERY

For drug delivery, the brain is a challenge from several perspectives. Firstly, with the aging population, the incidence of degenerative diseases in the brain would increase. Secondly, towards exogenous substances, the blood-brain barrier (BBB) is the best-ever gatekeeper in the body [146]. The luminal blood-brain barrier (BBB) is basically composed of tight junctions bound endothelia which serve to restrict the entry of hydrophilic and/or most high molecular weight therapeutics to the brain. Principal mechanisms responsible for the limited uptake of drugs by BBB include: (a) lack of pinocytosis, (b) absence of par acellular openings and (c) significant protein-mediated efflux. The high metabolic magnitude of cerebral endothelial cells and the deficiency in pinocytic vesicles can also result in limiting the exchange between the plasma and the CNS of anti-cancer agents [147]. At the interface, the endothelial barrier is precisely tight with the brain astrocytes and, in normal conditions, they can only be passed with the aid of endogenous BBB transporters that result in active efflux transport, carrier-mediated transport and/or receptor-mediated transport. However, the properties of the barrier and the restriction offered by it can be arbitrated intentionally or unintentionally by drug delivery [148]. For drug delivery into the brain, a physical association between the drug and the nanoparticles is necessary [149]. When the evaluation of nanoparticles with different surface characteristics was made, it was found that low concentrations of anionic nanoparticles and neutral nanoparticles have no effect on BBB integrity. On the other hand, higher concentrations of cationic and anionic nanoparticles have been toxic for the BBB. At lower concentrations, the range of anionic nanoparticles uptake by brain was greater to cationic or neutral formulations at similar concentrations. So, for the toxicity and brain distribution profiles, surface charges of nanoparticle must be considered [150]. Specifically, when nanoparticles were coated using polysorbate (Tween) surfactants, it has been observed that the drugs were transported across the blood-brain barrier [151]. The process of endocytosis has been suggested to be the possible mechanism for transport that occurs through the Low-Density Lipoprotein (LDL) receptor present on endothelial cells, after the lipoproteins adsorbed from the blood plasma to the nanoparticles [150]. Additional investigations reported the role of apolipoprotein-E for transport of drugs across BBB. Although the apolipoprotein-E variants which were not able to recognize lipoprotein receptors failed in the transportation of the drug across BBB [152]. It has been proposed that for the uptake of the drug by the brain, the recognition and interaction of nanocarrier with lipoprotein receptors on brain capillary endothelial cells were responsible.

By shielding certain drug features that prevent or limit their binding to cellular efflux systems like p-glycoprotein, the passage of BBB may also be attained. P-glycoprotein is a cellular transporter that is linked to drug removal from the cells. Also, it is an ATP-dependent efflux transporter that plays an important physiological role in limiting drug entry into the brain [153]. Poly(butyl) cyanoacrylate nanoparticles coated with surfactants have been used for the delivery of drugs to the CNS [154]. Paclitaxel (PX), a cytotoxic drug which is entrapped in acetyl alcohol/polysorbate nanoparticles (PX NP), has been evaluated in an *in situ* rat brain perfusion model where the entrapment effect was studied [155]. The observations suggested that the entrapping of paclitaxel by nanoparticles effectively increases the uptake of brain drugs. The toxicity towards p-glycoprotein was significant in expressing tumor cells. It has been assumed that PX nanoparticles limit the binding of paclitaxel to p-glycoprotein and subsequent efflux from the cells, which could consequently lead to higher tumor cell levels.

Other routes for reaching the brain, circumventing the BBB, may be *via* migration along the olfactory or trigeminal nerve endings after deposition on the olfactory mucosa in the nasal region [156]. Translocation of ultrafine 13C particles (35 nm) was detected by using this isotope measurement in the brain olfactory bulb after inhalation exposure. Also, other solid NPs like manganese oxide were shown to translocate to the brain by the olfactory route [157], based on the measurements of manganese in different parts of the brain. In order to increase the specific uptake *via* the inhalation route, nanoparticles have been functionalized by conjugation with bioactive ligands-lectins to the surface of poly (ethylene glycol)- poly (lactic acid) (PEG-PLA) nanoparticles. Wheat germ agglutinin (WGA) was used, which binds to N-Acetyl-D-glucosamine and sialic acid, both of which are abundantly present in the nasal cavity. There was a twofold increase in the brain uptake of such functionalized NPs [158]. However, it needs to be stated that both the passage of the BBB and the olfactory route only account for up to 2% nanoparticle uptake, and its efficacy with regard to drug delivery needs to make considerable increments before use.

FUTURE PROSPECTIVES

Nanotechnology has the potential to revolutionize a wide range of fields, from medicine and electronics to energy and materials science. Here are some of the key prospects of nanotechnology:

Medicine: Nanotechnology has the potential to transform the way we diagnose and treat diseases, by enabling targeted drug delivery, highly sensitive diagnostic tests, and innovative therapies such as gene editing and regenerative medicine.

Electronics: Nanotechnology can be used to create smaller, faster, and more energy-efficient electronic devices, such as ultra-high-density memory chips, more powerful batteries, and more efficient solar cells.

Energy: Nanotechnology can help to improve efficiency and reduce the cost of energy production, storage, and conversion, by enabling the development of new materials and devices such as fuel cells, supercapacitors, and photovoltaics.

Environment: Nanotechnology can be used to develop new materials and technologies for environmental remediation, pollution control, and sustainable agriculture, which can help reduce the impact of human activities on the environment.

Materials Science: Nanotechnology can be used to engineer new materials with unique properties and characteristics, such as super-strength, super-conductivity, and self-healing, which can be used in a wide range of applications from construction to aerospace.

However, as with any emerging technology, there are also challenges and risks associated with the development and application of nanotechnology, such as potential toxicity, ethical and regulatory issues, and the need for sustainable and responsible use. As a result, ongoing research and development in this area are needed to ensure that the benefits of nanotechnology can be realized in a safe, effective, and sustainable manner.

It is foreseen that future research in the field of medical science would certainly involve the use of nanoparticles, and nanotechnology would continue to advance in concern to scientific research in biomedical applications and many other areas of life sciences. Already, a lot has been achieved over a past few years when it comes to the achievement of the Nano field in medical sciences, including diagnostics, patient treatment and, systems of drug delivery and more is anticipated about the same. The area of drug delivery represents an imperative tool for pharmaceutical industries to expand drug marketing, because novel delivery systems can aid in repackaging classical drugs, thus offering an edge of competitiveness after the completion of the patent. Nanotechnology, being a multidisciplinary science, is particularly bringing the technologies of almost indistinctly small agents more and nearer to reality and eventually likely to affect precision medicine as well.

FUNDING

Rafat Ali was funded by ICMR as an SRF fellow under **Ref no-BMI/11/(35)/2020**.

ORCID

Armiya Sultan: https://orcid.org/0000-0001-5373-8824.

Rafat Ali: http://orcid.org/0000-0001-6324-7236

Nida Jamil Khan: https://orcid.org/0000-0002-1992-097X

ACKNOWLEDGEMENT

The authors are grateful to the Centre for Interdisciplinary Research in Basic Sciences (CIRBSc), Jamia Millia Islamia-110025, for providing the research infrastructure.

REFERENCES

[1] Buzea C, Pacheco II, Robbie K. Nanomaterials and nanoparticles: Sources and toxicity. Biointerphases 2007; 2(4): MR17-71. [http://dx.doi.org/10.1116/1.2815690] [PMID: 20419892]

[2] Duncan R. Polymer therapeutics: Nanomedicines in routine clinical use. 2005.

[3] Joseph T, Moore R. Drug delivery using nanotechnology technologies: markets \& competitive environment 2008.

[4] Boylan J, Swarbrick J. Encyclopedia of pharmaceutical technology. Marcel Dekker 2001.

[5] Panyam J, Labhasetwar V. Biodegradable nanoparticles for drug and gene delivery to cells and tissue. Adv Drug Deliv Rev 2003; 55(3): 329-47. [http://dx.doi.org/10.1016/S0169-409X(02)00228-4] [PMID: 12628320]

[6] Kroll RA, Pagel MA, Muldoon LL, *et al.* Improving drug delivery to intracerebral tumor and surrounding brain in a rodent model: A comparison of osmotic versus bradykinin modification of the blood-brain and/or blood-tumor barriers. Neurosurgery 1998; 43(4): 879-86. [http://dx.doi.org/10.1097/00006123-199810000-00090] [PMID: 9766316]

[7] Kreuter J, Ramge P, Petrov V, *et al.* Direct evidence that polysorbate-80-coated poly(butylcyanoacrylate) nanoparticles deliver drugs to the CNS *via* specific mechanisms requiring prior binding of drug to the nanoparticles. Pharm Res 2003; 20(3): 409-16. [http://dx.doi.org/10.1023/A:1022604120952] [PMID: 12669961]

[8] Zauner W, Farrow NA, Haines AMR. *In vitro* uptake of polystyrene microspheres: effect of particle size, cell line and cell density. J Control Release 2001; 71(1): 39-51. [http://dx.doi.org/10.1016/S0168-3659(00)00358-8] [PMID: 11245907]

[9] Desai MP, Labhasetwar V, Walter E, Levy RJ, Amidon GL. The mechanism of uptake of biodegradable microparticles in Caco-2 cells is size dependent. Pharm Res 1997; 14(11): 1568-73. [http://dx.doi.org/10.1023/A:1012126301290] [PMID: 9434276]

[10] Redhead HM, Davis SS, Illum L. Drug delivery in poly(lactide-co-glycolide) nanoparticles surface modified with poloxamer 407 and poloxamine 908: *in vitro* characterisation and *in vivo* evaluation. J

Control Release 2001; 70(3): 353-63.
[http://dx.doi.org/10.1016/S0168-3659(00)00367-9] [PMID: 11182205]

[11] Müller R, Maaben S, Weyhers H, Mehnert W. Phagocytic uptake and cytotoxicity of solid lipid nanoparticles (SLN) sterically stabilized with poloxamine 908 and poloxamer 407. J Drug Target 1996; 4(3): 161-70.
[http://dx.doi.org/10.3109/10611869609015973] [PMID: 8959488]

[12] Olivier JC. Drug transport to brain with targeted nanoparticles. NeuroRx 2005; 2(1): 108-19.
[http://dx.doi.org/10.1602/neurorx.2.1.108] [PMID: 15717062]

[13] Grislain L, Couvreur P, Lenaerts V, Roland M, Deprez-Decampeneere D, Speiser P. Pharmacokinetics and distribution of a biodegradable drug-carrier. Int J Pharm 1983; 15(3): 335-45.
[http://dx.doi.org/10.1016/0378-5173(83)90166-7]

[14] Couvreur P, Barratt G, Fattal E, Vauthier C, Vauthier C. Nanocapsule technology: A review. Crit Rev Ther Drug Carrier Syst 2002; 19(2): 99-134.
[http://dx.doi.org/10.1615/CritRevTherDrugCarrierSyst.v19.i2.10] [PMID: 12197610]

[15] Govender T, Stolnik S, Garnett MC, Illum L, Davis SS. PLGA nanoparticles prepared by nanoprecipitation: Drug loading and release studies of a water soluble drug. J Control Release 1999; 57(2): 171-85.
[http://dx.doi.org/10.1016/S0168-3659(98)00116-3] [PMID: 9971898]

[16] Peracchia MT, Gref R, Minamitake Y, Domb A, Lotan N, Langer R. PEG-coated nanospheres from amphiphilic diblock and multiblock copolymers: Investigation of their drug encapsulation and release characteristics1. J Control Release 1997; 46(3): 223-31.
[http://dx.doi.org/10.1016/S0168-3659(96)01597-0]

[17] Calvo P, Remuñan-López C, Vila-Jato JL, Alonso MJ. Chitosan and chitosan/ethylene oxide-propylene oxide block copolymer nanoparticles as novel carriers for proteins and vaccines. Pharm Res 1997; 14(10): 1431-6.
[http://dx.doi.org/10.1023/A:1012128907225] [PMID: 9358557]

[18] Chen Y, McCulloch R, Gray B. Synthesis of albumin-dextran sulfate microspheres possessing favourable loading and release characteristics for the anti-cancer drug doxorubicin. J Control Release 1994; 31(1): 49-54.
[http://dx.doi.org/10.1016/0168-3659(94)90250-X]

[19] Magenheim B, Levy MY, Benita S. A new *in vitro* technique for the evaluation of drug release profile from colloidal carriers : Ultrafiltration technique at low pressure. Int J Pharm 1993; 94(1-3): 115-23.
[http://dx.doi.org/10.1016/0378-5173(93)90015-8]

[20] Fresta M, Puglisi G, Giammona G, Cavallaro G, Micali N, Furneri PM. Pefloxacine mesilate- and ofloxacin-loaded polyethylcyanoacrylate nanoparticles: characterization of the colloidal drug carrier formulation. J Pharm Sci 1995; 84(7): 895-902.
[http://dx.doi.org/10.1002/jps.2600840721] [PMID: 7562444]

[21] Zha J, Roggendorf H. Sol-gel science, the physics and chemistry of sol-gel processing, Ed. by C. J. Brinker and G. W. Scherer, Academic Press, Boston 1990, xiv, 908 pp., bound?ISBN 0-12-134970-5.
[http://dx.doi.org/10.1002/adma.19910031025]

[22] Lee EJH, Ribeiro C, Longo E, Leite ER. Growth kinetics of tin oxide nanocrystals in colloidal suspensions under hydrothermal conditions. Chem Phys 2006; 328(1-3): 229-35.
[http://dx.doi.org/10.1016/j.chemphys.2006.06.032]

[23] Doria G, Conde J, Veigas B, *et al.* Noble metal nanoparticles for biosensing applications. Sensors 2012; 12(2): 1657-87.
[http://dx.doi.org/10.3390/s120201657] [PMID: 22438731]

[24] Tourinho PS, van Gestel CAM, Lofts S, Svendsen C, Soares AMVM, Loureiro S. Metal-based nanoparticles in soil: Fate, behavior, and effects on soil invertebrates. Environ Toxicol Chem 2012;

31(8): 1679-92.
[http://dx.doi.org/10.1002/etc.1880] [PMID: 22573562]

[25] Xu ZP, Zeng QH, Lu GQ, Yu AB. Inorganic nanoparticles as carriers for efficient cellular delivery. Chem Eng Sci 2006; 61(3): 1027-40.
[http://dx.doi.org/10.1016/j.ces.2005.06.019]

[26] Wong KKY, Liu XL. Nanomedicine: A primer for surgeons. Pediatr Surg Int 2012; 28(10): 943-51.
[http://dx.doi.org/10.1007/s00383-012-3162-y] [PMID: 22892910]

[27] Qian X, Peng XH, Ansari DO, *et al. In vivo* tumor targeting and spectroscopic detection with surface-enhanced Raman nanoparticle tags. Nat Biotechnol 2008; 26(1): 83-90.
[http://dx.doi.org/10.1038/nbt1377] [PMID: 18157119]

[28] Kang B, Mackey MA, El-Sayed MA. Nuclear targeting of gold nanoparticles in cancer cells induces DNA damage, causing cytokinesis arrest and apoptosis. J Am Chem Soc 2010; 132(5): 1517-9.
[http://dx.doi.org/10.1021/ja9102698] [PMID: 20085324]

[29] Gao H, Shi W, Freund LB. Mechanics of receptor-mediated endocytosis. Proc Natl Acad Sci 2005; 102(27): 9469-74.
[http://dx.doi.org/10.1073/pnas.0503879102] [PMID: 15972807]

[30] Nakielny S, Dreyfuss G. Transport of proteins and RNAs in and out of the nucleus. Cell 1999; 99(7): 677-90.
[http://dx.doi.org/10.1016/S0092-8674(00)81666-9] [PMID: 10619422]

[31] Xue H, Atakilit A, Zhu W, Li X, Ramos DM, Pytela R. Role of the α(v)β6 integrin in human oral squamous cell carcinoma growth *in vivo* and *in vitro*. Biochem Biophys Res Commun 2001; 288(3): 610-8.
[http://dx.doi.org/10.1006/bbrc.2001.5813] [PMID: 11676487]

[32] Wang AZ, Langer R, Farokhzad OC. Nanoparticle delivery of cancer drugs. Annu Rev Med 2012; 63(1): 185-98.
[http://dx.doi.org/10.1146/annurev-med-040210-162544] [PMID: 21888516]

[33] Mahapatra SS, Karak N. Silver nanoparticle in hyperbranched polyamine: Synthesis, characterization and antibacterial activity. Mater Chem Phys 2008; 112(3): 1114-9.
[http://dx.doi.org/10.1016/j.matchemphys.2008.07.047]

[34] Morales MP, Bomati-Miguel O, Pérez de Alejo R, Ruiz-Cabello J, Veintemillas-Verdaguer S, O'Grady K. Contrast agents for MRI based on iron oxide nanoparticles prepared by laser pyrolysis. J Magn Magn Mater 2003; 266(1-2): 102-9.
[http://dx.doi.org/10.1016/S0304-8853(03)00461-X]

[35] Scott BJ, Wirnsberger G, Stucky GD. Mesoporous and mesostructured materials for optical applications. Chem Mater 2001; 13(10): 3140-50.
[http://dx.doi.org/10.1021/cm0110730]

[36] Hartmann M. Ordered mesoporous materials for bioadsorption and biocatalysis. Chem Mater 2005; 17(18): 4577-93.
[http://dx.doi.org/10.1021/cm0485658]

[37] Safari J, Zarnegar Z. Advanced drug delivery systems: Nanotechnology of health design A review. J Saudi Chem Soc 2014; 18(2): 85-99.
[http://dx.doi.org/10.1016/j.jscs.2012.12.009]

[38] Slowing I, Viveroescoto J, Wu C, Lin V. Mesoporous silica nanoparticles as controlled release drug delivery and gene transfection carriers. Adv Drug Deliv Rev 2008; 60(11): 1278-88.
[http://dx.doi.org/10.1016/j.addr.2008.03.012] [PMID: 18514969]

[39] Vallet-Regi M, Rámila A, del Real RP, Pérez-Pariente J. A New Property of MCM-41: Drug Delivery System. Chem Mater 2001; 13(2): 308-11.
[http://dx.doi.org/10.1021/cm0011559]

[40] Cai Q, Luo ZS, Pang WQ, Fan YW, Chen XH, Cui FZ. Dilute solution routes to various controllable morphologies of MCM-41 Silica with a Basic Medium. Chem Mater 2001; 13(2): 258-63.
[http://dx.doi.org/10.1021/cm990661z]

[41] Yang H, Coombs N, Ozin GA. Morphogenesis of shapes and surface patterns in mesoporous silica. Nature 1997; 386(6626): 692-5.
[http://dx.doi.org/10.1038/386692a0]

[42] Xu AW. Neutral Templating Route to Unusual Mesostructured Silicas. J Phys Chem B 2002; 106(51): 13161-4.
[http://dx.doi.org/10.1021/jp026148h]

[43] Trewyn BG, Nieweg JA, Zhao Y, Lin VSY. Biocompatible mesoporous silica nanoparticles with different morphologies for animal cell membrane penetration. Chem Eng J 2008; 137(1): 23-9.
[http://dx.doi.org/10.1016/j.cej.2007.09.045]

[44] Li S, Shi , Hua , Chen , Ruan , Yan . Hollow Spheres of Mesoporous Aluminosilicate with a Three-Dimensional Pore Network and Extraordinarily High Hydrothermal Stability. Nano Lett 2003; 3(5): 609-12.
[http://dx.doi.org/10.1021/nl034134x]

[45] Chen Z, Niu D, Li Y, Shi J. One-step approach to synthesize hollow mesoporous silica spheres co-templated by an amphiphilic block copolymer and cationic surfactant. RSC Advances 2013; 3(19): 6767.
[http://dx.doi.org/10.1039/c3ra00058c]

[46] Zhu Y, Kockrick E, Ikoma T, Hanagata N, Kaskel S. An Efficient Route to Rattle-Type Fe_3O_4@SiO_2 Hollow Mesoporous Spheres Using Colloidal Carbon Spheres Templates. Chem Mater 2009; 21(12): 2547-53.
[http://dx.doi.org/10.1021/cm900956j]

[47] Lee J, Park JC, Bang JU, Song H. Precise tuning of porosity and surface functionality in Au@SiO_2 Nanoreactors for High Catalytic Efficiency. Chem Mater 2008; 20(18): 5839-44.
[http://dx.doi.org/10.1021/cm801149w]

[48] Zhao W, Lang M, Li Y, Li L, Shi J. Fabrication of uniform hollow mesoporous silica spheres and ellipsoids of tunable size through a facile hard-templating route. J Mater Chem 2009; 19(18): 2778.
[http://dx.doi.org/10.1039/b822444g]

[49] Min Y, Caster JM, Eblan MJ, Wang AZ. Clinical translation of nanomedicine. Chem Rev 2015; 115(19): 11147-90.
[http://dx.doi.org/10.1021/acs.chemrev.5b00116] [PMID: 26088284]

[50] Li C. Poly(l-glutamic acid)–anti-cancer drug conjugates. Adv Drug Deliv Rev 2002; 54(5): 695-713.
[http://dx.doi.org/10.1016/S0169-409X(02)00045-5] [PMID: 12204599]

[51] Bhatt R, de Vries P, Tulinsky J, *et al.* Synthesis and *in vivo* antitumor activity of poly(l-glutamic acid) conjugates of 20S-camptothecin. J Med Chem 2003; 46(1): 190-3.
[http://dx.doi.org/10.1021/jm020022r] [PMID: 12502373]

[52] Adams ML, Lavasanifar A, Kwon GS. Amphiphilic block copolymers for drug delivery. J Pharm Sci 2003; 92(7): 1343-55.
[http://dx.doi.org/10.1002/jps.10397] [PMID: 12820139]

[53] Nakanishi T, Fukushima S, Okamoto K, *et al.* Development of the polymer micelle carrier system for doxorubicin. J Control Release 2001; 74(1-3): 295-302.
[http://dx.doi.org/10.1016/S0168-3659(01)00341-8] [PMID: 11489509]

[54] Ghosh D, Pradhan AK, Mondal S, Begum NA, Mandal D. Proton transfer reactions of 4′-chloro substituted 3-hydroxyflavone in solvents and aqueous micelle solutions. Phys Chem Chem Phys 2014; 16(18): 8594-607.
[http://dx.doi.org/10.1039/c3cp52209a] [PMID: 24671355]

[55] He X, Wu X, Gao C, *et al.* Synthesis and self-assembly of a hydrophilic, thermo-responsive poly(ethylene oxide) monomethyl ether-block-poly(acrylic acid)-block-poly(N-isopropylacrylamide) copolymer to form micelles for drug delivery. React Funct Polym 2011; 71(5): 544-52. [http://dx.doi.org/10.1016/j.reactfunctpolym.2011.02.001]

[56] Barratt G. Colloidal drug carriers: achievements and perspectives. Cell Mol Life Sci 2003; 60(1): 21-37. [http://dx.doi.org/10.1007/s000180300002] [PMID: 12613656]

[57] Xiong XB, Falamarzian A, Garg SM, Lavasanifar A. Engineering of amphiphilic block copolymers for polymeric micellar drug and gene delivery. J Control Release 2011; 155(2): 248-61. [http://dx.doi.org/10.1016/j.jconrel.2011.04.028] [PMID: 21621570]

[58] Xu W, Ling P, Zhang T. Polymeric micelles, a promising drug delivery system to enhance bioavailability of poorly water-soluble drugs. J Drug Deliv 2013; 2013: 1-15. [http://dx.doi.org/10.1155/2013/340315] [PMID: 23936656]

[59] Kataoka K, Harada A, Nagasaki Y. Block copolymer micelles for drug delivery: Design, characterization and biological significance. Adv Drug Deliv Rev 2012; 64: 37-48. [http://dx.doi.org/10.1016/j.addr.2012.09.013] [PMID: 11251249]

[60] Kaditi E, Mountrichas G, Pispas S. Amphiphilic block copolymers by a combination of anionic polymerization and selective post-polymerization functionalization. Eur Polym J 2011; 47(4): 415-34. [http://dx.doi.org/10.1016/j.eurpolymj.2010.09.012]

[61] Chen Y, Liu L. Modern methods for delivery of drugs across the blood–brain barrier. Adv Drug Deliv Rev 2012; 64(7): 640-65. [http://dx.doi.org/10.1016/j.addr.2011.11.010] [PMID: 22154620]

[62] Yatvin MB, Weinstein JN, Dennis WH, Blumenthal R. Design of liposomes for enhanced local release of drugs by hyperthermia. Science 1978; 202(4374): 1290-3. [http://dx.doi.org/10.1126/science.364652] [PMID: 364652]

[63] Mura S, Nicolas J, Couvreur P. Stimuli-responsive nanocarriers for drug delivery. Nat Mater 2013; 12(11): 991-1003. [http://dx.doi.org/10.1038/nmat3776] [PMID: 24150417]

[64] Hoffman AS. Applications of thermally reversible polymers and hydrogels in therapeutics and diagnostics. J Control Release 1987; 6(1): 297-305. [http://dx.doi.org/10.1016/0168-3659(87)90083-6] [PMID: 25356472]

[65] MacEwan SR, Chilkoti A. Digital switching of local arginine density in a genetically encoded self-assembled polypeptide nanoparticle controls cellular uptake. Nano Lett 2012; 12(6): 3322-8. [http://dx.doi.org/10.1021/nl301529p] [PMID: 22625178]

[66] Oliveira AM, Oliveira PC, Santos AM, Zanin MHA, Ré MI. Synthesis and characterization of thermo-responsive particles of poly(hydroxybutirate-co-hydroxyvalerate)-b-poly(N-isopropylacrylamide). Braz J Phys 2009; 39(1a): 217-22. [http://dx.doi.org/10.1590/S0103-97332009000200015]

[67] Lee SH, Choi SH, Kim SH, Park TG. Thermally sensitive cationic polymer nanocapsules for specific cytosolic delivery and efficient gene silencing of siRNA: Swelling induced physical disruption of endosome by cold shock. J Control Release 2008; 125(1): 25-32. [http://dx.doi.org/10.1016/j.jconrel.2007.09.011] [PMID: 17976853]

[68] Yang HW, Hua MY, Liu HL, *et al.* Self-protecting core-shell magnetic nanoparticles for targeted, traceable, long half-life delivery of BCNU to gliomas. Biomaterials 2011; 32(27): 6523-32. [http://dx.doi.org/10.1016/j.biomaterials.2011.05.047] [PMID: 21645920]

[69] Zhang F, Braun GB, Pallaoro A, *et al.* Mesoporous multifunctional upconversion luminescent and magnetic "nanorattle" materials for targeted chemotherapy. Nano Lett 2012; 12(1): 61-7. [http://dx.doi.org/10.1021/nl202949y] [PMID: 22133237]

[70] Arias JL, Reddy LH, Othman M, *et al.* Squalene based nanocomposites: a new platform for the design of multifunctional pharmaceutical theragnostics. ACS Nano 2011; 5(2): 1513-21. [http://dx.doi.org/10.1021/nn1034197] [PMID: 21275408]

[71] Jenkins SI, Pickard MR, Granger N, Chari DM. Magnetic nanoparticle-mediated gene transfer to oligodendrocyte precursor cell transplant populations is enhanced by magnetofection strategies. ACS Nano 2011; 5(8): 6527-38. [http://dx.doi.org/10.1021/nn2018717] [PMID: 21721568]

[72] Kheirolomoom A, Mahakian LM, Lai CY, *et al.* Copper-doxorubicin as a nanoparticle cargo retains efficacy with minimal toxicity. Mol Pharm 2010; 7(6): 1948-58. [http://dx.doi.org/10.1021/mp100245u] [PMID: 20925429]

[73] Rapoport NY, Kennedy AM, Shea JE, Scaife CL, Nam KH. Controlled and targeted tumor chemotherapy by ultrasound-activated nanoemulsions/microbubbles. J Control Release 2009; 138(3): 268-76. [http://dx.doi.org/10.1016/j.jconrel.2009.05.026] [PMID: 19477208]

[74] Jin Q, Cai T, Wang Y, Wang H, Ji J. Light-Responsive Polyion Complex Micelles with Switchable Surface Charge for Efficient Protein Delivery. ACS Macro Lett 2014; 3(7): 679-83. [http://dx.doi.org/10.1021/mz500290s] [PMID: 35590768]

[75] Lu J, Choi E, Tamanoi F, Zink JI. Light-activated nanoimpeller-controlled drug release in cancer cells. Small 2008; 4(4): 421-6. [http://dx.doi.org/10.1002/smll.200700903] [PMID: 18383576]

[76] Yan H, Teh C, Sreejith S, *et al.* Functional mesoporous silica nanoparticles for photothermal-controlled drug delivery *in vivo.* Angew Chem Int Ed 2012; 51(33): 8373-7. [http://dx.doi.org/10.1002/anie.201203993] [PMID: 22777795]

[77] Liu YC, Le Ny ALM, Schmidt J, Talmon Y, Chmelka BF, Lee CT Jr. Photo-assisted gene delivery using light-responsive catanionic vesicles. Langmuir 2009; 25(10): 5713-24. [http://dx.doi.org/10.1021/la803588d] [PMID: 19435291]

[78] Tong R, Hemmati HD, Langer R, Kohane DS. Photoswitchable nanoparticles for triggered tissue penetration and drug delivery. J Am Chem Soc 2012; 134(21): 8848-55. [http://dx.doi.org/10.1021/ja211888a] [PMID: 22385538]

[79] Islam A, Yasin T. Controlled delivery of drug from pH sensitive chitosan/poly (vinyl alcohol) blend. Carbohydr Polym 2012; 88(3): 1055-60. [http://dx.doi.org/10.1016/j.carbpol.2012.01.070]

[80] Wang H, Xu F, Wang Y, Liu X, Jin Q, Ji J. pH-responsive and biodegradable polymeric micelles based on poly(β-amino ester)-graft-phosphorylcholine for doxorubicin delivery. Polym Chem 2013; 4(10): 3012. [http://dx.doi.org/10.1039/c3py00139c]

[81] Deng Z, Zhen Z, Hu X, Wu S, Xu Z, Chu PK. Hollow chitosan–silica nanospheres as pH-sensitive targeted delivery carriers in breast cancer therapy. Biomaterials 2011; 32(21): 4976-86. [http://dx.doi.org/10.1016/j.biomaterials.2011.03.050] [PMID: 21486679]

[82] Min KH, Kim JH, Bae SM, *et al.* Tumoral acidic pH-responsive MPEG-poly(β-amino ester) polymeric micelles for cancer targeting therapy. J Control Release 2010; 144(2): 259-66. [http://dx.doi.org/10.1016/j.jconrel.2010.02.024] [PMID: 20188131]

[83] Gao GH, Park MJ, Li Y, *et al.* The use of pH-sensitive positively charged polymeric micelles for protein delivery. Biomaterials 2012; 33(35): 9157-64. [http://dx.doi.org/10.1016/j.biomaterials.2012.09.016] [PMID: 23000386]

[84] Radovic-Moreno AF, Lu TK, Puscasu VA, Yoon CJ, Langer R, Farokhzad OC. Surface charge-switching polymeric nanoparticles for bacterial cell wall-targeted delivery of antibiotics. ACS Nano 2012; 6(5): 4279-87.

[http://dx.doi.org/10.1021/nn3008383] [PMID: 22471841]

[85] Wang XQ, Zhang Q. pH-sensitive polymeric nanoparticles to improve oral bio-availability of peptide/protein drugs and poorly water-soluble drugs. Eur J Pharm Biopharm 2012; 82(2): 219-29. [http://dx.doi.org/10.1016/j.ejpb.2012.07.014] [PMID: 22885229]

[86] Yang YQ, Zheng LS, Guo XD, Qian Y, Zhang LJ. pH-Sensitive micelles self-assembled from amphiphilic copolymer brush for delivery of poorly water-soluble drugs. Biomacromolecules 2011; 12(1): 116-22. [http://dx.doi.org/10.1021/bm101058w] [PMID: 21121600]

[87] Sung HW, Sonaje K, Liao ZX, Hsu LW, Chuang EY. pH-responsive nanoparticles shelled with chitosan for oral delivery of insulin: from mechanism to therapeutic applications. Acc Chem Res 2012; 45(4): 619-29. [http://dx.doi.org/10.1021/ar200234q] [PMID: 22236133]

[88] Özben T, Ed. Free Radicals, Oxidative Stress, and Antioxidants: Pathological and Physiological Significance. Boston, MA: Springer US 1998. [http://dx.doi.org/10.1007/978-1-4757-2907-8]

[89] Sun Y, Yan X, Yuan T, *et al.* Disassemblable micelles based on reduction-degradable amphiphilic graft copolymers for intracellular delivery of doxorubicin. Biomaterials 2010; 31(27): 7124-31. [http://dx.doi.org/10.1016/j.biomaterials.2010.06.011] [PMID: 20580429]

[90] Wang YC, Wang F, Sun TM, Wang J. Redox-responsive nanoparticles from the single disulfide bond-bridged block copolymer as drug carriers for overcoming multidrug resistance in cancer cells. Bioconjug Chem 2011; 22(10): 1939-45. [http://dx.doi.org/10.1021/bc200139n] [PMID: 21866903]

[91] Li Y, Xiao K, Luo J, *et al.* Well-defined, reversible disulfide cross-linked micelles for on-demand paclitaxel delivery. Biomaterials 2011; 32(27): 6633-45. [http://dx.doi.org/10.1016/j.biomaterials.2011.05.050] [PMID: 21658763]

[92] Ryu JH, Chacko RT, Jiwpanich S, Bickerton S, Babu RP, Thayumanavan S. Self-cross-linked polymer nanogels: A versatile nanoscopic drug delivery platform. J Am Chem Soc 2010; 132(48): 17227-35. [http://dx.doi.org/10.1021/ja1069932] [PMID: 21077674]

[93] Wilson DS, Dalmasso G, Wang L, Sitaraman SV, Merlin D, Murthy N. Orally delivered thioketal nanoparticles loaded with TNF-α–siRNA target inflammation and inhibit gene expression in the intestines. Nat Mater 2010; 9(11): 923-8. [http://dx.doi.org/10.1038/nmat2859] [PMID: 20935658]

[94] Yoon S, Kim WJ, Yoo HS. Dual-responsive breakdown of nanostructures with high doxorubicin payload for apoptotic anti-cancer therapy. Small 2013; 9(2): 284-93. [http://dx.doi.org/10.1002/smll.201200997] [PMID: 22930531]

[95] Dai J, Lin S, Cheng D, Zou S, Shuai X. Interlayer-crosslinked micelle with partially hydrated core showing reduction and pH dual sensitivity for pinpointed intracellular drug release. Angew Chem Int Ed 2011; 50(40): 9404-8. [http://dx.doi.org/10.1002/anie.201103806] [PMID: 21898731]

[96] Ta T, Convertine AJ, Reyes CR, Stayton PS, Porter TM. Thermosensitive liposomes modified with poly(*N*-isopropylacrylamide-*co*-propylacrylic acid) copolymers for triggered release of doxorubicin. Biomacromolecules 2010; 11(8): 1915-20. [http://dx.doi.org/10.1021/bm1004993] [PMID: 20690704]

[97] Fang W, Yang J, Gong J, Zheng N. Photo- and pH-Triggered Release of anti-cancer Drugs from Mesoporous Silica-Coated Pd@Ag Nanoparticles. Adv Funct Mater 2012; 22(4): 842-8. [http://dx.doi.org/10.1002/adfm.201101960]

[98] Zhuang J, Gordon MR, Ventura J, Li L, Thayumanavan S. Multi-stimuli responsive macromolecules and their assemblies. Chem Soc Rev 2013; 42(17): 7421-35.

[http://dx.doi.org/10.1039/c3cs60094g] [PMID: 23765263]

[99] Yang HY, Jang MS, Gao GH, Lee JH, Lee DS. Construction of redox/pH dual stimuli-responsive PEGylated polymeric micelles for intracellular doxorubicin delivery in liver cancer. Polym Chem 2016; 7(9): 1813-25.
[http://dx.doi.org/10.1039/C5PY01808K]

[100] Baeza A, Guisasola E, Ruiz-Hernández E, Vallet-Regí M. Magnetically Triggered Multidrug Release by Hybrid Mesoporous Silica Nanoparticles. Chem Mater 2012; 24(3): 517-24.
[http://dx.doi.org/10.1021/cm203000u]

[101] Nahire R, Paul S, Scott MD, *et al.* Ultrasound enhanced matrix metalloproteinase-9 triggered release of contents from echogenic liposomes. Mol Pharm 2012; 9(9): 2554-64.
[http://dx.doi.org/10.1021/mp300165s] [PMID: 22849291]

[102] Tomalia DA, Naylor AM, Goddard WA III. Starburst Dendrimers: Molecular-level control of size, shape, surface chemistry, topology, and flexibility from atoms to macroscopic matter. Angew Chem Int Ed Engl 1990; 29(2): 138-75.
[http://dx.doi.org/10.1002/anie.199001381]

[103] Kuchkina NV, Yuzik-Klimova EY, Sorokina SA, *et al.* Polyphenylenepyridyl Dendrons with Functional Periphery and Focal Points: Syntheses and Applications. Macromolecules 2013; 46(15): 5890-8.
[http://dx.doi.org/10.1021/ma401043u]

[104] Gitsov I, Lin C. Dendrimers : Nanoparticles with Precisely Engineered Surfaces. Curr Org Chem 2005; 9(11): 1025-51.
[http://dx.doi.org/10.2174/1385272054368448]

[105] Grayson SM, Fréchet JMJ. Convergent dendrons and dendrimers: from synthesis to applications. Chem Rev 2001; 101(12): 3819-68.
[http://dx.doi.org/10.1021/cr990116h] [PMID: 11740922]

[106] Gorman C. Dendrimers: Polymerization and Properties.Encyclopedia of Materials: Science and Technology. Elsevier 2001; pp. 2042-52.
[http://dx.doi.org/10.1016/B0-08-043152-6/00372-7]

[107] Ciolkowski M, Pałecz B, Appelhans D, Voit B, Klajnert B, Bryszewska M. The influence of maltose modified poly(propylene imine) dendrimers on hen egg white lysozyme structure and thermal stability. Colloids Surf B Biointerfaces 2012; 95: 103-8.
[http://dx.doi.org/10.1016/j.colsurfb.2012.02.021] [PMID: 22410344]

[108] Gurdag S, Khandare J, Stapels S, Matherly LH, Kannan RM. Activity of dendrimer-methotrexate conjugates on methotrexate-sensitive and -resistant cell lines. Bioconjug Chem 2006; 17(2): 275-83.
[http://dx.doi.org/10.1021/bc0501855] [PMID: 16536456]

[109] Siewiera K, Labieniec-Watala M. Ambiguous effect of dendrimer PAMAM G3 on rat heart respiration in a model of an experimental diabetes – Objective causes of laboratory misfortune or unpredictable G3 activity? Int J Pharm 2012; 430(1-2): 258-65.
[http://dx.doi.org/10.1016/j.ijpharm.2012.03.037] [PMID: 22486957]

[110] Yang W, Cheng Y, Xu T, Wang X, Wen L. Targeting cancer cells with biotin–dendrimer conjugates. Eur J Med Chem 2009; 44(2): 862-8.
[http://dx.doi.org/10.1016/j.ejmech.2008.04.021] [PMID: 18550227]

[111] Imae T, Hamaguchi S. Network of sodium hyaluronate with nano-knots junction of poly(amido amine) dendrimer. Carbohydr Polym 2012; 88(1): 352-60.
[http://dx.doi.org/10.1016/j.carbpol.2011.12.015]

[112] Konda SD, Wang S, Brechbiel M, Wiener EC. Bio-distribution of a 153 Gd-folate dendrimer, generation = 4, in mice with folate-receptor positive and negative ovarian tumor xenografts. Invest Radiol 2002; 37(4): 199-204.

[http://dx.doi.org/10.1097/00004424-200204000-00005] [PMID: 11923642]

[113] Kojima C, Kono K, Maruyama K, Takagishi T. Synthesis of polyamidoamine dendrimers having poly(ethylene glycol) grafts and their ability to encapsulate anti-cancer drugs. Bioconjug Chem 2000; 11(6): 910-7.
[http://dx.doi.org/10.1021/bc0000583] [PMID: 11087341]

[114] Gajbhiye V, Vijayaraj Kumar P, Tekade RK, Jain NK. PEGylated PPI dendritic architectures for sustained delivery of H2 receptor antagonist. Eur J Med Chem 2009; 44(3): 1155-66.
[http://dx.doi.org/10.1016/j.ejmech.2008.06.012] [PMID: 18760863]

[115] Pan S, Wang C, Zeng X, Wen Y, Wu H, Feng M. Short multi-armed polylysine-graft-polyamidoamine copolymer as efficient gene vectors. Int J Pharm 2011; 420(2): 206-15.
[http://dx.doi.org/10.1016/j.ijpharm.2011.08.036] [PMID: 21893180]

[116] Allen TM, Cullis PR. Drug delivery systems: entering the mainstream. Science 2004; 303(5665): 1818-22.
[http://dx.doi.org/10.1126/science.1095833] [PMID: 15031496]

[117] Gregory Gregoriadis E, Neerunjun D. Homing of liposomes to target cells. Biochem Biophys Res Commun 1975; 65(2): 537-44.
[http://dx.doi.org/10.1016/S0006-291X(75)80180-X] [PMID: 50067]

[118] Davis ME. Nanoparticle therapeutics: An emerging treatment modality for cancer, in Nanoscience and Technology. UK: Co-Published with Macmillan Publishers Ltd 2009; pp. 239-50.

[119] de Arajo Lopes SC, dos Santos Giuberti C, Ribeiro TG, dos Santos Ferreira D, Amaral Leite E, Cristina M. Liposomes as Carriers of anti-cancer Drugs.Cancer Treatment - Conventional and Innovative Approaches. InTech 2013.
[http://dx.doi.org/10.5772/55290]

[120] Puri A, Loomis K, Smith B, *et al.* Lipid-based nanoparticles as pharmaceutical drug carriers: from concepts to clinic. Crit Rev Ther Drug Carrier Syst 2009; 26(6): 523-80.
[http://dx.doi.org/10.1615/CritRevTherDrugCarrierSyst.v26.i6.10] [PMID: 20402623]

[121] Zhang L, Gu FX, Chan JM, Wang AZ, Langer RS, Farokhzad OC. Nanoparticles in medicine: therapeutic applications and developments. Clin Pharmacol Ther 2008; 83(5): 761-9.
[http://dx.doi.org/10.1038/sj.clpt.6100400] [PMID: 17957183]

[122] Murphy EA, Majeti BK, Barnes LA, *et al.* Nanoparticle-mediated drug delivery to tumor vasculature suppresses metastasis. Proc Natl Acad Sci 2008; 105(27): 9343-8.
[http://dx.doi.org/10.1073/pnas.0803728105] [PMID: 18607000]

[123] Ishida O, Maruyama K, Sasaki K, Iwatsuru M. Size-dependent extravasation and interstitial localization of polyethyleneglycol liposomes in solid tumor-bearing mice. Int J Pharm 1999; 190(1): 49-56.
[http://dx.doi.org/10.1016/S0378-5173(99)00256-2] [PMID: 10528096]

[124] Kim T, Afonin KA, Viard M, *et al. In Silico*, *In Vitro*, and *In Vivo* Studies Indicate the Potential Use of Bolaamphiphiles for Therapeutic siRNAs Delivery. Mol Ther Nucleic Acids 2013; 2(3): e80.
[http://dx.doi.org/10.1038/mtna.2013.5] [PMID: 23511334]

[125] Dexter AF, Middelberg APJ. Peptides as functional surfactants. Ind Eng Chem Res 2008; 47(17): 6391-8.
[http://dx.doi.org/10.1021/ie800127f]

[126] Arakawa K, Eguchi T, Kakinuma K. Highly Thermostable Liposome from 72-Membered Macrocyclic Tetraether Lipid: Importance of 72-Membered Lipid for Archaea to Thrive under Hyperthermal Environments. Chem Lett 2001; 30(5): 440-1.
[http://dx.doi.org/10.1246/cl.2001.440]

[127] Weiss-Wichert C, Smetazko M, Valina-Saba M, Schalkhammer T. A new analytical device based on gated ion channels: A peptide-channel biosensor. SLAS Discov 1997; 2(1): 11-8.

[http://dx.doi.org/10.1177/108705719700200104]

[128] Claussen RC, Rabatic BM, Stupp SI. Aqueous self-assembly of unsymmetric Peptide bolaamphiphiles into nanofibers with hydrophilic cores and surfaces. J Am Chem Soc 2003; 125(42): 12680-1. [http://dx.doi.org/10.1021/ja035882r] [PMID: 14558795]

[129] Kameta N, Minamikawa H, Masuda M, Mizuno G, Shimizu T. Controllable biomolecule release from self-assembled organic nanotubes with asymmetric surfaces: pH and temperature dependence. Soft Matter 2008; 4(8): 1681-7. [http://dx.doi.org/10.1039/b803742f] [PMID: 32907162]

[130] Schroeder A, Kost J, Barenholz Y. Ultrasound, liposomes, and drug delivery: principles for using ultrasound to control the release of drugs from liposomes. Chem Phys Lipids 2009; 162(1-2): 1-16. [http://dx.doi.org/10.1016/j.chemphyslip.2009.08.003] [PMID: 19703435]

[131] Brochu H, Polidori A, Pucci B, Vermette P. Drug delivery systems using immobilized intact liposomes: a comparative and critical review. Curr Drug Deliv 2004; 1(3): 299-312. [http://dx.doi.org/10.2174/1567201043334678] [PMID: 16305392]

[132] Zana R, Yiv S, Kale KM. Chemical relaxation and equilibrium studies of association in aqueous solutions of bolaform detergents. 3. Docosane-1,22-bis(trimethylammonium bromide). J Colloid Interface Sci 1980; 77(2): 456-65. [http://dx.doi.org/10.1016/0021-9797(80)90316-1]

[133] Lamprecht A, Ubrich N, Yamamoto H, *et al.* Biodegradable nanoparticles for targeted drug delivery in treatment of inflammatory bowel disease. J Pharmacol Exp Ther 2001; 299(2): 775-81. [PMID: 11602694]

[134] Sahoo SK, Sawa T, Fang J, *et al.* Pegylated zinc protoporphyrin: A water-soluble heme oxygenase inhibitor with tumor-targeting capacity. Bioconjug Chem 2002; 13(5): 1031-8. [http://dx.doi.org/10.1021/bc020010k] [PMID: 12236785]

[135] Gibaud S, Demoy M, Andreux JP, Weingarten C, Gouritin B, Couvreur P. Cells involved in the capture of nanoparticles in hematopoietic organs. J Pharm Sci 1996; 85(9): 944-50. [http://dx.doi.org/10.1021/js960032d] [PMID: 8877884]

[136] Niidome T, Yamagata M, Okamoto Y, *et al.* PEG-modified gold nanorods with a stealth character for *in vivo* applications. J Control Release 2006; 114(3): 343-7. [http://dx.doi.org/10.1016/j.jconrel.2006.06.017] [PMID: 16876898]

[137] Gupta AK, Gupta M. Synthesis and surface engineering of iron oxide nanoparticles for biomedical applications. Biomaterials 2005; 26(18): 3995-4021. [http://dx.doi.org/10.1016/j.biomaterials.2004.10.012] [PMID: 15626447]

[138] Edetsberger M, Gaubitzer E, Valic E, Waigmann E, Köhler G. Detection of nanometer-sized particles in living cells using modern fluorescence fluctuation methods. Biochem Biophys Res Commun 2005; 332(1): 109-16. [http://dx.doi.org/10.1016/j.bbrc.2005.04.100] [PMID: 15896306]

[139] Konan YN, Chevallier J, Gurny R, Allémann E. Encapsulation of p-THPP into nanoparticles: cellular uptake, subcellular localization and effect of serum on photodynamic activity. Photochem Photobiol 2003; 77(6): 638-44. [http://dx.doi.org/10.1562/0031-8655(2003)077<0638:EOPINC>2.0.CO;2] [PMID: 12870850]

[140] Panyam J, Zhou WZ, Prabha S, Sahoo SK, Labhasetwar V. Rapid endo-lysosomal escape of poly(DL-lactide- co glycolide) nanoparticles: implications for drug and gene delivery. FASEB J 2002; 16(10): 1217-26. [http://dx.doi.org/10.1096/fj.02-0088com] [PMID: 12153989]

[141] Bourges JL, Gautier SE, Delie F, *et al.* Ocular drug delivery targeting the retina and retinal pigment epithelium using polylactide nanoparticles. Invest Ophthalmol Vis Sci 2003; 44(8): 3562-9. [http://dx.doi.org/10.1167/iovs.02-1068] [PMID: 12882808]

[142] Akerman ME, Chan WCW, Laakkonen P, Bhatia SN, Ruoslahti E. Nanocrystal targeting *in vivo*. Proc Natl Acad Sci 2002; 99(20): 12617-21.
[http://dx.doi.org/10.1073/pnas.152463399] [PMID: 12235356]

[143] Ballou B, Lagerholm BC, Ernst LA, Bruchez MP, Waggoner AS. Noninvasive imaging of quantum dots in mice. Bioconjug Chem 2004; 15(1): 79-86.
[http://dx.doi.org/10.1021/bc034153y] [PMID: 14733586]

[144] Weissenböck A, Wirth M, Gabor F. WGA-grafted PLGA-nanospheres: preparation and association with Caco-2 single cells. J Control Release 2004; 99(3): 383-92.
[http://dx.doi.org/10.1016/j.jconrel.2004.07.025] [PMID: 15451596]

[145] Prinzen L, Miserus RJJHM, Dirksen A, *et al.* Optical and magnetic resonance imaging of cell death and platelet activation using annexin a5-functionalized quantum dots. Nano Lett 2007; 7(1): 93-100.
[http://dx.doi.org/10.1021/nl062226r] [PMID: 17212446]

[146] Boado RJ, Zhang Y, Zhang Y, Xia C, Wang Y, Pardridge WM. Genetic engineering of a lysosomal enzyme fusion protein for targeted delivery across the human blood-brain barrier. Biotechnol Bioeng 2008; 99(2): 475-84.
[http://dx.doi.org/10.1002/bit.21602] [PMID: 17680664]

[147] Reese TS, Karnovsky MJ. Fine structural localization of a blood-brain barrier to exogenous peroxidase. J Cell Biol 1967; 34(1): 207-17.
[http://dx.doi.org/10.1083/jcb.34.1.207] [PMID: 6033532]

[148] Koziara JM, Lockman PR, Allen DD, Mumper RJ. The blood-brain barrier and brain drug delivery. J Nanosci Nanotechnol 2006; 6(9): 2712-35.
[http://dx.doi.org/10.1166/jnn.2006.441] [PMID: 17048477]

[149] Tiwari S, Amiji M. A review of nanocarrier-based CNS delivery systems. Curr Drug Deliv 2006; 3(2): 219-32.
[http://dx.doi.org/10.2174/156720106776359230] [PMID: 16611008]

[150] Lockman PR, Koziara JM, Mumper RJ, Allen DD. Nanoparticle surface charges alter blood-brain barrier integrity and permeability. J Drug Target 2004; 12(9-10): 635-41.
[http://dx.doi.org/10.1080/10611860400015936] [PMID: 15621689]

[151] Kreuter J. Influence of the surface properties on nanoparticle-mediated transport of drugs to the brain. J Nanosci Nanotechnol 2004; 4(5): 484-8.
[http://dx.doi.org/10.1166/jnn.2003.077] [PMID: 15503433]

[152] Michaelis K, Hoffmann MM, Dreis S, *et al.* Covalent linkage of apolipoprotein e to albumin nanoparticles strongly enhances drug transport into the brain. J Pharmacol Exp Ther 2006; 317(3): 1246-53.
[http://dx.doi.org/10.1124/jpet.105.097139] [PMID: 16554356]

[153] Girardin F. Membrane transporter proteins: A challenge for CNS drug development. Dialogues Clin Neurosci 2006; 8(3): 311-21.
[http://dx.doi.org/10.31887/DCNS.2006.8.3/fgirardin] [PMID: 17117613]

[154] Alyautdin RN, Petrov VE, Langer K, Berthold A, Kharkevich DA, Kreuter J. Delivery of loperamide across the blood-brain barrier with polysorbate 80-coated polybutylcyanoacrylate nanoparticles. Pharm Res 1997; 14(3): 325-8.
[http://dx.doi.org/10.1023/A:1012098005098] [PMID: 9098875]

[155] Koziara JM, Lockman PR, Allen DD, Mumper RJ. Paclitaxel nanoparticles for the potential treatment of brain tumors. J Control Release 2004; 99(2): 259-69.
[http://dx.doi.org/10.1016/j.jconrel.2004.07.006] [PMID: 15380635]

[156] Oberdörster E. Manufactured nanomaterials (fullerenes, C_{60}) induce oxidative stress in the brain of juvenile largemouth bass. Environ Health Perspect 2004; 112(10): 1058-62.
[http://dx.doi.org/10.1289/ehp.7021] [PMID: 15238277]

[157] Elder A, Gelein R, Silva V, *et al.* Translocation of inhaled ultrafine manganese oxide particles to the central nervous system. Environ Health Perspect 2006; 114(8): 1172-8.
[http://dx.doi.org/10.1289/ehp.9030] [PMID: 16882521]

[158] Gao X, Tao W, Lu W, *et al.* Lectin-conjugated PEG–PLA nanoparticles: Preparation and brain delivery after intranasal administration. Biomaterials 2006; 27(18): 3482-90.
[http://dx.doi.org/10.1016/j.biomaterials.2006.01.038] [PMID: 16510178]

CHAPTER 20

Therapeutic Dynamics of Tannin Interaction and Significance in Precision Medicine

Mohammad Faheem Khan[1,2,*], **Waseem Ahmad Ansari**[2] and **Kajim Ali**[2]

[1] *Department of Chemistry, Era University, Lucknow-226003, UP, India*

[2] *Department of Biotechnology, Era's Lucknow Medical College & Hospital, Era University, Lucknow-226003, Uttar Pradesh, India*

Abstract: Personalized medicine is a targeted therapy that aims to provide people suffering from complex illnesses with tailored-made healthcare. Taking this into consideration, foods with diverse bioactive compounds have recently gained widespread scientific interest as alternatives to modern drugs for developing therapeutic agents against human diseases. Tannins are an important group of polyphenol compounds in foods that have both beneficial and anti-nutritional effects. As an anti-nutrient, they can reduce element bioavailability, and protein absorption, and inhibit enzymatic actions during metabolism. If tannin-rich foods are consumed in sufficient quantities and at the appropriate time, they may act similarly to natural drugs that ameliorate a range of metabolic disorders. Thus, the types of tannin-rich foods and the timing of consumption before or after meals should be considered for maximum physiological importance in maintaining human health. In this chapter, we compiled the different types of tannins and their food sources, as well as their beneficial and anti-nutrient effects on human health.

Keywords: Micronutrients, Macronutrients, Personalized medicine (PM), Polyphenols, Tannins, Tannins-rich foods.

INTRODUCTION

In the 21st century, personalized medicine (PM) is continuing to attract the attention of medical researchers and healthcare practitioners. PM is a novel concept in the medical sector that has the ability from mass targeting to the one-person target by providing effective, tailored therapeutic strategies on the basis of the genomic, and proteomic profile of an individual. PM provides both treatments

* **Corresponding author Mohammad Faheem Khan:** Department of Chemistry, Era University, Lucknow-226003, UP, India and Department of Biotechnology, Era's Lucknow Medical College & Hospital, Era University, Lucknow-226003, Uttar Pradesh, India; E-mail: faheemkhan35@gmail.com

Farzana Mahdi & Abbas Ali Mahdi (Eds.)

as well as preventive options. The assessment of proteogenomic along with mutations that give rise to resistance against treatment opens the doors for healthcare practitioners to decide which treatment is right for a particular person. Generally, it has been seen and happens that if there is no relief from one medication, then another medication is started. These types of trial-and-errors lead to side effects, drug interactions and worsen the disease state in the patients, which also affects the patient's mental health. To rule out the adverse effects of trial-and-error prescription specified treatment by PM approaches is more powerful. The development of PM will provide better treatment at a specific dose that will increase drug efficacy and minimize the patient's casualties [1]. The main focus of the PM is raise the advantages and prevent the risk to the patients by targeting the biological markers such as clinical, genetics, and genomic that intervene to develop therapeutic drugs [2]. Pharmacogenomics, pharmacoproteomics, and pharmacogenetics are major divisions of personalized medicine that have crucial roles in developing drugs and determining their efficacy on patients based on molecular diagnostics studies. In the current scenario, several biotechnological and pharmaceutical companies have announced personalized medicine will prime target to expand the individualized treatment for diseases in future [3]. In recent years, nutritional and lifestyle changes have gained attention in both developed and developing countries. Good nutrition is of utmost importance to maintain normal body function and to mitigate the dysfunction of metabolic pathways which are induced by various factors [4, 5].

Adequate nutrition provides both macronutrients and micronutrients to fulfil the physiological needs of human body. Macronutrients include carbohydrates, proteins, and fats that are necessary to provide cellular energy whereas micronutrients such as minerals and vitamins are needed for growth, development and metabolism for proper functioning of body [6]. Foods contain a complex system of both nutrients and non-nutrients components which are required for plants and animals because they have the abilities to modulate epigenetic, gene expression and protein functions [7, 8]. In plants foods, non-nutrients components are natural and synthetic compounds that can be beneficial, non-beneficial or even toxic. Natural compounds such as polyphenols, flavonoids, alkaloids and steroids have the beneficial effects for plants and human both. Among them, some of the group of compounds such as tannins, saponins, lectins and phytic acid may be considered as anti-nutrients because they cause adverse effect in human such as reduced bioavailability of elements and digestibility of protein if they are not taken at right time [9].

Tannins are the important class of polyphenols that provide beneficial effects such as anti-inflammatory, antioxidant, or anti-cancer properties [10]. Many of them are in foods like coffee, chocolate, olive and berries [11]. Anthocyanins, an important class of polyphenols are also responsible for berries colour such as red, blue, or purple color [12]. Non-extractable polyphenols form dietary fibers *via* polymerization reactions, which influence the gut health [13]. Lentils, and beans especially red kidney beans and black beans contain good number of polyphenols having antioxidant and anti-inflammatory activities [14]. Literature revealed that tannins might be good for human health if they are taken in particular quantities. Generally, they have beneficial effects but anti-nutrients effects cannot be ignored. Therefore, all the anti-nutrients effects of tannins should be studied before making any suggestion for possible consumption of those foods which are tannin rich. Thus, the aim of this chapter is to summarize the current knowledge based on tannins, their chemical structure, dietary sources and health benefits with adverse effects. The molecular mechanism of tannins in foods is also discussed in details, highlighting which food should be avoided or recommended for beneficial effects in human.

TANNINS: STRUCTURE AND CLASSIFICATION

Tannins are different types of polymeric compounds of phenols that are abundantly found in numerous plant-based foods and medicinal plants in their different parts such as fruits, leaves, seeds, stem and roots. Generally, tannins are of four types: (1) hydrolysable tannins, (2) condensed tannins, (3) pseudo-tannins, and (4) phlorotannins [15]. Hydrolysable tannins are synthesised from Shikimate pathway which is derived gallic acid metabolism. On hydrolysis, hydrolysable tannins *e.g.* gallotannins and ellagitannins yielded phenolic acids (*e.g.*, ellagic acid and gallic acid) along with carbohydrate (*e.g.* glucose) or their derivatives in basic units [16]. Condensed tannins, also known as proanthocyanidins, are polymers of the flavan-3-ols that yielded anthocyanidins *via* oxidation reactions. They are non-hydrolysable tannins. Condensed tannins are very complex in structure, which are formed by C-4 linkage of one catechin with C-6 or C-8 linkage of the adjacent monomeric catechin. Having catechin or epicatechin as building blocks of condensed tannins, they are from flavonol pathways originated [17]. Phlorotannins are oligomers of phloroglucinol, which are mainly found in algae. Phloroglucinol, an aromatic ring with 1, 3, 5 hydroxyl groups, is the constituted unit of various phlorotannins that undergo polymerisation at C1-C3 positions. Three distinctive classes of phlorotannins are fucols, phloroetols and fucophloroteols, which are made by coupling in between C-C, C-O-C, C-C and C-O-C units respectively. Pseudo tannins are polyphenols of gallic acid and falvan-3-ols units in their basic skeletons [18].

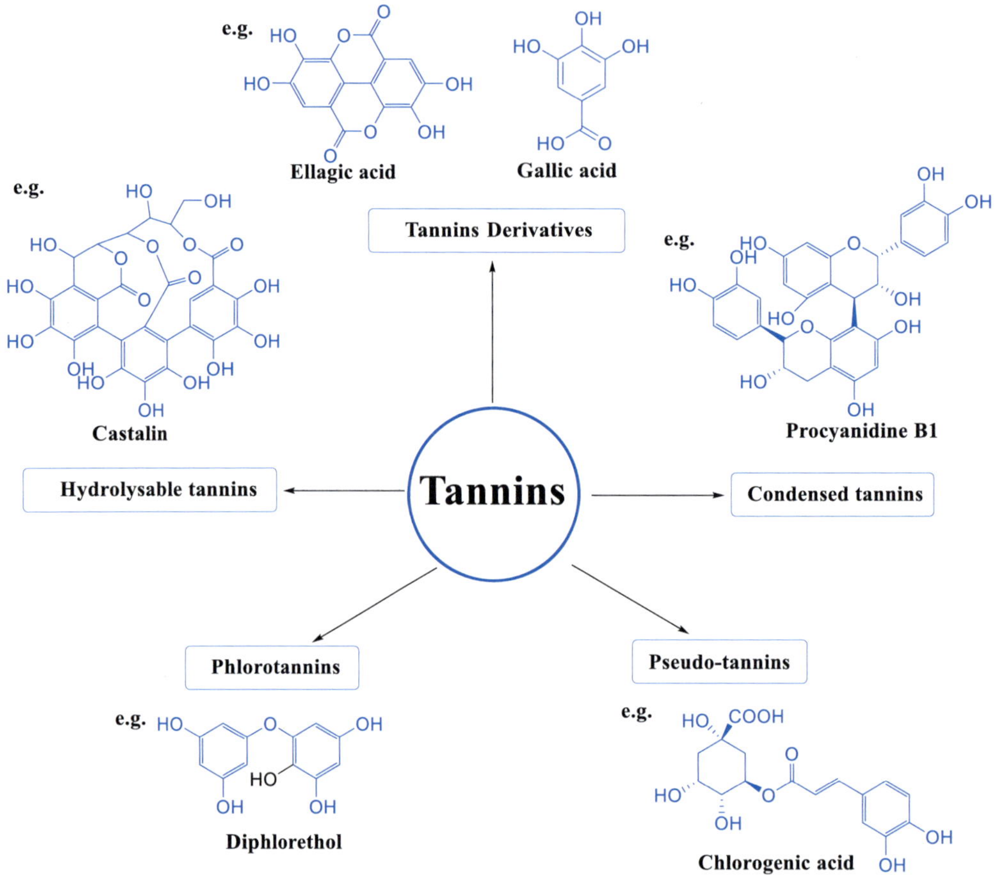

Fig. (1). Classifications of Tannins.

TANNINS: FOOD SOURCES

Tannins are astringent and bitter in taste that cause dryness to the tongue when someone consume the food containing high level of tannins. They have the abilities to precipitate the proteins and deactivate the enzymes. Thus, they impart both positive and negative effects in plant as well as human. The fruits, legume, vegetable, condiments and spices are well known for being good sources of tannins. Tannins are widely found in *Camellia sinensis* (tea), *Coffea arabica* (coffee), and *Theobroma coca* (cocoa). They are richest sources of tannins, which are responsible for their strong bitterness as well as astringent properties, so more strong tea or coffee means more tannin [19]. The fruits such as apple, grapes, peach, pomegranate, blueberries, raspberries, strawberries, and cranberries contain the significant number of tannins. The high concentration of tannins is also found in the skin and seeds of these fruits. The tannin content is highest while the fruits are mature and then decreases down as the fruits ages [20]. Unripe bananas (green) contain significant amounts of tannins but they decrease with age and thus ripe banana are lowers in tannin. The green bananas are often used for their resistance starch [21, 22]. The dry fruits such as hazelnuts, walnuts, peanuts, cashew, dates, and almonds also contain different types of tannins [23]. In almonds and walnuts, tannins are generally found in the skin that is why to eliminate the bitterness of these nuts, it is recommended to soak and then rinsing them before consumption. Cereals and legume like barley, millets, beans, cowpeas, kidney beans, and sweet peas are the common example of foods containing tannin in low amount whereas sorghum is well known as staple food in Asian and African countries that contain high amount of tannins [24]. Appreciable amount of tannins are also found in condiments and spices including cloves, cumin, thyme, coriander, tamarind, vanilla, chilies, and cinnamon *etc* [25]. Tannins are also found in beans and their content ranges from 0% to 2.0%, based on the type of bean. The good options of tannin containing beans are black grams, mung beans, kidney beans, and faba beans. Black eyed peas and pinto beans may also be good options for tannins but up to some extent [26].

TANNINS: POSITIVE AND NEGATIVE EFFECTS

Positive Effects

Many clinical studies revealed that proanthocyanidins compounds of grapes might be good for peoples suffering from Non-Proliferative Diabetic Retinopathy (NPDR), diabetes, hypertension and gingivitis problems. Such randomized, placebo-controlled clinical trials were found to link with the improvement of blood pressure, reduce the severity of hard exudate in NPDR patients, and prevent the bleeding from gums during gingivitis in dose-dependent manners from days to month's studies. These benefits highlighted the importance of tannins in human health [27 - 29]. There are many health benefits of tannic acid as evidenced by the literature. Tannic acid may prevent myocardial fibrosis, which is caused by the exaggerated activation of the β-adrenergic receptors and toll-like receptors (TLRs). Tannic acid also enhances the vasodilation of endothelial cells [30]. Several studies showed the anticancer effects of tannic acid because it inhibits the signaling such as EGFR/Jak2/STATs as well as inhibits the PKM2 glycolytic enzyme in cancer cell lines. In a study, tannic acid can prevent prostate cancer by inhibiting lipid metabolism in prostate cancer cells [31].

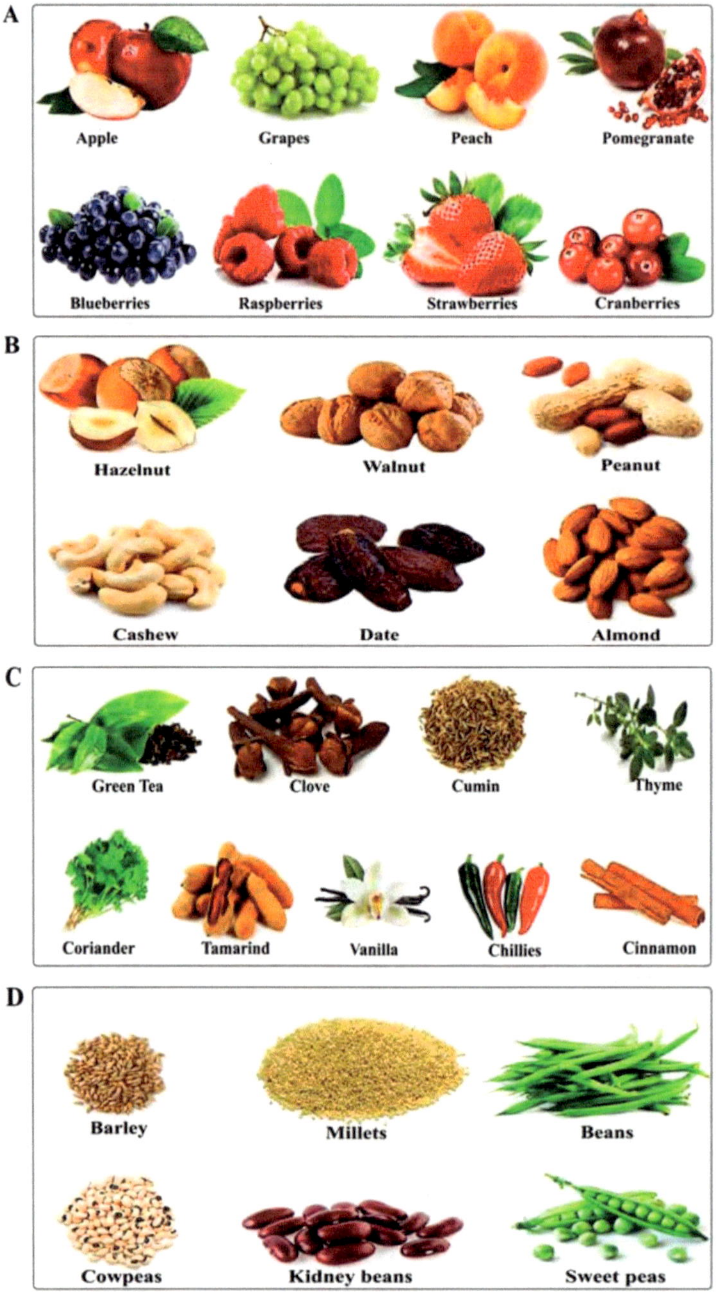

Fig. (2). Dietary sources of tannins **(A)** Fruits, **(B)** Dry fruits, **(C)** Herbs and condiments, and **(D)** Cereal, Beans and Peas.

Gallotannin is another important tannin with significant health benefits. Gallotannin prevent the formation of kidney stone because it interact with crystals of calcium oxalate monohydrate and prevent them to bind with the surface of renal endothelial cells. Being antioxidant agent, it can enhance the superoxide dismutase (SOD) enzyme activity and inhibit the monocyte chemoattractant protein-1 (MCP-1) and osteopontin protein expression. In a study, gallotannin can excrete out the excess concentration of creatinine [32]. Thus, ultimately, gallotannin might be helpful to the individuals who are affected by kidney failure problems. Overall, gallotannin rich foods should be recommended for those peoples. Corilagin, a gallotannin compound can prevent the ulcerative colitis by reducing pro-inflammatory markers like TNF-α, IL-1β, and IL-6 [33].

Negative Effects

There are many tannins found in tea where epigallocatechin gallate (EGCG) is one of the most important along with ellagitannins. Both the EGCG and ellagitannins are antioxidants, and anti-inflammatory as well as they reduce the growth or metastasis of cancer cells. However, several studies have shown that consumption of tea lowers down the serum hemoglobin level. Tannins content in tea interact with iron and prevent its absorption in the gut of individual person. Iron involves into synthesizing hemoglobin in the body and thus iron deficiency is one of the factors causing anemia. Therefore, anemic or iron-deficient persons can manage the problem by avoiding the consumption of tea with iron-rich foods [34]. On empty stomach, consumption of tea made by hard-boiling may cause nausea, which affects the digestive system because they may have a high level of tannins. Thus, to avoid such conditions, tea should not be recommended along with food because food contains protein and carbohydrates that interact with tannins to minimize their sensitivity to the digestive tract [35].

The gallotannins found in mango, grape, strawberry, raspberry, *etc.* show the iron complexing properties, which prevent the growth of food spoilage bacteria and Escherichia coli. Gallotannin causes negative health effects. Thus over eating of these fruits should be avoided if gut feeling is not good [36]. Although gallotannins exhibited antioxidative and antibacterial activities, they involve in precipitating the protein, inhibition of enzyme and metal chelation properties through forming hydrophobic as well as hydrophilic interactions. Study revealed that gallotannins interact with proteins namely α-amylase, pepsin, histone, bovine serum albumin, casein and gelatin, phospholipids such as L-α-lecithin, L-α-cephalin and sphingomyelin as well as sugars like glucose, maltose, maltotetraose, maltohexaose and starch. Such molecular interactions might result in a decrease in bioconversion, bioavailability of nutritional elements, and increase enzyme deactivation, which are useful in metabolism [37].

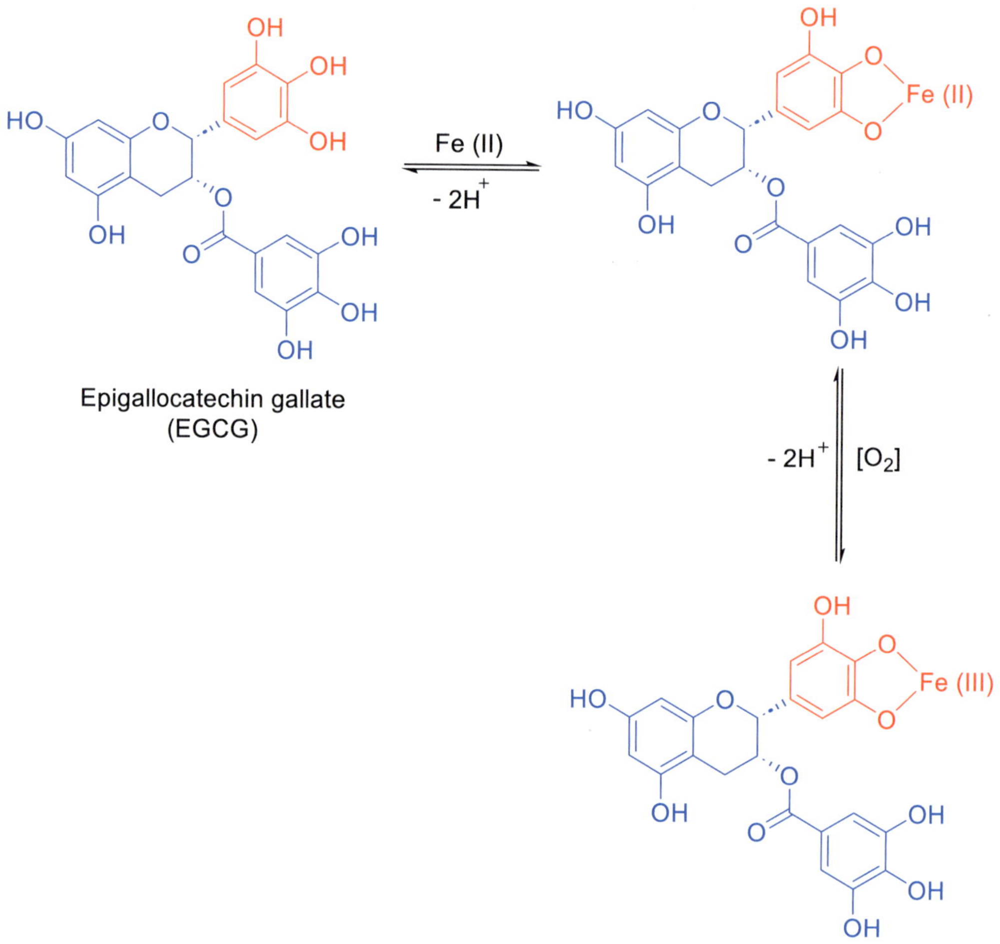

Fig. (3). The schematic diagram for molecular interaction of epigallocatechin gallate with iron.

In a study, it has been seen that pentagalloyl glucose, gallic acid, and ellagic acid were able to unbind the quaternary structure of bovine serum albumin when administered in the high concentrations of 100–500 μM. Therefore, higher concentrations of said compounds is major concern in albumin deficient individuals [38]. Thus, in disease conditions involving these proteins deficiency, gallotannins fruits should be avoided. α-glucosidase is a hydrolytic enzyme in carbohydrate metabolism that breaks down the dietary carbohydrate into monosaccharide units to be absorbed in circulatory blood. Suppression of this enzyme lead to retardation of glucose reabsorption and thus α-glucosidase inhibitors act as antidiabetic agents. Two ellagitannins (casuarictin and eugeniin) of clove buds exhibited the α-glucosidase, which is due to presence of a number of galloylation on glucose core. As a result, galloylation increases the enzyme inhibition action. Thus, clove buds might be recommended for diabetic patients [39].

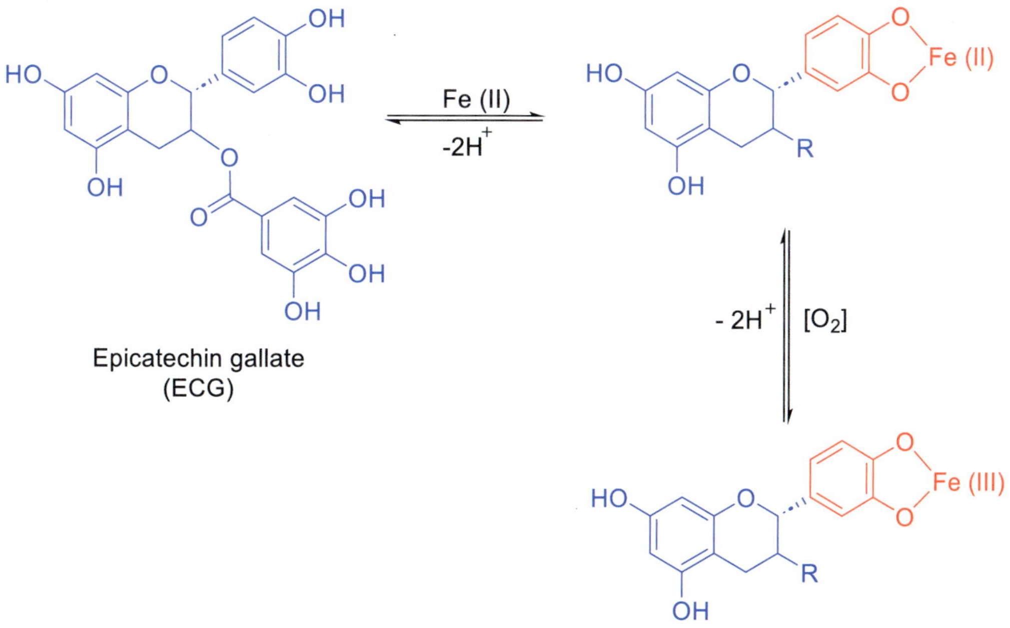

Fig. (4). The schematic diagram for molecular interaction of epicatechin gallate with iron.

Penta-O-galloyl-β-d-glucose (PGG) and tannic acid (TA) inhibited the pancreatic lipase enzyme. This enzymatic activity is due to presence of hydroxyl groups, which interact within the binding pockets of pancreatic lipase enzymes. Thus, the foods that contain PGG and TA are highly recommended to the individuals having high level of triglycerides for the prevention of hypolipidemic conditions [40].

Digestive enzymes play key roles to maintain the proper functioning of physiological processes. They greatly affect the human health and developing child if inhibited. Thus, they should work properly. Plant food like apples, grape, pomegranate, blue berry, cranberry, and cocoa contain some condensed types of tannins such as procyanidin, proanthocyanidins and ellagitannins that can interact with digestive enzymes like α-amylase, trypsin, and lipase and inhibit their actions. Therefore, consumption of these plant foods might be controlled in case of poor digestion. Along with foods, fruits that tannins should not be recommended [41].

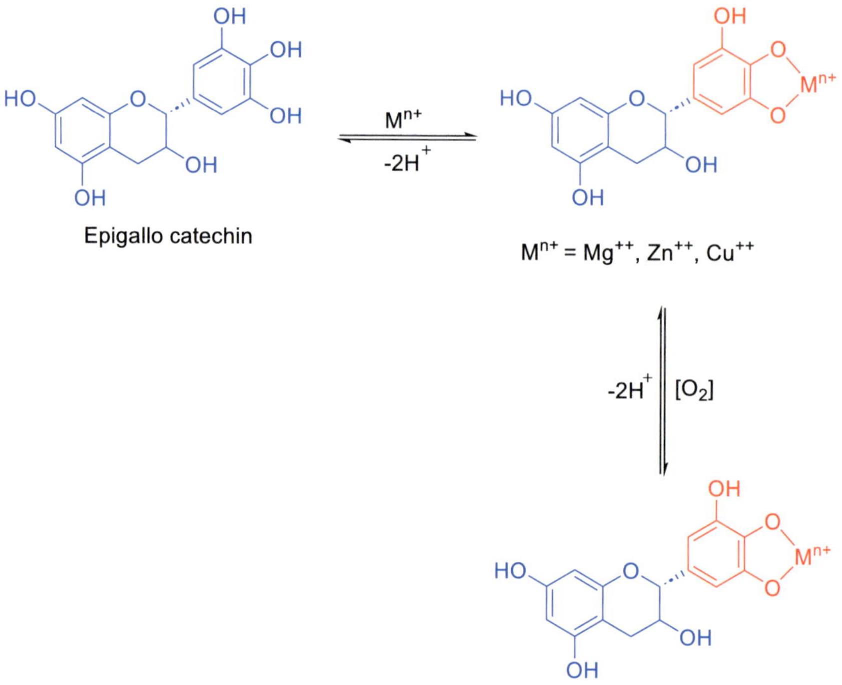

Fig. (5). The schematic diagram for molecular interaction of epigallo catechin with metal ions.

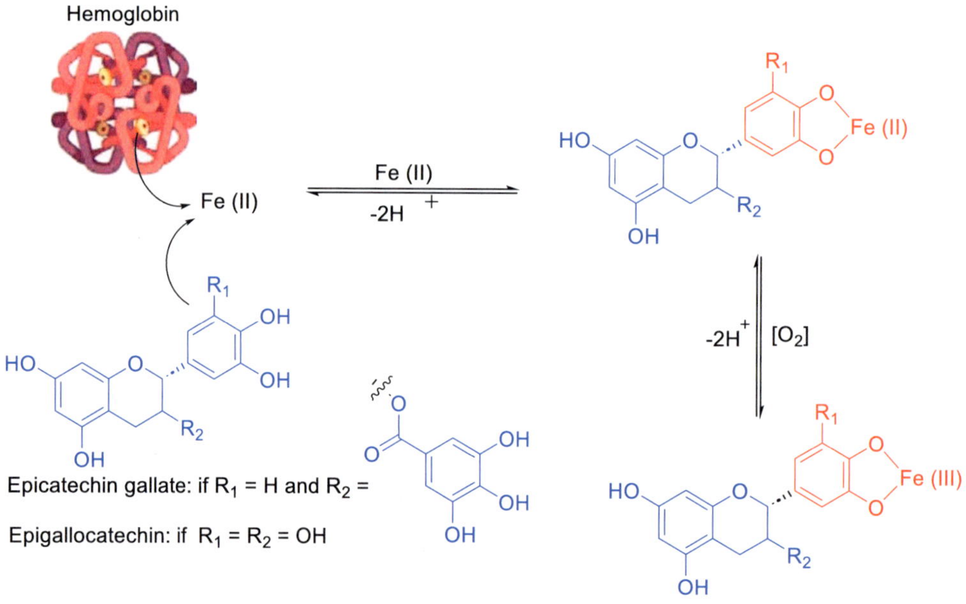

Fig. (6). The Schematic diagram for molecular interaction of tannins with hemoglobin.

FUTURE OUTLOOKS AND CONCLUSIONS

Tannins had both beneficial and antinutritional effects. Untimely and unbalanced consumption of tannin-rich foods causes anti-nutrient effects. It has been observed that tannin-rich foods have many beneficial effects, but their negative effects are due to the untimely consumption of that food, which contains a variety of other components. Tannins deplete elements (Zn^{2+}, Fe^{2+}, Cu^{+}, *etc.*) when consumed with other foods because tannins bind to the elements and excrete them without absorption in the gut. This is why tannins reduce the bioavailability of micronutrients. Furthermore, they cause the breakdown of protein structure and enzymatic activity, both of which are important in bodybuilding, and are thus responsible for poor growth in developing children. As a result, foods are unable to exert their therapeutic effects on people. Coordination between scientists, nutritionists, and clinicians is crucial for obtaining all possible beneficial and therapeutic effects from antinutrient compounds like food tannins. In the future, the accumulated results may encourage the development of a better strategy for reducing the negative effects of said compounds. These strategies may also clarify whether we need to consume tannin-rich foods or not, and if so, when we should consume them. Furthermore, in-depth molecular interactions in the field of food and nutrition should be investigated in laboratories as well as clinics. Thus, the potential benefits and drawbacks of food tannins must be thoroughly investigated in human subjects.

ACKNOWLEDGMENTS

We, authors, would like to express our sincere gratitude to the management of Era's Lucknow Medical College, Era University, Lucknow, and the American University of Barbados (AUB) for intramural fund and support for this work.

REFERENCES

[1] Najeeb Q. Personilized medicines versus era of " Trial and Error. J Pharm Biomed Sci 2012; 19(19): 1-5.

[2] Mathur S, Sutton J. Personalized medicine could transform healthcare. Biomed Rep 2017; 7(1): 3-5. [http://dx.doi.org/10.3892/br.2017.922] [PMID: 28685051]

[3] Shlyakhto E, Konradi A. Personalized medicine. History, Current state and future directions. Russian Journal for personalized medicines 2021; 1(1): 6-20.

[4] Witkamp RF. Nutrition to optimise human health—how to obtain physiological substantiation? Nutrients 2021; 13(7): 2155. [http://dx.doi.org/10.3390/nu13072155] [PMID: 34201670]

[5] Cena H, Calder PC. Defining a healthy diet: Evidence for the role of contemporary dietary patterns in health and disease. Nutrients 2020; 12(2): 334. [http://dx.doi.org/10.3390/nu12020334] [PMID: 32012681]

[6] Chen Y, Michalak M, Agellon LB. Importance of nutrients and nutrient metabolism on human health. Yale J Biol Med 2018; 91(2): 95-103.

[PMID: 29955217]

[7] Choi SW, Friso S. Epigenetics: A new bridge between nutrition and health. Adv Nutr 2010; 1(1): 8-16. [http://dx.doi.org/10.3945/an.110.1004] [PMID: 22043447]

[8] Hardy TM, Tollefsbol TO. Epigenetic diet: Impact on the epigenome and cancer. Epigenomics 2011; 3(4): 503-18. [http://dx.doi.org/10.2217/epi.11.71] [PMID: 22022340]

[9] Mennen LI, Walker R, Bennetau-Pelissero C, Scalbert A. Risks and safety of polyphenol consumption. Am J Clin Nutr 2005; 81(1) (Suppl.): 326S-9S. [http://dx.doi.org/10.1093/ajcn/81.1.326S] [PMID: 15640498]

[10] Das AK, Islam MN, Faruk MO, Ashaduzzaman M, Dungani R. Review on tannins: Extraction processes, applications and possibilities. S Afr J Bot 2020; 135: 58-70. [https://doi.org/10.1016/j.sajb.2020.08.008]. [http://dx.doi.org/10.1016/j.sajb.2020.08.008]

[11] Serrano J, Puupponen-Pimiä R, Dauer A, Aura AM, Saura-Calixto F. Tannins: Current knowledge of food sources, intake, bioavailability and biological effects. Mol Nutr Food Res 2009; 53(S2) (Suppl. 2): S310-29. [http://dx.doi.org/10.1002/mnfr.200900039] [PMID: 19437486]

[12] Khoo HE, Azlan A, Tang ST, Lim SM. Anthocyanidins and anthocyanins: colored pigments as food, pharmaceutical ingredients, and the potential health benefits. Food Nutr Res 2017; 61(1): 1361779. [http://dx.doi.org/10.1080/16546628.2017.1361779] [PMID: 28970777]

[13] Jakobek L, Matić P. Non-covalent dietary fiber - Polyphenol interactions and their influence on polyphenol bioaccessibility. Trends Food Sci Technol 2019; 83: 235-47. [https://doi.org/10.1016/j.tifs.2018.11.024]. [http://dx.doi.org/10.1016/j.tifs.2018.11.024]

[14] Ganesan K, Xu B. Polyphenol-rich dry common beans (Phaseolus vulgaris L.) and their health benefits. Int J Mol Sci 2017; 18(11): 2331. [http://dx.doi.org/10.3390/ijms18112331] [PMID: 29113066]

[15] Khanbabaee K, van Ree T. Tannins: Classification and definition. Nat Prod Rep 2001; 18(6): 641-9. [http://dx.doi.org/10.1039/b101061l] [PMID: 11820762]

[16] Vuolo M, Lima V, Maróstica M. Phenolic Compounds structure, classification, and Antioxidant power. Bioactive Compounds 2019; pp. 33-50. [https://doi.org/10.1016/b978-0-12-814774-0.00002-5]

[17] Rousserie P, Rabot A, Geny-Denis L. From flavanols biosynthesis to wine tannins: What place for grape seeds? J Agric Food Chem 2019; 67(5): 1325-43. [http://dx.doi.org/10.1021/acs.jafc.8b05768] [PMID: 30632368]

[18] Cuong X, Hoan N, Dong D, *et al.* Tannins: Extraction from Plants. Tannins - Structural Properties, Biological Properties and Current Knowledge 2020. [https://doi.org/10.5772/intechopen.86040]

[19] Hassanpour S, Maheri-Sis N, Eshratkhah B. Plants and secondary metabolites (Tannins), a review. Int J For Soil Eros 2011; 1(1): 47-53.

[20] Kumari M, Jain S. Screening of potential sources of tannin and its therapeutic application. International Journal of Nutrition and Food Sciences 2015; 4(2): 26. [https://doi.org/10.11648/j.ijnfs.s.2015040201.15]. [http://dx.doi.org/10.11648/j.ijnfs.s.2015040201.15]

[21] Ghag S, Ganapathi T. Banana and plantains: Improvement, nutrition, and health. In: Mérillon JM, Ramawat K, Eds. Bioactive Molecules in Food. 2019; pp. 1755-74. [https://doi.org/10.1007/978-3-319-78030-6_73] [http://dx.doi.org/10.1007/978-3-319-78030-6_73]

[22] Hoffmann Sardá FA, Giuntini EB, Gomez MLPA, *et al.* Impact of resistant starch from unripe banana

flour on hunger, satiety, and glucose homeostasis in healthy volunteers. J Funct Foods 2016; 24: 63-74.
[https://doi.org/10.1016/j.jff.2016.04.001].
[http://dx.doi.org/10.1016/j.jff.2016.04.001]

[23] Karamać M. Chelation of Cu(II), Zn(II), and Fe(II) by tannin constituents of selected edible nuts. Int J Mol Sci 2009; 10(12): 5485-97.
[http://dx.doi.org/10.3390/ijms10125485] [PMID: 20054482]

[24] Kumari M, Jain S. Tannins: An antinutrients with positive effect to manage diabetes. Res J Recent Sci 2012; 1(12): 70-3.

[25] Opara E, Chohan M. Culinary herbs and spices: their bioactive properties, the contribution of polyphenols and the challenges in deducing their true health benefits. Int J Mol Sci 2014; 15(10): 19183-202.
[http://dx.doi.org/10.3390/ijms151019183] [PMID: 25340982]

[26] Pedrosa MM, Guillamón E, Arribas C. Autoclaved and extruded legumes as a source of bioactive phytochemicals: A review. Foods 2021; 10(2): 379.
[http://dx.doi.org/10.3390/foods10020379] [PMID: 33572460]

[27] Odai T, Terauchi M, Kato K, Hirose A, Miyasaka N. Effects of grape seed proanthocyanidin extract on vascular endothelial function in participants with prehypertension: A randomized, double-blind, placebo-controlled study. Nutrients 2019; 11(12): 2844.
[http://dx.doi.org/10.3390/nu11122844] [PMID: 31757033]

[28] Moon SW, Shin YU, Cho H, Bae SH, Kim HK. Effect of grape seed proanthocyanidin extract on hard exudates in patients with non-proliferative diabetic retinopathy. Medicine (Baltimore) 2019; 98(21): e15515.
[http://dx.doi.org/10.1097/MD.0000000000015515] [PMID: 31124931]

[29] Díaz Sánchez RM, Castillo-Dalí G, Fernández-Olavarría A, *et al.* Torres-Lagare. A prospective, double-blind, randomized, controlled clinical trial in the gingivitis prevention with an oligoneric proanthocyanidin nutritional supplement. Mediators Inflamm 2017; 2017: 1-7. [https://doi.org/10.1155/2017/7460780].
[http://dx.doi.org/10.1155/2017/7460780]

[30] Tsai TY, Leong IL, Shiao LR, *et al.* Tannic acid, a vasodilator present in wines and beverages, stimulates Ca^{2+} influx via TRP channels in bEND.3 endothelial cells. Biochem Biophys Res Commun 2020; 526(1): 117-21.
[http://dx.doi.org/10.1016/j.bbrc.2020.03.078] [PMID: 32197839]

[31] Nagesh PKB, Chowdhury P, Hatami E, *et al.* Tannic acid inhibits lipid metabolism and induce ROS in prostate cancer cells. Sci Rep 2020; 10(1): 980.
[http://dx.doi.org/10.1038/s41598-020-57932-9] [PMID: 31969643]

[32] Lee HJ, Jeong SJ, Park MN, *et al.* Gallotannin suppresses calcium oxalate crystal binding and oxalate-induced oxidative stress in renal epithelial cells. Biol Pharm Bull 2012; 35(4): 539-44.
[http://dx.doi.org/10.1248/bpb.35.539] [PMID: 22466558]

[33] Xiao HT, Lin CY, Ho DHH, *et al.* Inhibitory effect of the gallotannin corilagin on dextran sulfate sodium-induced murine ulcerative colitis. J Nat Prod 2013; 76(11): 2120-5.
[http://dx.doi.org/10.1021/np4006772] [PMID: 24200352]

[34] Pebrina R, Nafilata I, Sunartono S, Aselina F. The relationship of drinking tea behavior with levels of hemoglobin in stikes guna bangsa yogyakarta students. Journal of Health 2019; 6(2): 126-31. [https://doi.org/10.30590/vol6-no2-p126-131].
[http://dx.doi.org/10.30590/vol6-no2-p126-131]

[35] Matthews CM. Steep your genes in health: drink tea. Proc Bayl Univ Med Cent 2010; 23(2): 142-4.
[http://dx.doi.org/10.1080/08998280.2010.11928604] [PMID: 20396424]

[36] Engels C, Knödler M, Zhao YY, Carle R, Gänzle MG, Schieber A. Antimicrobial activity of gallotannins isolated from mango (Mangifera indica L.) kernels. J Agric Food Chem 2009; 57(17): 7712-8.
[http://dx.doi.org/10.1021/jf901621m] [PMID: 19655802]

[37] He Q, Shi B, Yao K. Interactions of gallotannins with proteins, amino acids, phospholipids and sugars. Food Chem 2006; 95(2): 250-4.
[https://doi.org/10.1016/j.foodchem.2004.11.055].
[http://dx.doi.org/10.1016/j.foodchem.2004.11.055]

[38] Zhang L, Liu Y, Hu X, Xu M, Wang Y. Studies on interactions of pentagalloyl glucose, ellagic acid and gallic acid with bovine serum albumin: A spectroscopic analysis. Food Chem 2020; 324: 126872.
[http://dx.doi.org/10.1016/j.foodchem.2020.126872] [PMID: 32344347]

[39] Toda M, Kawabata J, Kasai T. Inhibitory effects of ellagi- and gallotannins on rat intestinal α-glucosidase complexes. Biosci Biotechnol Biochem 2001; 65(3): 542-7.
[http://dx.doi.org/10.1271/bbb.65.542] [PMID: 11330666]

[40] Moreno-Córdova. Elena, Arvizu-Flores A, Valenzuela-Soto E, García-Orozco K, Wall-Medrano A, Alvarez-Parrilla E, Ayala-Zavala J, Domínguez-Avila J, González-Aguilar G. Gallotannins Are Uncompetitive Inhibitors of Pancreatic Lipase Activity. Biophys Chem 2020; 264: 106409. [https://doi.org/10.1016/j.bpc.2020.106409].

[41] Barrett A, Ndou T, Hughey CA, *et al.* Inhibition of α-amylase and glucoamylase by tannins extracted from cocoa, pomegranates, cranberries, and grapes. J Agric Food Chem 2013; 61(7): 1477-86.
[http://dx.doi.org/10.1021/jf304876g] [PMID: 23289516]

SUBJECT INDEX

A

B

C

D

E

F

G

H

I

J

L

M

N

O

P

R

S

T

U

V

W

Made in the USA
Las Vegas, NV
04 November 2026

57438196R00333